STORIES OF STROKE

STORIES OF STROKE

KEY INDIVIDUALS AND THE EVOLUTION OF IDEAS

Edited by

LOUIS R. CAPLAN M.D.

Beth Israel Deaconess Medical Center

AISHWARYA AGGARWAL M.D.

John F. Kennedy Medical Center

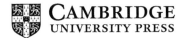
CAMBRIDGE
UNIVERSITY PRESS

CAMBRIDGE
UNIVERSITY PRESS

University Printing House, Cambridge CB2 8BS, United Kingdom

One Liberty Plaza, 20th Floor, New York, NY 10006, USA

477 Williamstown Road, Port Melbourne, VIC 3207, Australia

314–321, 3rd Floor, Plot 3, Splendor Forum, Jasola District Centre, New Delhi – 110025, India

103 Penang Road, #05–06/07, Visioncrest Commercial, Singapore 238467

Cambridge University Press is a part of the University of Cambridge.

It furthers the University's mission by disseminating knowledge in the pursuit of
education, learning, and research at the highest international levels of excellence.

www.cambridge.org
Information on this title: www.cambridge.org/9781316516676
DOI: 10.1017/9781009030854

© Cambridge University Press 2023

First published 2023

Printed in the United Kingdom by TJ Books Limited, Padstow Cornwall

A catalogue record for this publication is available from the British Library.

Library of Congress Cataloging-in-Publication Data
NAMES: Caplan, Louis R., editor. | Aggarwal, Aishwarya, editor.
TITLE: The story of stroke : key individuals and the evolution of ideas /
[edited by] Louis R. Caplan, Aishwarya Aggarwal.
DESCRIPTION: Cambridge, United Kingdom ; New York, NY : Cambridge University Press,
2022. | Includes bibliographical references and index.
IDENTIFIERS: LCCN 2022009559 (print) | LCCN 2022009560 (ebook) |
ISBN 9781316516676 (hardback) | ISBN 9781009030854 (epub)
SUBJECTS: MESH: Stroke–physiopathology | Stroke–history | Stroke–drug therapy |
Stroke Rehabilitation
CLASSIFICATION: LCC RC388.5 (print) | LCC RC388.5 (ebook) | NLM WL 356 |
DDC 616.8/1–dc23/eng/20220328
LC record available at https://lccn.loc.gov/2022009559
LC ebook record available at https://lccn.loc.gov/2022009560

ISBN 978-1-316-51667-6 Hardback

CONTENTS

List of Contributors   *page* ix

Why This Book Needed to Be Written   xiii

Preface   xix

PART I EARLY RECOGNITION

1 HIPPOCRATES AND EARLY GREEK MEDICAL PRACTICE   3

2 EARLY GRECO-ROMAN CONTRIBUTIONS   6

3 ISLAMIC AND MIDDLE EASTERN CONTRIBUTIONS   10

PART II BASIC KNOWLEDGE, SIXTEENTH TO EARLY TWENTIETH
CENTURIES: ANATOMY, PHYSIOLOGY, AND PATHOLOGY

4 ANDREAS VESALIUS   21

5 WILLIAM HARVEY: ON THE MOTION OF THE HEART
   AND BLOOD   25

6 THOMAS WILLIS: ANATOMY OF THE BRAIN AND
   ITS VASCULATURE   31

7 GIOVANNI MORGAGNI: EMPHASIS ON PATHOLOGY   37

8 APOPLEXY: IDEAS AND CONCEPTS, SEVENTEENTH TO
   TWENTIETH CENTURIES   42

9 ATLASES   55

10 BRAINSTEM SYNDROMES   64

11 JULES DEJERINE   72

12 ARTERIAL AND VENOUS ANATOMY   81

13 RUDOLF VIRCHOW   93

14 EARLY MEDICAL AND NEUROLOGICAL TEXTBOOKS   99

PART III MODERN ERA, MID-TWENTIETH CENTURY TO
THE PRESENT

TYPES OF STROKE

15 CAROTID ARTERY DISEASE   109

16 LACUNES   119

17 VERTEBROBASILAR DISEASE   127

18 ANEURYSMS AND SUBARACHNOID
   HEMORRHAGE   138

19 INTRACEREBRAL HEMORRHAGE   157

20 VASCULAR MALFORMATIONS   167

21 CEREBRAL VENOUS THROMBOSIS   174

22 ARTERIAL DISSECTIONS, FIBROMUSCULAR
   DYSPLASIA, MOYAMOYA DISEASE, AND
   REVERSIBLE CEREBRAL VASOCONSTRICTION
   SYNDROME   188

23 BLOOD DISORDERS   200

24 STROKE GENETICS   211

25 EYE VASCULAR DISEASE   226

26 SPINAL CORD VASCULAR DISEASE   238

SOME KEY PHYSICIANS

27 CHARLES FOIX   251

28 HOUSTON MERRITT AND CHARLES ARING   260

29 C. MILLER FISHER   265

30 LOUIS CAPLAN   280

IMAGING

31 CEREBRAL ANGIOGRAPHY   297

32 COMPUTED TOMOGRAPHY   304

33 MAGNETIC RESONANCE IMAGING   313

34 CEREBROVASCULAR ULTRASOUND   325

35 CEREBRAL BLOOD FLOW, RADIONUCLIDES,
   AND POSITRON EMISSION TOMOGRAPHY   338

36 CARDIAC IMAGING AND FUNCTION   352

37 STROKE-RELATED TERMS   358

38 EPIDEMIOLOGY AND RISK FACTORS   364

39 DATA BANKS AND REGISTRIES   370

40 PEDIATRIC STROKE   374

CARE

41 CARE OF STROKE PATIENTS   391

42 NEUROCRITICAL CARE   396

TREATMENT

43 CLINICAL STROKE TRIALS   413

44 HEPARIN   427

45 WARFARIN   434

46 DIRECT ORAL ANTICOAGULANTS   442

47 ASPIRIN   447

48 OTHER ANTIPLATELETS   455

49 OTHER MEDICAL TREATMENTS   465

50 NEUROPROTECTION   478

51 THROMBOLYSIS 491

52 TREATMENT OF CEREBRAL VENOUS THROMBOSIS 505

53 RECOVERY AND REHABILITATION 515

54 CAROTID ARTERY SURGERY 529

55 ANGIOPLASTY AND STENTING 541

56 ENDOVASCULAR TREATMENT OF ACUTE
ISCHEMIC STROKE 551

57 BRAIN ANEURYSM TREATMENT 562

58 MEDICAL AND SURGICAL TREATMENTS OF
INTRACEREBRAL HEMORRHAGE 577

59 TREATMENT OF VASCULAR MALFORMATIONS 590

PART IV STROKE LITERATURE, ORGANIZATIONS, AND PATIENTS

60 STROKE ORGANIZATIONS, JOURNALS, AND BOOKS 607

61 PROMINENT STROKE PATIENTS 610

Index 627

CONTRIBUTORS

Andrei V. Alexandrov (Chapter 34: Cerebrovascular Ultrasound),
Department of Neurology, University of Tennessee Health Science Center, USA

Adel A. Alhazzani (Chapter 3: Islamic and Middle Eastern Contributions)
College of Medicine, King Saud University, Riyadh, Saudi Arabia

Jean-Claude Baron (Chapter 35: Cerebral Blood Flow, Radionuclides, and Positron Emission Tomography)
Inserm, Paris, France

Mustafa K. Baskaya (Chapter 59: Treatment of Vascular Malformations)
University of Wisconsin School of Medicine, Madison, Wisconsin, USA

Ken Bauer (Chapter 46: Direct Oral Anticoagulants)
Beth Israel Deaconess Medical Center, Harvard Medical School, Boston, Massachusetts, USA

Alistaire Buchan (Chapter 50: Neuroprotection)
Acute Stroke Programme, Radcliffe Department of Medicine, Oxford University, Oxford, UK

Patricia Martins Canhão Rodrigues (Chapter 21: Cerebral Venous Thrombosis)
Hospital de Santa Maria, Lisbon, Portugal

Seemant Chaturvedi (Chapter 55: Angioplasty and Stenting)
University of Maryland, Baltimore, Maryland, USA

Jonathan Coutinho (Chapter 52: Treatment of Cerebral Venous Thrombosis)
Academisch Medisch Centrum Universiteit van Amsterdam, Amsterdam, Netherlands

Stephanie Debette (Chapter 24: Stroke Genetics)
University of Bordeaux and Bordeaux University Hospital, France

Michael DeGeorgia (Chapter 42: Neurocritical Care)
University Hospital, Western Reserve University, Cleveland, Ohio, USA

Gabrielle deVeber (Chapter 40: Pediatric Stroke)
Hospital for Sick Children, Toronto, Canada

Conrado J. Estol (Chapter 15: Carotid Artery Disease and Chapter 54 Carotid Artery Surgery)
Breyna, Heart and Brain Medicine, Buenos Aires, Argentina

Catarina Fonseca (Chapter 31: Cerebral Angiography and Chapter 36: Cardiac Imaging and Function)
Hopital St. Anne, Lisbon, Portugal

Mahmut Edip Gurol (Chapter 19: Intracerebral Hemorrhage)
Massachusetts General Hospital, Boston, Massachusetts, USA

Diogo Hausen (Chapter 56: Endovascular Treatment of Acute Ischemic Stroke)
Marcus Stroke & Neuroscience Center, Grady Memorial Hospital; Emory University School of Medicine; Atlanta, GA, USA

Roberto Heros (Chapter 59: Treatment of Vascular Malformations)
University of Miami, Miami, Florida, USA

Carlos S. Kase (Chapter 58: Medical and Surgical Treatments of Intracerebral Hemorrhage)
Department of Neurology, Emory University; Atlanta, Georgia, USA

Ismail A. Khatri (Chapter 3: Islamic and Middle Eastern Contributions)
King Saud bin Abdulaziz University for Health Sciences, Riyadh, Saudi Arabia

Katarzyna Krzywicka (Chapter 52: Treatment of Cerebral Venous Thrombosis)
Department of Neurology, Amsterdam University Medical Centers, Amsterdam, Netherlands

Michael S. Levy (Chapter 23: Blood Disorders)
Lahey Hospital and Medical Center, Burlington, Massachusetts, USA

Mahmoud Mohammaden (Chapter 56: Endovascular Treatment of Acute Ischemic Stroke)
Emory University, Atlanta, Georgia, USA

Adeolu Morawo (Chapter 55: Angioplasty and Stenting)
Creighton University, Francis, Nebraska, USA

Rubrachandran Murugesan (Chapter 57: Brain Aneurysm Treatment)
Boston Medical Center, Boston University, Boston, Massachusetts, USA

Ain Neuhaus (Chapter 50: Neuroprotection)
Acute Stroke Programme, Radcliffe Department of Medicine, Oxford
University, Oxford, UK

Norbert Nighoghossian (Chapter 16: Lacunes and Chapter 61: Prominent Stroke Patients)
Claude Bernard University, Lyon, France

Raul Nogueira (Chapter 56: Endovascular Treatment of Acute Ischemic Stroke)
Marcus Stroke & Neuroscience Center, Grady Memorial Hospital; Emory
University School of Medicine; Atlanta, GA, USA

Bo Norrving (Chapter 43: Clinical Stroke Trials)
Department of Clinical Sciences/Neurology, Lund University,
Lund, Sweden

Chris Ogilvy (Chapter 57: Brain Aneurysm Treatment)
Brain Aneurysm Institute, Beth Israel Deaconess Medical Center, Boston,
Massachusetts, USA

Vitor Oliveira (Chapter 31: Cerebral Angiography)
Hopital de Santa Maria, Lisbon, Portugal

David M. Pelz (Chapter 50: Neuroprotection)
Diagnostic Radiology, University Hospital, London, Ontario, Canada

Angela Richardson (Chapter 59: Treatment of Vascular Malformations)
Neurological Surgery, Indiana University, Indianapolis, Indiana, USA

Cameron John Sabet (Chapter 24: Stroke Genetics)
University of Pennsylvania, Philadelphia, Pennsylvania, USA

Anna Schneider (Chapter 50: Neuroprotection)
Acute Stroke Programme, Radcliffe Department of Medicine, Oxford
University, Oxford, UK

Sana Farhad Somani (Chapter 55: Angioplasty and Stenting)
University of Maryland, Baltimore, Maryland, USA

Barbara Voetsch (Chapter 23: Blood Disorders)
Lahey Hospital and Medical Center; Burlington, Massachusetts, USA

WHY THIS BOOK NEEDED TO BE WRITTEN

Bo Norrving, Professor of Neurology, Lund University, Sweden, Former Chair World Stroke Organization

Stroke is one of the leading causes of illness and disability worldwide. Despite its impact, stroke has for long been in the "shadow" of other diseases, much because there were no treatments available at all. Conceptions that it would never be possible to treat acute stroke because brain cells die within 5–10 minutes were common. Stroke happened by bad luck, out of the blue, and could not be prevented. Stroke patients had the lowest priority in emergency medicine.

All this changed a few decades ago, and by now stroke is one of the best examples of a disease where rapid recognition and treatment is key and dramatically changes the course of the disease. Stroke can be prevented, treated, and managed more effectively than almost any other disease. The history of stroke is a story of hard-won achievements, with chapters that are endlessly fascinating. It tells the story of visionary pioneers who developed new concepts and paved the way for the current public recognition of stroke. The history includes drama, passion, failures, and success.

The present book tells the full story of stroke for the first time, with contributions from many of those who were firsthand eyewitnesses in this long process. For me it is a privilege to contribute to this book, and I am looking forward to reading the chapters of the other authors. The book will surely be a standard reference in the history of medicine.

Jean-Claude Baron, Emeritus Professor of Stroke Medicine and consultant neurologist at Cambridge, UK; presently Consultant Institut National de la Santé et de la Recherche Médicale (INSERM), Paris, France

Knowing how present-day knowledge on diseases – particularly on stroke given the long-lasting nihilism – was acquired is essential to understanding the underlying mechanisms and in turn to manage each patient according to a personalized approach.

Professor Norbert Nighoghossian, Head of stroke department, University Claude Bernard, Lyon, France

I am passionate about the history of medicine and that is the reason for my participation in this book.

Seemant Chatervedi, Stewart J. Greenebaum Endowed Professor of Stroke Neurology, University of Maryland School of Medicine

I wished to contribute to the book for the following reasons: In order to move any scientific field forward, you need to understand which ideas have been tested and failed and which ideas have stood the test of time. I feel this book provides those with an interest in neurology and stroke a road map to the past and future for stroke prevention and treatment.

Jonathan Coutinho, Neurologist, Amsterdam University Medical Centers

When I was finishing up my PhD thesis on cerebral venous thrombosis in 2014, I reviewed the history of this condition because I wanted to understand which physicians had contributed the most to unraveling this rare disease. In this process, I stumbled upon a quote by Dr. Stansfield, who, in 1942, was one of the first who dared treating a patient with cerebral venous thrombosis – a condition that is often accompanied by intracerebral hemorrhages – with heparin. In light of our current evidence-based medicine, his case report may almost seem trivial, but without pioneers such as Dr. Stansfield, we would not have reached the level of understanding of this condition that we are currently at. Thus, when Dr. Caplan offered me the opportunity to contribute to his book and thereby highlight the importance of physicians like Dr. Stansfield, it did not take me long to decide.

Carlos Kase, Emeritus Professor and Chair of Neurology, Boston University Medical School; Consultant Neurologist, Emory University

To me, writing about the history of a disease is a way of recognizing and honoring those who, before us, contributed their knowledge to our current understanding of the condition.

Christopher Ogilvy, Professor of Neurosurgery, Harvard Medical School

While medical advances are being developed at logarithmic speed, it is critical to document and record the history and development of each subspecialty in the medical field. This is particularly true in the field of stroke diagnosis and management where the tools to diagnose and treat intracranial vascular problems have had many recent rapid advances. These advances would not have been possible without the careful and painstaking lines of investigation carried out by physicians and scientists to learn the pathophysiology of intracranial and extracranial vascular disease. Honest and complete documentation of the history of our knowledge of this disease is crucial for further movement forward.

Roberto C. Heros, Senior VP and Chief Medical Administrative Officer, Jackson Health System; Professor of Neurosurgery, University of Miami

I was delighted and very honored to be asked by Dr. Caplan to contribute to this book. Knowing well Dr. Caplan, his contributions to stroke, and his love of history, I have no doubt that this book will be a resounding success and will become a classic to be cherished by all with an interest in cerebrovascular diseases.

Michael DeGeorgia, Professor of Neurology, Case Western Reserve University School of Medicine

To make sense of how or why something happened, we need to retrace the factors that came together earlier. Using embryology as a metaphor: ontogeny recapitulates phylogeny. I was drawn to writing a chapter because I wanted to understand the evolution of neurocritical care. Only through studying history can we grasp how the past creates the present and informs the future.

Alastair Buchan, Neurologist and Professor of Stroke Research, University of Oxford

I wanted to contribute to the history book because my first experience of academic stroke care was as an elective student coming from Oxford, visiting Harvard, and working on the neurology ward at the Beth Israel, in the spring of 1980. I witnessed the next four decades that have seen brain and vessel imaging underpin a complete revolution in both prevention and interventional stroke care, one that now saves lives, reduces risk, and restores many of our patients to a full neurological recovery. We could not have imagined the way brain can be saved and deficits reversed in 1980.

I wanted to contribute to recording the key events over the last half century and give attribution to clinician scientists, by bringing a European flavor to a North American account of this transformation. In doing so I sought to recognize my many mentors and role models across many continents. I am mindful that neuroprotection remains an unmet need, so I look forward to contributing to a future second volume of this history, once that goal is achieved, hopefully before the decade is out.

Conrado Estol, Director, Breyna, Heart and Brain Medicine; Director, Stroke Unit, Guemes Clinic, Buenos Aires, Argentina

During the early years of my neurology residency in the 1980s at the Presbyterian Hospital in Pittsburgh, I was impressed that most neurologists seemed to be somewhat limited in the evaluation of patients with cerebrovascular disease. The exception was Oscar Reinmuth, chairman of the department, and also the editor of the Stroke *journal. My residency projects were based on stroke studies published by authors such as Lou Caplan and Mike Pessin. When I learned that they worked together in Boston,*

I applied for a stroke fellowship with them and was offered the position. Working with them and, above all, learning from them made me feel that I was being a part, albeit small, of history in the making. They stimulated and inspired me with a different view of the stroke patient and also with anecdotal evidence they had obtained directly from C. Miller Fisher during their own training at the Mass General Hospital. Following in their footsteps I was fortunate to be part of the team that treated one of the first patients in the world ever to receive tPA. I was also privileged in being able to attend the weekly brain-cutting sessions with Tessa Hedley-Whyte, E. P. Richardson, and Miller Fisher himself. During those years of intense learning – in which I was continually inspired by being given the right questions to ask – I reviewed and published the history of carotid artery surgery and the evolution, during the twentieth century, of the use of anticoagulants in cerebrovascular disease. As years go by, I now fully realize and appreciate even more the unique opportunity I had of sharing with these giants a small part in the history of stroke. It is a very special honor to contribute to a book edited by Dr. Louis Caplan on the history of stroke.

Adel Alhazzani, Professor of Neurology, College of Medicine, King Saud University

I have witnessed transformation of the treatment of stroke over the last two decades to become a preventable and treatable condition. I wanted to be part of telling the story of the evolution of knowledge about stroke and its treatment.

Gabrielle deVeber, Professor Emeritus, University of Toronto, Senior Scientist, Child Health Evaluative Sciences, Hospital for Sick Children Research Institute

I remember hearing in my adult neurology training that "you learn neurology stroke by stroke." The acute clinical nature of stroke, the precise localization of function with neuroanatomy, and the plasticity of the recovering brain fascinated me. In my career transition into child neurology I was stunned to see several children with stroke in my first year of practice. I saw that stroke in newborns and young children looked similar on brain imaging, but the mechanisms, manifestations, and trajectory of recovery were entirely different. Thus, treatments for stroke from adult studies could not be simply migrated to children. Over my career, childhood stroke emerged as its own subspecialty for the first time. Reaching back through the histories of adult stroke and pediatric cerebral palsy, and seeing the gradual converging of these two specialties over the past two centuries, I realized we are still part of an actively unfolding and dynamic story. I wanted this story to be told.

Patrícia Canhão, Assistant Professor, Faculty of Medicine University of Lisbon, Portugal

The history of cerebral venous thrombosis privileges us with very rich clinical reports, provides interesting considerations about etiology, puts forward modern therapeutic proposals, and excellently describes the progress in knowledge about the prognosis. It is a story told in different voices, by the actors of the different clinical scenarios in which CVT occurs. It is a success story that demonstrates how collaboration between researchers from multiple centers makes it possible to advance knowledge. Knowing part of this story is to understand more fully this disease of the venous side of the brain. This is the reason for my contributing a chapter to this book.

Victor Oliveira, Neurologist, Faculty of Medicine, University of Lisbon, Portugal

The history of cerebrovascular diseases in the last hundred years is made up of a sequence of achievements that completely overturned previous concepts. Advance in the understanding of its clinical manifestations, some of them subtle, and its pathophysiology, epidemiology, and treatments constitutes extraordinary progress with direct implications for a large number of patients around the world. Some doctors have left their names associated with milestones in that progression. Their works, personalities, and careers should be remembered not only as a tribute but also for the understanding of the history of medicine.

PREFACE

Every illness is not a set of pathologies but a personal story.
> —Anne Fadiman, *The Spirit Catches You and You Fall Down: A Hmong Child,*
> *Her American Doctors, and the Collision of Two Cultures* (New York: Farrar,
> Straus and Giroux, 1997)

There's always a story. It's all stories, really. The sun coming up every day is a story. Everything's got a story in it. Change the story, change the world.
> —Terry Pratchett, *A Hat Full of Sky* (New York: Harper Collins, 2000)

Behind every person, every idea, every event, every advance there is a story. In this book, we collect many of the stories that together tell some of the history of a medical condition: stroke.

Stroke is one of the most important and most feared conditions known to man. World history has been changed by stroke. Many important leaders in science, medicine, the arts, and politics have had their productivity cut prematurely short by stroke. Some of their stories are included in this book. Even more important is the threat that stroke poses to every individual. What could be more devastating than to lose the ability to move a limb, stand, walk, see, feel, think clearly, remember, read, write, speak, or understand language? Loss of function is often quick and totally unanticipated. Impairments may be permanent. Most individuals fear stroke more than any other disease, with the possible exception of cancer. Everyone would like to exit this life with their capabilities and mind intact, despite the inevitable aging of their bodies.

Clearly, the history of stroke needs to be written. Stroke is a very complex disorder. Multiple conditions and risk factors and developments in medical knowledge and technology relate intimately to the history of stroke. A detailed complete analysis of the evolution of knowledge about all these stroke-related factors would fill many large volumes. These volumes would constitute a reference valuable to scholars but would make rather tedious reading. Instead, we have striven herein to offer an eclectic, easily read, single volume that shares selected stories. We elected to focus on key individuals who were innovators, movers, and shakers who advanced the field further along. We also emphasized ideas – how they began, and how they then evolved up to the present day. We also chose to emphasize the twentieth century, especially the second half of the twentieth up to the end of the first quarter of the twenty-first century. This period saw the most dramatic and extensive changes in knowledge about stroke and in caring for stroke patients. The story of those advances has not been told. The senior editor was active during this period and, as a witness, could help deliver a firsthand account of progress and how it developed.

Many texts provide accounts of medical advances beginning with the ancients and Hippocrates. We include eclectically some of the early history that relates to the brain and to vascular disease, but it is not the emphasis of this volume.

We have asked individuals from different countries to contribute. They were chosen because of their knowledge about various aspects of stroke development. We have edited their contributions, sometimes extensively, to make them conform to the style and goals of the volume. We have also limited references to those that were essential and important. We kept the volume sparsely illustrated with figures in order to reduce the cost of publication and printing and to contain the cost for those who wish to purchase the book. Pictures and photographs of the individuals discussed are now readily available through the internet.

Louis R. Caplan MD
Aishwarya Aggarwal MD

PART I

EARLY RECOGNITION

CHAPTER ONE

HIPPOCRATES AND EARLY GREEK MEDICAL PRACTICE

Hippocrates is generally acknowledged to be the "Father of Medicine." He is usually portrayed in pictures and sculptures as a grandfatherly, bald man with a serious expression and a small well-trimmed beard. Much about him is unknown and much is myth.

Many schoolchildren have read Homer, the famous Greek poet, and his *Iliad* and *Odyssey*, which relate the tales of the ancient Greek gods. In the period after Homer, approximately 800–400 BCE, disease and illness were attributed to the gods, mostly a minor deity, Asclepius. Shrines to this god were erected; priests offered prayers at these shrines for restoration of health.

Around 400 BCE, a medical culture arose on the island of Cos, in the Aegean Sea within the Greek archipelago, that greatly departed from the supernaturally based precepts of the Aesculapian shrines. We know about this culture from a series of books, often dubbed the Hippocratic corpus [1–4]. The corpus of writings consisted of about 70 variegated texts written in the Ionic (Greek, meaning from Ionia) dialect using a wide variety of styles [3]. These are often collected as *The Genuine Works of Hippocrates* [5], *The Aphorisms of Hippocrates* [6], and *The Book of Prognostics* [7]. Although all are often attributed to one man, Hippocrates, much was certainly contributed by others. Hippocrates and his medical colleagues lived in a time of great intellectual activity and ferment in Greece. Hippocrates's life spanned those of Sophocles and Plato and intersected with Aristotle's. He was a contemporary of the statesmen Pericles and Cimon; of the playwrights Aeschylus, Sophocles, Euripides, and Aristophanes; and of the historians Herodotus and Thucydides [4].

Hippocrates and his followers taught that nature and natural causes explained health, illness, and diseases. Deviations from health were not the result of the action of gods. Natural causes could be discovered by careful observation. The task was difficult as emphasized in the most cited aphorism, "Life is short, the Art is long, opportunity fleeting, experience delusive, judgement difficult" [6]. The modus operandi of a physician was to observe the patient at the bedside. Hippocrates observed the patient carefully, wrote down a description of the symptoms, and taught his disciples at the bedside. Most importantly, the physician followed the course of the illness. A major focus was prognosis, for example, "in every disease it is a good sign when the patient's intellect is sound" [6]. Hippocrates emphasized professionalism. Physicians should interact with patients in a highly responsible and moral professional manner. We still revere this aspect by having students recite the Hippocratic oath at the beginning of medical school or when donning "white coats."

The writings of Hippocrates probably contain the first clear descriptions of stroke, and the first use of the term *apoplexy* [8,9]. Although "apoplexy" is not defined, its use within cases describes a very sudden loss of neurological function [9]. Hippocrates and his followers emphasized clinical observation and prognostic indicators. Hippocrates was a keen observer and urged careful observation and recording of phenomenology. The corpus contains many clear descriptions of cases. Hippocrates and his followers were mostly interested in predicting for the patient and family the outcome of an illness. In his aphorisms on apoplexy, Hippocrates wrote that apoplexy was most common between 40 and 60 years of age, and attacks of numbness might reflect "impending apoplexy" [8,10]: "To get over a strong attack of apoplexy is impossible, over a weak one, not easy." He astutely noted that "when persons in good health are suddenly seized with pains in the head and straightaway are laid down speechless and breathe with stertor, they die in seven days when fever comes on" [8,10]. This description of subarachnoid hemorrhage shows the Hippocratic emphasis on observation and prognosis. One of his descriptions was probably the first clinical description of aphasia. "A woman who lived on the sea-front was seized with a fever while in the third month of pregnancy.... On the third day, pain in the head, neck, and around the right clavicle. Very shortly, the tongue became unable to articulate and the right arm was paralyzed following a convulsion.... Her speech was delirious.... Fourth day speech was indistinct" [8].

In a case that described a wound to one side of the head, Hippocrates noted that paralysis affected the opposite side of the body [1]. Hippocrates observed that there were many blood vessels that were connected to the brain, most of which were thin, but two (the carotid arteries) were thick. The Greeks in the time of Hippocrates knew that interruption of these blood vessels could cause loss of consciousness, so they called these thick arteries *carotid* from the Greek word *karos* meaning deep sleep.

Hippocrates and his followers left a blueprint on how to practice medicine and how to interact with patients. That is their main legacy.

NOTES AND REFERENCES

1. Garrison FH. *An Introduction to the History of Medicine*, 4th ed. Philadelphia: WB Saunders, 1929, pp. 92–102.
2. McHenry LC. *Garrison's History of Neurology*. Revised and enlarged. Springfield, IL: Charles C. Thomas, 1969.
3. Nuland S. *Doctors: The Biography of Medicine*. Birmingham, AL: The Libraries of Gryphon Editions, 1988.
4. Major R. Hippocrates and the island of Cos. *Yale Journal of Biology and Medicine* 1941;14(1):1–11.
5. Adams F. *The Genuine Works of Hippocrates, Translated from the Greek*. Baltimore: Williams and Wilkins, 1939.
6. Adams F. *Aphorisms of Hippocrates*. London: Dodo Press, 2009.
7. Adams F, *Hippocrates: The Book of Prognostics*. London: Dodo Press, 2009.
8. Fields WS, Lemak NA. *A History of Stroke: Its Recognition and Treatment*. New York: Oxford University Press, 1989.
9. Engelhardt E. Apoplexy, cerebrovascular disease, and stroke. Historical evolution of terms and definitions. *Dementia Neuropsychologia* 2017;11:449–453.
10. Clark E. Apoplexy in the Hippocratic writings. *Bulletin of the History of Medicine* 1963; 37:301–314.

CHAPTER TWO

EARLY GRECO-ROMAN CONTRIBUTIONS

During the centuries after Hippocrates and before Galen, there were very few contributions concerning stroke. Most concerned observations that reflected on anatomy.

Aurelius Cornelius Celsus (25 BCE–50 CE) was a Roman writer who lived during the realms of Augustus and Tiberius. He was not a physician but was called an encyclopedist who accumulated and recorded vast quantities of information in *De medicina* [1–3]. This tome was divided into eight books, mostly consisting of long lists of various medications, weights, measures, and symbols. Management of injuries, skin conditions, and bone lesions predominated. Advice for management mostly referred to the writings and prescriptions of the Hippocratic corpus. Celsus classified "lesions harmful to the body" into five groups: (1) when something from without causes the lesion, e.g., a wound; (2) when some internal part becomes corrupted (diseased); (3) when some new formation has developed (he used the term *carcinoma*); (4) when something has grown bigger; and (5) when there is some defect [2]. Celsus commented on mydriasis and abnormalities of eye movement after an injury: "the eyeball cannot be directed at any object or be held at all steady but with no reason turns now this way now that and so does not afford a view of objects." Celsus uses the term *apoplexy* and indicated that paralysis could be limited to some body parts and need not be complete. He recognized bleeding under the skull and depressed skull fractures as affecting brain function. He is probably best known for describing the four characteristics of inflammation: "rubor et tumor cum calor et dolor" (redness, swelling, warmth, and pain) [2,4].

Rufus of Ephesus (110–180 CE) was a Greek physician and respected practitioner who wrote treatises on pathology, anatomy, and patient care [1,4–6]. He has been described as the medical link between Hippocrates and Galen. The description of the plague by Rufus includes the environment in which it flourished, the symptoms and physical signs, and the symptomatic treatments applied. At one time Ephesus had a population of 150,000 people. Medical care and public health were quite advanced. In Roman times, Ephesus contained temples that also functioned as hospitals, doctors who practiced according to the teachings of Asclepius, medical schools, and even public toilets. Although a follower of Hippocrates, Rufus often departed from that author's teachings. His writings dealt with the elderly, a topic neglected by prior writers. His teachings emphasized the importance of anatomy. He showed that nerves proceeded from the brain. He accurately described the optic nerves and their crossing, the optic chiasm. He divided the nerves that emanated from the brain into two classes, those of the senses and those of motion. He considered the heart to be the seat of life and responsible for the pulse felt in the limbs. He noted that the left ventricle was thicker than the right. Two of his books, *On the Names of the Parts of the Human Body* and *Case Histories*, are still available today.

Areteus of Cappadocia (120–180 CE) wrote a textbook on the practice of medicine [1,7–9]. The best-known book written by this Greek physician was *Of the Causes and Signs of Acute and Chronic Disease*. Like Hippocrates, he emphasized careful observation and recording of symptoms and signs. He noted the temperature, pulse, breathing rate, and the state of the pupils of each patient; he palpated the abdomen and internal organs. Areteus is credited with introducing the term *diabetes* into medicine. "Diabetes" is derived from the Greek word for "siphon," indicating the sufferer's intense thirst and excessive emission of fluids. He rendered the earliest clear account of this condition [10].

He described and separated apoplexy from paraplegia and paralysis. *Apoplexy* affected a number of functions, including a defect of understanding, motion, and sensation, while *paraplegia* was a localized disturbance of motion and touch in the arms or legs, and *paralysis* or *paresis* referred only to loss of motion. Loss of touch was anesthesia. He also wrote about the pupil and enlargement and constriction. He wrote that "should the apoplexy be severe, the patient is as good as dead, especially in the aged for they cannot survive the greatness of the illness combined with the misery of advanced life" [8,9]. Areteus noted that paralysis develops on the side opposite a head lesion but on the same side in a spinal lesion:

> If, therefore the commencement of the affection be below the head such as the membrane of the spinal marrow, the parts which are homonymous and connected with it are paralyzed: the right on the right side, the left on the left side. But if the head be primarily affected on the right side, the left side of the body will be paralyzed; and the right, if on the left side.

Areteus further explained: "The cause of this is the interchange in the origin of the nerves, for they do not pass along on the same side, the right on the right side, until their termination; but each of them passes over to the other side from that of its origin, decussating each other in the form of the letter X."

Paul of Aegenia (625–690) was a Byzantine Greek physician who wrote the *Medical Compendium in Seven Books* [11,12]. The intent was to contain all Western medical knowledge. The work was published in Venice, Italy, in 1528, and another edition appeared in Basel, Switzerland, in 1538. An English translation was published by Francis Adams in 1834 [5,6]. Paul commented on apoplexy without mention of the brain. His writings further stated: "Apoplectics lie speechless, motionless, and insensible, without fever. The precursors of this affection are sudden and acute pain of the head, distention of the jugular veins, vertigo, flashes as it were of light in the eyes, an inordinate coldness of the extremities, palpitation and difficult motion of the whole body" [12].

Greco-Roman physicians and writers thought of disease as an aberration of nature and natural forces and causes. Clinical observation was a method of diagnosis and prognosticating. Their reflections on brain anatomy and function came from carefully observing patients and their functioning. A major topic and concern was the physician-patient relationship.

These early writings contained mostly definitions of terms and observations concerning patients who developed apoplexy. They did not further knowledge concerning the causes or pathology of apoplexy, or the physiology of brain function.

NOTES AND REFERENCES

1. McHenry LC. *Garrison's History of Neurology*. Springfield, IL: Charles C. Thomas, 1969, pp. 15–17.
2. Celsus. *De medicina with an English translation by Walter George Spenser*. Cambridge, MA: Harvard University Press, 1961.
3. Fields WS, Lemak NA. *A History of Stroke*. New York: Oxford University Press, 1989, p. 4.
4. Lyons AS, Petrucelli RJ. *Medicine, an Illustrated History*. New York: Abradale Press, Harry N. Abrams, 1987, pp. 248–249.
5. Gersh CJ. Naming the body: A translation with commentary and interpretive essays of three anatomical works attributed to Rufus of Ephesus. Thesis, 2012. Handle: http://hdl.handle.net/2027.42/95946.
6. JHT. Editorial. Rufus of Ephesus. *JAMA* 1960;174:2070–2071.
7. Garcia-Albea Ristol E. Aretaeus of Cappadocia (2nd century AD) and the earliest neurological descriptions. *Revue Neurologique* 2009;48:322–327.
8. Aretus of Capadocia. *The Extant Works of Aretaeus the Capadocian*. Francis Adams Edition. London: Sydenham Society; Boston: Milford, 1856.
9. Aretus. *Of the Causes and Signs of Acute and Chronic Disease Translated from the Greek by T. F. Reynolds*. London: PF Pickering, 1837.

10. Laios K, Karamanou M, Saridaki Z, Androutsos G. Aretaeus of Cappadocia and the first description of diabetes. *Hormones (Athens)* 2012;11:109–113.

11. Paul of Aegina. Wikipedia. Available at https://en.wikipedia.org/wiki/Paul_of_ Aegina.

12. Paul of Aegina. *On Headache, Cephalea, Hemicrania, Phrenitis, Erysipelas of the Brain, Lethargy, Vertigo, Epilepsy, Apoplexy and Hemiplegia or Paralysis, Tetanus, Tremblings etc in the Seven Books of Paulus Aegineta Translated from the Greek by Francis Adams.* London: Printed for the Sydenham Society, 1844.

CHAPTER THREE

ISLAMIC AND MIDDLE EASTERN CONTRIBUTIONS

Quran (the holy book), prophetic traditions (sunnah) and Prophet Muhammad Peace Be Upon Him (PBUH) sayings (hadith) are the cornerstone of Islamic knowledge. Jurists and scholars later expanded on these foundations to build Islamic literature, not only about matters of prayers and submission, but also on day-to-day life affairs. Countless traditions and hadith deal with ailments and healing. Books that became a science of their own known as *Tibbul-Nabbi*; the Medicine of Prophet (PBUH), are based on these writings.

In the early days of Islamic medicine, work of at least seven different writers were titled as *Tibbul-Nabbi* describing the views of the Prophet (PBUH) on various aspects of medicine [1]. Among the most famous and detailed of these works is that by Ibn Qayyam Al-Juzziya. The work contains 277 chapters and discusses medications, various ailments, and other aspects of medicine such as medicolegal matters and hallmarks of competent doctors [1]. In addition to these works titled as *Tibbul-Nabbi*, later physicians and scientists wrote many treatises on medicine, some of which are preserved and translated into various languages. Others have perished with time, particularly after the destruction of large libraries by invaders. Several verses from the Quran and hadith deal with heart, blood vessels (the cardiovascular system), and blood [2].

Abu Ali Al-Hossein Ibn Sina (Avicenna) is the most well-known and recognized early Muslim philosopher, physician, and author. He wrote one of the most famous books in the history of Islamic medicine in 1025 CE.

Avicenna was born around 980 in Afshana, a village near Bukhara in present-day Uzbekistan. His father, Abdullāh, was a respected scholar. Avicenna had memorized the entire Quran by the age of 10. While still very young, he also studied Indian arithmetic, Islamic jurisprudence, and philosophy. The story is told that, as a teenager, he was greatly troubled by the *Metaphysics* of Aristotle, which he could not understand. During moments of baffled inquiry, he would leave his books, perform the requisite ablutions, and then go to a mosque and pray until he got some light or understanding. He used to study late into the night and at times would find solutions to his queries in dreams. He read through the *Metaphysics* of Aristotle 40 times, until the words were imprinted on his memory, but their meaning remained obscure. He rejoiced when a brief commentary by al-Farabi in a book that he bought from a bookstall for only three dirhams clarified Aristotle's text for him. He got involved in medicine at age 16, and not only learned medical theory, but also attended the sick, discovering new methods of treatment. He achieved full status as a qualified physician at age 18. He found medicine not to be a hard and thorny science, like mathematics and metaphysics, and he made great progress in medicine [3].

His major work, *al-Qanun fi'l tibb*, is commonly known as *The Canon of Medicine*. In this five-volume encyclopedia of medicine, Ibn Sina described vascular anatomy, including the role of the carotid arteries in supplying blood to the brain [4]. He also described major parts of the central and peripheral nervous systems, including the two cerebral hemispheres, their connection to the posterior regions of the brain, and extension into the spinal cord that gave rise to peripheral nerves [5].

One of the most cited and quoted early Muslim physicians was Abu Bakr Muhammed Ibn Zakria AlRazi (Rhazes) [6]. He was a Persian scholar, researcher, physician, and alchemist. He was probably the first to write separately on the diseases of children [6,7]. Rhazes preceded and was a major influence on Avicenna. He was born in in the ancient city of Rey, near Tehran. A musician during his youth, he later became an alchemist. He classified and categorized various substances. He also identified medical components of substances derived from plants, animals, and minerals [7]. He began to study medicine at age 30. Because of his expertise and reputation, he was appointed chief of the main hospital in Baghdad and became court physician. As a teacher of medicine, Rhazes attracted students of all backgrounds and interests and was said to be compassionate and devoted to the service of his patients, whether rich or poor. His medical works were translated and became known among medieval European practitioners. Some sections of his publications were used in the medical curriculum of Western universities for centuries. Rhazes wrote over 200 books and treatises on medicine, alchemy, philosophy, and religion. The best-known were *Liber almansoris*, a short general textbook on medicine in 10 chapters, and *Man la Yahduruhu al-Tabib* (For One without a Doctor), a medical book for the general public [6,7].

Other prominent Muslim physicians in the Islamic Golden Era included Abul Hasan Ali ibn Abbas Al Majusi (Haly Abbas), Abul Waleed Muhammad Ibn Ahmad Ibn Rushd (Averroes), Alauddin Abu al Hassan Ali ibn Hazmi (Ibn AlNafis), and Abu AlQasim Khalaf Ibn AlAbbas AlZahrawi (Albucasis). The time period and titles of their most famous books are summarized in Table 3.1. Some of the images available on various internet resources are shown in Figure 3.1.

Another very influential and often cited Middle Eastern physician and scholar was Moses ben Maimon (1138–1204), commonly known as Maimonides. He was born in 1138 in Cordoba, Spain. His father and many relatives were Jewish rabbis and scholars. At an early age, Maimonides developed an interest in sciences and philosophy. He read literature written by Greek philosophers that was accessible in Arabic translations, and became

TABLE 3.1. *Name, period, and books of some renowned Muslim physicians of Islamic Golden Era*

Arabic name	Latin name	Period	Title of the work (shown in *Arabic*, **English**, and ***Latin***)
Abu Bakr Muhammed Ibn Zakria AlRazi	Rhazes	854–925	*Kitab AlMansouri* **Book of Medicine Dedicated to Mansour** ***Liber de medicinaad Almansorem***
			Al-Kitab Al-Hawi **The Virtuous Life** ***Continens liber***
Abul Hasan Ali ibn Abbas Al Majusi	Haly Abbas	?–994	*Kitab Kamil as-Sina'a at-Tibbiya* **The Complete Art of Medicine** Also known as *Kitab AlMalakiy* **The Royal Book** ***Liber regalis***
Abu Ali Al-Hossein Ibn Sina	Avicenna	980–1037	*Al-Qanun fi'l tibb* **The Canon of Medicine**
			Kitab al-Shifa **The Book of Healing**
Abul Waleed Muhammad Ibn Ahmad Ibn Rushd	Averroes	1126–1198	*Al-Kulliyat fi'l tibb* **The General Principles of Medicine** ***Colliget***
Alauddin Abu al Hassan Ali ibn Hazmi al Qarshi al Dimashqi (ibn AlNafis)		1213–1288	*Al-Shamil fi'l tibb* **The Comprehensive Book on Medicine** *Sharah Tashrih AlQanun* **Commentary on the Canon**

Rhazes	Haly Abbas	Avicenna	Averroes	Ibn AlNafis	Maimonides
Abu Bakr Muhammed Ibn Zakria AlRazi	Abul Hasan Ali ibn Abbas Al Majusi	Abu Ali Al-Hossein Ibn Sina	Abul Waleed Muhammad Ibn Ahmad Ibn Rushd	Alauddin Abu al Hassan Ali ibn Hazmi al Qarshi al Dimashqi (ibn AlNafis)	Moses ben Maimon

3.1. Prominent Islamic and Middle Eastern physicians.

immersed in the sciences and learning of Islamic culture. Córdoba was captured in 1148, and the protected status of non-Muslims was abolished. Maimonides's family, along with most other Jews, chose exile. Maimonides may have feigned a conversion to Islam before escaping; however, this forced conversion was ruled legally invalid under Islamic law. Maimonides lived in Fez, Morocco, during the years 1166–1168. He ultimately settled in Fustat, Egypt, around 1168. His early years in Egypt were spent interpreting and writing religious texts [8,9].

Having achieved some medical training in Cordoba and Fez, he then began to vigorously and thoroughly study extant medical texts. He was able to gain widespread recognition for his medical knowledge and writings and was appointed court physician to the Grand Vizier al-Qadial Fadil, then to Sultan Saladin, after whose death he remained a physician to the Sunni Muslim Ayyubid dynasty. In 1193, Saladin died and his eldest son, al-Afdal Nur al-Din Ali, succeeded him. Maimonides's medical duties became even heavier. He described his day in a famous letter:

> I am obliged to visit him every day, early in the morning, and when he or any of his children or concubines are indisposed, I cannot leave Cairo but must stay during most of the day in the palace. It also frequently happens that one or two of the officers fall sick and I must attend to their healing. Every day, early in the morning, I go to Cairo and I do not return to Fostat until the afternoon. I dismount from my animal, wash my hands, go forth to my patients, and entreat them to bear with me while I partake of some light refreshment, the only meal I eat in twenty-four hours. Then I go to attend to my patients and write prescriptions and directions for their ailments. When night falls, I am so exhausted that I can hardly speak. [8]

In his medical writings, Maimonides emphasized moderation and a healthy lifestyle. He practiced holistic, patient-centered care and was an advocate of rehabilitative and occupational medicine. Maimonides's concept of "a healthy mind in a healthy body" was one of the earliest descriptions of psychosomatic medicine. He wrote that the physical well-being of a person was dependent on their mental well-being, and vice versa. He wrote about apoplexy, and one of his aphorisms was "One can prognosticate regarding a stroke, called apoplexy. If the attack is severe, he will certainly die but if it is minor, then cure is possible, though difficult ... the worst situation that can occur following a stroke is the complete irreversible suppression of respiration." His treatises became influential for generations of physicians. His greatest significance comes from his role as a transmitter across the divide from the ancient world to the emerging Arab and subsequently European scholarly world and from his role as a model physician [9].

WRITINGS ABOUT STROKE

Stroke, as we understand it today, is likely an evolution of the concept of apoplexy, which was described more than 2000 years ago by Hippocrates, Aristotle, and later Galen. Apoplexy referred to a clinical condition characterized by rapid loss of consciousness and various manifestations of brain dysfunction. The term *apoplexia* means struck down with violence or to strike suddenly [10]. The Greco-Roman concepts of stroke from the fifth century BCE to the second century BCE prevailed until about the eighth century CE, when Muslim physicians elaborated on and further refined their concepts of stroke [11,12]. They translated the work of Greco-Roman physicians and added their own observations. Stroke is referred to as *sekteh* in the works of Avicenna [13].

Clinical Features of Stroke

Some of the clinical features of stroke described by Avicenna included sudden onset without preceding symptoms, impairment of movement, lack of sensation, shallow breathing, absence of fever, feeble pulse, and dark, "vaporous" urine containing a branny or grainy sediment [11]. Unilateral weakness with or without premonitory symptoms of headache, dizziness, numbness of the limbs, and visual scotomas was also recognized [12]. Rhazes considered hemiplegia to be related to part of the brain (the parenchyma) and not just the ventricles [12]. Some literature suggests that Muslim physicians also recognized that speech was mostly affected when the right side of body was paralyzed and had some understanding of hemisphere dominance [11,12]. Similarly, facial palsy without paralysis of limbs was recognized as separate from stroke by Rhazes.

Stroke Etiology and Localization

Avicenna had tried to explain stroke using the mechanisms of "occlusion" and "repletion." In the occlusion mechanism he postulated contraction (head trauma?) or solidification of the brain due to excess cold. In this mechanism, there was no harmful material in the brain. In the explanation of repletion, he suggested presence of noxious material in the brain, either through swelling, tumor, or inflammation with fever; or repletion without swelling due to accumulation of one of the four humors in the brain [11]. The presence of this noxious material prevented the flow of animal spirit from the brain to the periphery, resulting in paralysis.

Avicenna attributed strokes to wet and cold nature, which in humoral theories may be related to people who are overweight [13]. Haly Abbas considered accumulation of thick phlegm or thick blood in the ventricles or cells as the cause of apoplexy or stroke. This probably was a description of hemorrhagic stroke [12]. Similarly, Avicenna attributed high blood humor as a potential cause of stroke, which may be associated with hypertension or hemorrhagic strokes, according to current understanding of stroke [13]. It is not clear if the Muslim physicians had access to autopsy specimens or merely speculated on these pathological mechanisms. Avicenna also considered total obstruction of the ventricles in severe strokes, and partial obstruction in less severe causes [12].

The question of the role of heart or brain as the seat of stroke remained during the beginning of the Muslim era until Averroes reached the concept that is closest to the current understanding of stroke. Ibn Rushd, often Latinized as Averroes, was a Muslim scientist and jurist who wrote about many subjects, including philosophy, theology, medicine, astronomy, physics, psychology, mathematics, Islamic jurisprudence and law, and linguistics. Averroes considered apoplexy to occur because of obstruction in the pathway (blood vessels) of spirits that passed from the heart to the brain [11]. Averroes posited that apoplexy (stroke) originated in arteries and the cerebral ventricles. This may have been the first conceptualization of obstruction in blood vessels leading to brain damage.

Treatment of Stroke

Avicenna described various ways of treating stroke in his book *The Canon of Medicine*. In the acute phase of stroke, he promoted venesection, or cupping, in the lower neck or upper back; enema (made of rose water, whey, and barley water); along with nasal application of aromatic agents that stimulated the central nervous system [12,13]. For the subacute phase, he added the use of laxatives, along with topical applications of various medicines and oils. In the chronic phase of stroke, he suggested emesis, purgatives, and gargles of various substances, along with massage [13]. Vegetables, fruits, and medicinal plants including citrus fruits, ginger, and beetroot were also prescribed [12,13]. Most of the medicinal plants described in the treatment of stroke were considered to have antioxidant and neuroprotective properties in herbal medicine [12,13]. Avicenna also discussed the quantity and quality of food for stroke patients. He wrote that drink with food could be harmful. He also suggested to not let patients sleep soon after meals. Both of these precautions can likely be explained by the risk of aspiration as we currently understand it. He also mentioned adequate rest, sleep, and some degree of exercise for these patients [11]. There is also mention of cautery in the chronic stage of stroke by Al-Zahrawi, known as Abulcasis, an Arab Andalusian physician, surgeon, and chemist. Albucasis favored four areas of cauterization on the head and one supplemental area of cautery on the abdomen [11].

Severity and Prognosis of Stroke

Some observations about respiratory status were associated with prognosis. Foaming from the mouth with strenuous breathing associated with apoplectic attack was considered a sign of fatal outcome by Rhazes [11]. Avicenna observed that respiration may be so shallow in apoplectic attack that it may be difficult to distinguish if the apoplectic victim was still comatose or dead. He suggested to postpone the funeral for 72 hours in such patients [11]. Patients who had paralysis associated with poor respiration and swallowing reflexes were considered to have poor prognosis by Avicenna, whereas those with preserved swallowing were considered to have a better prognosis. The patients who had severe headache with stroke were considered at risk of dying within 7 days [13]. The high mortality risk in strokes associated with severe headache may be related to patients who had subarachnoid hemorrhage but were not diagnosed as such.

CONCLUSIONS

Although some of Muslim physicians' work in the Islamic Golden Era had roots in Greco-Roman concepts, they clearly expanded on those concepts and made conclusions that fit more with current understanding of stroke. Similarly, Maimonides had one foot in Greco-Roman concepts and the other in Arab teachings and writings. Having no proven access to autopsy specimens, these physician scientists were able to explain stroke as a cerebrovascular disease in which the brain was afflicted by diseased vessels resulting in sudden catastrophic manifestations of stroke. They were able to categorize stroke severity and determine some stroke prognostic factors. The management strategies were limited but considered the complications of stroke, including aspiration, constipation, and physical disability. The knowledge provided by them remained the mainstay of medical concepts for almost a century from 700 CE to 1600 CE until the renaissance of European medicine.

NOTES AND REFERENCES

1. Elgood C. The medicine of the prophet. *Med. Hist.* 1962 Apr;6(2):146–153.

2. Loukas M, Saad Y, Tubbs RS, Shoja MM. The heart and cardiovascular system in the Qur'an and hadeeth. *Int. J. Cardiol.* 2010 Apr 1;140(1):19–23.

3. Avicenna, early life. Wikipedia. Available at https://en.wikipedia.org/wiki/Avicenna#Early_life (accessed on January 18, 2021).

4. Mazengenya P, Bhikha R. A critical appraisal of 11th century treatise by Ibn Sina (Avicenna) on the anatomy of the vascular system: Comparison with modern anatomic descriptions. *Morphologie.* 2018 Jun;102(337):61–68.

5. Mazengenya P, Bhikha R. The structure and function of the central nervous system and sense organs in *The Canon of Medicine* by Avicenna. *Arch. Iran Med.* 2017 Jan;20 (1):67–70.

6. Zarrintan S, Shahnaee A, Aslanabadi S. Rhazes (AD 865–925) and his early contributions to the field of pediatrics. *Child's Nervous Syst.* 2018;34:1435–1438. Modanlou HD. A tribute to Zakariya Razi (865–925 AD), an Iranian pioneer scholar. *Arch. Iran Med.* 2008;11:673–677.

7. Muhammad ibn Zakariya al-Razi. Wikipedia. Available at https://en.wikipedia.org/wiki/Muhammad_ibn_Zakariya_al-Razi.

8. Nuland SB. *Maimonides.* New York: Nextbook: Schocken, 2005. Rosner F. The life of Moses Maimonides, a prominent medieval physician. *Einstein Quart. J. Biol. Med.* 2002;19:125–128.

9. Rosner F. *The Medical Legacy of Moses Maimonides.* Hoboken, NJ: KTAV Publishing House, 1998. Rosner F. *Maimonides' Medical Writings, vol. 3: The Medical Aphorisms of Moses Maimonides.* Haifa: Israel Maimonides Research Institute, 1989.

10. Engelhardt E. Apoplexy, cerebrovascular disease, and stroke: Historical evolution of terms and definitions. *Dement. Neuropsychol.* 2017 Oct–Dec;11(4):449–453.

11. Karenberg A, Hort I. Medieval descriptions and doctrines of stroke: Preliminary analysis of select sources. Part II: between Galenism and Aristotelism – Islamic theories of apoplexy (800–1200). *J. Hist. Neurosci.* 1998 Dec;7(3):174–185.

12. Khuda I, Al-Shamrani F. Stroke medicine in antiquity: The Greek and Muslim contribution. *J. Family Community Med.* 2018 Sep–Dec;25(3):143–147.

13. Zargaran A, Zarshenas MM, Karimi A, Yarmohammadi H, Borhani-Haghighi A. Management of stroke as described by Ibn Sina (Avicenna) in *The Canon of Medicine.* *Int. J. Cardiol.* 2013 Nov 15;169(4):233–237.

PART II

BASIC KNOWLEDGE, SIXTEENTH TO EARLY
TWENTIETH CENTURIES

Anatomy, Physiology, and Pathology

CHAPTER FOUR

ANDREAS VESALIUS

Andreas Vesalius was born on December 31, 1514, in Brussels, Belgium. His father was an apothecary to members of the Hapsburg family. Others in his family were scholars or physicians, some also serving royalty. The family library was extensive, and, as a boy, Andreas was always reading. At age 15, Andreas left Brussels to study at the University of Louvain where he was taught Latin, Greek, philosophy, rhetoric, and some Hebrew. He earned a master of arts degree. Andreus had decided on a medical career, and since Louvain did not have an outstanding medical school, at age 18, he traveled to Paris [1–3]. The French medical school that he attended was dominated by reading and studying the writings of Galen. Vesalius did his first human cadaver dissections in Paris and became fascinated by anatomy. During his third year of study, war broke out in France. Vesalius returned to Belgium and finished his medical studies at the University of Louvain, earning a bachelor of medicine degree.

He traveled to Basel, Switzerland, where he was heavily influenced by the second edition of a book titled the *Paraphrase of Rhazes* written by a Persian physician. This may be when he had his first thought about publishing an anatomy book of his own. He then went to Venice where he began to search for an artist who might illustrate his anatomy text. There he was introduced, perhaps by Titian, to a young artist, Jan Stephan van Calcar, who was also originally from Belgium. Vesalius continued his medical studies in nearby Padua where he had bedside training. He was granted a doctor of medicine degree with distinction in December 1537. The day after his graduation he was appointed professor of surgery and anatomy and assigned the paltry salary of 40 florins per year.

The Renaissance flourished in Italy during the sixteenth century. The universities in Padua and Bologna were leaders in science and medicine. Leonardo da Vinci (1452–1519), and Botticelli (1445–1510) had preceded the medical career of Vesalius, but Michelangelo (1475–1564) and Titian (1488–1576) were still active. Leonardo's anatomical drawings may have stimulated Vesalius. Padua was an exciting place for students to learn and study art, science, and medicine. Among the educational policies of the University of Padua was the notion that faculty members were permitted, and even expected, to make innovations in the school's teaching methods. On the very first day of his appointment as professor, Vesalius began a series of cadaver dissections. In the past, the professor or a lecturer would sit on a high chair above the students and read the Galenic text in Latin while someone else performed a dissection below that the lecturer could not see. The stated purpose of these sessions was to prove the correctness of the Galenic writings. Instead of sitting above the action, however, Vesalius acted in the role of surgeon, lecturer, and demonstrator. He hung a skeleton near the dissection table for the students' reference and then began by sketching an outline of the bones on the skin surface of the cadaver. He prepared large charts to show the anatomy and what was known about function. He illustrated his teaching by dissections and even vivisections of small animals to demonstrate living organs or comparative anatomy. His lectures became very popular; he often attracted large audiences of students and colleagues.

After only a few months of dissection, Vesalius published six anatomical charts under the title *Tabulae anatomica sex*. The *Tabulae* were woodcut plates 19 × 13.5 inches in size. Three were drawings of the skeleton by Calcar; the other three were drawn by Vesalius, illustrating the arterial, venous, and portal circulations.

After many dissections Vesalius came to realize that Galen's descriptions were replete with errors and inaccuracies. Galen had dissected animals, not humans, and many structures described by Galen were absent in humans. One such structure was the so-called rete mirabile ("wonderful net"), a vascular structure at the base of the brain. Vesalius found this in sheep but not in human brains. Vesalius wrote about the modus operandi of dissecting cadavers that preceded him:

> The detestable procedure now in vogue [is] that one man should carry out the dissection of the human body, and another give the description of the parts. The lecturers are perched up aloft in a pulpit like jackdaws, and arrogantly prate about things they have never tried, but have committed to memory from the books of others, or placed in written form before their eyes. Thus everything is wrongly taught. [1]

In 1540, Vesalius was invited to teach in Bologna where he performed well-attended public dissections. Many were on human cadavers of executed criminals. Vesalius had ready access to recently dead bodies, and authorities often helped: The authorities in Padua were known to delay an execution until Vesalius was ready to dissect the body. Some of the stories may be apocryphal. For example, one story told of a bigamist who had murdered his first wife in order to simplify his domestic situation. He was found guilty by the authorities and was executed. As soon as the hangman's rope was removed from the body, the corpse was presented to Vaselius for public dissection and demonstration. Vesalius performed many dissections; as he cut, Calcar drew. They compiled the findings from nearly three years of observations into the prodigious book, *De humani corporis fabrica,* printed and published in Basel in 1543 by Johannes Oporinus. The word *fabrica* was chosen to mean "workings." The aim was to show how the human body and its parts appear and how the various parts function. The text of the *Fabrica* was organized into seven books; the books illustrated and discussed bones, muscles, blood vessels, nerves, abdominal and reproductive organs, chest structures, and the brain. The descriptive text was in Latin and was meant to be direct and conversational. Vesalius also published a summary of the book at the same time that was entitled the *Epitome.* This was a short version designed to be used in the classroom. Figures 4.1 and 4.2 show plates from Book 3 of the *Fabrica* illustrating the arterial circulation of the body and intracranial vasculature.

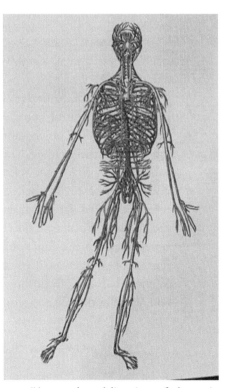

4.1. "A complete delineation of the entire great artery freed from all parts." Plate 45 from Book 3 of *De humani corporis fabrica.* From Saunders JBdeCM, O'Malley CD. *The Illustrations from the Works of Andreas Vesalius of Brussels.* New York: The Classics of Medicine Library Division of Gryphon Editions, 1993, p. 136, with permission.

After publication of the *Fabrica*, Vesalius performed his last public dissection in Padua in December 1543. Vesalius described the body as that of "a beautiful prostitute" taken by students from a tomb in a church. He had decided to become a clinical physician and so he collected his notes and manuscripts into a pile and torched them. He remarked that his intent was always to be a real doctor. The remainder of his life was very sad. He became physician to several royal courts but those he served mostly ignored his advice. When time allowed and travels took him to a city near a medical school, he dissected and demonstrated. While serving unsatisfactorily in the Spanish Court, he was informed that he was to be appointed to an illustrious professorship in Padua. Before he could assume that position, a ship he traveled on ran into a furious storm. The ship had to

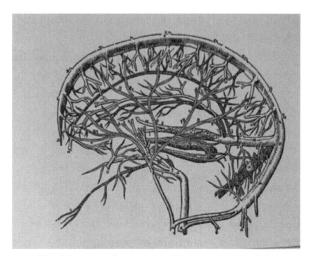

4.2. "In the present figure, a drawing is presented of the cerebral vessels laid bare, beginning with the arteries and veins before they have entirely entered the skull. However to prevent the numerous branches from obscuring everything, you will observe that the series of vessels of only one side has been drawn." From Saunders JBdeCM, O'Malley CD. *The Illustrations from the Works of Andreas Vesalius of Brussels.* New York: The Classics of Medicine Library Division of Gryphon Editions, 1993, p. 140, with permission.

make port on a small island where Vesalius became ill and died in 1564, at the age of 50.

The legacy of Andreas Vesalius is his modus operandi and his attitude toward acquisition of knowledge rather than his great book. He stressed the need for personal observations. Scientific knowledge grows by experimentation and activity rather than slavish adherence to prior writings and dogma. Students, physicians, and scientists should question prior statements and make conclusions based on their own observations and their own acquisition of information and data. William Harvey (Chapter 5), born about a decade after the death of Vesalius, followed his predecessor's practice of making detailed observations of the functioning of the heart and vascular system. Vesalius's illustrations of the vascular system and of the brain were a stimulus for Thomas Willis (Chapter 6) to further explore human anatomy and function. Vesalius and Willis both utilized accomplished artists to illustrate their dissections.

NOTES AND REFERENCES

1. Nuland S. The reawakening: Andreas Vesalius and the renaissance of medicine. In *Doctors: The Biography of Medicine*. New York: Vintage Books, 1988, pp. 61–93.
2. O'Malley CD. *Andreas Vesalius of Brussels, 1514–1564.* Berkeley: University of California Press, 1964.
3. Saunders JBdeCM, O'Malley CD. *The Illustrations from the Works of Andreas Vesalius of Brussels.* New York: The Classics of Medicine Library Division of Gryphon Editions, 1993.

CHAPTER FIVE

WILLIAM HARVEY

On the Motion of the Heart and Blood

BACKGROUND: GALEN AND HIS HUMORAL THEORY

Vesalius (Chapter 4) and William Harvey brought light into the study of human anatomy and physiology, medicine, neurology, and stroke during the sixteenth century. Before their contributions, Galenic writings, teachings, and proclamations had dominated medical practice for almost 1500 years. Galen was born in the Greek city of Pergamon in 130 CE. Galen introduced the principle that the sick could be properly treated only if physicians understood how the body works and how disease disturbs function [1]. To know the normal workings of the body, physician healers required a detailed knowledge of structure (human anatomy) and function (human physiology). Galen dissected mostly animals. His own proclamations and writings were not based on any scientific research. He was the major advocate of the humoral theory of disease. Illness was attributable to an imbalance of the four humors in the body: blood, phlegm, yellow bile, and black bile. Galen taught that blood was the dominant humor and he promoted the practice of bloodletting that held sway for centuries. The liver was the source of the blood. Blood was thought to be constantly manufactured in the liver's ample spongy depths made from the digested food brought there from the intestines. Treatments for most ailments were therefore designed to restore the balance of these humors and were comprised of enemas, emetics, and bloodletting [2].

Charles II (1630–1685) was bled profusely after a stroke. The practice of bloodletting was carried out well into the twentieth century. The name of the medical journal *Lancet* is based on the fact that a lancet – a sharp pointed, two-edged surgical instrument – was essential to practicing medicine at that time. Physicians carried lancets and fleams in their pockets and would perform venesections mostly involving the cubital veins. Other methods were cupping and leech therapy. Rows of patients would wait to be bled at their own request outside hospitals; it was believed that bleeding every spring brought vigor [3].

On December 14, 1799, at about 2 a.m. George Washington woke up with severe pain in the throat and difficulty breathing. He had gone horseback-riding in stormy weather the previous day and developed a sore throat. His physicians drew copious amounts of his blood, administered laxatives and emetics, and produced blisters on his throat to curtail inflammation. He was bled four times, and about 80 ounces of blood was drawn in 12 hours, amounting to about 40 percent of the total blood volume. He died that night. It is uncertain whether it was the disease or the treatment that led to his demise [4].

Today the idea of bloodletting to treat anything sounds absurd and unimaginable. Why for centuries was it not understood that bloodletting was harmful and not beneficial? This treatment was based on a major flaw in the understanding of human physiology. Galen believed that there were two different types of blood with distinct pathways. Venous blood was continuously produced in the liver from food and was absorbed by tissues and not returned to the heart. Arterial blood originated in the heart and was the source of vitality and, like venous blood, did not return to the heart. The circulation of the blood was not discovered until 1628 by William Harvey, and was entirely unexpected. Harvey was concerned that the discovery could jeopardize his medical practice [5,6]!

The sixteenth and seventeenth centuries were a time for enlightenment in medicine but also in the arts and humanities. Elizabethan England and Europe gave birth to Bacon, Cervantes, El Greco, Hobbes, Milton, Molière, Rembrandt, Vermeer, Shakespeare, and Spinoza, among others. In preceding centuries there was a feeling that everything was known that needed to be known and the wisdom of the ancients was unassailable and as holy as biblical scripture. Harvey and other scientists who followed sought the truth, not just from books but from experience and experimentation. The ultimate test of truth was that it could be demonstrated and confirmed and was convincing even to those who were skeptical.

WILLIAM HARVEY: EARLY LIFE AND TRAINING

William Harvey was born on April 1, 1578, in an English coastal town. He was the oldest among nine children; his family was prosperous. One of his brothers,

Eliab, who became quite wealthy, managed William's financial affairs so that William throughout life never had to worry about financial support [7]. William was quite short, had dark brown eyes and jet-black hair, and was full of nervous energy. He began his formal education at the King's School in Canterbury, whose statutes demanded that students should never use any language but Latin or Greek. Throughout his later life, he was an ardent student of the classical writers. He became fluent in Greek and Latin. At age 16, he enrolled in Caius College of Cambridge, an institution known for matriculating students interested in medicine. Each year there the bodies of two executed criminals were dissected in the presence of students. Harvey, like the great anatomist Vesalius, then enrolled in the University of Padua, Italy. In 1597, he attained his medical degree at the age of 19. He studied anatomy and physiology under Fabricius, who is credited with discovering valves within veins. Harvey late in life opined that the discovery of the one-way function of the valves – directing blood back to the heart – led him to his discovery of the circulation of blood [7]. Harvey returned to London in the year 1602 and became a member of the Royal College of Physicians where he gave annual anatomy lectures. He married Elizabeth Browne, the daughter of a physician, in 1604. He became an attending physician at Saint Bartholomew's Hospital and developed a flourishing private practice. He became one of the royal physicians to James I and later Charles I. During his early years of practice he found time to carry out anatomical and physiological research.

RESEARCH ON THE CIRCULATION OF BLOOD IN ANIMALS AND HUMANS

Dr. Harvey was determined to understand the physiology of the blood and circulation by independent, personal studies in animals and humans. He first set out to find the structure, function, and differences in the hearts of animals. He dissected over 80 different species of animals, including mollusks, fleas, bees, silkworms, fishes, turtles, snakes, geese, rats, dogs, cats, sheep, and deer. All this was done in his wife's kitchen [5]. When his wife's beloved parrot died, he dissected it too and discovered that it wasn't a male as was previously thought but a female who died due to a decaying egg in its oviduct. Harvey was barbaric and ruthless in conducting vivisections. He dissected living animals to study their beating hearts and was undaunted by their shrieking. In the rapidly beating hearts of most animals, he could not discern if the auricles contracted before the ventricles. To overcome this problem, Harvey observed the hearts of cold-blooded animals such as fish that beat at a slower rate; he waited as the warm-blooded animals died in front of him and their hearts became slower and slower. Through these experiments he observed that the auricles con-tracted first and ejected blood into the ventricles, which contracted later.

He proved to his own satisfaction that the heart contracts forcibly, and, as it contracts, it thrusts against the chest wall and at the same time the arteries dilate to receive the blood. He showed that once the blood leaves the ventricles, the valves prevent return of blood to the heart, so that the flow of blood is always toward the periphery. The function of the heart was to pump blood to the extremities, and the force transmitted was felt as pulsations in the arteries. He recognized that contraction of the left ventricle sent blood into the aorta and contraction of the right ventricle transmitted blood into the pulmonary artery [6].

Harvey's approach was not limited to observation but was supplemented by mathematics. Harvey measured the amount of blood in the left ventricle of a dog's heart and multiplied this approximate quantity with the number of heartbeats per minute. He calculated that the left ventricle ejected about three pounds of blood in half an hour, which was almost equal to the total blood volume of the animal. It was inconceivable that such a large amount of blood could be replaced by the blood produced in the liver or that it could be continually absorbed in the tissues. Harvey concluded that the blood had to have a specific movement in the body, that it was pumped by the heart into the arteries which carried it to the tissues, and that the veins brought it back to the heart from the tissues. The motion was thus "circular" [6].

He further substantiated the concept of circulation by occluding the single vein leading to the beating heart of a snake. He found that the heart became pale and shrank and stopped ejecting blood into the aorta. On releasing the occlusion, the heart regained color and again pumped blood into the aorta. He showed that, when a ligature was applied to a vein, the segment below it swelled while the segment above it collapsed, indicating the direction of flow toward the heart [6]. He also discerned the function of the valves in the veins – that they allow blood to flow in only one direction. He proved this by showing that a probe could be passed in a vein, in only one direction, the apparent direction of blood flow [8].

Anatomically, the arteries were placed deeper in the body, while the veins were superficial. Harvey applied a ligature on the arm of a human volunteer. The ligature was tight enough to occlude both the arteries and veins. He observed that the arm became pale, cold, and painful. The veins that were visible superficially collapsed. On loosening the ligature slightly, such that it allowed arterial blood flow but continued to occlude the vein, he observed that the arm and hand regained their color and became warm. The veins became distended with blood as the loosened ligature still prevented its further escape. Harvey established that the blood flowed from the arteries into the veins. He could not observe the connections as the microscope was yet to be discovered. In 1661, Marcello Malpighi, using a microscope, was able to detect the tiny vessels known as the capillaries, which connected the arteries to the veins [6].

Harvey concluded that while the heart is relaxing between contractions, it is passively filled with blood from the body. The conduit into the right heart is via two large veins (the superior and inferior venae cavae), and the path into the left atrium is from the pulmonary veins. Harvey concluded that the circuit was complete. The blood enters the right heart from the venae cavae, is driven through the lungs by contraction of the right ventricle, returns to the left atrium, and from there to the left ventricle, which pumps blood into the aorta and from there into the rest of the body [6].

An observation by a Spanish-born French physician and religious philosopher, Michael Servetus, preceded Harvey's work. Servetus noted that, contrary to Galen's writings, transmission of the blood from the right ventricle of the heart to the left ventricle does not take place through pores in the middle wall of the heart, but rather by means of a great contrivance that pumps blood forward from the right ventricle toward the lungs for its oxygenation, and transfuses it afterward to the left ventricle of the heart [9,10]. This statement appeared in a religiously oriented treatise, which subsequently was one factor that got Servetus burned at the stake for heresy. It is unclear if Harvey was aware of this statement.

Harvey's discovery of the circulation of blood refuted Galen's physiology and the therapeutics based on it. He very cautiously ensured the support of his colleagues at the Royal College and convinced them by demonstrations, over a period of nine years, before publishing his work [8]. Harvey's famous book *De motu cordis* (On the motion of the heart and the blood) was published in 1628, in the city of Frankfurt. After publication, he faced considerable criticism from European contemporaries for his discovery [5].

Harvey wrote a letter to the President and Fellows of the College of Physicians that was included as a preface to this book. "I profess both to learn and to teach anatomy, not from books but from dissections; not from the positions of philosophers but from the fabric of nature" [5].

After publication of *De motu cordis*, Harvey directed his attention to the development of embryos. He accumulated evidence with his naked eye and a simple lens. His observations were published in a book in 1651 entitled *De generatone animalium* [11]. William Harvey died of a stroke in the year 1657.

NOTES AND REFERENCES

1. Nuland S. The paradox of Pergamon, Galen. In *Doctors: The Biography of Medicine*. New York: Alfred A. Knopf, 1988, pp. 31–60.
2. Porter R. *The Greatest Benefit to Mankind: A Medical History of Humanity from Antiquity to the Present*. London: HarperCollins, 1997.
3. Cohen J. A brief history of bloodletting. History. Available at www.history.com/news/a-brief-history-of-bloodletting.

4. Bloodletting and blisters: Solving the medical mystery of George Washington's death. PBS NewsHour. 2014. Available at www.pbs.org/newshour/show/bloodletting-blis ters-solving-medical-mystery-george-washingtons-death.

5. Royal College of Physicians. How William Harvey discovered the circulation of the blood and why he regretted it. Available at www.youtube.com/watch?v= ZR8LmpfkXhQ.

6. Friedman M, Friedland GW. William Harvey and the circulation of blood. In *Medicine's 10 Greatest Discoveries*. New Haven, CT: Yale University Press, pp. 18–36.

7. Nuland S. "Nature herself must be our advisor": William Harvey's discovery of the circulation. In *Doctors: The Biography of Medicine*. New York: Alfred A Knopf, 1988, pp. 120–144.

8. Friedland G. Discovery of the function of the heart and circulation of blood. *Cardiovasc. J. Afr.* 2009 May;20(3):160.

9. Servetus and the circulation of the blood. Michael Servetus Institute. Available at https://miguelservet.org/servetus/circulation.htm.

10. Servetus M. *Christianismi restitutio totius ecclesiae apostolicae est ad sua limina vocatio, in intyegrum rstituta cognitione, fidei Christi, iustificationis nostrae, regenerationis baptismi, et coenae domini manducationis. restitutio denique nobis regno coelesti, Babylonis impiae captivate soluta, et Antichristo cum suis penitus destrcucto.* M.D. Llll, 734 pages MVS. Book V (pp. 168–173) contains the famous paragraph of the pulmonary circulation system.

11. Ribatti D. William Harvey and the discovery of the circulation of the blood. *J. Angiogenesis Res.* 2009;1:3.

CHAPTER SIX

THOMAS WILLIS

Anatomy of the Brain and Its Vasculature

Thomas Willis was born on January 27, 1621, in a small village within Great Bedwyn, UK, a prosperous wool town that housed between 1,500 and 2,000 inhabitants. He was the oldest child among three sons and three daughters. When he was 10, his mother died. Thomas walked two miles each day to and from Sylvester's Academy, a local private school that had a reputation for providing a classical education in Latin and Greek. When he was 16, he began to matriculate at the University of Oxford as a servitor to Dr. Thomas Iles, a canon of Christ Church. Servitors were usually bright lads from humble circumstances who performed menial tasks in exchange for free housing and tuition [1–3]. Ms. Iles, though not a trained physician, practiced medicine and was described as a knowing woman in physic and surgery who performed many cures [1]. Willis spent ample time with her during his tutelage. Willis graduated as a bachelor of Arts in 1639, and three years later, after more attendance at lectures and teaching, he received a master of arts degree. Thomas intended to be ordained as an Anglican clergyman.

His entry into medicine was attributable to an accident of the times. During a civil war that began shortly after his graduation, a severe epidemic (possibly typhus) led to the death of his father and his stepmother. He had to give up thoughts of a church career. He returned home, now being responsible for managing two farms and for parenting and educating his younger siblings. A half year after the civil war ended in 1646, Willis graduated with a bachelor of medicine degree. This degree usually required three years of residential study after a master of arts diploma, but these requirements were waived because of a shortage of physicians.

At first his practice from his clinical rooms at Christ Church was meager. Willis had time for learning and research. His lifetime shortly followed the reign of Queen Elizabeth in England. Creativity in art, literature, and science flourished in Elizabethan England. William Shakespeare, Edward Spenser, Christopher Marlowe, and Ben Jonson were all active before and some during Willis's lifetime. Oxford became a center for learning and creativity. In 1648 Willis became an active member of a group of Trinity College "natural philosophers" who were actively engaged in clinical research in the tradition of William Harvey. "The Invisible College," also called "the Philosophical College" was an informal group established by several scientifically minded individuals of Oxford who met every Thursday to perform experiments and share knowledge [4]. Among the group were Thomas Willis, philosopher and physicist Robert Boyle, mathematician John Wallis, architect and anatomist Christopher Wren, economist and physician Sir William Petty, prominent physician Thomas Sydenham, philosopher John Locke, and physician Richard Lower. The group is considered one of the predecessors of the Royal Society of London. Here Willis gained his experimental aptitude and met with brilliant minds like Wren and Boyle.

As his practice grew, he developed a strict schedule [2]. He paid a curate schoolmaster to read prayers at 6 o'clock in summer and 7 o'clock in winter. After attending this religious service he started his day's work by giving free treatment and advice to the sick poor who came to his home. He then set out with his coachman on clinical rounds of consultations for the wealthy sick and to visit apothecaries for medicines. At 5 o'clock he attended another religious service and, after dinner, made notes on patients seen during the day, replied to the inquiries of colleagues, continued his research and writing, and made himself available for night calls. He became the most successful practitioner in the Oxford region.

WILLIS IS MOSTLY REMEMBERED FOR FOUR CONTRIBUTIONS AND ATTRIBUTES

1. Willis organized and led a consortium of scientists and investigators who collaborated on medical and other research. After becoming acquainted with various members of the invisible Oxford college, he organized his own, smaller group of collaborators. This group included the physicists Robert Boyle and his associate the architect and scientist Robert Hooke, the architect illustrator and inventor Christopher Wren, and the physicians Thomas Millington and Richard Lower.

Robert Boyle, the famous physicist who showed that the volume of a gas is inversely proportional to its pressure (Boyle's law), was a significant contributor to the group. He introduced the concept of preservation of tissues. He suggested the use of alcohol to preserve the human body after he noticed that wine preserved fish from stinking and going bad. This technique was adopted by Willis and colleagues for the preservation of brains for dissection. Boyle studied the effect of viper poison in dogs. With Wren, he devised the technique of intravenous injection that Willis used for injecting dye into the arteries within the skull. As dye flowed through the lumen of the blood vessels, it traced the entire vasculature of the brain and demonstrated connections and anastomoses.

Robert Hooke was originally employed by Boyle to construct an air pump. Hooke discovered his law of elasticity, which stated that stretching of a solid body such as wood or metal was proportional to the force applied to it. This law laid the basis for studies of stress and strain and for understanding properties of elastic materials. Hooke was later appointed curator of experiments to the Royal Society of London and was elected a fellow of that society.

Richard Lower was first a student of Willis who became one of his research associates after acquiring his MD degree. Lower formed part of an informal research team, performing laboratory experiments at the University of Oxford. He was a pioneer of experimental physiology. His major work, *Tractatus de corde*, published in 1669, was concerned with the functions of the heart and lungs [5]. Lower traced the circulation of blood as it passed through the lungs and learned that it changed when exposed to air. Lower was the first to observe the difference in arterial and venous blood. He also investigated how cerebrospinal fluid was formed and how it circulated. These experiments led to a study of hydrocephalus, a condition characterized by increased fluid in the cavities of the brain. He is mostly remembered for giving the first blood transfusions. He showed it was possible for blood to be transfused intravenously from animal to animal and from animal to man. In November 1667, he worked with Edmund King, another student of Willis, to transfuse sheep's blood into a mentally ill man. Lower advanced science but also believed that individuals could be helped, either by the infusion of fresh blood or by the removal of old blood. It was difficult to find people who would agree to be transfused, but an eccentric scholar, Arthur Coga, consented and the procedure was carried out by Lower and King before the Royal Society on November 23, 1667 [6].

Sir Christopher Wren was an English anatomist, astronomer, geometer, and mathematician-physicist, as well as one of the most highly acclaimed English architects in history. He is best remembered as the architect of St. Paul's Cathedral in London. Willis wrote, "Dr. Wren was pleased out of his singular humanity, wherewith he abounds, to delineate with his own skillful hands many Figures of the Brain and Skull, whereby the work might be more exact" [7]. Wren was the major illustrator of Willis's anatomy text and atlas. Wren was 30 years old when he began working with the group. He performed animal experiments including surgically removing the spleen from a dog [1]. At that time there was no precedent for making injections into blood vessels of humans or animals. Wren designed a technique for cutting down on the hind leg of a dog, identifying a vein, introducing a cylindrical pipe-like object into the vein, and injecting various substances [1]. This was a prelude to Lower's later transfusions and Willis's injections into the vessels supplying the brain in cadavers.

2. Willis is mostly known for his brain dissections and his clear illustration with Wren of the anatomical circle (polygon) of arteries at the very base of the brain, forever memorialized as the "Circle of Willis." Studying the anatomy of the brain was a difficult task at that time for it decayed rapidly; the prevalent approach to its dissection had several limitations. The earlier anatomists did not extract the brain as a whole but dissected it in slices after opening the skull. Willis along with his colleagues removed the intact brain from the vault, enabling them to better study the vascular structure of the brain. Willis, Wren, and Lower, an anatomist of tremendous dexterity and precision, elucidated the anatomical structure of the brain. In 1664 Willis published his book *Cerebri anatome cui accessit nervorum descriptio et usus* (The Anatomy of the Brain and Nerves) [7]. In *The Practice of Physick*, Willis described the experiment that showed the connection through the circle at the base of the brain between the two sides of arteries that supplied the brain (Figure 6.1):

> The Vessels interwoven within the thin Meninx or Pia mater are Arteries and Veins. The arteries are four, viz, two Carotides and two Vertebrals. Out of either side of the tunnel, the ends of the cut Carotodick Arteries shew themselves, the trunks of which ascending upwards, are presently diffused from either side into the anterior and posterior or fore and hinder branch. Either pair of these inclining one towards the other, are mutually conjoined: moreover, the posterior branches so joined, are united with the Vertebral branches (growing together first into one trunk).

Willis was not the first to describe the circle. Galen had referred to a "rete mirabile" at the base of the brain, but this structure was later shown to exist only in animals. Fallopius, Casserio, Vesling, and Wepfer had all previously described the configuration of arteries but none had experimentally deduced the function of this anastomotic configuration [8,9].

3. Willis and his coworkers were the first to emphasize collateral circulation, through the anastomotic circle and through other channels:

> Let the Carotodick Arteries be laid bare on either side of the Cervix on the hinder part of the head, so that their little tubes or Pipes, about half an

inch long, may be exhibited together to the sight; then let a dyed liquor, and contained in a large Squirt or Pipe, be injected upwards in the trunk of one side, after once or twice injecting, you shall see the tincture or dyed liquor to descend from the other side by the trunk of the opposite Artery.

Willis related the anatomical structure of the circle to its function. He autopsied a man who had died of a mesenteric tumor but was neurologically asymptomatic and reported his findings:

When his skull was opened we beheld those things belonging to the head, and found, the right carotid artery, rising within the skull plainly bony or rather stony, its cavity being almost wholly shut up so that the influx of blood being denied by this passage, it seemed wonderful, wherefore this sick person had not died before of an apoplexy: which indeed he was so far from, that he enjoyed to the last moment of his life, the free exercise of his mind and animal functions. Nature has substituted a sufficient remedy against the danger of apoplexy; as the Vertebral artery on the same side, in which the carotid was occluded became thrice as big as both its pipes on the other side.

In another patient who had an arterial occlusion, Willis reasoned that the remaining large vessels flowing toward the arterial circle at the base of the brain were able, by way of their "mutual conjoining," to "supply or fill the channels and passages of all the rest." Willis conducted an experiment with Wren. They tied both the carotid arteries of a spaniel and found the dog to be completely asymptomatic. Later when they opened its head, they found that all the vessels were filled with blood, demonstrating the connections and compensation by the vertebral arteries.

4. Willis is also given credit by some for first describing warnings prior to the development of a stroke. These warnings are now generally referred to as transient ischemic attacks (TIAs). The passage cited is rather ethereal but this type of writing is typical for Willis in his books about the practice of medicine [10,11]: " the irradiation of the spirits is wont to be interrupted with little clouds, as it were, scatterred here and there but in the former, the same is forthwith wholly darkened and undergoes total eclipse." Undoubtedly, the writings and illustrations of Willis and his co-researchers concerning the anatomy and functions of the brain and the vessels that nourished it had profound effects on physicians and scientists who followed. Often lost sight of is the example that Willis set as a role model for subsequent physicians and researchers. Dewhurst reflected on the reasons behind Willis's economic and professional success:

From the beginnings of his career, he had organized his life extremely well. Willis had the discernment to select able and loyal assistants to whom he delegated many routine tasks in chemistry and anatomy enabling him to accomplish so much writing and research while consciously attending his many patients. Outwardly pious, modest, and unassuming, Thomas Willis was essentially a tireless, bold, and speculative genius.

Three centuries later, C. Miller Fisher's modus operandi would mirror that of Willis [12].

NOTES AND REFERENCES

1. Zimmer C. *Soul Made Flesh: The Discovery of the Brain and How It Changed the World.* New York: William Heinemann (Random House), 2004.
2. Dewhurst K. *Willis's Oxford Lectures.* Oxford: Sanford Publications, 1980.
3. O'Connor JPB. Thomas Willis and the background to *Cerebri anatome. J. R. Soc. Med.* 2003 Mar;96(3):139–143.
4. Evans R. The Invisible College (1645–1658). Technical Education Matters. December 12, 2010. Available at https://technicaleducationmatters.org/2010/12/12/the-invisible-college-1645-1658/.
5. Lower R. *Tractatus de corde: Item de motu et colore sanguinis.* London: John Redmayne for James Allestry, 1669.
6. Fastag E, Varon J, Sternbach G. Richard Lower: The origins of blood transfusion. *J. Emerg. Med.* 2013;44:1146–1150.
7. Willis T. *Cerebri anatome: Cui accessit nervorum descriptio et usus.* London: J. Flesher, 1664.
8. Fields WS, Lemak NA. *A History of Stroke: Its Recognition and Treatment.* New York: Oxford University Press, 1989.
9. Lo WB, Ellis H. The circle before Willis: A historical account of the intracranial anastomosis. *Neurosurgery.* 2010 Jan;66(1):7–18; discussion 17–18.
10. Willis T. Instructions and prescripts for curing the apoplexy. In Portage S (ed.), *The London Practice of Physic.* London, 1679.
11. Willis T. *Instructions and Prescripts for Curing the Apoplexy. The London Practice of Physic or the Whole Practical Part of Physic.* 1679.
12. Caplan LR. *C. Miller Fisher: Stroke in the Twentieth Century.* New York: Oxford University Press, 2020.

CHAPTER SEVEN

GIOVANNI MORGAGNI

Emphasis on Pathology

How to approach care of patients? Galen's idea of humors, miasma, and natural influences affecting health and disease held sway for centuries. The methods of science – observation, hypothesis generation, experimentation, careful review of results, and then, revision of hypotheses and concepts – began to take hold in various academic centers in Europe and Asia during an age of enlightenment. Andreus Vesalius had shown how the study of human anatomy should be conducted (Chapter 4). William Harvey had shown how knowledge about human physiology should be approached (Chapter 5), and Thomas Willis had reinforced the need for a scientific approach to anatomy and experimentation as an important predecessor to caring for patients (Chapter 6). But it was Giovanni Battista Morgagni who put the final nail in the coffin of the Galenian approach to medicine. Morgagni emphasized examination of the body after death, to determine *pathology*, as a critical way of identifying disease and contributing importantly to knowledge. Anatomy, physiology, and pathology were the triad of disciplines that lead to the understanding of disease.

Giovanni Morgagni was born on February 25, 1682, in the small northern Italian town of Forlì. When he was 16, Morgagni went to the nearby city of Bologna to study medicine and philosophy. There he came under the influence of the renowned anatomist Antonio Valsalva, who had been a pupil and disciple of Marcello Malpighi, a physician and biologist known for his study of microscopic anatomy. After receiving his medical degree, in

1701 the 19-year-old Morgagni became Valsalva's assistant during the next six years [1,2]. During this time he performed postmortem examinations and kept notes about his cases. More than a year of graduate study followed. Morgagni then returned to his hometown of Forlì to become a practicing physician. The years that he spent practicing medicine in a small town were very productive and were an important influence on his later career. By all accounts he became a very successful practitioner and a sought-after consultant. He was described as tall, handsome, affable, and able. He married Paola Verzeri, the daughter of a noble family of the town. He missed the academic environment that he had trained in, and in 1711, he was invited to Padua to become a junior professor of theoretical medicine.

After four years of teaching and dissection he was named professor of anatomy at the University of Padua. This was the oldest and most esteemed chair at the university. The previous chairmen included Vesalius, Fallopius, and Fabricius. Morgagni continued to consult on patients, but his main activities were necropsy examinations and teaching pathology and anatomy. He also read avidly. He was familiar with Francis Bacon's writing on science and of Vesalius's work. One tome with which he became very familiar was written by Theophilus Bonetus, a Genovese anatomist. This book, entitled *Sepulchretum sive anatomia practica ex cadaveribus morbo denatis*, was customarily referred to as the *Sepulchretum anatomicum*. The long title and subtitle further conveyed the contents: *Repository of Anatomy Practiced on Corpses Deceased of Disease, Which Reports the Histories and Observations of All Alterations of the Human Body and Reveals the Hidden Causes*. Indeed, anatomy deserves to be called the foundation of real pathology and proper treatment of disease, even the inspiration of old and recent medicine [1,2]. Bonetus assembled from available writings material from 3,000 cases in which clinical histories, autopsies, and commentaries were available. The first edition contained writings from more than 450 authors in 1,700 pages of text. An enlarged edition edited by Mangetus appeared in the year 1700 [3].

Morgagni was stimulated by the *Sepulchretum*, especially by its emphasis on pathology as the way to understand disease. He became increasingly aware of its flaws, however, which included inadequate and inaccurate observations, misquotes, and misinterpretations. Early in his career he flirted with the idea of rewriting or editing the text. Ultimately, he decided it was better to publish his own collection of cases.

Morgagni assiduously collected cases in which there was information about the history of illness before death and a necropsy examination. When Morgagni was 79 years old, he finally published the cases that he had been collecting into a book, *De sedibus et causis morborum per anatomen indagatis* (The Seats and Causes of Disease Investigated by Anatomy). This great tome, customarily referred to as *De sedibus*, is organized in the form of 70 letters written to a young man. Supposedly, this young man was someone Morgagni had encountered during the years of the collection. Morgagni described the individual as being "much given to the study of the sciences and particularly to that of medicine" [1,4]. The purported receiver of the letters was a student and an academician. In *De sedibus* he explained that Professor Valsalva had urged him to render a new edition of published writings, including the *Sepulchretum*. He expected that Morgagni would write "in as familiar a manner as I would" [4]. Morgagni said that instead he would engage in a trial of letters, which, if found to be suitable, he would publish as his own book. Morgagni wrote in his preface to *De sedibus*:

> I began, upon returning to Padua to make a trial of that nature by sending some letters to my friend. And that he was pleased with them appears from two circumstances: the first, that he was continuously soliciting me to send him more and more after that, till he drew me on so far as the seventieth; the second, that when I begg'd them of him, in order to revise their contents he did not return them, till he made me promise that I would not abridge any part therof. [4, p. 11]

This so-called trial, in retrospect, may have been a literary way to explain his decision to write a monograph rather than redoing or editing the work of others. The first book in *De sedibus* contained 27 letters and was entitled "Of Disorders of the Head." The first five letters concerned apoplexy, which, Morgagni wrote, could be of a sanguineous or serum nature. Morgagni's style was conversational, a master teacher revealing to readers the observations, insights, and inferences after a lifetime of experience. I quote one of the cases that was among those that described the "sanguinous apoplexies":

> A great man, a Cardinal . . . was of a moderate nature, or somewhat taller, of a full fleshy habit and a florid colour . . . was also subject to the gout.. . . When he was five and fifty years of age, having liv'd for two months in a mountainous country, on which the south winds generally blew, and the air of which he had at other times found extremely inimical to him, and being also troubled with cares and anxieties of mind . . . he fell into a vertiginous disorder . . . and a propensity to sleep. Within about twenty days, the vertiginous disorder return'd and brought a vomiting with it . . . and after that a violent pain in the head. The day following, all sense of feeling and power of motion was lost in the left part of his body, and he lay as if overcome with profound sleep. [4, pp. 22, 23]

On the tenth day he died and Morgagni performed the necropsy. "The brain was flaccid; and in the left ventricle was a little serum but the right contain'd more than two ounces of coagulated blood" [4, p. 23]. This was likely the first reported case of hypertensive encephalopathy followed by a large intracerebral hemorrhage.

The fourth letter was among the cases that "treats of the serous apoplexy" A man of 63 " was afflicted with heavy pains in his head . . . and a dullness in his senses." His father had died of an apoplexy. He had a large amount of edema in his legs. He first developed weakness of his right limbs and later developed weakness of the right face and aphasia. "He was again stricken speechless, yet shew'd that he understood everything which was said, and even sometimes brought forth a word but with great difficulty of utterance, and a low voice.. . . On the fifth day of this kind of apoplectic disorder, he died" [4, pp. 62, 63].

At necropsy his left cardiac ventricle was large, the brain was soft (not further described) and had large ventricles filled with serum: "both the carotid and vertebral arteries shew'd everywhere, in their internal coats, white and firm corpuscles . . . most of them were almost of the nature of a cartilage only, wheras some approach'd nearly to that of bone" [4, p. 63].

Morgani clearly distinguished fatal cases of apoplexy due to hemorrhage, some bleeding within and some outside the brain, from those in which bleeding was not found at necropsy but where there was an abundance of serous fluid in the head. Although some of the serous cases had cardiac disease and carotid and vertebral artery disease at necropsy, he did not identify brain infarction as the cause of the "serous apoplexies." That connection was to come much later in history when myocardial infarction and brain infarction became known entities during the twentieth century. Morgagni gave credit to his professor and mentor Valsalva, for discovering that lesions in one cerebral hemisphere gave signs of abnormality in life on the contralateral side of the body.

Morgagni was a practicing consultant during his entire career. As his fame spread, he was called to see important patients throughout Italy and Europe. He emphasized detailed description of symptoms during life as well as the nature, family history, and the physical and psychological environment of the patient. The symptoms drew attention to the disorder of an organ, and activities or illnesses and familial propensities provided clues to the nature and cause of dysfunction of that organ or organs. Pathology provided the answer to the cause of the disorder affecting that organ. This information would, he hoped, be useful for present and future physicians in caring for their patients.

Morgagni was one of the earliest true biological scientists. His method was that of observation, hypothesis generation, experimentation, recording of data, and cautious generation of inferences based on repeated, reproducible studies. He was a very patient man, waiting until observations and inferences were clear before publishing his monumental work.

By all accounts Morgagni was a highly respected and revered patriarch during his life. Morgagni and his wife Paola had a very large family: twelve daughters, three sons, and many grandchildren. *De sedibus* was widely read. Morgagni became revered during the ensuing years as the leading sage of medical science. Morgagni's wife Paola died in September 1770. In 1771 Morgagni had a stroke. His teachers and predecessors Valsalva and Malpighi had also succumbed to stroke. Morgagni died in the same house where he had raised his family. A plaque there reads "Giamb Morgagni, after founding pathological anatomy, died here on December 6, 1771" [1].

A triad of keen minds and their writings, Vesalius, Harvey, and Morgagni cleared the way for scientific research on medicine, neurology, and stroke during the ensuing decades and centuries.

NOTES AND REFERENCES

1. Nuland SW. *Doctors: The Biography of Medicine*. New York: Vintage Books, 1995, pp. 145–170.
2. McHenry LC. *Garrison's History of Neurology*. Springfield, IL: Charles C. Thomas, 1969.
3. Schutta HS, Howe HM. Seventeenth century concepts of "apoplexy" as reflected in Bonet's "Sepulchretum." *J. Hist. Neurosci.* 2006;15(3):250–268. DOI: 10.1080/09647040500403312.
4. *De sedibus et causis morborum per anatomen indagatis. The Seats and Causes of Diseases Investigated by Anatomy by Giambattista Morgagni*. London: A. Millar and T. Cadell, 1769.

CHAPTER EIGHT

APOPLEXY

Ideas and Concepts, Seventeenth to Twentieth Centuries

Sudden or protracted loss of bodily motion and functions has fascinated physicians throughout history. Coma, stupor, and paralysis are difficult conditions to ignore, especially when they develop suddenly. Apoplexy was a term introduced (possibly by Hippocrates) before the common era for such diverse bodily states. Since then many physicians have written about apoplexy: its definitions, concepts, phenomenology, examples, purported mechanisms, epidemiology, causes, and outcomes. I (LRC) will herein be eclectic, mentioning some contributions briefly but emphasizing individuals and ideas that had more important content and lasting influence.

JOHANN JAKOB WEPFER

Johann Jakob Wepfer was born in Schaffhausen, Switzerland, on December 23, 1620. His father was a merchant, magistrate, and judge. Among his secondary school teachers was Johannes Fabricius, who taught him natural history and instilled a passion in him for observing living things and nature. In 1637 Wepfer left Schaffhausen for Strasbourg and then to Padua, where he studied at the Faculty of Medicine and Pharmacy. In 1647 he received the doctorate in medicine at Basel. He returned to his native city of Schaffhausen where he became municipal physician in 1648. He remained there as physician and scientist during his entire career. Schaffhausen had no university and so Wepfer never occupied a faculty chair, but he attracted students and followers.

He became a highly respected physician and consultant and the private physician of several German princes, including the Duke of Wurtemberg [1,2].

Wepfer followed the clinical evolution of an illness, carefully noting all the symptoms. He sought to confirm hypotheses generated from his human studies by performing experiments on animals. He systematically studied poisons with particular attention to toxic substances found in plants. He analyzed the pharmacological effects of an alkaloid derived from hemlock and described the effects of hemlock poisoning [1]. He also studied mercury poisoning. He indicated the danger for workers with this metal who fail to take the proper precautions [1].

When Wepfer became municipal physician of Schaffhausen, he was given the right to perform autopsies. He performed meticulous dissections on cadavers. He studied the anatomy of blood vessels and of the brain and he described the pathology that he found. A major research interest was the brain. Being a skilled experimentalist, he devised new techniques. He was the first to color cervical vessels by injecting dye. His anatomical observations were published in a tome entitled *Historia anatomica de puella sine cerebro nata*, published in 1665 [3]. His classic work concerning apoplexy and other brain conditions, *Observationes anatomicae ex cadaveribus eorum, quos sustulit apoplexia, cum exercitatione de eius loco affecto*, was first published in 1658 and reprinted many times. In this book, he discussed many original observations based on his anatomical dissections [4].

Wepfer described the appearance of the internal carotid artery in the siphon and the course of each intracranial artery. Some intracranial arteries were described as being as hard and like stone. Blockage of the carotid or vertebral arteries was recognized as a cause of apoplexy, the obstruction preventing entry of sufficient blood into a portion of the brain. Wepfer was the first to clearly show that hemorrhage into and around the brain was an important cause of apoplexy. Wepfer distinguished two types of apoplexy: in one form, the supply of blood to the brain was obstructed or precluded, and in the other (hemorrhage), animal spirits escaped [3,4].

Wepfer included in his treatise the findings in four patients with hemorrhage, subarachnoid and intracerebral. A sample case report is an example of his writings. Wepfer described a fatal subarachnoid hemorrhage but did not find the aneurysm responsible [5]:

> Johann Jacobus Reiter Kenzinga-Brisgojus, age about 45 years with a slender build, endowed with yellow curly hair, naturally strong of honest parents. He suffered from extensive gouty arthritis. In the year 1655, the seventh day of November ... he did much of everything – assisted the Most Reverend Lord Abbott in the carrying out of sacraments; later that day, the Abbott by chance found him prostrate upon the ground, insensible to shouts, to shaking and pinching.... I arrived in half an hour, I saw him livid from pallor, deprived of all sensation and animate motion, with

nostrils cold to the touch. His pulse strong, full quick, soon after weaker, smaller and more frequent, his breathing more laborious, soon it became irregular, and many times appeared about to cease from within.... At the tenth hour before midday his body was shaken albeit by a movement and much sputum white viscid, tenacious passed from his mouth, but indeed no blood: after this more and more his strength began to weaken and his extremities to become more cold. The first hour after midday he ceased to live. I opened the head: the skull removed and the dura mater being cut into pieces much blood flowed from the space between this and the thin meninges, copiously.... Nor truly had the blood collected solely at the base of the brain, but covered it all over the top both anteriorly and posteriorly, indeed it had forced itself into nearly all the windings of the brain, as many as there are: extravasated blood totaled two pounds.... The whole brain, ventricles and surface were contaminated by blood in large amounts and crumbly; ... I was able to find no ruptured vein or artery. This however is certain, no external violence cause, be it a blow, be it a fall was the cause of such ruptures of the blood vessels; to settle this point with his haircut and skin washed off he showed not the slightest trace of any contusion whatever. [5]

OTHER SEVENTEENTH-, EIGHTEENTH-, AND EARLY NINETEENTH-CENTURY WRITINGS ON APOPLEXY

Gregor Nymann of Wittenberg, Germany, published the first monograph on apoplexy in 1619 [2,6]. Nymann was an anatomist and pathologist who followed the general dissection technique of Costanzo Varolio, a professor of anatomy in Bologna and a physician to the Pope. Varolio suggested dissecting the brain from the base region [7]. Nymann opined that an apoplectic attack could occur if vessels were occluded. The blockage would deprive the brain of vital spirits [2,6].

Francois Bayle (1622–1709), in his treatise on apoplexy that was published in 1677, also recognized that intracranial arteries were often calcified and contained plaques in their linings [8].

William Cole, a British physician and contemporary of Thomas Sydenham and John Locke, wrote an essay on apoplexy that was published in 1689. He first cited the writings of Thomas Willis and Johann Wepfer. He then asserted that apoplexy was a disorder of the brain. He called attention to the blood and may have been one of the first physicians to identify thrombi, which he thought were secretions from the vessels somehow related to inflammation. Cole's English is often ambiguous (similar to Willis's) and open to interpretation [9]:

The Nature of the distemper may be deduced. And it seems to me probable, that it consists indeed in the defect of that matter, which should be supplied to the nerves for the exercise of the animal functions, but occasioned from the vitiated organization of the parts and vessels of the Brain, from whence a due secretion (which I have heretofore endeavoured to make probable to be here performed by a simple colature in the Cortical glandules) of the nervous liquor out of the bloud cannot be made, but that, either from the forementioned distention of the sanguiferous vessels, the secretory ducts cannot readily admit the matter to be separated; the confusion of the masse, emergent upon such a congestion, prohibiting a regular secession; or else the grosser substance of the bloud, not moved as 'twas wont, being brought to the beginnings of the nerves, must needs obstruct them, and so cause an immediate cessation of motion in all parts below, as well as, by disturbing the regular motion of the spirits in the Brain, hinder the exertion, not only of the Intellectual, but also sensitive faculties. [9]

The idea that thrombi were the result of inflammation and injury and represented secretions from the vessels themselves was an idea that persisted until the time of Rudolph Virchow during the mid-nineteenth century [10–12]. John Hunter, a well-known surgeon who wrote toward the end of the eighteenth century, noted the frequency of inflammation affecting veins after phlebotomy and surgery. Often the veins became thrombosed. Hunter opined that venous clots formed as an exudate from the walls of vessels, and, if adhesions did not form, thrombi could be swept into the circulation and carried by the bloodstream into distant parts [11,12]. Clotting was attributable to inflammation of vessel walls in the venous and arterial systems. Jean Cruveilhier, a prominent French anatomist and pathologist, echoed this same concept concerning the origin of thrombi during the early nineteenth century [12,13].

Domenico Mistichelli, a professor of medicine at the University of Pisa, published a treatise on apoplexy in 1709. He remarked that it was a well-known fact in his time that disease of one cerebral hemisphere caused abnormalities on the opposite side of the body. He included in his treatise an illustration of the decussation of the pyramidal tracts in the brainstem [2,14].

Thomas Kirkland, a British surgeon and physician, was a writer who published his opinion on a wide variety of topics. His treatise on apoplexy was published in 1792 [15]. His reason for publishing a commentary on apoplexy was dissatisfaction with concepts and especially treatments espoused by earlier authors. He recognized an "apoplectic diathesis" in some individuals. Some of his apoplexy patients had irregular pulses. Some apoplexies could be minor and not preceded or accompanied by loss of consciousness. "The disease now before us [apoplexy] is an instantaneous relaxation of the muscles and tendons uncontrollable by the will.... Sometimes the disorder makes its onset with apoplectic symptoms and leaves an hemiplegia behind." One patient he described as follows: "A gentleman was seized with a giddiness in his head, and fell down, but after some time his senses returned and he was found to have lost the entire use of one side" [15]. Kirkland described patients and emphasized treatment with purging, bleeding, and emetics.

John Cheyne (1777–1836), a prominent Irish physician, wrote an influential treatise on apoplexy that was published in 1812 [16]. Cheyne was born and educated in Edinburgh and served in the Scottish Army as a surgeon before moving to Dublin, Ireland, where he spent his entire career as a highly respected consultant physician. He was a practical man who sought to share his experiences and observations, rather than an experimenter or academician. Cheyne sought to separate the phenomenology of lethargy from apoplexy. Cheyne included in his treatise detailed clinical descriptions of patients, as they would be encountered socially in their usual attire, and the appearance of brains at necropsy. After reviewing the history of writings on apoplexy and its treatment (emetics, bloodletting, purges, external applications, etc.), Cheyne described 23 cases of apoplexy. A few plates illustrated the "morbid appearances" of the brains. Cheyne described brain softening and both intracerebral and subarachnoid hemorrhages. In patients who survived for some time, Cheyne found cavities filled with rusty yellowish serum within the brain at necropsy. Cheyne surmised that the cavities were lined by a membrane that was able to absorb red blood cells. One patient described by Cheyne had a pontine hematoma:

Case IX described a "carpenter, 35 years of age, phlegmatic, pale, muscular, not habitually intemperate, and of a costive habit of body, [who] died on the night of June 1, 1808." He had severe headaches, and, after one such headache, he vomited and soon after "became insensible." About an hour later, his breathing became irregular and he was deeply comatose, and soon dead. Cheyne described this man's brain as follows: "In dissecting the base of the brain, there was discovered, formed by rupture in the substance of the pons varolii a collection of dark clotted blood, in an irregular cavity, having a ragged surface and communicating with the fourth ventricle which was full of blood" [16].

After presenting the cases, he wrote a commentary based on his experience and that of prior authors that he cited. He announced his aim in describing the cases: "My chief objects are to fix the cases in the student's mind by pointing out the most remarkable feature of each and to explain some of the concomitant circumstances of apoplexy.... A clinical treatise should be of a descriptive nature" [16].

His concepts of causation were often muddled and overly broad but contained some important observations. He considered apoplexy to be "generally the effect of intemperance and improper indulgences." He divided apoplexy into cases based on primary causes, in which the seat of the disease exists within the cranium, and sympathetic, when the "disease appears connected with an original affection of the thorax or abdomen." He noted that "apoplexy often arises from interrupted circulation to the lungs." He also mentioned disease of the stomach and liver as prominent causes. "Inordinate contractions of the heart ... have preceded apoplexy and are probably connected with the disease" [16].

The next major writing on nervous disease and apoplexy was by John Cooke, an erudite British physician. He served as a physician and teacher at the London Hospital between 1784 and 1807. He became ill and resigned his position as acting physician but proceeded to write a treatise on nervous system diseases. The first volume, *On Apoplexy*, was published in 1820 [17]. His treatise represented a review of topics rather than new observations. He read widely and cited many physicians and philosophers, including Socrates, Hippocrates, Plato, Aristotle, Galen, Vesalius, Descartes, Wepfer, Willis, Locke, Morgagni, Kirkland, Hunter, Galvani, and Cheyne. His aim was stated clearly in the preface:

> The more real service may be rendered to medicine by the illustration of what is already known on the subject, than by any attempts to promulgate new theories or new modes of practice.... I have taken considerable pains in endeavoring to collect, to arrange, and to communicate in plain clear language, a variety of useful observations from the best authors, both ancient and modern, respecting the principal diseases of the nervous system. [17]

Cooke was critical concerning the present state of knowledge. After 150 pages of text in which he laboriously and eruditely cited and discussed the writings and opinions of physicians, anatomists, and philosophers, he pens a very honest and telling conclusion:

> From this slight sketch ... a general notion of the opinions, both of the ancients and moderns, respecting the nature and uses of the nervous system, may be formed; and hence it appears, that, notwithstanding the laborious investigations of the subject by philosophers in various ages of the world, the physiology of the nervous system, as to many particulars remains involved in impenetrable obscurity. The sensible qualities of the organs of the nervous system, the form, size, colour, relative situation, protuberances, cavities, and divisions of the various substances contained within the cranium and spine have been accurately described; but no satisfactory explanation has been given of their intimate nature, and of the manner in which they immediately act in producing sensation and motion. The most minute examination of the brain and nerves has thrown no light on this mystery. [17]

In his treatise on apoplexy he reviews sequentially what others had written about the morbid appearance at autopsy, causes, distinctive subtypes, diagnosis, prognosis, and treatment. He was skeptical about a serous cause and thought most apoplexies were due to bleeding. He opined that hydrocephalus was an important component or sequela of many apoplexies.

John Abercrombie, a Scottish physician and philosopher, contributed a more detailed clinical classification of apoplexy in his text published in 1828 [18]. He was very familiar with the writings of Cheyne; Léon Rostan [19], a French pathologist and physicist; and Antoine Étienne Renaud Augustin Serres [20], a French anatomist and physiologist, citing their publications in his text. His writings were concerned with the mechanism of apoplexy. He emphasized the heterogeneity of the clinical and pathological findings in patients with apoplexy. Abercrombie used the presence of headache, stupor, paralysis, and outcome to separate apoplectics into three clinical groups. In the first group, which he termed "primary apoplexy," the onset was sudden, unilateral paralysis; rigidity and stupor were present; and the outcome was poor. These patients probably had large intracerebral hemorrhages or large brain infarcts. In the second group, patients had the sudden onset of headache, vomiting, and either faintness or falling but no paralysis. Undoubtedly, these patients had subarachnoid hemorrhages. In the third group, there was unilateral paralysis, often with abnormal speech, but neither stupor nor headache was present. This group must have had smaller infarcts or parenchymatous hemorrhages. Abercrombie speculated on etiologic mechanisms, mentioning spasm of vessels, interruption of the circulation, and rupture of diseased vessels causing hemorrhage [18].

Abercrombie described prodromal symptoms that often precede a severe apoplectic attack:

> The apoplectic attack is generally preceded by symptoms indicating some derangement of the circulation in the brain. The most remarkable of these are: headache, giddiness ... violent pulsations of the arteries ... by loss of recollection and incoherent talking ... by affections of the sight, double vision and temporary blindness ... we also frequently observe indistinct articulations and other partial paralytic affections. These are sometimes confined to one limb; sometimes affect the eyelids ... and frequently impair the muscles of the face, producing a slight distortion of the mouth. These symptoms, and others of a similar kind, mark the tendency to the apoplectic state, and often appear for a considerable time before the attack actually takes place. [18]

Abercrombie used the French term *ramollissements* (softenings), probably in reference to the writings of Rostan, to refer to soft regions that he found in the brain at autopsy:

> Ramollissements of the cerebral substance is analogous to gangrene in other parts of the body.... This appears to be a disease of the aged.... I alluded to the extent of the disease of the arterial system of the brain in advanced life; and there appears to be considerable probability that this

may be the source of the ramollissement.... The disease of the arteries consists of ossification with thickening and contraction ... it corresponds precisely with the state of the arteries which we know to produce gangrene in other parts of the body particularly in the toes and feet of old people. [18]

Abercrombie performed an autopsy in a patient who two months previously had become hemiplegic and speechless:

On opening the head there appeared a remarkable depression on the upper part of the left hemisphere of the brain, about two inches in length and somewhat less in breadth the dura mater sinking into it to the depth of about half an inch. On removing the dura mater, the substance of the brain at this place was to a great extent broken down, soft and pulpy; and this appearance extended along nearly the whole upper part of the left hemisphere. [18]

Abercrombie may have been the first to describe the clinical picture in patients with epidural hemorrhage: "Extravasation on the surface of the brain from external injuries. The patient recovers from the immediate effects of the injury, walks home, and after some time, perhaps an hour or two, becomes oppressed and at last comatose. The extravasated blood ... removed by the operation of trephine, the coma disappears" [18].

Sir George Burrows, a British physician, gave the Lumleian lectures delivered at the Royal College of Physicians in London during 1843 and 1844. The lectures and additional information were published in 1846 in a treatise, *On the Disorders of the Cerebral Circulation* [21]. Burrows was a practicing physician whose major interest, activities, and reputation concerned insanity. His treatise on the brain and apoplexy was based mainly on his review of prior literature and his own hypotheses. He began the treatise by reviewing the experiments and writings of Drs. Monro [22] and Kellie [23] in order to refute their conclusion. The Monro-Kellie doctrine states that the sum of the volumes of brain, cerebrospinal fluid, and intracranial blood is constant. An increase in one causes a decrease in one or both of the remaining two. Burrows emphasizes that Monro and Kellie infer that the amount of blood in the head is nearly constant: "The quantity of blood within the head must be the same at all times whether in health or disease, in life or after death" [21,22]. Burrows then cites pathological reports that indicate that the brain vessels are often congested and filled with blood at necropsy. He relies heavily on necropsies of individuals who had died by hanging to support his opinions. In contrast to Monro and Kellie's doctrine, he emphasized that the amount of blood in the head can and does often increase, at times dramatically so. "The quantity of blood within the cranium, so far from being a constant quantity is, on the contrary, as variable as in other parts of the body" [21].

He opined that:

> In the vast majority of cases of apoplexy, coma is attributable to pressure
> induced by brain congestion.. . . I therefore infer that in the large number
> of cases of apoplexy accompanied with extravasation of blood, the coma
> is to be attributed to antecedent or coexisting cerebral congestion, while
> the paralysis which is more durable is dependent upon the limited local
> mischief produced by extravasation. [21]

Congestion causes pressure on the brain and alters function. The remedy he
espouses is to try to reduce the amount of blood in the head. This could be
done by venesection or by using a rotatory machine that drives blood from the
head. If that does not work, then a ligature should be placed around the
common carotid artery in the neck. Burrows was skeptical of the entity of
serous causes of apoplexy. He opined that, when hemorrhages were not found
at necropsy, the congestion and increase of blood in the head that existed
before the serous effusion had been depleted by the time of necropsy.

Burrows concludes his treatise by emphasizing the importance of heart
disease in understanding apoplexy and many other conditions. He notes that
valvular disease and cardiac hypertrophy are often found at necropsy in patients
with apoplexy and other conditions. He does not proffer opinions on the
mechanism of the interrelationship between heart and brain disease.

> The influence of structural diseases of the heart upon the brain is not
> confined to the production of apoplexies and attacks of hemiplegia, but
> many other disorders which are characterized by a variety of symptoms
> indicative of disturbance of circulation in the head . . . recurring attacks of
> vertigo, headaches, rushing of blood to the head, of epistaxis, somno-
> lency, nervous irritability, and even insanity may often be traced to the
> operations of cardiac disease. [21]

During the time of Burrows's medical practice and before, blood pressure
was not measured and hypertension was not recognized or treated. The
frequency of brain hemorrhage was undoubtedly higher than in present times,
and may have been more common than brain infarction. The pathological
findings in patients with apoplexy who did not have brain or intracranial
hemorrhage were not well characterized, although "serous effusions" and
ramollissements were described by some. In many, no definite causative
pathology was described. Burrows's espousing of vigorous venesection and
ligature of the common carotid artery were unfortunate and set back treatment
of apoplectic patients for nearly a century.

Sir John Liddell was a Scottish medical doctor and head physician of the
Royal Navy. He authored a treatise on apoplexy published in 1873 [24].
Liddell was a very active clinician who also performed autopsies on his patients.

He also saw infants and children. Liddell began by reflecting on the word "apoplexy": "The term is derived from the Greek word which signifies to strike to earth, to knock down; hence the term stroke is sometimes used as expressing the same idea." He reviews data that showed that most apoplexies occur in older individuals, especially between 60 and 70 years of age. He attributes this to degenerative changes in the heart, aorta, and blood vessels, as well as excessive imbibition of alcohol. A chapter on cerebral hemorrhage includes many clinical- and necropsy-confirmed cases of intracerebral hemorrhage. Liddell clearly describes brain embolism as a cause: "There are cases of cerebral embolism where a cerebral artery of large size becomes suddenly occluded by a clot of blood or plug of fibrine swept into it by the torrent of the circulation from some distant part."

Liddell includes in his treatise a chapter on embolism. A typical case is that of a 34-year-old woman who suddenly became paralyzed on her left side and died five days later:

> The right middle cerebral artery just at its commencement was plugged up by a small nodule of firm whitish fibrinous-looking substance; right corpus striatum much softened; right cerebral hemisphere generally contained less than the normal quantity of blood and was softer than normal in consistency. The mitral valve was much diseased, the auricular surface of the large cusp being beset with large warty excrescences of adherent blood-stained fibrin. The right common iliac artery was also obstructed. [24]

Liddell was impressed that somehow emotions, stress, and disease of other organs could cause apoplexy. He discusses nervous apoplexy: "hemiplegia of left side induced probably by intestinal irritation through reflex nervous action." Sections on cerebral gout and cerebral rheumatism described patients with gout or joint inflammation who had apoplectic attacks.

A unique component of Liddell's treatise is a chapter on infantile apoplexy. He noted that "infants perish of apoplexy much oftener than is generally supposed." Some children had perinatal hemorrhages. Other chronically or acutely ill children developed coma likely from toxi-metabolic or infectious causes that Liddell included among his infantile apoplectic cases.

HISTORICAL CONTRIBUTIONS OF THESE WRITINGS ON APOPLEXY

Sudden loss of function with stupor, with and without paralysis, was a common condition that often led to death or severe disability. It was a condition hard to ignore. The term "apoplexy" was generally applied, although Liddell noted that "stroke" was another term in use for the condition. Writers had difficulty separating apoplexy that we now define as caused by vascular disease from other general brain conditions and from toxi-metabolic causes. Terms such as "reflex apoplexy" and "sympathetic apo-plexy" were used as well as "cerebral gout" and "cerebral rheumatism" to infer that the cause lay in systemic organs and general conditions and not within the brain.

The epidemiology of apoplexy was commented on. Most instances of apoplexy were in older adults, aged 50–70. Intemperance was an important cause. Many had minor attacks and systemic illnesses before developing a severe apoplectic attack.

In most instances, a cause was identified only when necropsies were performed and hemorrhages were found. Necropsies were often performed by physicians who had seen the patient during the apoplectic condition. Examination of the cadavers was performed soon after death. Only descriptions of the gross appearance of the brain were included; no microscopic examinations were reported. Hemorrhages both intracerebral and subarachnoid were well described, and nearly all writers recognized "sanguinous apoplexies." The designation "serous apoplexies" was applied when no gross bleeding was found at necropsy. Some writers believed that even these cases were somehow related to bleeding and congestion and that blood was absorbed before necropsy. French physicians and Abercrombie wrote about softening "ramollissements," which represented areas of old infarction.

Recently acquired brain ischemia was not well recognized at necropsy since the gross appearance of the brain did not show well demarcated infarction and no microscopy was performed. Liddell in one case noted that "the surface of a section was pale, moist, shining and rather exsanguinated in appearance." Some of the non-hemorrhagic cases described were likely cardiac arrest with prolonged brain hypoperfusion. This caused no focal abnormality and the true nature of the insult would be apparent only after microscopic examination.

Wepfer, Abercrombie, and Liddell wrote about hardening, stenosis, and obstruction of arteries within the skull, but most writers did not comment on the relationship of these changes to apoplexy. Wepfer and Abercrombie recognized that these local abnormalities caused blockage of blood flow and that the lack of blood flow caused damage to brain tissue beyond the blockage. Some writers described thrombi, but the pathophysiology of thrombus formation was not discussed. Toward the end of the century, Virchow was the first to analyze the mechanisms of thrombus formation. Liddell wrote about cerebral embolism and was aware that thrombi often formed elsewhere and were taken up by the circulation and went to the brain, blocking major arteries. This represented one cause of apoplexy. Liddell also described the cardiac pathology found at necropsy, mostly rheumatic and infective. He related heart disease to apoplexy, although he did not comment on the mechanism except in some cases of cerebral embolism.

Rudolph Virchow, an anatomical and experimental pathologist, would during the later years of the nineteenth century clarify much of the pathophysiology of brain ischemia and infarction (Chapter 13 discusses Virchow's contributions).

NOTES AND REFERENCES

1. Wepfer, Johann-Jakob. Encyclopedia.com.
2. McHenry L. *Garrison's History of Neurology*. Springfield, IL: Charles C. Thomas, 1969.
3. Wepfer J-J. *Historia anatomica de puella sine cerebro nata* (1665). *Historiae apoplecticorum*. 1658. English translation from *Bagvili's Practice of Physik*, London, 1704; cited in Major RH. *Classic Descriptions of Disease*, 3rd ed. Springfield, IL: Charles C. Thomas, 1945, pp. 474–477. Blane G. History of cases of disease in the brain, with an account of the appearances upon examination after death and some general observations on complaints of the head. *Tr. Soc. Improvement M. & Chir. Knowledge* 1800;2:192–212.
4. Wepfer J-J. *Observationes anatomicae ex cadaveribus eorum, quos sustulit apoplexia, cum exercitatione de eius loco affect*. Schaffhausen, 1658.
5. Pierce JM. Johann Jakob Wepfer (1620–1695) and cerebral haemorrhage. *J. Neurol. Neurosurg. Psychiatry* 1997;62(4):387.
6. Nymann G. *De apoplexia tractus*, 2nd ed. Wittebergae: JW Finceli, 1670.
7. Varolio C. *De neruis opticis, nonnullisque aliis praeter commune opinionem in humano capite observatis*. Frankfurt: Ioannem Wechelum & petrum, Fischerum, 1591.
8. Bayle F. *Tractatus de apoplexia*. Toulousse: B. Guillemente, 1677.
9. Cole W. *A Physico-Medical Essay Concerning the Late Frequency of Apoplexies*. Oxford: Printed at the Theatre, 1689. Reprinted by The Classics of Neurology & Neurosurgery Library. New York: Gryphon Editions, 1995.
10. This idea is discussed in more detail in Chapter 13 on Virchow.
11. Hunter J. *A Treatise on the Blood, Inflammation, and Gunshot Wounds*. London: George Nicol, 1794.
12. Fisher CM. The history of cerebral embolism and hemorrhagic infarction. In Furlan A (ed.), *The Heart and Stroke*. Berlin: Springer-Verlag, 1987, pp. 3–16.
13. Cruveilhier J. *Anatomie pathologique du corps humain*. Paris, 1829, vol. 1, chapter 11, p. 7.
14. Mistichelli D. *Trattato dell apoplessia*. Rome: A. de Rossi alla Piazza di Ceri, 1709.
15. Kirkland T. *A Commentary on Apoplectic and Paralytic Affections and on Diseases Connected with the Subject*. London: William Dawson, 1792.
16. Cheyne J. *Cases of Apoplexy and Lethargy with Observations upon the Comatose Diseases*. London: J. Moyes printer, 1812.
17. Cooke J. *A Treatise on Nervous Diseases, vol. 1: On Apoplexy Including Apoplexia Hydrocephalica*. London: Longman, Hurst, Rees, Orme and Brown Publishers, 1820. Reprinted as part of the Classics of Neurology and Neurosurgery Library. Birmingham, AL: Gryphon Editions, 1984.
18. Abercrombie J. *Pathological and Practical Researches on Diseases of the Brain and the Spinal Cord*. Edinburgh: Waugh and Innes, 1828. Reprinted as part of the Classics of Neurology and Neurosurgery Library. New York: Gryphon Editions, 1993.
19. Rostan L. *Recherhes sur le ramollissement du cerveau. Ouvrage dans lequel on s'efforce de distinguer les diverses affections de ce viscère par de signes caractéristiques*. Paris: Bechet, 1823.

20. Serres AERA. Sur les maladies organique du cervelet: Des apoplexies cerebellerises. *J. Physiol. Exp. Path.* 1822;2:172;249; Serres AERA. New divisions of apoplexies. *Phil. J. Med. Phys. Sci.* 1824 (multiple articles).

21. Burrows G. *On the Disorders of the Cerebral Circulation and on the Connection between Affections of the Brain and Diseases of the Heart.* London: Longman, Brown, Green, and Longmans, 1846. Reprinted as part of the Classics of Neurology and Neurosurgery Library. New York: Gryphon Editions, 1994.

22. Monro A. *Observations on Structure and Functions of the Nervous System.* Edinburgh: Creech and Johnson, 1783.

23. Kellie G. Appearances observed in the dissection of two individuals; death from cold and congestion of the brain. *Trans. Med-Chir. Soc. Edinburgh* 1824;1:84.

24. Liddell J. *A Treatise on Apoplexy, Cerebral Hemorrhage, Cerebral Embolism, Cerebral Gout, Cerebral Rheumatism, and Epidemic Cerebro-Spinal Meningitis.* New York: WM Wood, 1873. Reprinted as part of the Classics of Neurology and Neurosurgery Library. Birmingham, AL: Gryphon Editions, 1990.

CHAPTER NINE

ATLASES

The origin of illustrated anatomy treatises dates to the Renaissance. They became popular after Andreas Vesalius's *De humani corporis fabrica* was published in 1543. It was after a quarter of the millennium that illustrated pathological treatises became a medical genre with Eduard Sandifort's *Museum anatomicum*, published in 1793 [1].

Anatomy was the study of healthy body parts, which could be seen as many times as the investigator wanted, and there were many early comparable treatises available. In contrast, some rare pathological cases occurred only once in a lifetime of a physician. There were no early comparable treatises in pathology. The investigators relied on occasional publications of articles in scientific and medical journals for comparison. An anatomy treatise could be completed by the dissection of a small number of bodies, but for documenting various pathological lesions at different sites, a larger number of bodies had to be dissected. Vesalius produced his anatomy treatise at the age of 28, whereas Morgagni was nearly 80 when he published his pathological treatise *De sedibus,* for which he relied on material assembled during his entire professional career and on reports collected by his teacher Valsalva [1].

Since the Renaissance, artists were trained in anatomical drawing and focused on the harmony, beauty, and proportion of the human body. The illustrations had an aesthetic appeal. In contrast, illustrations of pathology highlighted the disruption and destruction of harmony, beauty, and proportion. Artists were not trained to study the diseased body parts nor were they often found in hospitals or morgues drawing ulcers, tumors, or tubercles. The conditions of the specimens changed rapidly after death with regard to structure, texture, and color, and the artists had to act quickly in order to make their illustrations reliable. While preservation techniques allowed the accumulation of a large number of preparations, they also affected texture and obliterated color and so were problematic [1].

Various printing techniques also evolved during the decades around 1800. Those based on traditional black ink were woodcut, cross-hatching, stipple engraving, mezzotint, and aquatint. Different methods were used to add color. The simplest was to pay low-ranked artists to hand-color each plate, usually not more than a few hundred. Early in the eighteenth century Jacob Christoph Le Blon, inspired by Newton's theory, devised a method for color printing involving three plates, each with a separate color: red, blue, and yellow. A modification of the method was the addition of a fourth plate for black. A different technique called *à la poupée* involved only one plate to which different colors were applied selectively in different areas using a cloth or a paintbrush [1].

An important advancement was the development of lithography. Lithography was a planographic printing process that made use of the immiscibility of grease and water. The process was discovered in 1798 by Alois Senefelder of Munich, who used a porous Bavarian limestone for his plate (hence lithography, from Greek *lithos*, "stone"). The secret of lithographic printing was closely held until 1818, when Senefelder published *Vollständiges Lehrbuch der Steindruckerey* (A Complete Course of Lithography). Lithography originally used an image drawn with oil, fat, or wax onto the surface of a smooth, level lithograph limestone plate. The stone was then treated with a mixture of acid and gum arabic, etching the portions of the stone that were not protected by the grease-based image. When the stone was later moistened, these etched areas retained water. An oil-based ink could then be applied that would be repelled by the water and would stick only to the original drawing. The ink would finally be transferred to paper by means of a special press. This printing technique was used by Jean Cruveilhier, James Hope, and Robert Carswell [1–3].

In this chapter, we focus on the salient features of the famous atlases by Robert Hooper, Richard Bright, Jean Cruveilhier, and Robert Carswell. These atlases have contributed to the understanding of various neurological and cerebrovascular conditions.

ROBERT HOOPER

Robert Hooper (1773–1835) was born in Uxbridge, London, and qualified from St. Andrews University in 1805. He was a physician at Marylebone

Infirmary, a popular lecturer, and a prolific medical writer. In 1799, he published an essay on intestinal worms, *Observations on the Structure of the Intestinal Worms of the Human Body*, which contained striking aquatint illustrations based on microscopic observations. He published *Anatomical Plates of the Bones and Muscles Reduced from Albinus, for the Use of Students in Anatomy, and Artists* in 1802. His *Morbid Anatomy of the Human Brain* was published in 1826 and a second enlarged edition appeared in 1828. In 1832, he published *Morbid Anatomy of the Human Uterus and Its Appendages* [1].

The *Morbid Anatomy of the Human Brain* was the first neuropathological atlas and was based on more than 4,000 autopsies performed over a period of thirty years [4,5]. It consisted of 15 engraved delineations, representing the morbid states and changes most frequently observed in the brain and its membranous coverings. The parts were represented at their natural size and were beautifully colored after their natural appearance, with great attention to rules of art. Hooper identified five categories of diseases: (1) inflammation and its effects, (2) tumors, (3) diseased structures and unnatural appearances without tumefaction, (4) morbid collections of fluids secreted between membranes and in the cavities, and (5) extravasated fluids [4].

The first and second engravings presented beautiful specimens of inflammation of the dura mater. In the third and fourth, inflammation of the pia mater and arachnoid membrane was illustrated. The fifth showed osseous deposits in the membranes; the sixth, tubercles; and the seventh, tumors of the dura mater. The eighth presented a fine view of the effects of inflammation and the pulpy softening (ramollissement) in different stages; the ninth, cerebral abscess. A hematoma in the tenth and a scrofulous growth of the cerebellum in eleventh. The twelfth consisted of white, black, and bony tumors of the brain, diseases of the choroid plexus, and the pineal gland. The thirteenth contained an encysted tumor in the middle lobe on the right side; and the fourteenth exhibited a transverse section of a brain containing globular cysts [4].

The fifteenth involved the vascular system. It depicted extravasation of blood from rupture of a vessel in its substance, forming an apoplectic cavity [4] (Figure 9.1).

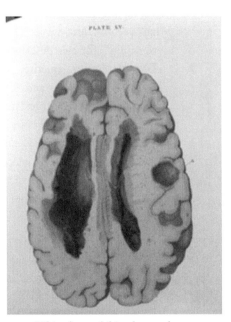

9.1. "This plate exhibits the usual appearance which the brain presents when blood is extravasated from the spontaneous rupture of a vessel in its substance. In the centre of the right hemisphere is an apoplectic cell between the middle of the corpus striatum and the external and lateral surface of the brain. The contents were a sanguineous fluid, partly coagulated" [4].

RICHARD BRIGHT

Richard Bright (1789–1858), the son of a wealthy Bristol banker, did his schooling in Bristol and Exeter. He went to Edinburgh University in 1808. Bright went on an expedition to Iceland, where he focused on zoology, botany, and mineralogy and made several sketches. He studied at Guy's Hospital, London, as well as Edinburgh, where he gained his MD with a thesis on contagious erysipelas in 1813. Bright then embarked on two continental tours and visited several centers and anatomical museums, including Leiden, Vienna, and the University Hospital at Pest. In 1815, he tended to the wounded after the Battle of Waterloo. During his second continental journey he visited the Paris hospitals and met René Laennec, who had just invented the stethoscope. Bright had a deep interest in the visual arts and was an accomplished draftsman of landscapes and natural and medical specimens. He also collected books on the history of print making. In 1816, Bright became a licentiate of the Royal College of Physicians and in 1820 was elected a Fellow of the Royal Society. He became an assistant physician at Guy's Hospital in 1820 and a full physician at Guy's in 1824. Along with Thomas Addison and Thomas Hodgkin, Bright founded the famous "Guy's Triumvirate" [1,5]. His research into the causes and symptoms of kidney disease led to his identifying what became known as Bright's disease. He is considered the "father of nephrology" for this description [6].

Bright's famous treatise, *Reports of Medical Cases, Selected with a View to Illustrate the Symptoms and Cure of Diseases by a Reference to Morbid Anatomy*, appeared in two volumes, in 1827 and 1831. In the second volume, titled *Diseases of the Brain and Nervous System Together with a Concise Statement of the Diseased Appearance of the Brain and Its Membranes*, he dealt with a wide range of neurological disorders. It was due to the suggestion of the eminent surgeon Sir Astley Cooper that he decided to focus on diseases of an individual organ, instead of bringing together dissertations on individual diseases of separate organs in volume 2. Volume 2 was published in two parts: part 1 included section I, inflammation of the brain and its membranes, acute hydrocephalus, and delirium tremens; and section II, apoplexy, paraplegia, concussion, chronic hydrocephalus, and spina bifida. Part 2 included hysteria, chorea, palsy from mercury, neuralgia, epilepsy, tetanus, and hydrophobia [7].

Bright used the clinicopathological method in his research. His observations were accurate, and his descriptions were supplemented with intricate illustrations of pathological specimens. He divided 310 cases of brain diseases into three sections: inflammation, pressure, and irritation. He attributed interrupted brain function mainly to an increase in pressure caused by intracranial hemorrhages, space-occupying lesions, vascular congestion, inflammation, intracranial effusion of "serum," changes in vascular pressure, defective circulation, concussion, or a state of torpor in the action of the nerves themselves. He arranged the section on pressure into 11 groups of cases: the first three contained cases of apoplexy, and the remaining were cases of brain tumors, lead paralysis, and chronic hydrocephalus [6].

Bright did not use current terminology to identify various types of intracranial hemorrhages – that is, subarachnoid, subdural, epidural, and intracerebral hemorrhages – but his cases were arranged based on the autopsy findings that highlighted the important differences between the various types of bleeds. He also showed that diseases of the heart, large vessels, lungs, and the kidneys were risk factors for apoplexy. Bright was also a pioneer in the doctrine of cerebral localization. He pointed out that damage to the cerebral cortex was associated with epileptic seizures. He noted the association between a severe sudden headache and subarachnoid hemorrhage. He provided illustrations of arteriovenous malformations and a ruptured middle cerebral artery aneurysm. He provided an early description of the syndrome of pathological laughing and crying and correlated it with bilateral lesions in the regions of the basal ganglia. His clinical observations also suggested that the areas of the brain controlling speech and upper extremity movements are close to each other [6].

JEAN CRUVEILHIER

Jean Cruveilhier (1791–1874) was born in Limoges, France, and was the son and grandson of surgeons. He wished to enter priesthood in his youth, but his father persuaded him to enter medical studies. In 1810, he moved to Paris from Limoges and commenced his medical studies under the famous surgeon Guillaume Dupuytren. He received his degree in 1816 and settled in Limoges. In 1823, he was appointed professor of surgery at Montpellier through the influence of Dupuytren. In 1825, he returned to Paris as professor of descriptive anatomy. In 1826 he revived the Anatomical Society, which had been founded by Dupuytren but had become inactive just a few years later. In 1836, Cruveilhier was appointed to the first chair of pathological anatomy in Paris. The chair was introduced along with a museum containing pathological preparations, wax models, and drawings, established with a 200,000-franc donation from Dupuytren. In addition to his work in pathology at the Charité and particularly at Salpêtrière, he was involved in a highly active clinical practice in Paris [1,8–10].

Jean Cruveilhier is the author of the two-volume atlas *L'Anatomie pathologique du corps humain*, which appeared in 40 installments over a period of 14 years. It is considered a fascinating storehouse of cases of the nervous system. His illustrations are aesthetically appealing and are unique in all the literature of pathology for their clarity and accuracy of presentation. He is known for his views on the role of phlebitis and inflammation in general disease processes.

He also provided an early description of several conditions such as peptic ulcer disease, multiple sclerosis, and progressive muscular atrophy [8]. A large number of anatomical structures and diseases bear his name: Cruveilhier's plexus, Cruveilhier's joint, Cruveilhier-Baumgarten disease, Cruveilhier's fossa, Cruveilhier's fascia, Cruveilhier disease, Cruveilhier atrophy, Cruveilhier tumor, Cruveilhier ligaments, and Cruveilhier ulcer [10,11].

Cruveilhier's injections of mercury into the blood vessels and the bronchial system bore out the theory of phlebitis, which, he said "dominates the whole of pathology." This theory was later disproved by Virchow, who came up with the concept of embolism [10]. In addition to illustrations, Cruveilhier added extensive clinical material for most of the cases and summarized those with his own comments on patients' histories, physical findings, and autopsies. His organization is such that certain patterns useful in arriving at diagnoses can be made. He emphasized correlating autopsy findings with events in the history and clinical examination. His clinical acumen distinguished him from the other contemporary illustrators. He was capable of organizing different findings of a patient in such a way as to arrive at a diagnosis based on neuroanatomy and neurophysiology [8].

He classified spinal cord lesions into four categories: (1) paraplegia by alteration of the cord itself, (2) paraplegia by compression, (3) paraplegia by inflammation, and (4) false paraplegia due to rigidity of joint. He stated the distinction between extrinsic and intrinsic lesions to be important as extrinsic lesions could benefit from surgical intervention. The extent of his interest in spinal cord diseases can be seen with his illustrations of cases of Pott's disease, hydatid cyst, apoplexy in the cord, and subluxation of C1 and C2. He also included cases of congenital and neonatal malformations such as hydrocephalus, spina bifida, and meningomyelocele. There is also one case of congenital absence of the cerebellum [8].

He included cases of patients with paraplegia in whom a "grey degeneration or transformation" was found throughout the spinal cord, brain stem, and cerebellum. The lesions were small, multiple, and denser than the tissue of the spinal cord. He felt that this was a new disease entity. These cases are considered the earliest description of multiple sclerosis [8].

In the first half of the nineteenth century, cerebrovascular disease was divided into two types: hemorrhage and infarction; the concept of embolism was not appreciated. Cruveilhier attempted to distinguish between red and white infarcts based on clinical and pathological criteria. His clinical distinction, although not applicable today, was based on his opinion that hemorrhagic lesions had a more abrupt onset in their clinical presentation than softening. He felt that in hemorrhage the motor system was principally affected, while in softening, mental changes were also noted [8].

Cruveilhier made the diagnosis of a very large apoplectic cavity in the left thalamus with probable communication of the clot with the lateral ventricle.

These were the findings at autopsy; also found was an old cystic lesion in the region of the insula. He explained that thalamic hemorrhage was the most frequent lesion in cases with sudden onset of profound hemiplegia, and the communication with the ventricle resulted in coma and unresponsiveness. The loss of consciousness at the onset of the illness pointed toward a grave prognosis. He explained that the old lesion indicated a prior hemorrhage that was not fatal due to its location. He was aware that the clinical course of patients with apoplexy depended more on the location and size of the lesion than on differences in the disease processes [8].

He also distinguished brain stem hemorrhage that was characterized by sudden collapse of the patient, complete loss of movement and sensation, and rapid death. He cautioned that every rapid demise of this sort was not due to a pontine hemorrhage. Cruveilhier, like Rostan, noted the frequency of left ventricular hypertension in cases of cerebral apoplexy, which we know today is a result of hypertension [8].

Cruveilhier also discussed cerebral tumors along with lesions such as tuberculomas and abscesses. Harvey Cushing called attention to the accuracy of Cruveilhier's observations on brain tumors. He included Cruveilhier's reports and reproduced his illustrations in his works on acoustic neuromas (1917) and meningiomas (1938), nearly a century later [8].

ROBERT CARSWELL

Robert Carswell (1793–1857) was born in Paisley, near Glasgow, Scotland. He was a son of a printmaker and was exposed to artistic productions from an early age. He began his medical studies at the University of Glasgow. His artistic skills brought him to the notice of Dr. John Thomson of Edinburgh, one of the foremost physicians of the day. In the early 1820s, Thomson sent his son William with Carswell to France to study, draw, and paint fresh pathological specimens in color. He spent two years working in the hospitals in Paris and Lyons. He returned to Scotland and took his MD degree at Marischal College, Aberdeen, in 1826. He returned to Paris and resumed his studies of morbid anatomy under the celebrated physician Pierre C. A. Louis. In 1828, he was nominated to become the first professor of pathological anatomy at the new University College, London. However, before beginning his teaching duties, he was commissioned to prepare a collection of pathological drawings for the university. He remained in Paris until 1831, by which time he had completed over 1,000 watercolors of diseased structures [1,12].

On his arrival in London, Carswell took up his duties as a professor and was also appointed as physician to the University College Hospital. He published his famous work *Pathological Anatomy: Illustrations of the Elementary Forms of Disease* in 1838. He described the reason for undertaking the publication as follows [12,13]: "The great difficulty, and frequently the impossibility, of comprehending even the best descriptions of the physical or anatomical characters of diseases, without the aid of coloured delineations, induced me to undertake the publication of the present work" [13].

He dedicated his book to James Jeffray, his professor of anatomy and physiology at the University of Glasgow, and recalled Jeffray's approbation of his "coloured delineations" of "the healthy and diseased appearances of the human body" [13]. The volume's contents were arranged according to pathological states under the headings of Inflammation, Analogous Tissues, Atrophy, Hypertrophy, Pus, Mortification, Haemorrhage, Softening, Melanoma, Carcinoma, and Tubercle [12,13]:

Carswell is regarded as the first illustrator of the lesions of multiple sclerosis. Out of the 1,034 paintings, 99 are of the brain and spinal cord and plate 4, figure 4.4, in the atlas is of the spinal cord, pons, and medulla, titled "Brown Transparent Discolouration without Softening of the Spinal Cord," depicting a condition he said was "a peculiar diseased state of the cord and pons variolii." There were both fresh and old scars, which he thought were due to deficiency of blood supply. There were little clinical details other than that the patient was paralyzed. He indicated that he saw two examples of this pathology; he had not examined either of the patients, but illustrated one of them [14].

Carswell was also responsible for making the first colored pictures of the pathology in Hodgkin disease. Thomas Hodgkin recognized these while leafing through Carswell's "unrivalled" collection of drawings and displayed them when he read his classic paper on the subject in London in 1832 [12].

Under the section "Haemorrhage," Carswell described the various causes and physical characteristics of brain hemorrhage. His atlas contained illustrations of cerebral apoplexy in various stages [13]. Carswell was the first to prove that ramollissement was a necrotic process driven by cerebro-arterial obstruction. He also highlighted carotid artery disease as a cause for cerebral injury [15]. He wrote that

> if the obliteration has taken place in the carotid or one of its principal divisions within the cranium, the greater part or the whole of a hemisphere may be softened.... When effusion takes place, it is probably the consequence of rupture of the obliterated vessels, or of some of the smaller ones having remained pervious and yielding to the increased momentum of the blood. [13]

Published anatomy and pathology atlases became generally available. By the middle of the nineteenth century, physicians, especially those who did not perform autopsies, could visualize the pathology in the organs of the body. Various brain pathologies were well shown. There is no better example of the adage "a picture is worth a thousand words" than the visual advance that atlases made.

NOTES AND REFERENCES

1. Meli DB. *Visualizing Disease: The Art and History of Pathological Illustrations*. Chicago: University of Chicago Press, 2018.

2. Lithography. Wikipedia. Available at https://en.wikipedia.org/w/index.php?title= Lithography&oldid=972927973.

3. Lithography/printing. *Encyclopedia Britannica*. Available at www.britannica.com/technology/lithography.

4. Hooper R. *The Morbid Anatomy of the Human Brain Being Illustrations of the Most Frequent and Important Organic Diseases to Which That Viscus Is Subject*. London: Longman, Rees, Orme, Brown, and Green, 1828.

5. Rose FC. *History of British Neurology*. Singapore: World Scientific Publishing Co., 2011.

6. Schutta HS. Apoplexy in Richard Bright's (1789–1858) reports of medical cases. *J. Hist. Neurosci.* 2020 Jun 22:1–23.

7. Bright R. *Reports of Medical Cases, Selected with a View of Illustrating the Symptoms and Cures of Diseases by a Reference to Morbid Anatomy*. London: Longman, Rees, Orme, Brown, and Green, 1831.

8. Flamm ES. The neurology of Jean Cruveilhier. *Med. Hist.* 1973 Oct;17(4):343–355.

9. de Saint-Maur PP. The birth of the clinicopathological method in France: The rise of morbid anatomy in France during the first half of the nineteenth century. *Virchows Arch.* 2012;460(1):109–117.

10. Kosif R. Jean Cruveilhier and his explorations. *World J. Res. Rev.* 2019;8(4):29–31.

11. Cruveilhier J. *Anatomie pathologique du corps humain: Descriptions avec figures lithographiees et caloriees des diverses alterations morbides dont le corps humanin est susceptible*. Paris: JB Bailliere, 1835–1842.

12. Robert Carswell, *Carswell's Illustrations of the Elementary Forms of Disease*. Glasgow University Library Special Collections Department Book of the Month. October 2003. Available at www.gla.ac.uk/myglasgow/library/files/special/exhibns/month/oct2003.html.

13. Carswell R. *Pathological Anatomy: Illustrations of the Elementary Forms of Disease*. London: Longman, 1838.

14. Murray TJ. Robert Carswell: The first illustrator of MS. *Int. MS J.* 2009 Sep;16 (3):98–101.

15. Munster AB, Thapar A, Davies AH. History of carotid stroke. *Stroke* 2016 Apr 1;47(4): e66–e69.

CHAPTER TEN

BRAINSTEM SYNDROMES

During the second half of the nineteenth century and early years of the twentieth century, clinicians described instances of focal brainstem lesions at various levels. The intent was to learn the location and function of various nuclei and tracts. Some lesions were due to infarcts and hemorrhages. Others were caused by tumors, infections, or other nonvascular processes. These focal lesions were usually named after the first describers. Herein are notable examples.

LATERAL MEDULLARY INFARCTION: WALLENBERG SYNDROME

Although one of the last published eponymous lesions, reports by Wallenberg described the anatomy, function, and vascular mechanism in the most detail. His name and syndrome are most familiar to neurologists and stroke specialists.

Adolph Wallenberg was a practicing physician in Danzig, Poland. He also performed neuroanatomical research [1,2]. His knowledge of anatomy allowed him to predict the location of his original patient's brain lesion. Wallenberg wrote four papers on lateral medullary infarcts [3]. Wallenberg knew the original patient, a 38-year-old ropemaker whom he had seen during prior medical encounters. He had first examined the patient in 1889 for appendicitis and had seen him for cardiovascular symptoms, tachycardia, dyspnea, and a pounding pulse, which Wallenberg attributed to "fatty degeneration of the heart" [1–3]. The patient drank alcohol and smoked heavily. At autopsy, he had a very large heart and extensive atherosclerosis. Hypertension and premature atherosclerosis had been present for years.

On the evening of September 9, 1893, the patient suddenly developed violent vertigo and intense pain in the left eye that spread to the entire left side of the face. Vertigo subsided. He could not swallow and his voice became hoarse. Wallenberg examined the patient the next day and found the following: (1) horizontal and vertical nystagmus, (2) hyperesthesia of the entire left face and a decreased left corneal reflex, (3) loss of pain and temperature sense on the right side of the face and body, (4) weakness of the left palate, (5) left vocal cord paralysis, and (6) left limb ataxia.

The patient became able to walk but leaned to the left, requiring the help of two people for support. Sensation on the right side of the face normalized and the left facial hyperesthesia became analgesia. The patient developed a roaring in the ears, and a loud systolic bruit became audible in the neck that was loudest at the right carotid artery bifurcation. This may be the earliest report of clinical detection of a carotid bruit. Two months after the stroke, Wallenberg demonstrated the findings at a meeting of the Danzig Medical Society, and the original report appeared March 21, 1894, about six months after the patient's stroke [1–3].

Wallenberg relied on his own anatomical knowledge, the vascular studies of Duret [4], and published case reports (some with necropsies) to predict the location and extent of the brain softenings and vascular etiology of the syndrome. Wallenberg began by focusing on the persistent findings, ignoring those that were transient. He emphasized the combination of left vocal cord paralysis and left palatal paralysis to indicate involvement of the "left accessory nerve" and to localize the lesion to the left half of the medulla extending from its caudal limit at the upper level of the pyramidal decussation to the vagus or lower glossopharyngeal levels more rostrally [1–3]. The facial and body sensory findings and the ataxia further localized the lesion to the lateral medulla and possibly the left cerebellum. His final anatomical prediction was precise:

> We are dealing with an insult on the left side of the medulla. It begins just above the pyramidal decussation. It passes through the accessory olive and the inferior olive more rostrally. Laterally it destroys the entire medulla to the pia mater. Rostrally and medially it reaches the ascending lemniscus, damages the restiform body and ultimately also the cerebellum. There is no evidence to indicate that the disease crossed to the right side of the medulla. [1–3]

Wallenberg speculated on the cause of the stroke, considering the possibilities of hemorrhage, thrombosis, and embolism. He reasoned that hemorrhage was unlikely because the patient survived. The sudden onset of symptoms favored embolism as the mechanism of the stroke. He localized the recipient site of the embolus to the left posterior inferior cerebellar artery (PICA). Wallenberg found in his dissections that PICA gave off "2–5 fine feeders to the roots of the bulbar division of the accessory nerve and the vagus fibers. Branches entered the substance of the medulla in the region of the descending trigeminal tract and nucleus. These ran medially and fed the medial portion of the olive" [2]. Wallenberg speculated on the cause of the bruit, mentioning carotid artery narrowing as one possibility. "For all I know, the bruit may have been caused by blood rushing through a narrowed portion of the vessel into a wider portion" [3]. Unfortunately, the carotid arteries in the neck were not described in the later necropsy report.

Six years after his original stroke, the patient had several dizzy spells on two successive days and noted right-hand weakness. He did not consult a physician. As he undressed for bed, he suddenly collapsed and died. Wallenberg performed the autopsy himself and reported the pathological findings in detail [3]. The arteries at the base of the brain showed "irregular thickened calcified areas with occasional bumpy prominences." The rostral basilar artery and the intracranial vertebral arteries (ICVAs) were very stenotic. The left PICA was very stenotic at its origin from the left ICVA, and the left PICA was occluded 2 centimeters after its origin. Wallenberg described the findings in sections from the upper cervical cord through the brainstem. The location and extent of the infarct in the left lateral medulla was exactly as he had predicted. Since Wallenberg's report the lateral medullary syndrome has often been labeled the *PICA syndrome*. In the original patient described by Wallenberg, the infarct was most likely attributable to severe stenosis of the ipsilateral ICVA, not PICA.

Adolph Wallenberg was appointed chief of the internal medicine and psychiatric divisions of the Danzig City Hospital when Danzig was an independent free city. When the Nazi regime came to power in Danzig in 1938, Wallenberg, a Jew, was forced to leave his home and his job in the hospital. He fled to Holland and then England and from there came to the United States in 1943. He lived in the Chicago region during the remainder of his life.

The very first case of the lateral medullary syndrome had been reported more than eight decades earlier by Marcet in 1811 [5]. This report concerned Dr. Gaspard Vieusseux, an eminent physician from Geneva, Switzerland, who had a stroke in January 1808. Vieusseux was so puzzled and impressed by his own abnormal sensory experiences that he traveled to London in 1810 to present his unusual case to the Medical and Chirurgical Society of London. Marcet, the secretary of the society, recorded and edited the presentation, and published his report in the society proceedings [5]. On December 29, 1807, Dr. Vieusseux developed an unusual and severe pain in his left gum and jaw. On January 4, the pain in the gum recurred and was accompanied by an extremely acute pain in the left eye. He then developed severe vertigo, which he colorfully described as "a peculiar and inexpressible perturbation in all his sensations," a giddiness that affected his vision and "occasioned feelings similar to those produced by a ship violently agitated." He vomited, lost his voice, had difficulty swallowing fluids, and felt that his left side was weak. He examined himself and found that "the whole of his right side was so insensible that he could be scratched or pinched without experiencing any pain and that this insensibility abruptly terminated at a line dividing the whole body in a vertical direction" [5]. The sensations of heat and cold were totally different on his right side, but he was puzzled to find that he had not lost the perception of touch on that side. The left side of the head and face were also insensible to pricking or scratching over the left forehead, nose, lips, chin, and ear. He also noted that his left eye was partially shut and that the left corner of his mouth was drawn downward. The right side of the face felt normal as did the left side of his body and limbs. His left leg dragged slightly when he walked. During the next weeks, his dysarthria and difficulty swallowing improved but he developed hiccups. "His intellectual faculties remained quite unimpaired so that he could accurately observe the whole succession of symptoms" [5].

Wallenberg clearly was not the first to describe the lateral medullary syndrome. In addition to the report by Marcet, which included no anatomical data or even speculation about the localization of the lesion, in 1881, H. Senator, a neurologist working at the Charitè hospital in Berlin, described a patient with lateral medullary infarction [6], and two years later wrote on the differential diagnosis of brain infarcts including those in the medulla [7]. Wallenberg cited the reports of Senator, which appeared in the same journal as Wallenberg's case report. Wallenberg's scholarship and the detail of his reports and analyses were excellent examples of the clinicopathological method and certainly warranted his eponymous linkage with the lateral medullary syndrome. Original patients had lesions that involved vestibular nuclei, the spinal nucleus of V and its tract, restiform body, nucleus ambiguous, spinothalamic tract, quintothalamic tract, and descending sympathetic fibers. Later studies showed that small regions within the dorsolateral and ventrolateral medulla produced partial lateral medullary syndromes.

Physicians began to describe patients with medullary lesions that involved the medial medulla, a territory fed by different vertebral artery branches than the lateral medulla. These patients had contralateral hemiparesis, often sparing the face, and slight posterior column symptoms on the side of the hemiparesis, and some had tongue weakness. In 1902, Joseph Jules Francois Félix Babinski, a very respected neurologist, and Jean Nageotte, an anatomist and histologist, demonstrated the findings in a patient and later reported three patients who had prominent features of the lateral medullary syndrome combined with contralateral weakness and contralateral pyramidal tract signs [7–9]. They introduced the term "lateropulsion" to describe pulling and veering to the ipsilateral side when walking. Only one of their patients had a necropsy, which showed a lesion involving both the lateral and medial medulla on one side, causing a hemimedullary syndrome. The findings included ipsilateral limb ataxia, nystagmus, sensory deficits of the face, ptosis and pupillary meiosis, weakness of the soft palate larynx and tongue, and contralateral weakness and sensory loss. Since then infarcts involving one half of the medulla have been labeled the Babinski-Nageotte syndrome.

PONTINE LESIONS (MILLARD GUBLER AND FOVILLE AND RAYMOND SYNDROMES)

In 1856, in a series of publications, Dr. Adolphe Gubler showed definitively that lesions that affected the ventral portion of the pons on one side caused an ipsilateral facial paralysis and a contralateral hemiplegia [10,11]. Gubler was professor of medicine and director of the central outpatient clinic in Paris [10]. Gubler wrote: "We now summarize the symptoms produced in our cases of pontine lesions, documented or inferred. Intelligence was unaltered in all cases … the limbs were always paralyzed on the side opposite the lesion … there is no paralysis at all on the side of the face corresponding to the hemiplegia and the limbs on the side of the facial paralysis are normal" [11].

August Millard, who was 25 years old and had just graduated from medical school, wrote a letter to the journal that published Gubler's papers [10,12], informing the journal that he had, a year before, published a similar case, a patient with a pontine hemorrhage who had crossed hemiplegia [13]. The name Millard Gubler syndrome became attached to the syndrome despite the fact that Gubler's role was much more definitive than Millard's. The lesion in the ventral pons affected the fibers of the facial nerve as they exited and the cortico-spinal tract fibers in the basis pontis before they crossed. If the facial nucleus or dorsal portion of the nerve were affected, the ipsilateral sixth nerve would also be involved.

In 1858, Achille Louis Foville, a professor of physiology first in Rouen and later in Clarenton, published a report on a patient with a unilateral dorsal pontine lesion [10,14]. Fourteen years previously, Foville had authored a treatise on the physiology and pathology of the nervous system [13]. He had found a patient with alternating hemiplegia due to an apoplectic attack who "displayed a singular and little-known affection of eye movement" [12]. When Foville published his report, the patient was still alive. Foville wrote: "The case lacks anatomical documentation and my comments are designed primarily to draw your attention to the problem for your further study of similar cases" [14]. The patient had a left facial paralysis and right hemiplegia. "When he attempted to look to the left, either conjugately or with each eye alone, the globes moved to the midline but no further" [14]. The right gaze was normal.

Foville localized the lesion to the dorsal portion of the lower pontine tegmentum where the VII nerve nucleus and proximal nerve fibers course around the sixth nerve nucleus in the area of a conjugate gaze center (later labeled the paramedian pontine reticular formation (PPRF) lateral gaze center). He commented on control of lateral eye movement: "nature controls conjugate movements in much the same way as a man driving a team of horses. He unites the reins in each hand so a single movement will turn both horses to the left or right" [14,15]. Jean Baptiste-Octave Landry in the very next report in the same journal, described a patient with a right sixth nerve paralysis and left facial and body hemiparesis and sensory loss from a lesion shown at necropsy to involve the rostral pons [10,16]. This case is cited as among the first to first illustrate the difference between lower motor neuron and upper motor neuron function. The abducens weakness was a direct effect of injury to the nucleus or fibers of the sixth nerve, while the crossed facial and body paresis were related to as yet uncrossed descending cortico-facial and cortico-spinal fibers in the pons rostral to the facial nucleus. Fulgence Raymond, Charcot's successor as chair of neurology at the Faculty of Medicine in Paris, later discussed localization of a lesion that would cause an ipsilateral sixth nerve paralysis and a crossed hemiplegia sparing the face [10,17]. This came to be labeled Raymond's syndrome, although he did not report a confirmed case with a single pontine lesion. Raymond discussed the location of corticobulbar descending fibers so that such a lesion would have to involve the caudal pons.

MIDBRAIN LESIONS (WEBER AND BENEDIKT SYNDROMES)

Sir Hermann David Weber, a German-born physician, practiced medicine in London. He was knighted for espousing open-air treatment of tuberculosis. In 1863 he reported a patient who had had rheumatic fever and symptoms of heart failure. The 52-year-old man suddenly felt faint; a surgeon examined him and found "a complete paralysis of the right side from the face to the toes, ptosis of the left upper eyelid, squinting, and the pulse weak and irregular" [10,18]. Two days later Weber examined the patient and elaborated on the eye signs. The left pupil was more dilated than the right. "A more accurate examination of the eyes shows that the right obeys the will while the left is entirely motionless except in the horizontal direction inwards, outwards ... there exists on the left side paralysis of the third nerve and immunity of the fourth and sixth nerves" [10,18]. The patient died five weeks later and a hemorrhagic infarct involved the midbrain in the area of the cerebral peduncle and the emerging third nerve. Since then Weber's syndrome is cited as consisting of an ipsilateral third nerve palsy and a contralateral hemiparesis.

In 1889, Moritz Benedikt (1835–1920), a Hungarian-Austrian neurologist, described a patient during a lecture delivered in his native German language in

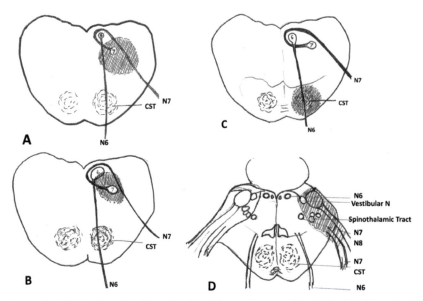

10.1. Artist's drawings (Dr. Linda Davis) of the syndromes of A .Millard-Gubler, B. Foville, C. Raymond,D. Gasperini CST= Corticospinal tract' N= Cranial Nerve

Paris. That patient had a Weber syndrome plus ipsilateral ataxia. At necropsy the patient had a tuberculoma that involved the cerebral peduncle and the red nucleus as well as the fibers of the exiting third nerve [10,19].

These observations further awakened interest in brain anatomy and function. There was little interest, except in the case of Adolph Wallenberg in the vascular cause. There was no treatment.

NOTES AND REFERENCES

1. Caplan LR. *Vertebrobasilar Ischemia and Hemorrhage: Clinical Findings, Diagnosis, and Management of Posterior Circulation Disease.* Cambridge: Cambridge University Press, 2014.
2. Wilkins RH, Brody IA. Neurological classics XXX. Wallenberg's syndrome. *Arch. Neurol.* 1970;22:379–382. Wolf M. Wallenberg's syndrome. In *The Classical Brain Stem Syndromes.* Springfield, IL: Charles C. Thomas, 1971, pp. 113–136.
3. Wallenberg A. Acute bulbaraffection (Embolie der art. cerebellar post. inf.sinistr.?). *Arch. Psychiat. Nervenkr.* 1895;27:504–540. Wallenberg A. Anatomischer befund in einem als "acute bulbar affection (embolie der art. cerebellar post. inf. sinistra?)" beschreibenen falle. *Arch. Psychiat. Nervenkr.* 1901;34:923–959. Wallenberg A. Verschluss der arteria cerebelli inferior posterior sinistra. *Neurologische Zentralblatt* 1915;34:236–247. Wallenberg A. Verschluss der arteria cerebelli inferior posterior dextra (mit sektionbefund). *Deutsche Zeitschrift f Nervenheilk* 1922;73:189–212.
4. Duret H. Sur la distribution des arteres nouricièrres du bulb rachidien. *Arch. Physiol. Norm. Path.* 1873; 5:97–113. These studies are discussed further in Chapter 12.
5. Marcet A. History of a singular nervous or paralytic affection attended with anomalous morbid sensations. *Medico-Chir. Trans.* 1811;2:215–233.

6. Senator H. Apoplectische bulbarparalyse mit wechselstandiger empfindungslahmung. *Arch. Psychiat. Nervenkr.* 1881;11:713–726.

7. Senator H. Zur diagnostik der heiderkrankungen in der Brücke und dem verlingerten marks. *Arch. Psychiat. Nervenkr.* 1883;14:618–643.

8. Babinski J, Nageotte J. Hémiasynergie, latéropulsion et myosis bulbaires avec hémianesthesie et hémiplégie croisées. *Rev. Neurol. (Paris)* 1902;10:358–365. Babinski J, Nageotte J. Lésions syphilitiques des centres nerveux. Foyers de ramollissement dans le bulbe. Hémiasynergie, latéropulsion et myosis bulbaires avec hémianesthésie et hémiplégie croisées. *Nouv. Iconogr. Salpêtriere* 1902;15:492–512.

9. Dejerine J. *Semiologie des affections du système nerveux.* Paris: Masson, 1977, p. 214. Contributions are discussed in Chapter 11.

10. Wolf M. *The Classical Brain Stem Syndromes.* Springfield, IL: Charles C. Thomas, 1971.

11. Gubler A. Alternating hemiplegia, a sign of pontine lesion, and documentation of the proof of the facial decussation. *Gazette hebdomadaire de médicine et chirurgie* 1856;3;740–754, 789–792.

12. Millard A. To the editor in chief. *Gazette hebdomadaire de médicine et chirurgie* 1856;3;811–816.

13. Millard A. Case of pontine hemorrhage. *Bulletins de la société anatomique* 1855;30:204–209; 1856;31:206–221.

14. Foville AL. Note on a little-known paralysis of eye muscles and its relation to the anatomy and physiology of the pons. *Bulletin de la societé anatomique de Paris* 1858;33:373–405.

15. Foville AL. *Traité complet de l'anatomie, de la physiologie et de la pathologie du système nerveux cérébro-spinal.* Paris: Fortin Macron, 1844.

16. Landry JB-O. *Bulletin de la société anatomique de Paris* 1858;33:406–410.

17. Raymond F. Concerning a special type of hemiplegia. Lecture of January 11, 1895. In *Lecons sur les maladies nerveux 1894–1895,* Première série. Paris: Riklin and Souques, 1896, pp. 365–383.

18. Weber H. A contribution to the pathology of the crura cerebri. *Medico-Chirurgical Transactions of the Royal Medical and Chirurgical Society* 1863; 46 (second series 28):121–139.

19. Benedikt M. *Le bulletin medicale* 1889;3:547–548. A lecture transcribed by Dr. Léon Leibowitz and translated by Dr. Gallois; Benedikt, M. Zur Lehre von der Lokalisation der Gehirn fuctionen. Wiener Klinik, 1883, pp 101–159.

CHAPTER ELEVEN

JULES DEJERINE

Jules Joseph Dejerine was born in 1839 in Geneva, Switzerland [1–5]. Although his parents, who were originally from France, had only modest means, they encouraged their son to pursue his studies. In 1871, he went to Paris in a third-class train compartment intending to study medicine. He carried with him a brief introduction to Vulpian [1]. Edmé Félix Alfred Vulpian was one of the most influential French physicians at that time. Vulpian soon became a full professor of medicine; he was elected to the Académie Nationale de Médecine and the Académie des Sciences and later became dean of the Paris Faculty of Medicine [6]. Dejerine became a pupil of Vulpian's at the Hôpital de la Pitié-Salpêtrière. The influence of and the relationship with Vulpian were the strongest and most enduring during his entire career. Dejerine also attended the lectures of Brown-Sequard and later became one of his friends.

In 1879, Dejerine became senior registrar (*chef de clinique*) at the Hôpital Bicêtre. He was given the appointment of hospital consultant (*Médecin des Hôpitaux de Paris*) in 1882. Dejerine became an associate professor after completing a competitive exam and a dissertation thesis in 1886 on the heredity of nervous system diseases. He was by many accounts a gifted and intuitive clinician and an outstanding teacher who attracted many students to his laboratory. After a memorable and "heated interview" with Charcot, he was nominated as assistant professor (*professeur agrégé*). In 1887, he became chief consultant at the Hôpital Bicêtre Hospital and he organized and established a laboratory in pathology. He remained at Bicêtre for eight years. Already well known and respected internationally, he was visited there by Sir Charles Sherrington and other international neuroscientists and clinicians.

While working with Vulpian, Dejerine had encountered Augusta Marie Klumpke, a brilliant young medical student, and in 1888 they married. They had met in 1880 at Charité Hospital, where Dejerine was chief resident and she was a junior assistant in practical training. Augusta was born in San Francisco, California, in 1859 [1]. When she was 11, she settled down with her mother, four sisters, and a brother near Lausanne, Switzerland. Her father remained in San Francisco. She was encouraged by her mother to pursue medical studies. The family moved to Paris. In 1882, Klumpke became the first woman to win an externship, a hospital position without residence at a hospital, shortly after women won the right to compete. As an extern at Hotel Dieu, she diagnosed a case of brachial plexus palsy with ocular sympathetic palsy (Dejerine-Klumpke's paralysis) and in 1885 subsequently published an article in the *Revue de Médicine*. This won her an Academy of Medicine prize but not an internship because women were not yet allowed to compete. She gradually ascended within the Paris Hospital system and became the first woman to become Interne des Hôpitaux in France in 1886–1887. The appointment awarded was despite pressure exerted by male members of the faculty. The Minister of Health and influential medical colleagues, among whom were Vulpian and Charcot, supported her appointment. She had in 1885 already published papers on radicular palsies of the lower brachial plexus (later known as Klumpke's palsy) and on Horner's syndrome.

With their marriage in 1888, Klumpke (now Madame Dejerine-Klumpke) and Dejerine became lifelong collaborators who became experts in nervous system anatomy and pathology. They published widely: 195 articles by Dejerine and 56 neurological articles by Klumpke-Dejerine. Their texts were often anonymously and skillfully illustrated by Dejerine-Klumpke. Dejerine's work focused on anatomical and anatomical-pathological studies conducted mainly with his wife. These led to the publication of the *Anatomie des centres nerveux* [7] and the *Sémiologie des affections du système nerveux* in 1914 [8]. Essential for the anatomical studies were the use of Golgi's and other recently described staining methods and the use of the principle of secondary degeneration to localize various fiber tracts. In addition to his laboratory work, Dejerine made important clinicopathological correlations. He was known to be an excellent clinician and teacher. He explained symptoms and signs in simple, direct language. He was thorough and kind to patients. Figure 11.1 shows Dejerine making a hospital ward round with his staff.

In 1895, Dejerine moved to the Salpêtrière Hospital where he spent the next 23 years. In 1899, Dejerine was among the 17 founding members of the French Neurological Society, among whom 13 were pupils of Charcot.

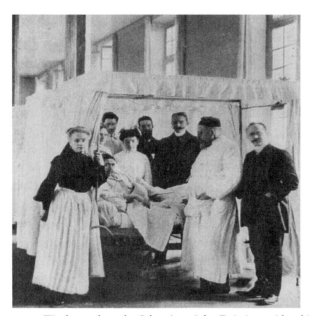

11.1. Ward rounds at the Salpetriere. Jules Dejerine, with white robe and black hat, is the imposing figure standing on the right. Reprinted with permission from Dejerine J, Gaukler E. *Les manifestations fonctionelles des psychoneuroses*. Paris: Masson et Cie, 1911.

In 1901, he became professor of the history of medicine and surgery and, in 1907, professor in internal medicine. In 1911, he was appointed to the chair in nervous system diseases in the Faculty of Medicine of Paris. Dejerine was the third occupant of the world's first chair of neurology at La Salpêtrière. The chair was previously occupied by Fulgence Raymond, who in 1894 succeeded the famous and charismatic Jean-Martin Charcot.

CONTRIBUTIONS TO NEUROLOGY IN GENERAL

Dejerine's two-volume book on semiology contained innumerable anatomic-clinical descriptions of the symptoms and clinical findings in patients with lesions throughout the nervous system [8]. Dejerine had an interest in higher brain functions and in the anatomical basis of aphasia and disorders of language. He studied the spinal cord and authored a book on the spinal cord with Andre Thomas [9]. He was interested in muscle and nerve diseases. Later in life he became interested in psychological disturbances, as had Charcot. Dejerine collaborated with many colleagues and his name still is attached to some syndromes and conditions: the Dejerine-Roussy syndrome, found in lesions of the ventro-lateral thalamus with Gustave Roussy; Dejerine-Sottas disease, a progressive hereditary form of hypertrophic neuropathy along with Jules Sottas; Dejerine-Thomas olivopontocerebellar atrophy, a sporadically occurring form of chronic progressive ataxia with André Thomas; and the

Landouzy-Dejerine syndrome, an autosomal dominant hereditary form of muscular dystrophy with Louis Théophile Joseph Landouzy.

STROKE-RELATED CONTRIBUTIONS

In his semiology book Dejerine described the findings in patients with focal brainstem lesions. In a section of the first volume of the *Semiology* entitled *Troubles de la motilité*, Dejerine and Madame Dejerine-Klumpke include 16 figures that depict focal, presumably vascular, lesions in the brainstem. All of these drawings show the lesions within the brainstem in black. The important anatomical structures within that brainstem level are noted. The figures all include the face and upper torso of a man. Regions of sensory and motor loss are indicated on the figures. In some figures, small drawings show the mouth and pharynx to indicate tongue and pharyngeal weakness. Figure 11.2 shows one such example in a patient whose lesion involves a large portion of the right hemimedulla.

It is unclear from the writing whether Dejerine found examples of these syndromes in his pathological material, became aware of many of the syndromes from the writing of others, or simply projected the likely clinical findings based on his knowledge of the anatomy and functions of various brain structures. His text does cite the writings of those who had published the findings accompanying some brainstem lesions. An example is the hemimedullary syndrome illustrated in Figure 11.2. Joseph Babinski and Jean Nageotte are usually given credit for describing the syndrome of infarction involving both the medial and lateral medulla on one side [10]. They reported on three patients, all of whom had prominent features of the lateral medullary syndrome combined with slight contralateral weakness and contralateral pyramidal tract signs. They attributed the condition to syphilis. Only one of their patients had a necropsy that showed the hemimedullary infarct.

An important and lasting anatomico-clinical contribution was the description of a vascular syndrome involving the lateral portion of the thalamus. Dejerine and Roussy described the findings in patients with infarcts in the ventro-postero-lateral portion of the thalamus, which they designated *le syndrome thalamique* [11]. Clinical findings came from two cases reported previously by Dejerine and Egger and from three reported by colleagues. The pathologic findings of three of these cases were reviewed for the first time. All signs were contralateral to the thalamic infarcts and included a rapidly regressing slight hemiparesis; a more prominent and persistent sensory abnormality affecting both "superficial" (touch, pain, and temperature) and "deep" (articular and proprioceptive) sensory modalities affecting the face, limbs, and trunk; contralateral limbs that were hypotonic and uncoordinated, a finding the authors related to the sensory loss; abnormal spontaneous movements

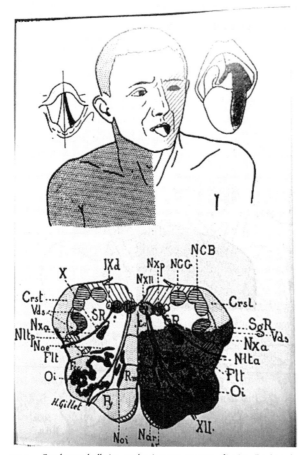

11.2. *Syndrome bulbaire antéro-interne et retro-olivaire*. Lesion involving the left hemimedulla, causing weakness of the left tongue and palate; Horner's syndrome and pain and temperature sensory loss on the left face; and hemisensory loss and hemiplegia involving the right side of the body. From *Sémiologie des affections du système nerveux*, with Augusta Marie Dejerine-Klumpke. Paris: Masson & Co., 1914 (1977 edition, Paris Masson), p. 214, *figure 50, with permission.*

usually small, of the hand and limbs occasionally with an undulating, rhythmic character at times resembling tremor; and pain and dysesthesia that developed later on the hemianesthetic side. Dejerine and Roussy did not comment on the vascular anatomy of the supply to that area of the thalamus or the location and nature of the vascular lesion.

The other major vascular contribution of Dejerine surrounds a single case [12,13]. The history and clinical findings were described and illustrated in detail. This clinico-anatomical study supports the value of thorough, detailed, single case reports ($n = 1$) that yield important general information.

A very intelligent 68-year-old businessman (identified as Courrière in Dejerine's *Anatomy* text) on October 25, 1887, realized that he could not read, even a single word. He consulted a noted Parisian ophthalmologist, Dr. Landolt, who found a right hemiachromatopsia and other abnormalities within the right visual hemifield. He referred the patient to Professor Dejerine. Landolt noted that his visual acuity was 8 out of 10, but he could not read any letters on the Snellen chart. He could outline their form but not name them. He copied them and likened the A to a trestle, the Z to a serpent, and the P to an earring. He copied letters "as if it was a technical drawing examining each stroke to assure the exactitude of the design" (*ecriture servile*). Previously, he had had warning spells of transient right leg and right arm numbness. He then suddenly discovered that he could not read. When Dejerine examined him, he had no limb motor or sensory signs.

He spoke fluently without error and understood spoken speech normally. His memory functions were normal. He named objects normally, even pictures of instruments in a catalogue. He identified his own morning newspaper by its form but could not read its name. He could name no written letters. The only written material he could read was his own name. He could not read isolated letters but could identify them by name by tracing their contours with his finger. When Dejerine moved his hand in a trajectory forming the letters he could name them. Initially, he could read individual numbers but had difficulty calculating. Later he could read numbers and calculate even complex arithmetic tasks.

A trained musician, he could no longer read musical symbols but could write a scale or particular notes to command. He continued to be able to sing and play his instrument well and play new songs that he heard. His writing was preserved, but if interrupted he could not continue his thought and could not read what he had written.

During the next four years Dejerine followed him carefully. Courrière was active and very successful in business, gambled successfully in cards, played new pieces of music, and had no difficulty when going to unaccustomed regions of Paris. Courrière never regained the ability to read. On January 5, 1892, he suddenly developed paraphasic speech and could no longer write. He died 11 days later.

At postmortem examination, Dejerine found an old shrunken infarction in the left occipital lobe, occipital white matter and the splenium of the corpus callosum in the distribution of the left posterior cerebral artery, and a fresh infarction of the left angular gyrus (Figure 11.3). The patient had rheumatic heart disease and had developed sequential embolic brain infarcts in the left cerebral hemisphere.

This single, well-studied case and a previous case led Dejerine to separate and define two clinical syndromes in which reading was defective (*cécité verbal*, or verbal blindness): alexia without agraphia (pure alexia) and alexia with

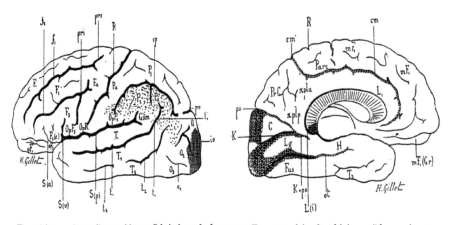

Fɪɢ. 80. — **Cas Courrière.** Cécité verbale pure. Topographie des lésions. Plaque jaune

11.3. Drawing of the brain autopsy findings in the case of Courrière. The left drawing shows the convex surface of the left cerebral hemisphere The right drawing is a sagittal midline section. The old lesion is indicated in black. The recent infarct is shown on the left figure using black dots. From Dejerine J, Dejerine-Klumpke AM. *Anatomie des centres nerveux*, vol. 2. Masson, 1980, p. 110, figure 80.

agraphia. A year earlier Dejerine had published a single case report of a man who suddenly lost the ability to read and write (alexia with agraphia) [13,14]. Examination showed a right hemianopia. At autopsy the only lesion was an old infarct (the patient died eight years after the stroke) involving the inferior three-quarters of the angular gyrus and surrounding white matter. From these two cases, Dejerine proposed that the left angular gyrus contained "a visual memory center for words." Patients with a lesion in this region (the site of the most recent brain infarct in Courrière and also in the prior case) had great difficulty with reading, writing, and spelling, although spoken language was well preserved. The patients behaved as if they were illiterate. In contrast, patients with alexia without agraphia had lesions in the left occipital lobe that affected the representation of their right visual field in the calcarine cortex and adjacent white matter. The older lesion in Courrière also involved fibers entering and within the splenium of the corpus callosum where visual information from the right cerebral hemisphere visual radiation was transferred to the left cerebral hemisphere. Courrière was seeing words using his right brain and his left visual field. He could not transmit this visual information to his visual memory center for words, located in the left angular gyrus region, and so could not read the words. Because, at that time, his angular gyrus was operative, he could speak normally and write. Figure 11.4 shows Dejerine's diagram of the alexia without agraphia syndrome. This abnormality was later dubbed by Norman Geschwind a disconnection syndrome in which lesions of white matter tracts blocked communication from one center to another, creating specific cognitive and behavioral syndromes [14].

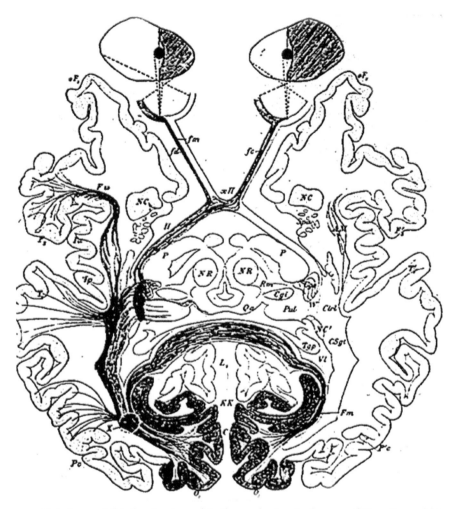

11.4. Dejerine used this drawing to explain the mechanism in the case of Courrière and his inability to read words.

NOTES AND REFERENCES

1. Schurch B, Dollfus P. The "Dejerines": An historical review and homage to two pioneers in the field of neurology and their contribution to the understanding of spinal cord pathology. *Spinal Cord* 1998;36:78–86.
2. Bassetti C, Jagella EC. Joseph Jules Dejerine (1849–1917). *J. Neurol.* 2006;253:823–824.
3. Joseph Jules Dejerine (1849–1917) *JAMA* 1969;207(2):359–360.
4. Gauckler E. *Professeur J. Dejerine 1849–1917* (in French). Paris: Masson & Co., 1922.
5. Zabriskie EG. *Joseph Jules Dejerine (1849–1917)*. Founders of Neurology. Springfield, IL: Charles C. Thomas, 1953, pp. 271–275.
6. Bogousslavsky J, Walusinski O, Moulin T. Alfred Vulpian and Jean-Martin Charcot in each other's shadow? From Castor and Pollux at La Salpêtrière to neurology forever. *Eur. Neurol.* 2011;65:215–222.
7. Dejerine J, with Augusta Marie Dejerine-Klumpke. *Anatomie des centres nerveux*, 2 vols. Paris: Rueff & Co., 1895, 1901.

8. Dejerine J, with Augusta Marie Dejerine-Klumpke. *Sémiologie des affections du système nerveux*. Paris: Masson & Co., 1914.

9. Dejerine J, Thomas A. *Traité des maladies de la moelle épinière*. Paris: JB Baillière, 1902.

10. This paper and other previously reported brainstem syndromes are discussed in Chapter 10. Babinski J, Nageotte J. Hémiasynergie, latéropulsion et myosis bulbaires avec hémianesthesie et hémiplégie croisées. *Rev. Neurol. (Paris)* 1902;10:358–365. Babinski J, Nageotte J. Lésions syphilitiques des centres nerveux. Foyers de ramollissement dans le bulbe. Hémiasynergie, latéropulsion et myosis bulbaires avec hémianesthésie et hémiplégie croisées. *Nouv. Iconogr. Salpêtriere* 1902;15:492–512.

11. Dejerine J, Roussy G. Le syndrome thalamique. *Rev. Neurol.* 1906;12:521–532. Caplan LR, DeWitt LD, Pessin MS, Gorelick PB, Adelman LS. Lateral thalamic infarcts. *Archives of Neurology* 1988;45:959–964.

12. Dejerine JJ. Contribution à l'étude anatomo-pathologique et clinique des différentes variétés de cécité verbale. *Mémoires de la Société de Biologie* 1892;44:61–90.

13. Geschwind N. Disconnexion syndromes in animals and man. *Brain* 1965;88:237–294, 585–644.

14. Dejerine JJ. Sur un cas de cécité verbale avec agraphie, suivi d'autopsie. *CR Société du Biologie* 1891;43:197–201.

CHAPTER TWELVE

ARTERIAL AND VENOUS ANATOMY

Knowledge of the anatomy of the vessels that supply and drain the brain was clearly crucial for advances in diagnosis and treatment. Many anatomical studies were performed by neurologists and neurosurgeons who were also clinicians. Some research focused on single arteries or single brain territories. Highlighted herein are some of the researchers and their contributions.

GENERAL VASCULAR ANATOMY CONTRIBUTIONS DURING THE EARLY TWENTIETH CENTURY

Henri Duret

Henri Duret was born in the township of Condé-sur Noireau in northern Normandy on July 7, 1849. After matriculating at the Marist College, he studied at Caen medical school. At the outbreak of the Franco-Prussian War of 1870–1871 he served as a surgeon-aide and later received the Legion of Honor for his service. After returning to Paris, Duret pursued the competitive academic surgery course in Paris and reached the rank of *chef de clinique* for the professor of surgery [1]. His early training began in the laboratory of Jean-Martin Charcot and Alfred Vulpian at the Salpêtrière Hôpital. Using injections of colored gelatin into vessels at necropsy, Duret was the first to describe the distribution of supply arteries to the human cerebral cortex and brainstem. His descriptions correlated the territories irrigated with infarcted zones and the neurological deficits that resulted [2]. By also studying different mammals, he showed that it was possible to discern in the fetus a common pattern of blood supply to the brain. By exploring the smallest blood vessels he proposed the notion of "nourishing arteries," a type of vessel that had been previously neglected [1]. These tiny vessels emerged from large- or medium-sized arteries and penetrated the brain from the circle of Willis, up to the basal ganglia, and from the basilar artery trunk into the brainstem tracts and nuclei. Duret described a system of anastomoses between the pial arterioles that could partly account for recovery from cortical lesions. He focused his 1878 thesis on experimental studies of brain trauma and localized the origin of disturbances in alertness and function to the brainstem [3]. He linked these disturbances to microhemorrhages affecting the tegmentum of the midbrain and pons that are now known as Duret hemorrhages.

Duret also studied voluntary motor functions in the cerebral cortex in experimental animals. He mastered a technique for producing well-circumscribed cortical lesions. He also used a specially devised curette for creating deep lesions with minimal trauma. Another innovation was to use faradic instead of galvanic currents to stimulate the cerebral cortex. This work supported the concept of an integrated somatosensory cortex and drew attention to the possibility of partial recovery from the effects of cortical lesions, in contrast to deeper lesions that produced permanent impairments.

In 1885 Duret was appointed professor of surgery in the developing Catholic University in Lille, together with the chairmanship of the surgical services of the Hôpital de la Charité. He served there for three terms as dean of the faculty of medicine.

Charles Edward Beevor

Charles Edward Beevor was born in London in 1854, the eldest son of Charles Beevor, a surgeon. He was educated at Blackheath Proprietary School and University College, London, qualifying in medicine in 1878 [4]. After holding house officer appointments at University College Hospital and the National Hospital for the Paralysed and Epileptic at Queens Square, he studied in Vienna, Leipzig, Berlin, and Paris. Beevor returned to London in 1883 to take up the appointment of assistant physician at Queen Square. Two years later he was elected assistant physician to the Great Northern Central Hospital, and both hospitals later promoted him to physician status. Devoting himself to neurology, he worked with Victor Horsley for four years on problems of cerebral localization, the topic of his Croonian Lectures at the Royal College of Physicians in 1907. He published the valuable *Handbook on Diseases of the Nervous System* in 1898 and gave the Lettsomian Lectures before the Medical Society of London in 1907 on the diagnosis and localization of cerebral tumors

[4]. His most important research was his description of the arterial supply to all parts of the brain, which filled a gap in contemporary anatomical knowledge [5].

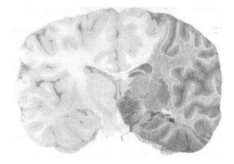

12.1. Coronal sections of the brain made through the tuber cinereum and the genu of the internal capsule. The supply areas of the anterior (dark gray at bottom right of figure adjacent to the midline), middle (very large, triangular-shaped dark gray area, especially outlining the gyri), anterior choroidal (very light gray), and posterior cerebral (very dark gray at bottom right of figure) arteries are shown on the right of the figure. From Compston A. The cerebral arterial supply by Charles E Beevor MD, FRCP. *Brain* 1908;30:403–425. *Brain* 2013;136:362–367, with permission.

Alistaire Compston, the editor of *Brain*, opined that Beevor's depictions of the vascular supply of the cerebral hemispheres were methodologically innovative and the results definitive [6]. Beevor's vascular studies were performed during a seven-year period in which he injected nearly 100 human necropsy specimens. His technique involved preparing colored solutions by dissolving pigments in gelatin and straining the mixture through flannel. Beevor immersed the brains in a water bath kept at 40–50°C and flushed the vessels to remove blood. Each of the five main arteries – the posterior communicating and anterior choroidal branches of the internal carotid artery and the anterior, middle, and posterior cerebral arteries – was injected separately with a different colored solution. He also injected separately the basal and cortical distributions of each main artery. In other observations he injected the five arteries together. The arteries were then ligated and the brain hardened and fixated in formaldehyde, potassic nitrate, potassic acetate, water, and a saturated aqueous solution of alum for one month before sections were cut in the horizontal, sagittal, and coronal planes. Figure 12.1 shows one specimen.

Beevor had a long and fruitful clinical career. He was a man of exceptional modesty and simplicity of character, very self-critical, and gifted musically and artistically. He lectured in the United States in 1908. He is known by most neurologists for calling attention to Beevor's sign, found in patients with selective weakness of the lower abdominal muscles, involving movement of the navel toward the head when the neck is flexed [7].

Charles Foix

Drs. Duret and Beevor made their major contributions to knowledge about arteries supplying the brain during their early careers while devoted to this research. They injected colored substances into arteries and followed their branching and their supply. Their later careers were devoted to clinical work: Duret to neurosurgery and Beevor to clinical neurology. In contrast, Charles Foix performed his studies of the brain-supplying arteries while at the peak of his clinical activities. He was a master clinician who examined patients in detail at the bedside and studied their brains at necropsy. Chapter 24 in this volume is devoted to Foix and his career and his contributions. Foix and his colleagues used the clinical-pathological method of analyzing the brain and vascular findings at autopsy and correlating the findings with the clinical symptoms and signs found when the patients were examined after the stroke had occurred. They did not inject the various arteries but dissected the branches at the necropsy table. Foix and his colleagues published many reports during a whirlwind four-year period between 1923 and 1927 on the blood supply to the cerebral hemispheres – the anterior, middle, anterior choroidal, and posterior cerebral arteries – and to the brainstem regions – the pons, medulla oblongata, and the thalamus [8]. Branches of these arteries with their special zones of supply were well illustrated with comments on the symptoms and signs in patients with restricted infarctions in these territories.

CONTRIBUTIONS THAT CLARIFIED THE VASCULAR ANATOMY OF PORTIONS OF THE ARTERIAL SYSTEMS OR SINGLE ARTERIES

Alexander Kolisko: Anterior Choroidal Artery

Alexander Kolisko was an Austrian pathologist who was born in Vienna in 1857. He earned his medical doctorate at the University of Vienna and then became an assistant at the pathological anatomy institute of the university [9]. In 1898 he was appointed professor of forensic medicine and in 1916 professor of pathologic anatomy at the University of Vienna. His major contribution was focused on the anterior choroidal artery. In 1891, Kolisko reported the results of necropsy studies using injection techniques to determine the territory of the anterior choroidal artery [10]. He showed that the anterior choroidal artery supplied the posterior two thirds of the posterior limb of the internal capsule, the retrolenticular fibers posterior to the internal capsule, the medial aspect of the globus pallidus, the uncus, the posterior portion of the optic tract, the tail of the caudate nucleus, the lateral choroid plexus, and exceptionally superficial areas of the thalamus.

Johann Otto Leonhard Heubner: Recurrent Artery of Heubner

Johann Otto Leonhard Heubner (1843–1926) was a German internist and pediatrician. He studied medicine and spent his early career at the University of Leipzig. He founded a children's hospital and clinic in Leipzig, and in 1891 was appointed to the chair of pediatrics at the university. In 1894 he moved to Berlin where he became director of the children's clinic and polyclinic at the Charité Hospital. Heubner is considered one of the fathers of pediatric medicine [11]. He performed necropsies and investigated the anatomy of the vascular supply of the brain. He published an early description of arteritis related to syphilis. In 1874 he used injections to study the vasculature of the cerebral hemispheres and identified the recurrent artery of Heubner, which typically originates from the junction of the A1 and A2 segments of the anterior cerebral artery [12].

John Sebastian Bach Stopford: Arterial Supply of the Pons and Medulla

John Sebastian Bach Stopford (1888–1961) was a British physician and neurologist. In 1906 he entered the Medical School of Manchester University. He graduated MB, ChB, with honors in 1911, winning the Dumville Surgical Prize and the Bradley Memorial Surgical Scholarship at the Manchester Royal Infirmary [13]. After a resident position at Rochdale Infirmary, he joined the department of anatomy of Manchester University as junior demonstrator in anatomy in 1912. Seven years later he was appointed professor of anatomy. In 1913 he was awarded the Tom Jones Memorial Scholarship in Surgery. In 1915 he was awarded the MD degree, receiving the Gold Medal for his thesis on the arterial supply of the pons and medulla [14]. During the next few years, he published extensively on the arterial supply of the hindbrain and its variability. His first long report reviewed the writings concerning these arteries prior to his own studies. The second report described his own anatomical studies. He used a technique similar to that of Beevor, injecting each artery with a colored gelatin preparation. In the third report, he correlated the vascular anatomy with regions of infarction and the clinical syndrome resulting from the vascular lesions that affecting them [15].

His appointment early in the First World War as neurologist to the Second Western General and the Grangethorpe hospitals stimulated him to pursue clinical work and led to the publication of a series of papers on cutaneous and deep sensibility arising from his observations of peripheral nerve injuries. In 1920 he was awarded an MBE (Member of the Order of the British Empire) in recognition of his work among the wounded of the First World War; he was knighted in 1941. He also held honorary degrees: in science of the universities of Cambridge, Dublin, and Leeds and in Law of the universities of Durham, Liverpool, and Manchester [13].

Albert Wojciech Adamkiewicz: The Great Spinal Artery of Adamkiewicz

Albert Wojciech Adamkiewicz (1850–1921) was a Polish pathologist. Born in Zercow, Poland, Adamkiewicz earned his medical doctorate in 1873 from the University of Breslau [16]. Between 1879 until 1892, he was the chief of general and experimental pathology at the Jagiellonian University in Cracow, Poland. From 1879 to 1892, Adamkiewicz and Henryk Kadyi, an assistant in the anatomy lab and later professor of anatomy, independently and together studied the blood supply of the spinal cord. Between 1881 and 1889 they published the results of their work [17,18]. They used a novel method of injection for which the Cracow laboratory was famous. They injected the vessels with putty-like substances composed of zinc white, linseed oil, ammonia, mercury sulfate, and carmine sediment (as a red, or "arterial" dye), as well as Prussian blue (for vein staining). Other liquid substances used in injecting capillary vessels were enriched with paraffin oil or carbon disulfide. One of the major, largest, and most variable arteries studied was the arteria radicularis anterior magna. Adamkiewicz documented the variable origin, course, and supply of this vessel that has since his studies universally been dubbed the artery of Adamkiewicz. The artery originates from the aorta and enters the spinal canal through an intervertebral foramen. Most often it enters on the left from T9 to L1, but it can enter on either side from T5 to L4. The artery supplies the anterior spinal artery, which courses along the anterior surface of the lower thoracic, lumbar, and sacral spinal cord.

After his anatomical studies, he relocated to Vienna where he practiced medicine at Rothschild Hospital. His later scientific reports focused on neurology, in particular, the vasculature of the nervous system, as well as on histology and the theory of neoplastic tumor development. He wrote most of his reports in German and Polish, but also several articles in French and Latin [15].

Lois Adele Gillilan: Veins and Arteries of the Spinal Cord and Brainstem

Lois Adele Gillilan was an American physician and neuroanatomist. She matriculated at Mt. Holyoke College, obtained a master's degree at Vassar, and an MD degree at the University of Pittsburgh in 1947. She was, by all accounts, a meticulous researcher and a revered teacher and mentor. Her early anatomical research was performed at the University of Pennsylvania. She then moved to the University of Kentucky where she remained for the remainder of her career. She is remembered mostly for her depiction of the veins draining the brainstem, cerebellum, and spinal cord and the arterial supply of these regions [19]. An example of her technique was to inject the veins of the isolated spinal cords of humans and primates with a blue pigment in a vehicle of aqueous gum acacia or aqueous 7 percent gelatin. Her vascular anatomical research incorporated the entire neuraxis, and she strove to correlate the vascular anatomical results with the clinical neurological findings [20].

Gerard Percheron: The Artery of Percheron

Gerard Percheron (1930–2011) was a practicing neurologist and prolific researcher at the Institute Nationale de la Sante et de la Recherche Medicale (INSERM) in France. His interest in the thalamus and its blood supply eventually led him to identify an anatomic variation in its vascular supply [21]. The artery of Percheron describes a rare variation of the paramedian thalamic-mesencephalic arterial supply in which a single blood vessel arises from the posterior cerebral arteries and distributes to both paramedian thalami.

Percheron received a doctoral degree from Rouen Medical School. He then moved to Paris to begin his training as an internist at the Salpêtrière Hospital, where he became highly interested in research dealing with thalamic vascularization. He completed a thesis on this subject in 1966 and thereafter continued to write about thalamic blood supply [22]. His fascination with the thalamic arterial structure and lesions continued, and he found himself inclined more toward research than clinical practice.

Henry M. Duvernoy: Arteries and Veins of the Brainstem

Henry M. Duvernoy was a French physician who was born in 1931. He attended the Besançon medical school and had further training in Strausberg. He then returned to Besançon to join the anatomy department. His father, Maurice Duvernoy, was also an anatomist and was the director of the medical school of Besançon. Henry M. Duvernoy became the head of the anatomy laboratory of the medical school of Besançon and served as chief until 1999 when he retired. He did not see patients but spent full time on anatomical research. His anatomic research focused on brain anatomy, in particular, micro-vascularization. He published several beautifully illustrated atlases, mostly of the major supply arteries and veins of the human brainstem, their small branches, and their zones of supply [23]. Duvernoy also published several editions concerning hippocampal anatomy [24].

Vittorio Luigi Bernasconi and Valentino Cassinari: The Artery of Bernasconi and Cassinari

The mellifluous sound, "the artery of Bernasconi–Cassinari" rolls off the tongue, endearing this vessel to neurologists and neurosurgeons. Vittorio Luigi Bernasconi (1921–2016) was a neuroradiological consultant at the Military Hospital, Padova, Italy, in 1941–1942. Valentino Cassinari (1926–2014) was a neurosurgeon. After working as an assistant at the Maggiore Hospital in Milan, he became the head of the neurosurgery department in Bergamo, Italy, from 1964 to 1993. In 1956 Bernasconi and Cassinari noticed in the carotid angiograms of five out of seven patients with tentorial meningiomas a thin, unusual artery that they judged to be of specific value in the recognition of such lesions. This vessel most often arises from the cavernous segment of the internal carotid artery and may be referred to as the medial or marginal tentorial artery of Bernasconi–Cassinari [25].

MICROSURGICAL NEUROANATOMY OF THE VASCULAR
SUPPLY OF THE BRAIN

With the advent of the dissecting microscope, it became even more essential than in the past to recognize the anatomy of arteries and their branches, especially those that could be damaged during vascular neurosurgery.

Mahmut Gazi Yaşargil

Mahmut Gazi Yaşargil (born in 1925), a Turkish-born medical scientist and neurosurgeon, was a pioneer in the development of microneurosurgery for treatment of cerebrovascular lesions, including aneurysms and arterio-venous malformations (AVMs). After attending Ankara Atatürk Lisesi and Ankara University in Ankara, Turkey, he studied medicine at the Friedrich Schiller University of Jena, Germany. From 1953 until his retirement in 1993 he was first resident, then chief resident (under Professor Hugo Krayenbühl), and then professor and chair of the department of neurosurgery at the University of Zurich and the Zurich University Hospital [26]. After returning from a two-year microsurgery fellowship in Raymond M. P. Donaghy's neurosurgery department in Burlington, Vermont, Yaşargil developed microsurgery with enthusiasm. In 1999 he was honored as "Neurosurgery's Man of the Century 1950–1999" at the annual meeting of the Congress of Neurological Surgeons. He operated on previously inoperable patients using his unique microsurgical techniques.

He performed laboratory research that analyzed the precise anatomy of arteries that branched off the larger intracranial arteries. He illustrated the vascular anatomy in his many tomes of *Microneurosurgery* [27]. He performed 7,500 intracranial operations in Zurich. He used his own microsurgical techniques to avoid injury to branching arteries during aneurysm surgery. In 1994, Yaşargil accepted an appointment as professor of neurosurgery at the College of Medicine, University of Arkansas for Medical Sciences, in Little Rock, Arkansas.

Albert Loren Rhoton Jr.

Albert Loren Rhoton Jr. (1932–2016) was an American neurosurgeon who specialized in microsurgical neuroanatomy. He developed and introduced microsurgical techniques that improved the safety and effectiveness of neurosurgery, including the use of the surgical microscope. He also designed some of the commonly used microneurosurgical instruments. Rhoton grew up in a log cabin without plumbing or electricity in rural eastern Kentucky. His family moved to Akron, Ohio, during World War II where his father was a rubber chemist. He graduated from the Washington University School of Medicine in 1959 and then completed two years of training at Columbia-Presbyterian Medical Center in New York City, one year in general surgery and the other in neurological surgery. He returned to Washington University and completed his neurosurgery residency at Barnes Hospital under Dr. Henry Schwartz in 1964. He remained at Washington University for a one-year NIH research fellowship in neuroanatomy during which time he began to use the surgical microscope in his research work [28]. He recognized its potential to improve surgery and to take brain and vascular anatomy to a greater level of detail. Rhoton began as a staff neurosurgeon at the Mayo Clinic in Rochester, Minnesota, in 1966. He joined the University of Florida in 1972 as professor of surgery and the chairman of the department of neurological surgery.

In 1975, soon after opening his lab, Rhoton established the five-day microvascular and dissection courses to train neurosurgeons primarily in the use of the operative microscope. The courses consisted of three-day rat anastomosis practice and a two-day dissection of the human cadaveric sphenoid and temporal bones,. For more than 10 years, the five-day courses made a crucial contribution to the training of hundreds of neurosurgeons and residents from all over the world. In 2014 Rhoton became the director of the Neuro-Microanatomy Lab at the McKnight Brain Institute. Rhoton and his associates and fellows, at one time or another, used the microscope to study and illustrate all of the major intracranial arteries [29].

NOTES AND REFERENCES

1. Feinsod M, Soustiel JF. Henri Duret (1849–1921). *J. Neurol.* 2011; 258, article number 1732.

2. Duret H. Sur la distribution des artères nourricières du bulbe rachidien. *Arch. Anat. Physiol. Norm. Pathol.* 1873;5:97–114. Duret H. Recherches anatomiques sur la circulation de l'encéphale. *Arch. Anat. Physiol. Norm. Pathol.* 1874;6:60–91. Duret H. Recherches anatomiques sur la circulation de l'encéphale. 3. Artères corticales ou des circonvolutions cérébrales. *Arch. Anat. Physiol. Norm. Pathol.* 1874;6:316–353. Duret H. Recherches anatomiques sur la circulation de l'encéphale. *Archives de physiologie normale et pathologique* 1874;1:664–693, 917–957.

3. Duret H. *Études expérimentales et cliniques sur les traumatismes cérébreaux.* Paris: Delahaye, 1878.

4. Charles Edward Beevor, Royal College of Physicians. Available at https://history .rcplondon.ac.uk/inspiring-physicians/charles-edward-beevor.

5. Beevor CE. The cerebral arterial supply. *Brain* 1907;30:403–425. Beevor CE. On the distribution of the different arteries supplying the human brain. *Philos. Trans. R. Soc. Lond.* [Biol.] 1909;200:1–55.

6. Compston A. From the archives. The cerebral arterial supply. By Charles E Beevor MD, FRCP. Brain 1908;30:403–25. *Brain* 2013;136:362–367.

7. Pearce JM. Beevor's sign. *Eur. Neurol.* 2005;53(4):208–209.

8. Caplan LR. Charles Foix, the first modern stroke neurologist. *Stroke* 1990;21:348–356. Foix C, Hillemand P. Irrigation de la protuberance. *C R Soc. Biol. (Paris)* 1925;92:35–36. Foix C, Hillemand P. Les arteres de l'axe encephalique jusqu'au diencephale inclusivement. *Rev. Neurol. (Paris)* 1925;41:705–739. Foix C, Masson A. Le syndrome de l'artere cerebrale posterieure. *Presse Med.* 1923;31:361–365. Foix C. Hillemand P. Les syndromes de l'artere cerebrale anterieure. *Encephale* 1925;20:209–232. Foix C, Levy M. Les ramollissements sylviens. *Rev. Neurol. (Paris)* 1927;43:1–51.

9. Alexander Kolisko. Wikipedia. Available at https://en.wikipedia.org/wiki/Alexander_Kolisko.

10. Kolisko A. *Ueber die Beziehung der Arteria choroidea anterior zum hinteren Schenkel der inneren Kapsel des Gehirns.* Wien: Alfred Holder, 1891.

11. Pearce JM. Heubner's artery. *Eur. Neurol.* 2005;54(2):112–114. Haroun RI, Rigamonti D, Tamargo RJ. The recurrent artery of Heubner: Otto Heubner's description of the artery and his influence on pediatrics in Germany. *J. Neurosurg.* 2000;93 (6):1084–1088.

12. Heubner O. *Die Leutische Erkrankung der Hinarterien.* Liepzig: Vogel, 1874.

13. Le Gros Clark WE, Mansfield CW. John Sebastian Bach Stopford, Baron Stopford of Fallowfield 1888–1961. *Biogr. Mem. Fellows R. Soc.* 1961;7:271–279.

14. Stopford JSB. The arteries of the pons and medulla. Thesis, Manchester University, 1915.

15. Stopford JSB. The arteries of the pons and medulla oblongata. *J. Anat. Physiol.* 1916;50:131–163. Stopford JSB. The arteries of the pons and medulla oblongata: Part II. *J. Anat. Physiol.* 1916;50:255–280. Stopford JSB. The arteries of the pons and medulla Part III. *J. Anat.* 1917;51(3):250–277.

16. Skalski JH, Zembala M. Albert Wojciech Adamkiewicz: The discoverer of the variable vascularity of the spinal cord. *Ann. Thor. Surg.* 2005;80:1971–1975.

17. Adamkiewicz A. Über die mikroskopischen Gefäße des menschlichen Rückenmarkes. Trans. Int. Med. Contr., 7th Sess., London 1, 155–157 (1881). Adamkiewicz A. Die Blutgefäße des menschlichen Rückenmarks. 1. Die Gefäße der Rückenmark-substanz. Sitz. ber. Akad. Wiss. Wien, Math.-nat. Kl. 84, 469–502 (1881). Adamkiewicz A. Die Blutgefäße des menschlichen Rückenmarks. H. Die Gefäße der Rückenmarks-oberfläche. Sitz. ber. Akad. Wiss. Wien, Math.-nat. Kl. 85, 101–130 (1882).

18. Kadyl H. Über die Blutgefäße des menschlichen Rückenmarks. *Anat. Anz.* 1886;1:304–314. Kadyi H. *Über die Blutgefäße des menschlichen Rückenmarks.* Lemberg: Gubrynowicz u. Schmidt, 1889.

19. Gillilan LA. Angioarchitecture of the human brainstem. *Anat. Rec.* 1955;121:299–312. Gillilan LA. The arterial and venous blood supply of the human spinal cord. *Anat. Rec.* 1957;127:466. Gillilan L. The arterial blood supply of the human spinal cord. *J. Comp. Neurol.* 1958;110:75–103. Gillilan LA. Veins of the spinal cord. Anatomic details; suggested clinical applications. *Neurology* 1970;20:860–868. Gillilan LA. The arterial and venous blood supplies to the cerebellum of primates. *J. Neuropath. Exp. Neurol.* 1969;28(2):295–307. Gillilan LA. The correlation of the blood supply to the human brainstem with clinical brainstem lesions. *J. Neuropath. Exp. Neurol.* 1964;23:78–108.

20. Gillilan LA. Visualization of the principal arteries of the human central nervous system. *Anat. Rec.* 1952;112:477. Gillilan LA. Significant superficial anastomoses in the arterial blood supply to the human brain. *J. Comp. Neurol.* 1959;112:55–74. Gillilan LA.

Potential collateral circulation to the human cerebral cortex. *Neurology* 1974;24:941–948. Gillilan LA. General principals of the arterial blood vessel patterns to the brain. *Transactions ANA* 1957;65–68.

21. Agarwal N, Chaudhari A, Hansberry DR, Prestigiacomo CJ. Redefining thalamic vascularization vicariously through Gerald Percheron: A historical vignette. *World Neurosurg.* 2014;81(1):198–201. Percheron G. The anatomy of the arterial supply of the human thalamus and its use for the interpretation of the thalamic vascular pathology. *Z. Neurol.* 1973;205(1):1–13.

22. Percheron G. Étude anatomique du thalamus de l'homme adulte et de sa vascularisation artérielle (avec un atlas). Thèse médicale. La Salpêtrière, 1966. Percheron G. Arteries of the human thalamus. I. Artery and polar thalamic territory of the posterior communicating artery. *Rev. Neurol.* 1976;132(5):297–307. Percheron G. Arteries of the human thalamus: II. Arteries and paramedian thalamic territory of the communicating basilar artery. *Rev. Neurol.* 1976;132(5):309–324.

23. Duvernoy H. *Human Brainstem Vessels.* Springer, 1978; 2nd ed., 1999. Duvernoy H. *The Superficial Veins of the Human Brain: Veins of the Brain Stem and of the Base of the Brain.* Springer, 1975. Duvernoy H. *Human Brainstem Vessels.* Springer, 1978; 2nd ed., 1999. Duvernoy H. *The Human Brain Stem and Cerebellum: Surface, Structure, Vascularization and Three-Dimensional Sectional Anatomy with MRI.* Springer, 1995. Duvernoy H. *The Human Brain: Surface, Three-Dimensional Sectional Anatomy with MRI, and Blood Supply.* Springer, 1991, 2nd ed. Springer, 1999.

24. Duvernoy H. *The Human Hippocampus: An Atlas of Applied Anatomy.* Springer, 1974.

25. Bernasconi V, Cassinari V. Un segno carotidografico tipico di meningioma del tentorio. *Chirurgia* 1956;11(3):586–588. Bernasconi V, Cassinari V. Angiographical characteristics of meningiomas of tentorium. *Radiol. Med.* 1957;43:1015–1263. Bernasconi V, Cassinari V, Gori G. Diagnostic value of the tentorial arteries of the carotid siphon (angiographic study of a case of falcotentorial angioma). *Neurochirurgia (Stuttgart)* 1965;62:67–72.

26. Gazi Yaşargil. Wikipedia. Available at https://en.wikipedia.org/wiki/Gazi_Yaşargil. Stienen MN, Serra C, Stieglitz LH, Krayenbühl, N, Bozinov O, Regli L. UniversitätsSpital Zürich: 80 years of neurosurgical patient care in Switzerland. *Acta Neurochir. (Wien)* 2018;160(1):3–22. Flamm ES. Professor M. Gazi Yasargil: An appreciation by former apprentice. *Neurosurgery* 1999;45(5):1015–1018.

27. Yasargil, MG. *Microneurosurgery Tomo I: Microsurgical Anatomy of the Basal Cisterns and Vessels of the Brain, Diagnostic Studies, General Operative Techniques and Pathological Considerations of the Intracranial Aneurysms.* Thieme, 1985.

28. Matsushima T, Matsushima K, Kobayashi S, Lister R, Morcos JJ. The microneurosurgical anatomy legacy of Albert L. Rhoton Jr., MD: An analysis of transition and evolution over 50 years. *J. Neurosurg.* 2018;129(5):1331–1341. Fernandez-Miranda JC. Prof. Albert L. Rhoton, Jr.: His life and legacy. *World Neurosurg.* 2016;92:590–596. Matsushima T, Kobayashi S, Inque T, Rhoton AS, Vlasak AL, de Oliveira E. Albert L. Rhoton Jr., MD: His philosophy and education of neurosurgeons. *Neurol. Med. Chir. (Tokyo)* 2018;58(7):279–289.

29. Rhoton AL. *Cranial Anatomy and Surgical Approaches.* Philadelphia: Lippincott Williams & Wilkins, 2003. Perlmutter D, Rhoton AL Jr. Microsurgical anatomy of the anterior cerebral-anterior communicating-recurrent artery complex. *J. Neurosurg.* 1976;45:259–272. Zeal AA, Rhoton AL Jr. Microsurgical anatomy of the posterior cerebral artery. *J. Neurosurg.* 1978;48:534–559. Fine AD, Cardoso A, Rhoton AL Jr.

Microsurgical anatomy of the extracranial-extradural origin of the posterior inferior cerebellar artery. *J. Neurosurg.* 1999;91:645–652. Fujii K, Lenkey C, Rhoton AL Jr. Microsurgical anatomy of the choroidal arteries: Lateral and third ventricles. *J. Neurosurg.* 1980;52:165–188. Gibo H, Carver CC, Rhoton AL Jr, Lenkey C, Mitchell RJ. Microsurgical anatomy of the middle cerebral artery. *J. Neurosurg.* 1981;54:151–169. Hardy DG, Peace DA, Rhoton AL Jr. Microsurgical anatomy of the superior cerebellar artery. *Neurosurgery* 1980;6:10–28.

CHAPTER THIRTEEN

RUDOLF VIRCHOW

Toward the end of the eighteenth century, interest turned to thrombi found within vessels. Morgagni opined that most thrombi found within vessels at necropsy developed after death but that intravascular clotting could occur during life [1,2]. Baillie wrote in 1793 that "it was known to every person acquainted with the animal economy that the blood coagulated in the vessels of the living body" [1,3]. He called attention to clots that formed in vessels after ligatures were placed and within dilated arteries.

John Hunter, a surgeon and one of the most colorful and influential figures of this period, provided his observations and opinion about clot formation. William Hunter is described as an elegant gentlemanly physician, while his younger brother John is characterized as a brush, feisty, rough-hewn firebrand of activity [4]. In the middle of the eighteenth century John arrived in London "as an outspoken, high spirited youth whose good intentions were often frustrated by his insensitivity to the feelings of the ordinary mortals around him" [4]. He chose surgery as his craft. (Even in those days surgeons were thought to have limited communication and interpersonal skills compared to physicians.) John Hunter was also a naturalist who wanted to explore in depth the anatomy and function of animals and humans. He was an experimentalist who believed and taught that surgeons should pursue science as well as a practical craft. One of his best-known experiments was to inoculate himself by dipping a lancet into purulent gonorrheal discharge and injecting it into his own penis. The symptoms of gonorrhea developed followed soon thereafter by manifestations of syphilis [5].

Much of his career was dedicated to understanding inflammation. His treatise on this topic was finished just before his death [6]. He studied various types of tissue injuries and their repair. Hunter used the term "inflammation" to refer to the process by which diseased parts recover. He noted the frequency of inflammation affecting veins after phlebotomy and surgery. Often veins became thrombosed. Hunter opined that venous clots formed as an exudate from the walls of vessels, and, if adhesions did not form, thrombi could be swept into the circulation and carried by the blood stream into distant parts [6,7]. Following the teaching of Hunter, clotting was attributable to inflammation of vessel walls in both the venous and arterial systems [7].

During the first portion of the nineteenth century, Jean Cruveilhier, an influential French anatomist and pathologist, carried Hunter's concepts of blood clotting even further. He maintained that all inflammation was basically a capillary phlebitis: "La phlebite domine toute la pathologie" [8]. He noted that thrombosis developed in veins whose walls appeared normal; coagulation within veins was the earliest sign of phlebitis. Clotting within arteries or heart chambers was the earliest manifestation of arteritis. Thrombi within vessels were formed from an exudate often admixed with the formed cellular elements of the blood.

RUDOLF VIRCHOW AND EXPERIMENTAL PATHOLOGY

The Hunterian concept of the inflammatory cause of blood clot formation held sway until the middle of the nineteenth century and the work of German pathologist Rudolf Ludwig Karl Virchow. Virchow was born on October 13, 1821, in Schievelbein, eastern Pomerania (today Poland) as the only child of a working-class family. His father was a farmer who also was the treasurer of Schievelbein. Virchow studied at the community school and took private lessons. By age 13 he had mastered Latin. He became fluent in German, Dutch, Latin, Greek, Italian, Hebrew, English, Arabic, and French. Virchow initially wanted to pursue theology, but he chose medicine because he considered his voice too weak for preaching [9,10]. In 1839, he received a military scholarship to learn medicine at Friedrich-Wilhelms Institute in Berlin, a unit within the University of Berlin whose main purpose was to train medical officers for the Prussian Army. Virchow studied under Johannes Peter Müller, an eminent neurophysiological researcher. Müller's experiments on nerve conduction proved that the dorsal roots of the spinal cord carried information about sensation and that the anterior roots controlled movement. His studies improved the understanding of sensory mechanisms of vision and hearing. On receiving his degree, Virchow wrote to his parents that he had received it from the "world's most famous physiologist." In fact, Müller's *Handbuch der Physiologie* (Handbook of Physiology) was referred to as the physiologist's bible. Virchow wrote a thesis on corneal manifestations of rheumatic disease under Müller [11].

After receiving his medical degree, Virchow was appointed intern at the Charité Hospital in Berlin in 1843. He enjoyed his work on the wards but was more drawn to the work of the pathologist Robert Froriep, from whom he learned to use a microscope. Virchow acquired the belief that medical progress can be made by making clinical observations, experimenting on animals, and studying pathological anatomy at the microscopic level [11].

Virchow's initial studies were on blood. In 1845, he published his first case report on "leukemia," a term he coined to describe the presence of cancerous white cells in the blood. After refusal of the editors of various journals to publish two of his papers, in 1846 Virchow, along with his colleague Benno Ernst Heinrich Reinhardt, founded a new journal: *Archiv für pathologische Anatomie und Physiologie und für klinische Medizin* (Archives of Pathological Anatomy and Physiology and of Clinical Medicine). The journal published research of the highest quality as manuscripts with outdated, untested, or speculative and dogmatic ideas were rejected. The journal was later renamed to *Virchow's Archiv* and is still published by the European Society of Pathology [11].

In 1848, Virchow was employed to study the typhus epidemic in Upper Silesia. Virchow's recommendations to control the epidemic were not better hygiene or sanitation but political freedom and social and educational reforms for the people. His political ideas infuriated the government and he was forced to move from Berlin to Würzburg, where he spent the next seven years. His exile was productive as he devoted his time to studying cells and contributing to cell theory. He popularized the epigram *Omnis cellula e cellula* (All cells arise from preexisting cells). It was during this period that he studied venous thrombosis. In 1856, Virchow returned to the Charité Hospital in Berlin as the director of the newly built pathological institute [11].

Virchow's work on thrombosis began when he was tasked by his professor Robert Froriep to study the assertion made by Cruveilhier that inflammation caused coagulation. Virchow questioned the evidence supporting this idea. He showed experimentally that the lining of an artery was very resistant to irritants and that the arterial wall never poured an exudate into the lumen. He showed that clotting within an artery required perturbation of the intima of the vessel. His early experimentation concerned mainly the development of pulmonary thrombosis. His postmortem findings led to the conclusion that thrombi he observed had not originated in the pulmonary vasculature but were similar to larger thrombi in other distant vessels such as those of the leg; the concave surface of the pulmonary clot fitted the leg thrombus perfectly, "like a cap."

To prove his hypothesis, Virchow began injecting substances such as cadaveric thrombi, coagulated blood, and berries into the jugular veins of dogs to represent thrombi traveling from the leg. Many of his experimental dogs developed respiratory distress following the procedure, proving that blood could transport foreign substances to the lungs [12].

In a remarkable series of observations and experiments, Virchow analyzed the relationship between thrombi and infarction, locally and at a distance. Among 76 necropsies performed in 1847, Virchow found thrombi in extremity veins in 18 patients and within the pulmonary arteries in 11 [12]. He reasoned that the bloodstream emanating from these veins must have been the conduit for transportation of the thrombi to distant sites such as the arteries of the lung. Virchow then used animal experiments to study the fate of foreign materials placed in veins. He later sought and found obstruction of brain, splenic, renal, and limb arteries at necropsy in patients who had cardiac valve disease and left atrial thrombi. Virchow showed systematically that in situ thrombosis and embolism were the cause of infarction and that the process was unrelated to inflammation, the predominant theory at that time. Virchow called this phenomenon "embolism" and the detached clots "emboli." Inflammation, he believed, was a secondary process due to the chemical changes in the thrombus. Prior to Virchow's work, regions of brain softening (encephalomalacia, ramollissements) were not understood to represent infarction related to death of tissue attributable to insufficient blood supply [11].

Virchow studied blood clotting in vitro. The nature of fibrin clots was not understood at the time. When fresh blood was stirred with a glass rod that was intermittently wiped clean to remove fibrin and the blood was then left to stand, it would not clot. The blood would settle with red cells at the bottom, a white layer above, and serum on top. He concluded that fibrin could not be detected in fresh blood. He proposed that it existed as an inactive precursor for which he introduced the term "fibrinogen." Virchow also observed that clots were formed around an introduced foreign body, which he explained to be the consequence of irritation of the vessel wall, increased tendency of the blood to clot, or obstruction to the flow of blood. These concepts formed the basis of *Virchow's triad* of vascular thrombosis: (1) stasis of blood in a vessel, (2) injury to the wall of the blood vessel especially the endothelium, and (3) an abnormality in the balance between blood procoagulant and anticoagulant factors. Before Virchow's studies and reports, blood factors and thrombosis were given little attention [12].

Virchow also investigated cerebral embolism and considered it to be the most common cause of "ischemic" (his term) apoplexy. Virchow thus reclassified apoplexy as "sanguinea" (i.e., with an intracerebral hemorrhage) and "ischaemica" (due to occlusion as with emboli). The most common sites of cerebral embolism were found to be the middle and anterior cerebral arteries, the carotid arteries, and the vertebral arteries. Virchow described the association of carotid thrombosis with ipsilateral blindness. He found the lumens of the ophthalmic and central retinal arteries to be patent and extrapolated the source of the embolus to be the carotid artery [13].

Virchow revived the term "arteriosclerosis" (first used by Lobstein) and described it as a "simple fat metamorphosis" that led to the development of thrombi in the carotid arteries [13].

In his three-volume treatise on blood vessels, Virchow described different types of intracranial malformations such as telangiectatic venous malformations, arterial malformations, arteriovenous malformations, and cystic angiomas. Vascular malformations could cause spontaneous intracranial hemorrhages [11].

Virchow was not only a brilliant pathologist but also a physician, anthropologist, and politician. He contributed enormously to the understanding of diseases, and some of his other contributions include the description of Virchow's node, Virchow-Robins space, and the phagocytic nature of the neuroglia cells in encephalomalacia. He also described tumors of the spinal cord and discovered the substance "amyloid." Virchow also contributed to parasitology, forensic medicine, and anthropology [11].

Virchow continued to influence medicine internationally until his death. Virchow was so active and fearless that he jumped off a running streetcar at age 81. Unfortunately, he developed a hip fracture that never healed and died of heart failure eight months later [9,14].

NOTES AND REFERENCES

1. Fisher CM. The history of cerebral embolism and hemorrhagic infarction. In Furlan A (ed.), *The Heart and Stroke*. Berlin: Springer-Verlag, 1987, pp. 3–16.

2. Morgagni GB. *The Seats and Causes of Diseases Investigated by Anatomy*. Trans. B. Alexander. London: Miller and Cadell, 1769.

3. Baillie M. Of uncommon appearances of disease in blood-vessels. *Transactions Society for the Improvement of Medical and Chirurgical Knowledge* 1793;1:119–137.

4. Nuland S. Why the leaves changed colors in the autumn: Surgery, science and John Hunter. In *Doctors: The Biography of Medicine*, 2nd ed. New York: Vintage Books, 1995, pp. 171–199.

5. Hunter I. Syphilis in the illness of John Hunter. *J. Hist. Med.* 1953;8:249–262.

6. Hunter J. *A Treatise on the Blood, Inflammation, and Gunshot Wounds*. London: George Nicol, 1794.

7. Fisher CM. The history of cerebral embolism and hemorrhagic infarction. In Furlan A (ed.), *The Heart and Stroke*. Berlin: Springer-Verlag, 1987, pp. 3–16.

8. Cruveilhier J. *Anatomie pathologique du corps humain*. Paris, 1829, vol. 1, chapter 11, p. 7.

9. Walter E, Scott M. The life and work of Rudolf Virchow 1821–1902: "Cell theory, thrombosis and the sausage duel." *J. Intensive Care Soc.* 2017 Aug;18(3):234–235.

10. Nuland S. The fundamental unit of life: Sick cells, microscopes, and Rudolf Virchow. In *Doctors: The Biography of Medicine*, 2nd ed. New York: Alfred A. Knopf, 1995, pp. 304–342.

11. Safavi-Abbasi S, Reis C, Talley MC, Theodore N, Nakaji P, Spetzler RF, et al. Rudolf Ludwig Karl Virchow: Pathologist, physician, anthropologist, and politician. Implications of his work for the understanding of cerebrovascular pathology and stroke. *Neurosurg. Focus* 2006 Jun 15;20(6):E1.

12. Dickson BC. Venous thrombosis: On the history of Virchow's triad. *Univer. Toronto Med. J.* 2004;166–171.

13. Fisher M. The history of stroke and cerebrovascular disease. In *Handbook of Clinical Neurology*, vol. 92 (3rd series). Amsterdam: Elsevier, 2009, pp. 3–23.

14. Ackerknecht EH. *Rudolf Virchow: Doctor, Statesman, Anthropologist.* Madison: University of Wisconsin Press, 1953.

CHAPTER FOURTEEN

EARLY MEDICAL AND NEUROLOGICAL TEXTBOOKS

During the first half of the twentieth century, most physicians obtained information about medical conditions and their diagnosis and management from textbooks. The great majority of stroke patients were cared for by primary care physicians and internists. No physicians specialized in stroke. Few neurologists were consulted. A review of some major popular internal medical and neurological textbooks yields a glimpse into knowledge about stroke and its cause at that time.

INTERNAL MEDICAL TEXTS

Osler's Textbook of Medicine

William Osler was by far the most well-known and respected physician and internal medicine specialist in the world in the years before and after the turn of the twentieth century. His textbook, revised and republished often, was likely on the bookshelf of most practitioners. Osler was especially interested in nervous system disease. In his 1903 *Textbook of Medicine*, 249 of the 1,150 pages (22%) were devoted to the nervous system but only 26 were devoted to affections of the blood vessels and three to spinal cord vascular disease [1].

There was very little discussion about conditions such as hypertension, diabetes, high cholesterol, and atherosclerosis, which later became well recognized forerunners and causes of stroke and cerebrovascular disease.

Hypertension was not listed in the index. No section was solely devoted to hypertension, although it is clear that Osler was well aware of the condition. In a few sentences that comment on causes of left ventricular cardiac hypertrophy, valve lesions are emphasized, but he notes hypertension as a cause "all states of increased arterial tension induced by the contraction of the smaller arteries under the influence of certain toxic substances which as Bright suggested by affecting the minute capillary circulation render greater action necessary to send the blood through the distant subdivisions of the vascular system" [1]. At that time there was no direct way to measure blood pressure clinically. The sphygmomanometer was invented by Samuel von Basch in 1881 [2]. Scipione Riva-Rocci introduced a more user-friendly version in 1896. Harvey Cushing in 1901 brought an example of the Riva-Rocci's device to the United States, modernized it, and popularized it within the medical community. In 1905, Nikolai Korotkov, a Russian physician, included diastolic blood pressure measurements [2].

The section on diabetes mellitus was very short. Criteria for diagnosis were that "the form of sugar eliminated in the urine be grape sugar, that it must be eliminated for weeks, months, or years and that the excretion of sugar must take place after the ingestion of moderate amounts of carbohydrate" [1]. Treatment was dietary only. Insulin had not yet been discovered.

Regarding arteriosclerosis: "A condition of thickening, diffuse or circumscribed, beginning in the intima ... the process leads in the larger arteries to atheroma and to endarteritis deformans and seriously interferes with the normal functions of various organs.... As an involution process arteriosclerosis is an accompaniment of old age and is the expression of the natural wear and tear to which the tubes are subjected" [1].

In the portion of the nervous system chapter devoted to affections of the blood vessels, there were brief discussions of subarachnoid hemorrhage and intracerebral hemorrhage. More attention was given to embolism and thrombosis as causes of brain softening. The term "infarction" was not used. Embolism was attributed to valve disease, mostly mitral stenosis, which was more common in women than men, and infectious endocarditis. Concerning thrombosis, Osler comments that clotting of blood in the cerebral vessels "occurs: 1) about an embolus 2) as a result of a lesion of the arterial wall (either endarteritis with or without atheroma or, particularly the syphilitic arteritis, 3) in aneurysms both course and military, and 4) very rarely as a direct result of abnormal conditions of the blood" [1]. Osler mentions warnings before a stroke but does not elaborate on nature and timing.

In a section entitled treatment of cerebral hemorrhage and softening, Osler suggests:

> The patient should be placed on his back ... kept absolutely quiet, and
> measures immediately taken to reduce the arterial pressure. Of these the

most rapid and satisfactory is venesection. With a small pulse of low tension and signs of cardiac weakness it is contraindicated. The chief difficulty is determining whether the apoplexy is really due to hemorrhage or to thrombosis or embolism since in the latter ... bleeding probably does harm. [1]

Osler includes a few pages devoted to thrombosis of cerebral sinuses and veins and to hemiplegia in young children.

NELSON'S LOOSE-LEAF MEDICAL TEXT

Texts that could be kept in a notebook and updated regularly became popular. Nelson's version was among the most purchased and used. There were eight separate volumes, each multiauthored and regularly updated. Volume 6 was devoted to the nervous system. Among the 728 pages of text, in that volume, 14 were devoted to meningovascular syphilis and 8 to a chapter on cerebral softening, written by Dr. Charles Foix and translated by Walter Kraus. The chapter began with brief comments on causes. Embolism was a recognized mechanism in patients with mitral stenotic valve lesions. Thrombosis was attributed to syphilis in the young and atherosclerosis in older individuals. Softenings were also found in patients with serious infections and cachexia. "It has been claimed that increase in the amount of fibrin and a slowing of the circulation bring about the condition [thrombosis]. These theories are far from being proved." Foix discussed the gross and microscopic pathology and the usual locations and concludes, "The prognosis of softening is relatively favorable as to life but relatively grave as to function" [3].

There are no chapters or discussion of hypertension or brain hemorrhage. There is a discussion on management in patients with hemiplegia.

HARRISON'S *PRINCIPLES OF INTERNAL MEDICINE*

The first edition of what would become the veritable "bible" of internal medicine was first published in 1950 [4]. The first edition of 1554 pages did not have a section on disorders of nervous function. It contained 48 pages that briefly described various neurological conditions, among which 10 pages were devoted to diseases of the blood vessels of the brain and spinal cord.

NEUROLOGY TEXTS

British Texts

The most popular neurological texts used in the United States were written by British neurologists. Those written by Sir William Gowers [5], S. A. Kinnier

Wilson (and edited by Alexander Ninian Bruce after Wilson's death) [6], and Lord Russel Brain [7] were the most popular. A relatively small amount of space was devoted to cerebral vascular disease: 4.5 percent in Brain's text, 6 percent in Gowers text, and 8.2 percent in Wilson and Bruce's. All emphasized localization within the brain and clinical symptoms and signs.

Gower's textbook was first published before the turn of the century [5]. Fourteen pages were devoted to anemia and hyperemia (pallor and congestion in the brain at necropsy), probably referring to the opinion of Burrows [8] (discussed in Chapter 8) that too much blood or too little were major causes of apoplexy. Softenings were attributed to syphilis, atheroma, and blood disorders and to embolism from mitral stenosis and infective endocarditis. Hypertension was not mentioned as a cause of brain hemorrhage except when blood pressure rose abruptly during muscular effort. Rest was the major treatment. In patients with hemorrhage, purgatives and venesection were used, but Gowers cautioned against indiscriminate use of bloodletting [5].

Brain's neurology text emphasizes localization and clinical signs [7]. This text was published long after sphygmomanometers were in general use. Malignant hypertension is noted in the index, and there were three pages of discussion of hypertensive encephalopathy. Brain notes, "The commonest cause of intracerebral arterial haemorrhage is rupture of an atheromatous artery in an individual suffering from high blood pressure. The rise in blood pressure is usually due to primary hyperpiesia" [7]. "Primary hyperpiesia" referred to chronically elevated blood pressure without a defined cause. Brain added: "Haemorrhage does not necessarily occur even when the blood pressure is very high unless vascular hypertrophy has given place to degeneration" [7]. Brain attributed bleeding to chronic vascular injury, while later research and experience showed that the opposite was true – that a sudden rise in blood pressure was a more common cause than chronic hypertension [9]. The treatment of patients with hemorrhage should include rest, an icebag on the head, purgatives, and venesection. Surgical drainage could be considered in some cases.

Wilson and Bruce also include sections on cerebral anemia and hyperemia. Brain hemorrhage is attributed mostly to vascular degeneration; atheroma, occluded vessels, embolism, syphilis, and blood disorders are the most important etiologies. "Essential hyperpiesis should not be omitted – that state of heightened blood pressure without evidence of cardiac, renal or arterial disease at times familial and possibly due to adreno-thyroidal disturbance" [6]. Wilson did not favor venesection but used it in some cases. He espoused mostly lifestyle modification: "When signs of increasing strain on a diseased cerebral vascular system are manifest, risk of apoplexy may be reduced by diet, regime, suitable drugs, by disallowance of alcohol and heavy smoking. Mental excitement and physical stress, sudden or prolonged are alike forbidden; the 'simple life' is advocated" [6]. Wilson discussed arteriospasm: "however seductive the angiospastic theory, it is not the only one capable of throwing light on sudden interference with cellular nutrition. Yet it would apply more easily than others to the occurrence of transient cerebral symptoms in those whose vascular system is not diseased or undergoing involution" [6].

American Texts

The four most read American neurology texts were written by William A Hammond (six editions, 1872–1876 [10]), Charles A. Mills (1898 [11]), Charles Loomis Dana (10 editions, 1892–1925 [12]), and Israel S. Wechsler (eight editions, 1927–1958 [13]). All had brief sections devoted to vascular disease that emphasized clinical localization and symptoms and signs. Diagnosis and treatment did not importantly differ from Osler's text.

Other European Texts

Herman Oppenheim began his career at the Charité Hospital in Berlin. In 1891 he opened a successful private hospital in Berlin and, in 1894, authored a textbook on nervous system disease [14] that soon became standard in Germany and was published in several editions and languages. The 2,267-page textbook published in 1923 contained 80 pages on circulatory conditions, but more space was devoted to neuroses. There were two other large, multi-authored German neurology textbooks, edited by Lewandowsky [15] and Bumke and Foerster [16]. Early editions had little coverage of cerebrovascular disease. By 1936, volume 11 in the Bumke-Foerster edited book contained a 280-page chapter on cerebrovascular disease written by Munich neurologist Friedrich Hiller and colleagues [16,17].

The most read French neurology text was edited by followers of Jean Martin Charcot [18]. The material consisted of lectures delivered by Charcot in reference to cases presented. None in the 1877 edition involved cerebrovascular disease.

NOTES AND REFERENCES

1. Osler W. *The Principles and Practice of Medicine*. New York: D. Appleton and Company, 1903.
2. Sphygmomanometer. Wikipedia. Available at https://en.wikipedia.org/wiki/Sphygmomanometer.
3. *Nelson Loose-Leaf Living Medicine, vol. 6: Diseases of the Nervous System*. New York: Thomas Nelson & Sons, 1928, pp. 511–518.
4. Harrison TR, Beeson PB, Resnik WH, Thorn GW, Wintrobe MM, eds. *Principles of Internal Medicine*. Philadelphia: Blakiston, 1950.

5. Gowers WR. *Manual of Diseases of the Nervous System (American Edition).* Philadelphia: P. Blakiston, Son & Co., 1888. Reprinted in The Classics of Neurology & Neurosurgery Library, Division of Gryphon Editions, Birmingham, AL, 1989.

6. Wilson SAK, Bruce AN. *Neurology.* London: Edward Arnold, 1940. Reprinted in The Classics of Neurology & Neurosurgery Library, Division of Gryphon Editions, Birmingham, AL, 1989.

7. Brain WR. *Diseases of the Nervous System.* London: Oxford University Press, 1940.

8. Burrows G. *On Disorders of the Cerebral Circulation and on the Connection between Affections of the Brain and Diseases of the Heart.* London: Longman, Brown, Green, and Longmans, 1846. Reprinted as part of the Classics of Neurology and Neurosurgery Library, New York: Gryphon Editions, 1994.

9. Caplan LR, Kase C. Intracerebral hemorrhage. In Caplan L (ed.), *Stroke: A Clinical Approach.* Boston: Butterworth-Heinemann, 1994.

10. Hammond WA. *A Treatise on Diseases of the Nervous System,* 6th ed. New York: D. Appleton, 1876.

11. Mills CK. *The Nervous System and Its Diseases: A Practical Treatise on Neurology for the Use of Physicians and Students.* Philadelphia: JB Lippincott, 1898.

12. Dana CL. *Text-book of Nervous Diseases for the Use of Students and Practitioners of Medicine,* 8th ed. New York: William Wood & Company, 1915.

13. Wechsler IS. *A Textbook of Clinical Neurology,* 7th ed. Philadelphia: WB Saunders, 1952.

14. Oppenheim H. *Lehrbuch der Nervenkrankheiten.* Berlin: Verlag von S Karger, 1923.

15. Lewandowsky M. *Handbuch der Neurologie,* vol. 5. Berlin: Springer, 1910–1914.

16. Bumke O, Foerster O, eds. *Handbuch der Neurologie, vol. 11: Speziekke Neurologie III. Erkrankungen des Rückenmarks uund Gehirns I Traumatische präsenile und senile erkrankungen zirkulationsstörungen.* Berlin: Verlag von Julius Springer, 1936.

17. Koehler PJ, Stahnisch FW. Three twentieth-century multiauthored neurological handbooks – A historical analysis and bibliometric comparison. *J. History Neurosci.* 2014;23(1):1–30.

18. Charcot JM. *Lectures on the Diseases of the Nervous System.* Trans. George Sigerson. London: Sydenham Society, 1877.

PART III

MODERN ERA, MID-TWENTIETH CENTURY
TO THE PRESENT

TYPES OF STROKE

CHAPTER FIFTEEN

CAROTID ARTERY DISEASE

Carotid artery occlusion and the occurrence of ocular and hemispheric signs became recognized during the latter years of the nineteenth century. Surgical ligations of the carotid artery were attempted during the twentieth century. A prevalent notion at the time was that intracranial vasospasm of small vessels precipitated by extracranial carotid disease caused the symptoms. For this reason, the most popular treatment for carotid disease was sympathectomy. C. M. Fisher first suggested that "bypassing" the occluded carotid artery segment could preclude clinical manifestations. His contributions were a quantum leap in understanding the mechanisms of carotid stroke. More than half a century after his landmark publication, treatment of carotid artery stenosis is still debated.

CAROTID ARTERY DISEASE: 1600–1900

During the seventeenth century, Francois Bayle was probably the first to report a correlation between the presence of plaques in the cerebral arteries and the occurrence of "apoplexy." Kussmaul in 1872 correlated occlusion of the extracranial carotid and ipsilateral monocular visual alterations [1]. Gowers in 1875 reported a 30-year-old man with rheumatic mitral valve disease who had simultaneous emboli found in the central retinal and the middle cerebral arteries [2]. The contributions during this period reflected astute observations.

CAROTID ARTERY DISEASE: 1900–1950

Hans Chiari in Prague in 1905 noted the presence of different degrees of occlusion at the carotid bifurcation that led him to propose that "thrombus in the area of the carotid bifurcation may embolize to the cerebral arteries explaining neurological symptoms" [3]. Hans Chiari was born in 1851 in Vienna, Austria. His father and brother were physicians [4]. Chiari studied medicine in Vienna, where he was an assistant to Carl von Rokitansky. In 1878 he received his habilitation in pathological anatomy, and, within a few years, he became an associate professor at the University of Prague. He later relocated to the University of Strasbourg. His medical contributions related to findings at autopsy. In addition to carotid artery disease he became well known for his recognition of abnormalities at the cranio-spinal junction (Chiari malformations) and for liver abnormalities (Budd-Chiari syndrome).

His interest in vascular disease was triggered by one patient in whom an embolic source was not found in the heart; but upon opening the carotid artery he found a thrombus attached to an ulcer in the carotid wall. He found the missing fragment occluding an intracranial vessel. This was the first account of artery to artery embolism as a mechanism of stroke. Chiari emphasized the importance of evaluating the carotid arteries in the neck in patients with stroke and personally studied 400 cases, finding occlusion of the carotid bifurcation in seven [3].

In 1906, Sir William Gowers recognized that "softening of the brain" resulted from arterial occlusion, that clinical manifestations for the same artery were variable, and that hemiplegia commonly preceded coma [5]. Ramsay Hunt in 1914 correlated the presence of an occluded carotid artery with ipsilateral blindness, optic disease pallor, and contralateral hemiparesis [6]. James Ramsay Hunt was a very prominent American physician and neurologist [7]. He was born in Philadelphia and received his MD degree from the University of Pennsylvania School of Medicine in 1893. He went abroad and studied in Paris, Vienna, and Berlin and returned to the United States to practice neurology in New York City, first at Cornell and later at Columbia Medical Schools. During World War I, he became a lieutenant colonel in the Army Medical Corps and served in France as the director of neuropsychiatry. He was consulting physician at several New York hospitals, and was appointed professor of neurology at Columbia in 1924. He served as president of the American Neurologic Association in 1920. Hunt coined the term "intermittent cerebral claudication" in patients with different degrees of arterial stenosis or occlusion and the status of collateral circulation. He suggested palpating the carotid artery pulse in the neck of patients with "softening of the brain."

The Portuguese neurologist Egas Moniz (Nobel laureate, 1949) performed the first successful cerebral angiography in a 20-year-old man with a pituitary tumor [8]. Moniz injected 30 percent sodium iodide directly into the carotid. X-rays were taken simultaneously with the injections and opacification of the vessels was seen. He performed almost 200 angiograms and decided to change contrast to Thorotrast because iodine caused convulsions in many patients. Unfortunately, Thorotrast was associated with thrombosis of the artery. Moniz had previously practiced extensively in cadavers and without success in a few patients with brain tumors.

In 1936, Sjoqvist reported the first case diagnosed with angiography of an occluded carotid artery [9]. In 1937, Moniz reported four patients with carotid artery occlusion in the neck. His aim was to study tumors by assessing vessel displacement. He had little interest in vascular disease. Angiography remained unpopular until the 1950s because of the high rate of complications associated with the contrast agents used – strontium and thorium dioxide (Thorotrast) – and the need for surgical cutdown. In 1942 Hultquist reported a 3 percent incidence of thrombosis in a pathological study after examining the entire carotid circulation among 1,400 autopsies [10]. Despite having ample data, he did not correlate pathological and clinical findings.

In 1944, Krayenbuhl and Weber reported 16 patients with carotid artery thrombosis with total occlusion in 11 [11]. The patients were studied with angiography and then at autopsy. The authors erroneously thought that the cause was Buerger's disease. C. M. Fisher thought this was one of the most relevant studies performed until that time and was sorry that limited communications precluded collaboration among different researchers. Fisher had dinner with Weber on many occasions, although he never mentioned the work with Krayenbuhl on carotid artery disease.

From Chiari to Hultquist there was an important advance in knowledge of carotid artery stroke mechanisms. Progress was limited because angiographic evaluation and confirmation of carotid disease was either not available or considered dangerous. Recognition at necropsy of carotid artery disease was delayed for decades in the United States because these vessels were preserved by undertakers for embalming bodies before burial.

CAROTID ARTERY DISEASE: 1950–1970

In 1951, H. C. Johnson and A. E. Walker found six carotid artery occlusions among 500 patients studied angiographically [12]. They suggested that carotid occlusion was more common than reported. They contributed to the notion that carotid thrombosis caused a reflex spasm in intracranial vessels, explaining the transient nature of some clinical phenomena. Until Miller Fisher proposed bypassing the occluded arterial segment in the neck in the early 1950s, treatment of carotid disease was excision or ligation of the artery to prevent dislodgement of thrombotic fragments as emboli to the brain.

Fisher had a clear idea that both embolic and hemodynamic mechanisms, depending on the different degrees of carotid artery disease and associated collateral circulation, operated as the basis for transient ischemic attack (TIA) and stroke [13]. He could not foresee that the surgical treatment he had proposed would remain essentially unchanged for the next 60 years. Fisher was convinced that the extracranial carotid should be the culprit of many strokes since he frequently found thrombosis of the carotid artery in the neck but could not find a case of in situ middle cerebral artery occlusion. He puzzled about strokes in patients who did not have the usual aortic or cardiac sources of embolism. He recognized that most pathologists did not study the carotid artery in the neck.

Fisher reported eight patients with occlusion of the internal carotid artery. Brain infarctions were preceded by transient symptoms in seven. One of the patients told Dr. Fisher that "something was wrong" since "the weakness involves the left arm but it was my right eye that went blind" [13]. The patient died during a weekend, and when Fisher found about this after returning from a weekend away, he went to the funeral parlor, asked the family for permission, and extracted the carotid artery for pathological analysis. He was also a neuropathologist. This was the first patient in whom Dr. Fisher confirmed occlusion of the carotid artery in the neck. He clearly established that transient monocular blindness – using the term he coined to differentiate this phenomenon from hemianopsia – and the hemispheric symptoms hemiplegia and aphasia were typical clinical manifestations of carotid artery disease.

In 1961, Robert Hollenhorst described bright plaques occluding the retinal arterioles [14]. Among 235 patients with occlusive carotid disease, 27 had orange and yellow plaques observed with ophthalmoscopy at the bifurcation of retinal arterioles. In some patients these particles moved to distal bifurcations or fragmented and disappeared. In a few patients undergoing endarterectomy, the plaques appeared during surgery. They did not occlude retinal vessels and were believed to be cholesterol crystals dislodged from the aorta or innominate or carotid arteries.

Fisher, who had recently moved from Canada, was surprised to find that there was a law for embalming bodies through the carotid arteries in the United States, making difficult to study these vessels postmortem. An embolic source in the neck could explain strokes in patients who did not have a cardiac, aortic, or intracranial thrombotic source. He wrote: "Unexplained cerebral embolism may arise from thrombotic material lying in the carotid sinus," clearly alluding to an artery-to-artery embolic mechanism [13].

In his further experience with carotid artery occlusion, Fisher reported that among more than 400 autopsies, he found a 9.5 percent incidence of severe carotid artery disease in one or both arteries [15]. He proposed that stenosis could cause similar symptoms to occlusions, that some patients had no symptoms despite severe disease. He confirmed the presence of distal occlusions, establishing the concept of artery-to-artery embolism [13,15]. He posited that "long infarctions" running from the frontal to the occipital lobes in the distal middle cerebral artery (MCA) and anterior cerebral artery (ACA) branches could occur ipsilaterally to severely stenotic arteries accurately describing border-zone ischemia. In 1969, J. P. Mohr (one of Fisher's stroke fellows) reported "distal field infarctions" referring to border-zone or watershed ischemia attributable to severe hypotension [16]. The same mechanism could operate in severe carotid stenosis and occlusion, frequently causing brachial paresis dubbed "man-in-the-barrel syndrome" – since the person is unable to move both arms but could move the legs as if trapped in a barrel – when the ischemia was bilateral.

Fisher understood that atherosclerosis was the pathological process of carotid disease and called attention to frequently associated coronary heart disease, claudication, and absent leg pulses. Studying the cerebral vessels was facilitated when Sven-Ivar Seldinger in Stockholm introduced a catheter method to avoid surgical exposure of the artery.

HEMODYNAMIC VERSUS EMBOLIC MECHANISMS OF CAROTID ARTERY STROKE: 1970 TO THE PRESENT

The 1976 Stroke Princeton conference on cerebrovascular disease was the setting of a discussion that shed light on understanding carotid stroke mechanisms [17]. During one of the sessions, Peritz Scheinberg, chairman of the conference, asked Dr. Fisher: "Dr. Fisher, could I presume upon you to give us perhaps five reasons why TIAs are not embolic?" Fisher answered: "I have for some time kept track of observations that are difficult to reconcile with fibrin-platelet emboli as the mechanism and have assembled 30-odd items, and here I am referring predominantly to recurrent TIAs lasting 10 minutes or less." He then enumerated all these reasons, among which some are mentioned here. Dr. Fisher argued that it is highly unlikely that same-size platelet-fibrin emboli would form, enter arteries with turbulent flow, and end up recurrently in the same vascular territory. He argued that even with laminar flow emboli will unlikely follow the same course. Ulcerations of carotid plaques did not cause stereotyped or even different recurrent TIAs. Patients who had fundoscopic examinations while having transient monocular blindness did not have plaques in the retinal arterioles. Conventional embolism caused TIAs that last longer than the 0.5–2 minutes observed in some patients. Occasionally, transient monocular blindness (TMB) can occur simultaneously with contralateral hemiparesis, something unlikely for a TIA. In personally observed cases, the marching numbness in fingers and hand cleared and reappeared in a way atypical for embolism. On exercising, a patient with bilateral carotid artery occlusion had symptoms. Another patient had multiple TIAs with medication-induced postural hypotension. A string sign in a dissection is often associated with TIAs even when a thrombus is not seen. Dr. Fisher concluded that his arguments did not mean that multiple TIAs could not be embolic. Strokes in the territory of the middle and anterior cerebral arteries could be caused by thrombi dislodged from an extracranial lesion in the internal carotid artery, the so-called artery-to-artery embolism. The alternative was that severely decreased blood flow perfusion caused by a stenotic or occluded extracranial carotid artery resulted in a so-called hemodynamic mechanism.

MECHANISMS OF ACUTE CAROTID STROKE

Michael Pessin et al. in 1977 studied 95 patients who had only transient carotid territory symptoms and underwent angiography [18]. After a neurology residency in Colorado, Pessin was a stroke fellow of J. P. Mohr at Massachusetts General Hospital and then a stroke neurologist at the New England Medical Center in Boston. He died suddenly and prematurely at age 55. In 52 patients Pessin and colleagues found only hemispheric symptoms; 33 had isolated monocular blindness; and 10 had both clinical manifestations. A severe extracranial stenosis was found in 50 percent of patients and intracranial occlusions in 14 percent. Patients with hemispheric TIAs lasting an hour or longer had no associated severe carotid stenosis, but those patients who had both hemispheric and retinal episodes had severe carotid stenosis. They concluded that "there were several distinct groups of patients with carotid transient ischemic attacks" [18]. Pessin and Mohr et al. advanced their observations by correlating the angiographic and clinical findings in 64 patients with stroke in the carotid territory and extracranial carotid artery disease [19]. They identified two different groups: in one, angiography revealed evidence of embolic occlusion of intracranial vessels in the territory of a stenosed or occluded extracranial artery. Most of these patients had moderate to large strokes that were not preceded by TIAs. This group represented an artery-to-artery embolism mechanism. The second group of patients showed delayed cerebral perfusion, had no evidence of intracranial embolism, and strokes – which were mostly moderate – were heralded by multiple TIAs. The latter represented a hemodynamic mechanism.

Embolic mechanism did not provide warning of stroke occurrence and so prevention was difficult. Embolic strokes were larger than those caused by a hemodynamic mechanism. Pessin et al. also recognized the importance of collateral flow in the pathogenesis of stroke, although they could not assess this variable. They mentioned that asymptomatic occlusion of the carotid artery was not uncommon. Importantly, the study also recognized that when angiography was delayed, the intracranial occlusion would not be detected because the body's fibrinolytic system dissolved the embolus.

Pessin concluded that waiting for the occurrence of TIAs was not acceptable since poor outcome occurred in up to 50 percent of patients, and so "the evaluation and treatment of asymptomatic extracranial carotid artery occlusive disease may be critical in reducing stroke" [19]. These among other observations prompted the organization of the future carotid surgery trials in asymptomatic patients. It would take a few decades to show that medical treatment of asymptomatic carotid disease was at least as good as surgery – or stenting – to prevent TIAs and stroke.

Later, Louis Caplan and Michael Hennerici provided evidence that the two mechanisms, hemodynamic hypoperfusion and embolism, often coexisted and were complementary. Hypoperfusion facilitated thrombus formation. Particles of thrombi broke often and flowed distally. Diminished flow reduced washout of these emboli [20].

CAROTID ARTERY PULSE PALPATION AND AUSCULTATION

Prior to modern ultrasound and carotid artery imaging, the eyes, ears, and fingers were used to detect and quantify carotid disease. Auscultation of a bruit in the neck was identified as a reliable indicator of stenosis when the residual lumen of the carotid artery was less than 3 millimeters. In those patients and in patients with carotid artery occlusion it was also possible to auscultate an ipsilateral or contralateral ocular bruit. In patients with an occluded carotid artery, a bruit was sometimes present over the contralateral artery in the neck.

Fisher recognized that an absent pulse upon palpation of the carotid in the neck was suggestive of occlusion [21]. An absent temporal artery pulse suggested common carotid artery occlusion. A rough estimate of decreased retinal artery perfusion pressure could be obtained by gently pressing the side of the ocular globe with a finger or dynamometer until the disappearance of blood flow in the retina. Palpation of facial arteries (angular, brow, cheek [ABC]) was useful in patients with carotid occlusion when collateral circulation in dilated branches of the external carotid artery carried flow to the orbit and internal carotid circulation. Caplan proposed the "frontal artery sign" as an indicator of ophthalmic artery flow reversal suggestive of stenotic disease in the proximal internal carotid artery [22]. The medial forehead is irrigated by the frontal and supraorbital arteries, which are branches of the ophthalmic artery. Careful, alternate occlusion of these arteries shows reversal in the flow of the frontal artery, revealing a more proximal vascular deficit in the carotid territory.

CAROTID PLAQUES AND STENOSING AND NONSTENOSING LESIONS

The characteristics of carotid artery plaques were explored first pathologically and later by ultrasound and advanced computed tomography (CT) and magnetic resonance imaging (MRI). Anthony M. Imparato et al. in 1979 studied endarterectomy specimens and found that most had intraplaque hemorrhages, atheromatous debris, and thrombi with or without ulceration [23]. Plaques started as fibrointimal thickening that progressed to different pathological states, among which hemorrhage was the most frequent. Other authors confirmed these findings and correlated the onset of symptoms with the occurrence of plaque hemorrhage.

MRI, CT, and pathological plaque studies have assessed plaque characteristics that increase vulnerability and stroke risk. Alterations in the fibrous cap, neo-vascularization, release of pro-inflammatory and pro-coagulant factors, calcification, plaque load, degree of stenosis, echolucency, plaque irregularity, intraplaque hemorrhage, and plaque embolism documented with transcranial doppler became recognized.

Fisher and Ojemann performed a valuable clinic-pathological correlation study of carotid plaques removed at surgery [24]. Patients included 34 with multiple TIAs, 23 with transient monocular blindness, 33 asymptomatic, and 51 with persisting neurological symptoms. Their endarterectomy specimens provided 1,000–3,000 eight-micron slices, and intraplaque hemorrhage, ulceration, and thrombus were evaluated. TIAs and transient monocular visual loss were correlated with very tight carotid stenosis (less than 1 millimeter lumen) but not with mural thrombus, ulceration, or plaque hemorrhage. Asymptomatic patients did not have severe stenosis and patients with stroke often had occlusions. Large rounded cavities in plaques sometimes had a smooth lining of normal epithelium and did not meet criteria for eroded ulcers. This is an important contribution showing that ulcer is a microscopic diagnosis when there is lack or disruption of a normal endothelium.

In 2010 J. David Spence and Daniel Hackam proposed treating arteries instead of risk factors [25]. They implemented a method of measuring carotid artery plaque load (measured with surface area or volume) and reported that this value was a strong predictor of stroke, myocardial infarction, and death. After adjusting for different variables, patients that were in the highest quartile of plaque load had a three to four times greater risk for all vascular events compared to those in the lowest quartile. In 2015, the Bioimage study led by Valentin Fuster confirmed that plaque load was as good as coronary calcium measured with multi-slice CT studies in predicting vascular events [26]. Arterial plaque load measurement provides a reliable indicator of individualized vascular risk. Spence and Hackam concluded that "treating atherosclerosis without measuring plaque would be like treating hypertension without measuring blood pressure."

Did nonstenosing plaques account for many embolisms of uncertain origin and cryptogenic strokes [27]? Among carotid arteries with less than 50 percent stenosis, there was a difference in occurrence of stroke between plaques considered "vulnerable" (high lipid content or intraplaque hemorrhage) and those that were stable. Small fragments dislodged from nonstenosing plaques, especially those with vulnerable plaques, were an important unappreciated cause of stroke.

NOTES AND REFERENCES

1. Kussmaul A. Zwi Falle spontaner allmaliger Verschliessung grosser Halsarterienstamme. *Deutsch. Klin.* 1872;24:461–465.

2. Gowers WR. On a case of simultaneous embolism of central retinal and middle cerebral arteries. *Lancet* 1875;2:794–796.

3. Chiari H. Uber das Verhalten des Tielungswinkels der Carotis communis bei der Endarteritis chronica deformans. *Verhandl. deutschpath. Gesellsch.* 1905;9:326–330.

4. Hans Chiari. Wikipedia. Available at https://en.wikipedia.org/wiki/Hans_Chiari.

5. Gowers WR. *A Manual of Diseases of the Nervous System*, 2nd ed., vol. 2. Philadelphia: Blakiston's Sons and Co., 1906, pp. 421–429. Gowers's textbook of neurology is discussed in Chapter 14.

6. Hunt JR. The role of the carotid arteries in the causation of vascular lesions of the brain, with remarks on certain special features of the symptomatology. *Am. J. Med. Sci.* 1914;147:704–771.

7. James Ramsay Hunt. Wikipedia. Available at https://en.wikipedia.org/wiki/James_Ramsay_Hunt.

8. Moniz E, Lima A, de Lacerda R. Par thrombose de la carotide interne. *Presse Med.* 1937;45:977. Moniz's contributions are discussed in detail in Chapter 31.

9. Sjöqvist O. Über intrakranielle Aneurysmen der Arteria carotis und deren Beziehung zur ophthalmoplegischen Migräne. *Nervenarzt* 1936;9:233–241.

10. Hultquist GT, Jena GF. Uber Thrombose und Embolie der Arteria carotis und hierbei vorkommende Gehirnstorungen. Quoted in Fisher CM, Adams RD. Observations on brain embolism with special reference to the mechanism of hemorrhagic infarction. *J. Neuropathol. Exp. Neurol.* 1951;10:92–93.

11. Krayenbühl H, Weber G. Die Thrombose der Arteria carotis interna und ihre Beziehung zur Endangiitis obliterans v. Winiwarter-Buerger. *Helvet. Med. Acta* 1944;11:289–333.

12. Johnson HC, Walker AE. The angiographic diagnosis of spontaneous thrombosis of the internal and common carotid arteries. *J. Neurosurg.* 1951;8:631–639.

13. Fisher CM. Occlusion of the internal carotid artery. *Arch. Neurol. Psychiatry* 1951;65:346–377. Miller Fisher and his career and contributions is the topic of Chapter 29. His contributions are discussed at length in Caplan LR. *C. Miller Fisher: Stroke in the 20th Century*. New York: Oxford University Press, 2020. More detail about his carotid artery contributions are contained in Estol CJ. Dr C. Miller Fisher and the history of carotid artery disease. *Stroke* 1996;27(3):559–566.

14. Hollenhorst RW. Significance of bright plaques in the retinal arterioles. *JAMA* 1961;178:123–129.

15. Fisher CM. Occlusion of the carotid arteries: Further experiences. *Arch. Neurol. Psychiatry* 1954;72:187–204.

16. Mohr J. Distal field infarction. *Neurology* 1969;19:279.

17. Fisher CM. The microembolic theory of transient ischemic attacks. In Scheinberg P (ed.), *Proceedings of the 10th Princeton Conference for Cerebrovascular Diseases*. New York: Raven Press, 1976, pp. 50–53.

18. Pessin MS, Duncan GW, Mohr JP, et al. Clinical and angiographic features of carotid transient ischemic attacks. *N. Engl. J. Med.* 1977;296:38–362.

19. Pessin MS, Hinton RC, Davis KR, et al. Mechanisms of acute carotid stroke. *Ann. Neurol.* 1979;6:245–252.

20. Caplan LR, Hennerici M. Impaired clearance of emboli (washout) is an important link between hypoperfusion, embolism, and ischemic stroke. *Arch. Neurol.* 1998;55:1475–1482. Caplan LR, Wong K-S, Gao S, et al. Is hypoperfusion an important cause of strokes? If so, how? *Cerebrovasc. Dis.* 2006;21:145–153.

21. Fisher CM. Facial pulses in internal carotid artery occlusion. *Neurology* 1970;20:476–478.

22. Caplan LR. The frontal artery sign: A bedside indicator of internal carotid occlusive disease. *N. Engl. J. Med.* 1973;288:1008–1009.

23. Imparato AM, Riles TS, Gorstein F. The carotid bifurcation plaque: Pathologic findings associated with cerebral ischemia. *Stroke* 1979;10:238–245.

24. Fisher CM, Ojemann RG. A clinico-pathologic study of carotid endarterectomy plaques. *Rev. Neurol. (Paris)* 1986;142:573–589.

25. Spence DJ, Hackam DG. Treating arteries instead of risk factors: A paradigm change in management of atherosclerosis. *Stroke* 2010;41:1193–1199.

26. Baber U, Mehran R, Sartori S, et al. Prevalence, impact, and predictive value of detecting subclinical coronary and carotid atherosclerosis in asymptomatic adults: The BioImage study. *J. Am. Coll. Cardiol.* 2015 Mar 24;65(11):1065–1074.

27. Kamel H, Navi BB, Merkler AE, et al. Reclassification of ischemic stroke etiological subtypes on the basis of high-risk nonstenosing carotid plaque. *Stroke* 2020;51:504–510.

CHAPTER SIXTEEN

LACUNES

CHARCOT AND MARIE AND COLLEAGUES

Jean-Martin Charcot (1825–1893) is generally acclaimed as the father of modern clinical neurology. Charcot rose within the ranks of the Paris Hospital systems, and in 1872 was appointed professor of pathological anatomy at the University of Paris. He worked and taught at the Pitié-Salpêtrière Hospital for 33 years. His reputation as a teacher and lecturer drew students and colleagues from all over Europe. He established a neurology clinic at Salpêtrière, the first of its kind in Europe. Charcot mostly focused on clinical symptoms and signs and neurological phenomenology. His writings did not contain material about cerebrovascular disease [1]. Charcot established neurology as an important medical discipline in Europe and throughout the world. One of his most well-known and influential successors in the chair of neurology in Paris was Pierre Marie, a principal figure in bringing lacunar infarction to the attention of the medical community at the turn of the twentieth century.

Marie like Charcot rose within the Paris hospital system. He established a neurological unit at the Bicêtre Hospital where he did his most important work. Marie is known for his original descriptions of thyrotoxicosis, acromegaly, hereditary cerebellar ataxia, and peroneal atrophy. Marie was a large and imposing figure. Often referred to as "Le Grand Père," he ran his unit with an iron hand. Marie had an allergy to formalin, so viewed pathological specimens through a glass plate.

The French term *lacune* (derived from the Latin *lacuna*, a tiny hole, pit, or cavity) denotes a small, cystic cavity in the brain substance. The clinical findings in patients with lacunes were first described by Jean Ferrand in a thesis while working in the laboratory of Pierre Marie [2], and by Marie himself [3]. They noted the usual locations of these lacunes within the cerebral hemispheres and the brainstem. Paralysis of the limbs on one side of the body, hemiplegia, was the major finding in patients who had developed recent lacunes. The clinical condition of multiple lacunes was termed *état lacunaire* (lacunar state) by Marie and was characterized by slurred speech, difficulty swallowing and an abnormal small-stepped gait. Marie noted that these lacunar cavities were infarctions caused by insufficient supply of blood or could represent dilated perivascular spaces: "Progressive vascular lesions induce the rupture or the occlusion of one or a few small branches, and cause one or a few lacunes, for we know that in the deepest parts of the brain the vessel distribution is terminal i.e., there is little or no anastomoses, so that any territory the nutritive vessel of which is occluded, is unavoidably doomed to necrobiosis" [3,4].

INITIAL DESCRIPTION OF LACUNES

The first description of lacunes appeared many years before Marie and Ferrand [5–7]. The original description of lacunes was by Amedée Dechambre [5], an intern at the Salpêtrière Hospital in Paris who worked under the French pathologist Jean Cruveilhier. Apoplexy was considered at the time a uniformly fatal disease and Dechambre provided clinicopathological observations of stroke survivors. His report "Memoir on the Curability of Cerebral Softening" appeared in the *Gazette Médicale de Paris* on May 19, 1838. Dechambre found at autopsy "a number of small lacunes of variable size and form." He concluded that lacunes result from liquefaction and partial reabsorption in the center of the cerebral softening. Five years later, Maxime Durand-Fardel (1816–1899) [6], the father of gerontology in France, independently confirmed Dechambre's observations and posited the pathogenesis of lacunes in his book *Traité du Ramollissement du Cerveau*, published in Paris in 1843 [7]. Durand-Fardel's is one of the first books on ischemic stroke ever published. He made no reference to the previous description of lacunes by Dechambre. Durand-Fardel clearly distinguished lacunes from dilatations of the perivascular spaces (*état criblé*).

C. MILLER FISHER

The topic of lacunes lay fallow and virtually unexplored until Miller Fisher began his research half a century after Marie's and Ferrand's publications. Fisher systematically examined 1,000 or more thinly cut serial sections of brain specimens. In one study, among 1,042 brains studied at autopsy, 114 (11%) had lacunar infarcts, often multiple [8]. The commonest locations were deep within the brain: the internal capsule, basal ganglia, thalamus, and pons, the same locations as hypertensive intracerebral bleeds. Recent infarcts represented small regions of brain softening. Older lesions were cavities ranging from 1 to 17 millimeters in size. Often, strands of fibrillary connective tissue traversed the cavities. He studied the small penetrating arteries and arterioles that supplied these small deep infarcts and found segmental occlusions within them [9]. He dubbed the pathology "segmental arterial disorganization" and also applied the term "lipohyalinosis," indicating that fatty material (lipid) was included and that the wall took on a glassy (hyaline) appearance. Lipid material and connective tissue called fibrinoid thickened the wall of the small arteries, causing encroachment on the vascular lumen. For Fisher lacunar infarctions were defined by the vascular process responsible: lipohyalinosis, an alteration of the arteriolar wall directly related to high blood pressure; fibroid necrosis observed in severe arterial hypertension; and microathema within the origins of penetrating arterial branches.

Fisher and Caplan described another vascular lesion that caused small deep infarcts [10]. The initial designation for this alternate pathology was "basilar branch infarcts" since the pathology was found in studying branches of the basilar artery. This pathology also involved branches of the main arteries supplying the cerebral hemispheres and was labeled "intracranial branch ather-omatous disease" [11]. Fisher reported and analyzed the different syndromes that were found in patients with these lacunar infarcts [12]. The four main syndromes that he opined could reliably be attributed to lacunar infarction were: (1) Pure motor hemiplegia: paralysis of the face and upper and lower limbs without sensory deficit, visual field abnormalities, or cognitive impairment. The lesion is located along the corticospinal tract, most often in the posterior limb of the internal capsule or the pons. (2) Pure sensory stroke: paresthesias or numbness involving one side of the body and limbs without motor, visual, or cognitive deficits. The lesion is most often found in the ventrolateral thalamus. (3) Ataxic hemiparesis: weakness and ataxia on one side of the body. The lesion is in the pons or posterior limb of the internal capsule. (4) Dysarthria-clumsy hand syndrome: slurred speech and distal upper limb clumsiness, sometimes supplemented by opercular elements, dysphagia, central facial paralysis, and tongue deviation. The lesion is mainly localized to the internal capsule, less often in the corona radiata or pons [12].

LATER DESCRIPTION OF THE PATHOLOGY

The neuropathology of lacunes was further clarified by Jacques Poirier and Christian Derouesné [13,14]. They emphasized that the macroscopic cavities (lacunes) had different microscopic appearances corresponding to various pathologic processes. They divided lacunes into three categories: Type I lacunes correspond to old, small brain infarcts; these were irregular anfractuous cavities devoid of any lining epithelium that contained macrophages and small parenchymatous fragments, usually surrounded by marked astrocytic gliosis. Type II lacunes were old, small hemorrhages easily recognized by the presence of hemosiderin-laden macrophages and iron pigmentation within their walls. Type III lacunes were due to dilatation of the perivascular space. These were round, very regular cavities that always contained one or two sections of an artery with a patent lumen and usually normal walls. The cavity was lined by a single layer of epithelial cells that corresponded to the leptomeningeal cells forming the normal lining of the perivascular spaces [13,14].

NEUROIMAGING OF LACUNAR INFARCTS

Prior descriptions and research were based on clinic-pathological analyses. Since few patients died of an acute lacunar infarction, pathological specimens were only available years after the index stroke, making clinicopathological correlations difficult. When CT and later MRI became widely available during the last quarter of the twentieth century, it became possible to perform clinical-imaging analyses. MRI was able to localize small deep infarcts and small hemorrhages better than CT. It was now possible to separate using neuro-imaging small deep infarcts (lacunes) from cortical and cortical-subcortical infarcts and hemorrhages. Atlases [15] and reviews led to analyses of risk factors, predominant location of infarcts, and the addition of new clinical syndromes [16]. Researchers led by Joanna Wardlaw of Edinburgh defined standards for reporting of the neuroimaging findings [17] and analyzed the various evolutions of acute small deep infarcts [18].

MULTIPLE LACUNAR INFARCTS AND ACCOMPANYING WHITE MATTER PATHOLOGY

Marie, in his original report, discussed the findings in patients with a recent lacunar infarct as well as patients with multiple lacunar infarcts, which he dubbed *état lacunaire* [3]. Otto Binswanger, a prominent German neuropathologist, wrote an article that appeared in 1894 in three installments in a German weekly clinical newspaper for practicing physicians [19]. Binswanger discussed the clinical and pathological findings in patients with syphilitic general paralysis of the insane (GPI), a commonly diagnosed condition at that time. He contrasted the findings to other disorders that also caused mental and physical deterioration. He clearly separated GPI from arteriosclerotic vascular dementias. Encephalitis subcorticalis chronica progressiva (ESCP) was characterized pathologically by "pronounced atrophy of the white matter, either confined to one or more gyri of the brain or in several sections of the hemisphere" [19]. The cerebral ventricles were enlarged, especially the posterior horns, and the cerebral cortex was spared. Microscopic examination showed extensive atrophic or fatty degeneration of the small arterial and venules. Alois Alzheimer, in 1902, referred to Binswanger's reports and further elaborated on the pathology that included numerous foci of severe gliosis in the cerebral white matter, the internal capsule, lenticular nuclei, thalamus, and pons [20]. He attributed these to atherosclerosis of long, deep vessels causing atrophy of the white matter. Franz Nissl, another famous neuropathologist, described patchy loss of white matter with gliosis in a man with dementia of 10 years' duration [21]. Nissl described the vascular changes in more detail than had prior authors: severe and often extreme thickening of vascular walls. Jerzy Olszewski, a Canadian neuropathologist, called the condition "subcortical arteriosclerotic encephalopathy" and emphasized extensive hyalinization, intimal fibrosis, and splitting of the internal elastic laminae in the small arteries and arterioles of the basal ganglia and cerebral white matter [22]. The lumens of small vessels were severely narrowed and, occasionally, completely occluded. Louis Caplan and William Schoene reported a further series of pathologically confirmed cases that they labeled Binswanger disease [23].

These reports were based on necropsy-confirmed cases and preceded modern neuroimaging. When CT and later MRI became available, it became possible to diagnose chronic perforating artery disease (Binswanger's) during life [24]. The usual age of onset was between 55 and 75 years. Men and women were equally affected. Most patients had a history or evidence of hypertension. Patients had had acute strokes, often with symptoms and signs conforming to one of the lacunar syndromes. They also developed the subacute onset of focal neurologic signs that often progressed during days. Some had seizures, especially during the subacute progression of signs. Stepwise and gradual progression of neurologic motor, cognitive, and behavioral deficits accrued during a period of 5–10 years. The clinical course was often characterized by periods of stabilization, plateaus, and sometimes periods of improvement. Neurological examination showed pyramidal tract signs. extrapyramidal type abnormalities, an abnormal small stepped gait, pseudobulbar signs, apathy, inertia, disinterest, abulia, poor judgment, lack of insight, and altered affective responses and variable deficits in memory, language, and visuospatial functions [24].

MRI in these patients showed patchy, irregular periventricular white matter attenuation; irregular focal periventricular lesions that extended into the subjacent white matter; white matter lesions in the corona radiata and centrum semiovale not continuous with periventricular abnormalities; multiple lacunar infarcts; enlargement of Virchow-Robin spaces; hydrocephalus; and often multiple microbleeds within the deep regions of the cerebral hemispheres [24].

During the 1990s and early twenty-first century, genetic disorders including cerebral autosomal dominant arteriopathy with subcortical infarcts and leukoencephalopathy (CADASIL) [25] and cerebral autosomal recessive arteriopathy with subcortical infarcts and leukoencephalopathy (CARASIL) [26] were decribed and characterized. They shared many clinical and imaging features with the previously described Binswanger cases, but these genetic conditions usually had earlier onset of clinical and MRI abnormalities and there were other affected family members. In CADASIL the defining microscopic feature was the deposition of granular osmophilic non-amyloid staining material within the vascular basal lamina on electron microscopy. In CARASIL the small arteries were thickened by fibrous intimal proliferation, severe hyalinosis, and the intima and/or the internal elastic membrane was often split. White matter abnormalities were similar to those found in Binswanger patients and often deep lacunar infarcts were present. The white matter abnormalities often preceded clinical signs, clinical strokes, and discrete infarcts.

Damaged vascular walls in patients with hypertension, pseudoxanthoma elasticum, CADASIL, CARASIL, cerebral amyloid angiopathy, and other conditions led to small deep infarcts and small hemorrhages (microbleeds). The extensive white matter abnormalities were more difficult to explain. The posited causes of these white matter abnormalities included tandem stenosis/occlusion of adjacent penetrators causing ischemia in larger regions than one vessel and hypertensive crisis with resultant chronic brain edema. Recent studies have shown that the cause is more likely to be chromic leakage of fluid outside diseased small blood vessels causing perivascular edema [27]. Gliosis then develops in areas of edema, creating the imaging changes and explaining softening of tissue at necropsy. Diseased small vessel walls contain abnormal metalloproteinases that allow perivascular leakage [27–29]. Matrix metalloproteinases disrupt the blood-brain barrier by degrading tight junction proteins found within the vascular walls.

NOTES AND REFERENCES

1. Charcot JM, Goetz CG. Charcot, the clinician: The Tuesday lessons: Excerpts from nine case presentations on general neurology delivered at the Salpêtrière Hospital in 1887–88. In Charcot JM. *Lectures on the Diseases of the Nervous System*. Trans. George Sigerson. London: Sydenham Society, 1877.
2. Ferrand J. Essai sur l'hemiplegie des vieillards: les lacunes de desintegration cerebrale. Thesis, University of Paris, 1902.
3. Marie P. Des foyers lacunaires de désintégration et des différents autres états cavitaires du cerveau. *Revue de Médeciné (Paris)* 1901;21:281–298. Marie P. *Travaux et mémoires*, vol. 2. Paris: Masson et Cie, 1928, pp. 72–89.

4. Hauw J-J. The history of lacunes. In Donnan G, Norrving B, Bamford J Bogousslavsky, J (eds.), *Lacunar and Other Subcortical Infarcts*. Oxford: Oxford University Press, 1995, pp. 3–15.

5. Dechambre A. Mémoire sur la curabilité du ramollissement cérérebral. *Gaz. Méd. Paris* 1838;6:305–314.

6. Durand-Fardel M. Memoire sur une alteration particuliere de la substance cérébrale. *Gaz. Méd. Paris* 1842;10:23–26, 33–38.

7. Durand-Fardel M. *Traite des ramollisements du cerveau*. Paris: Bailliere, 1843.

8. Fisher CM. Lacunes, small deep cerebral infarcts. *Neurology* 1965;15:774–784.

9. Fisher CM. The vascular lesion in lacunae. *Transactions of the American Neurological Association* 1965;90:243–245. Fisher CM. The arterial lesions underlying lacunes. *Acta Neuropathologica* 1969;12:1–15.

10. Fisher CM, Caplan LR. Basilar artery branch occlusion: A cause of pontine infarction. *Neurology* 1971; 21:900–905. Fisher CM. Bilateral occlusion of basilar artery branches. *J. Neurol. Neurosurg. Psychiatry* 1977;40:1182–1189 (discussed further in Chapters 29 and 30).

11. Caplan LR. Intracranial branch atheromatous disease: A neglected, understudied and underused concept. *Neurology* 1989;39:1246–1250.

12. Clinical syndromes are discussed in Chapter 26 and are reported in Fisher CM. Pure motor hemiplegia of vascular origin. *Arch. Neurol.* 1965;13:30–44. Fisher CM. Pure sensory stroke involving face, arm, and leg. *Neurology* 1965;15:76–80. Fisher CM. Thalamic pure sensory stroke: A pathologic study. *Neurology* 1978;28:1141–1144. Fisher CM. Pure sensory stroke and allied conditions. *Stroke* 1982;13:434–447. Fisher CM. A lacunar stroke, the dysarthria-clumsy hand syndrome. *Neurology* 1967;17:614–617. Fisher CM, Cole M. Homolateral ataxia and crural paresis, a vascular syndrome. *J. Neurol. Neurosurg. Psychiatry* 1965;28:48–55. Fisher CM. Ataxic hemiparesis. *Archives of Neurology* 1978;35:126–128. Fisher FM. Capsular infarcts. *Arch. Neurol.* 1979;36:65–73.

13. Poirier J, Derouesné C. Le concept de lacune cérébrale de 1838 à nos jours. *Rev. Neurol. (Paris)* 1985;141:3–17.

14. Poirier J, Derouesné C. Cerebral lacunae: A proposed new classification (letter). *Clin. Neuropathol.* 1984;3:266.

15. Besson G. Les infarctus lacunaires, evaluation clinque et par l'imagerie par resonance magnetique. Thesis, University of Grenoble, 1989.

16. Fisher CM. Lacunar infarcts – A review. *Cerebrovasc. Dis.* 1991;1:311–320. Donnan GA, Norrving B, Bamford JM, Bogoussslavsky J. *Lacunar and Other Subcortical Infarctions*. Oxford: Oxford University Press, 1995. Norrving B. Evolving concept of small vessel disease through advanced brain imaging. *J. Stroke* 2015;17(2):94–100.

17. Wardlaw JM, Smith EE, Biessels GJ, Cordonnier C, Fazekas F, Frayne R, et al. Neuroimaging standards for research into small vessel disease and its contribution to ageing and neurodegeneration. *Lancet Neurol.* 2013;12:822–838.

18. Loos CMJ, Makin SDJ, Staals J, Dennis MS, van Oostenbrugge RJ, Wardlaw JM. Long-term morphological changes of symptomatic lacunar infarcts and surrounding white matter on structural magnetic resonance imaging. *Stroke* 2018;49(5):1183–1188.

19. Binswanger O. Die abgrenzung der allgemeinen progressiven paralyse. *Klin. Wochenschr.* 1894;49:1103–1105; 1895;50:1137–1139; 1895;52:1180–1186. Blass JP. Hoyer S, Nitsch R. A translation of Otto Binswanger's article, "The delineation of the generalised progressive paralyses." *Arch. Neurol.* 1991;48:961–972.

20. Alzheimer A. Die Seelenstorungen auf arteriosklerotischer grundlage. *Z. Psych.* 1902;59:695–711. Alzheimer A. Neue arbeiten uber die dementia senilis und die auf atheromatoser gefasserkrankungen basierenden gehirnerkrankungen. *Monatsachr. Psych. Neurol.* 1898;3:101–115.

21. Nissl F. Zur kasuistic der artenoskleriotischen demenz. ein fall von sogenannten "encephalitis subcorticalis." *Z. Neurol. Psychiatr.* 1920;19:438–443.

22. Olszewski J. Subcortical arteriosclerotic encephalopathy. Review of the literature on the so-called Binswanger's disease and presentation of two cases. *World Neurol.* 1962;3:359–375.

23. Caplan LR, Schoene WC. Clinical features of subcortical arteriosclerotic encephalopathy (Binswanger disease). *Neurology* 1978;28:1206–1215.

24. Caplan LR. Binswanger's disease revisited. *Neurology* 1995;45:626–633.

25. Tournier-Lasserve E, Joutel A, Melki J, et al. Cerebral autosomal dominant arteriopathy with subcortical infarcts and leukoencephalopathy maps to chromosome 19q12. *Nat. Genet.* 1993;3:256–259. Joutel A, Corpechot C, Ducros A, et al. Notch3 mutations in CADASIL a hereditary adult-onset condition causing stroke and dementia. *Nature* 1996;383:707–710.

26. Yanagawa S, Ito N, Arima K, Ikeda S. Cerebral autosomal recessive arteriopathy with subcortical infarcts and leukoencephalopathy. *Neurology* 2002;58:817–820.

27. Rosenberg GA, Sullivan N, Esiri NM. White matter damage is associated with matrix metalloproteinases in vascular dementia. *Stroke* 2001;32:1162–1168. Wardlaw JM, Doubal FN, Valdes-Hernandez M, et al. Blood-brain barrier permeability and long-term clinical and imaging outcomes in cerebral small vessel disease. *Stroke* 2013;44 (2):525–527.

28. Regenhardt RW, Das AS, Lo EH, Caplan LR. Advances in understanding the pathophysiology of lacunar stroke: A review. *JAMA Neurol.* 2018;75(10):1273–1281.

29. Caplan LR. Microbleeds. *Circulation* 2015;132:479–480.

CHAPTER SEVENTEEN

VERTEBROBASILAR DISEASE

EARLY ANATOMICAL AND CLINICAL-PATHOLOGICAL STUDIES

The first important attention given to disease of the posterior circulation was likely by a Swiss pathologist and physician Johan Jacob Wepfer [1]. He followed the example of Vesalius and performed meticulous necropsy examinations. He described the results of his dissections in his magnum opus on apoplexy, published in 1658 [2]. He described the appearance and the course of the intracranial arteries and recognized blockage of the carotid and vertebral arteries caused by disease of the arterial walls as a cause of apoplexy, the obstruction preventing entry of sufficient blood into a portion of the brain. He described the anatomy of the intracranial vertebral arteries as follows:

> As regards the vertebral arteries, they emerge from the nearest foramen, that great orifice through which the spinal marrow descends. They advance to the sides of the medulla oblongata.... When they reach that place where the sixth pair of nerves (IX, X, XI, XII) arises, the right and left branches are joined and form a single channel (basilar artery) and remain united along the whole marrow tract.

The next time attention was given to the posterior circulation was by clinicians and researchers in Europe during the second half of the nineteenth century and early twentieth century. They were mostly interested in brain and vascular anatomy and in anatomic-physiologic correlations. The so-called classic brainstem syndromes, all eponymic and named after the original describers of the syndromes, were studied by authors who were fascinated by the anatomy and functions of the brainstem. Recognized still today are these various constellations of findings as the syndromes of Benedikt, Claude, Millard-Gubler, Babinski-Nageotte, Foville, and Wallenberg, among others [3]. Reviews of these reports showed that many lesions were not vascular; the underlying arterial lesions and vascular pathology were rarely studied or commented on. The brainstem with its dense, packed heterogeneous and complex anatomy was of particular interest. Focal lesions limited to one location in the midbrain, pons, or medulla provided insight into the anatomy and physiology of the brainstem. Of special utility in localization were crossed syndromes in which cranial nerve abnormalities involved one side of the head, while long tract motor or sensory or extrapyramidal-cerebellar abnormalities involved the limbs and trunk on the opposite side of the body. The Millard-Gubler syndrome of ipsilateral facial palsy and contralateral hemiparesis was an example. Since there was no way during that time to identify the causative vascular lesion during life, and no treatment was known or available even if the cause was known, there was no interest in stroke etiology or the mechanism of ischemia in patients with brainstem or cerebellar infarcts.

VASCULAR LESIONS WITHIN THE POSTERIOR CIRCULATION

The first detailed study of the clinical, pathological, and etiological aspects of brainstem infarction was by the German physician Adolf Wallenberg. During a period of 27 years, Wallenberg published four reports on infarction of the lateral medulla: a detailed analysis of the clinical findings in one patient, the necropsy findings in that patient, a single case report of another patient, and the clinical and pathological findings in the fifteenth patient he had studied [4]. Wallenberg had first seen the original patient, a ropemaker, in 1889 for appendicitis. In 1993, the patient developed severe vertigo, intense pain in the left eye, difficulty swallowing, and hoarseness. Wallenberg reported a detailed clinical neurological examination that showed horizontal and vertical nystagmus, abnormal pain and temperature sensation in the left face and right face and body, weakness of the left palate, paralysis of the left vocal cord, and left limb ataxia. Wallenberg wrote: "We are dealing with an insult on the left side of the medulla. It begins just above the pyramidal decussation. It passes through the accessory olive and the inferior olive more rostrally. Laterally it destroys the entire medulla to the pia mater. Rostrally and medially it reaches the ascending lemniscus damaging the restiform body and ultimately also the cerebellum."

Six years after the initial report, the patient had another acute stroke and died. Wallenberg performed the autopsy himself and described and illustrated the location and extent of the medullary infarct. The vertebral arteries were severely diseased and the left posterior inferior cerebellar artery was occluded.

Anatomists and researchers working during the early part of the twentieth century became interested in the blood vessels that supply the brain, including the brainstem and cerebellum. Duret [5] in France and Stopford [6] in England meticulously dissected the arteries that supply the brainstem. Particularly prolific in performing studies that clarified arterial anatomy was Charles Foix, who worked in the clinics and pathology laboratories at the Salpêtrière hospital in Paris [7]. Foix and his colleagues defined the distribution and localization of brain infarcts ("ramollissements") and the corresponding neurological abnormalities that they caused during life. They also sought to clarify the anatomical distribution of the arterial supply to these areas. During four short years, between 1923 and 1927, Foix and his colleagues defined the arterial distribution of the posterior cerebral artery including the branches to the thalamus, and the supply of the pons, and the medulla oblongata [7]. Foix noted the common pattern of irrigation of all parts of the brainstem by paramedian, short circumferential, and long circumferential arteries.

Probably the single most important and influential communication regarding posterior circulation ischemia was the report on basilar artery occlusion by Charles Kubik and Raymond Adams, published in 1946 [8]. This report was one of the most complete and most detailed clinical-pathological studies of any vascular syndrome. Kubik and Adams did not publish the very first report of occlusion of the basilar artery; there had been prior reports. The report of Kubik and Adams was very important and influential because of the large size of the series (18 patients), the meticulous dissection and illustration of the brain lesions at the various brainstem levels, as well as delineation of the vascular occlusion and the details of the clinical findings.

At the time of their report, Kubik and Adams were both neuropathologists working in the necropsy laboratories at the Massachusetts General Hospital and the Boston City Hospital in Boston, as well as being active on the neurology wards of the hospitals. The authors examined some of the patients during life and later reviewed their clinical charts. The extent and location of the thrombosis correlated well with the areas of brainstem infarction, and usually only a portion of the basilar artery was occluded (Figure 17.1). The infarcts were mostly confined to the territories of the paramedian and short circumferential pontine arteries. Seven of the 18 basilar artery occlusions were embolic. The symptoms in most patients began abruptly and all cases were fatal (or else the patient would not have reached their laboratory in the morgue). The clinical symptoms and signs during life included dizziness, altered consciousness, dysarthria, paresthesias, pseudobulbar palsy, hemiplegia or quadriplegia, pupillary and oculomotor abnormalities, facial paralysis, and visual loss, which correlated well with the brainstem and posterior hemispheral structures involved. The authors emphasized that recognition of these signs should allow for accurate antemortem diagnosis of basilar artery occlusion.

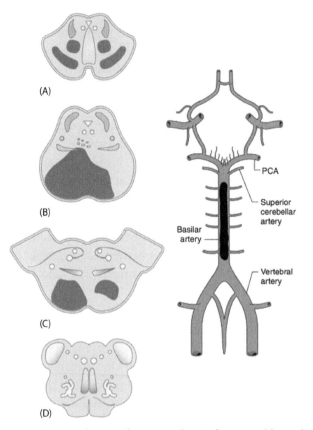

17.1. Cartoon showing the pons with an infarct caused by occlusion of the basilar artery: (A) midbrain, (B) upper pons, (C) lower pons, and (D) medulla. Based on the work of Kubik and Adams [8].

E. C. Hutchinson and P. O. Yates systematically dissected and examined the cervicocranial arteries in the neck [9]. They found a high frequency of occlusive disease in the cervical vertebral arteries near their origins from the subclavian arteries. Vertebral artery occlusive disease in the neck seemed to parallel carotid occlusive disease, leading Hutchinson and Yates to coin the term "carotico- vertebral" stenosis [9]. Later, C. Miller Fisher also emphasized the importance of occlusive disease involving the vertebral arteries in the neck, which often involved these vessels bilaterally [10].

Description of the subclavian steal syndrome added more weight to the growing evidence that extracranial occlusive disease was common. The report by Martin Reivich and colleagues called attention to patients with periodic attacks of dizziness and vertigo, sometimes precipitated by arm exercise, who had occlusive lesions involving the subclavian artery proximal to the vertebral artery origin [11]. Angiography and blood flow studies showed that blood coursed from the contralateral subclavian artery up the vertebral artery to reach the cranium and then traveled retrograde down the vertebral artery ipsilateral to the subclavian artery stenosis or occlusion. Ultimately, the retrograde vertebral artery flow went into the ischemic arm. Later, Michael Hennerici and colleagues showed that reversed vertebral artery flow was common in patients with subclavian artery occlusive disease but rarely produced important neurological symptoms or signs [12].

During the 1950s, clinicians had become alerted to the presence of transient ischemic attacks (TIAs) by Miller Fisher. They had also become aware of the usual symptoms and signs in patients who were later proven to have fatal basilar artery occlusions by Kubik and Adams [8]. During the 1950s and 1960s, a series of articles was written by American and British clinicians about patients with posterior circulation TIAs. When studied during life by angiography, there was a high frequency of severe vertebrobasilar occlusive lesions. The lesions involved mostly the basilar artery, but the cervical and intracranial portions of the vertebral arteries were also often stenosed or occluded. The syndrome of intermittent TIAs involving the posterior circulation was dubbed "vertebro-basilar insufficiency" (VBI) by neurologists at the Mayo Clinic in Rochester, Minnesota – Clark Millikan, Robert Siekert, and Jack Whisnant – and by British clinicians [13]. Influenced greatly by the report of Kubik and Adams on necropsy-proven cases of basilar artery occlusion, clinicians during the middle of the twentieth century widely believed that severe occlusive disease of the intracranial posterior circulation arteries was a very serious, often mortal disease. During this era, the popular drug that was being used for occlusive vascular disease was warfarin. Anticoagulation had been used in patients with thrombophlebitis and pulmonary embolism, myocardial infarction, and rheumatic valve disease with systemic and brain embolism. Warfarin seemed to be worth trying for occlusive vascular disease. Using this reasoning, Millikan, Siekert, and Richard Shick, from the Mayo Clinic, published an important and very influential paper on the use of warfarin anticoagulation to treat patients with VBI [14]. Patients with the clinical symptoms and signs of VBI (angiography was not often used) were given warfarin in an uncontrolled observational study. Some patients stopped having attacks and many had no or minimal strokes. Believing that the disease was usually fatal or disabling without treatment, the authors believed that warfarin was clearly effective and indicated to treat patients with symptoms suggesting VBI.

By the middle of the 1960s there was widespread belief in the medical and neurological community that posterior circulation TIAs and ischemic strokes could be readily diagnosed clinically; that transient attacks and insufficiency states could be explained by hemodynamic factors; and that anticoagulation with heparin-warfarin therapy was an effective treatment. Angiography was considered not to be indicated, although a few anecdotal studies later showed the ability of angiography to clarify the nature of the underlying vascular disease and prognosis in isolated instances. Patients with posterior circulation ischemia were usually given heparin and warfarin unless contraindicated. Few investigations were performed. This situation remained until modern brain and vascular imaging including magnetic resonance imaging (MRI), magnetic resonance angiography (MRA), and computed tomography angiography (CTA) became widely available during the last years of the twentieth century.

Many years later, in the Warfarin-Aspirin for Symptomatic Intracranial Disease (WASID) trial of patients with severe intracranial atherosclerosis, there was no significant difference in preventing new strokes between aspirin and warfarin [15]. The study drugs were begun often weeks after the last ischemic event. Warfarin was difficult to control; patients maintained within the target therapeutic international normalized ratio (INR) range of warfarin performed better than patients treated with 1,300 milligrams of aspirin per day. In those treated with warfarin whose INR levels were below the target range, more infarcts developed, and more hemorrhages developed in those above the target INR range. There were too few patients with severe (>80%) intracranial vertebral (107 patients) or basilar artery stenosis (112 patients) to render meaningful conclusions about treatment of these specific occlusive lesions [15].

Although the mechanism of TIAs was uncertain, opinion during the middle years of the twentieth century favored hemodynamic, general circulatory mechanisms. Derek Denny-Brown put forth the hypothesis that intermittent spells of ischemia were explained by circulatory perturbations, and he called the temporarily inadequate blood flow "insufficiency." Denny-Brown hypothesized that carotid and vertebrobasilar insufficiency was a "physiological, potential hemodynamic state in which reversible hemodynamic crises could be elicited by any factor that impaired the collateral circulation" [16]. Hemodynamic crises could be transient or partially or completely reversible, depending on the length and severity of the pathophysiological cause. Denny-Brown reviewed the anatomical, physiological, and experimental data that favored his hypothesis. His own tilt table experiments, which used electro-encephalogram (EEG) monitoring of patients with clinical "insufficiency," more often than not failed to provoke attacks or EEG changes.

CLINICOPATHOLOGIC AND CLINICAL-IMAGING STUDIES DURING THE SECOND HALF OF THE TWENTIETH CENTURY

The advent of modern brain and vascular imaging (MRI, MRA, and CTA) and safer catheter angiography facilitated study of various clinical posterior circulation syndromes. Clinicians and researchers in the United States, Europe, and Asia studied and reported clinical syndromes related to involvement of specific locations within the posterior circulation–supplied brain regions and caused by various stroke subtypes. These studies included reports about lateral and medial medullary infarcts, cerebellar infarcts, top of the basilar syndrome, basilar artery occlusion, thalamic infarcts, pontine lacunar infarcts causing pure motor hemiparesis, ataxic hemiparesis, and dysarthria-clumsy hand syndrome, lateral tegmental pontine syndrome, basilar branch occlusion, midbrain infarcts, and posterior cerebral artery territory infarcts [17]. A registry of over 400 patients with posterior circulation infarcts and TIAs showed the frequency of various symptoms and signs, vascular lesions, and outcomes [18].

VERTEBROBASILAR TERRITORY BRAIN HEMORRHAGES

The first recognition and description of a posterior circulation hemorrhage was in a treatise on apoplexy published in 1812 by Irish physician John Cheyne [19]. A patient described by Cheyne had a pontine hematoma. Case 14 was a "carpenter, 35 years of age, phlegmatic, pale, muscular, not habitually intemperate." He had severe headaches, and after one such headache, he vomited and soon after "became insensible." About an hour later, his breathing became irregular and he was deeply comatose, and soon dead. Cheyne described this man's brain as follows: "In dissecting the base of the brain, there was discovered, formed by rupture in the substance of the pons varolii, a collection of dark clotted blood, in an irregular cavity, having a ragged surface and communicating with the fourth ventricle which was full of blood" [19].

In 1903, Charles Dana, then professor of neurology at Cornell University in New York, reviewed prior reports and his own personal experience, and summarized the clinical aspects of pontine hemorrhages and infarcts [20]. Dana reviewed the brain and vascular anatomy of the pons. Among 2,288 hematomas found at necropsy, 205 (9%) were pontine [20]. Dana described the typical patient:

> Some prodromal headache and malaise for a few days ... then he falls suddenly as if by a lightning stroke, into a coma, usually very profound. There are twitching of the face or of the limbs or both ... the pupils are contracted to a pinpoint ... there is convergent strabismus or conjugate deviation of the eyes. The limbs are at first stiff but tone may be reduced later and the reflexes increased. The patient can not be aroused but can be made to vomit ... the patient dies in 6 to 20 hours usually with paralysis of respiration. [20]

Dana listed the "syndrome of the pons" as: (1) headache, malaise, vomiting; (2) sudden profound coma; (3) face and limb twitching; (4) small pupils, convergent strabismus, or conjugate eye deviation; (5) slow irregular respirations; (6) irregular pulse; (7) dysphagia; (8) paralysis of all limbs, or crossed paralysis; (9) gradual rise of temperature; and (10) death within 24 hours [20].

Some pontine hematomas described in the nineteenth century were accompanied by supratentorial hemorrhages. Separation of primary pontine hematomas from secondary, pressure-related lesions did not occur until the twentieth century. Henry Duret produced brainstem hemorrhages experimentally by injecting fluids into the supratentorial tissues of dogs [21]. Duret then showed that the secondary hemorrhages in the midbrain and pons, now referred to as Duret hemorrhages, were caused by sudden intracranial supratentorial pressure that distorted and compressed the brainstem and its vessels, causing the latter to stretch and tear [21].

Although most authors continued to emphasize the abrupt onset of symptoms, Kornyey, in a remarkable single case report, described the gradual, inexorable progression of symptoms and signs in a young man whose pontine hematoma occurred and developed under observation [22]. The patient was a 39-year-old man sent to the hospital in Hungary where Kornyey practiced for treatment of severe malignant hypertension. While his history was taken, the patient reported numbness and tingling of the hands followed by restlessness, dysphagia, and loss of hearing. His blood pressure was measured at 245/170 mmHg. While being observed, he developed bilateral sixth nerve palsies, dysarthria, deafness, and left hemiparesis. Then small pupils, quadriplegia, and coma developed. Within two hours after walking into the clinic, he had died of a pontine hematoma [22].

CT and later MRI allowed for detection of smaller pontine hemorrhages that were previously not identified. The classic large central pontine hematomas were the result of rupture of the large paramedian pontine artery penetrators. The next syndrome that was recognized was lateral tegmental hematomas that arose from rupture of arteries penetrating into the lateral tegmentum as branches of long circumferential arteries, especially the superior cerebellar arteries. These lesions caused a contralateral hemisensory loss due to involvement of the sensory lemniscus formed in the pons from merging of the lateral spinothalamic tract and the medial lemniscus. Ataxia and oculomotor abnormalities were also often present but paresis was absent or minimal. Later, smaller lateral tegmental hematomas were described that caused only contralateral sensory abnormalities. Small basal hematomas arising from small paramedian arteries and short circumferential penetrators could cause pure motor hemiparesis or ataxic hemiparesis, causing similar signs as patients with lacunar infarcts.

Another common region of posterior circulation bleeding was in the cerebellum. Childs in 1858 reported the first American patient, a 19-year-old woman who developed a cerebellar hemorrhage while shaking her head vigorously to amuse a child [23]. In 1942, Mitchell and Angrist reported 15 patients with spontaneous cerebellar hemorrhage and also reviewed the 109 cases reported to that time [24]. "Coma as a prominent symptom far overshadowed all other findings" and was present in 64 of the 124 patients (52%). The next most common symptoms were vomiting and headaches.

Dizziness was present in only 16 patients (13%) and ataxia in 11 (9%) [24]. In 1960, Wylie McKissock and his London colleagues reported 34 patients with cerebellar hemorrhage who had been under the care of one surgeon (McKissock) [25]. Hypertension was the commonest cause but six patients in the series had angiomas and two had aneurysms. The outcome was very poor since 19 of the 28 surgically treated patients died. The authors were pessimistic about clinical recognition of cerebellar hemorrhage: "The neurological signs presented by these patients were in the main singularly unhelpful. Localizing signs could not be elicited in those patients who were unconscious except that most of them had constricted and non-reactive pupils and periodic respirations. In the conscious patients, signs of cerebellar dysfunction were present in less than half" [25].

Miller Fisher and colleagues, in an important benchmark 1965 report, emphasized clinical findings that would improve clinical recognition of cerebellar hemorrhage [26]. They described three patients in detail. In an addendum, added after the paper had been accepted, the authors mentioned that they had since seen eight other patients in whom the rules derived from the original three patients and outlined in the paper had allowed the diagnosis of cerebellar hematomas, which were confirmed at surgery [26]. Vomiting was a constant feature; inability to stand or walk especially unaided was a reliable and very consistent sign; ipsilateral sixth nerve palsy and conjugate gaze palsy were very common; hemiparesis or hemiplegia was not observed, but often there was bilateral increased deep tendon reflexes and Babinski signs [26]. Headache, neck stiffness, limb ataxia, dysarthria, and dizziness were variable findings. The authors urged surgical exploration when the clinical signs were typical. Large clinical series of patients with cerebellar hemorrhages corroborated the frequency of the symptoms and signs reported by Fisher et al.

CT and MRI allowed for the diagnosis of smaller cerebellar hematomas. Most involve the cerebellar hemispheres, especially the white matter in the region of the dentate nucleus in the territory of the superior cerebellar arteries. Some also arise more caudally from posterior inferior cerebellar artery (PICA) territory branches. Occasionally, hemorrhages arise in the vermis and compress the fourth ventricle and the medullary and pontine tegmentum.

Although bleeding into the thalamus was another common site of posterior circulation hemorrhage, separation of the clinical symptoms and signs from those found in patients with putaminal and basal ganglionic hemorrhages did not occur until Fisher's discussion during a 1959 meeting of the Houston Neurological Society [26,27]. Fisher emphasized the presence of vertical gaze paralysis, position of the eyes downward at rest as if the patient is peering at the tip of the nose, constricted pupils, and sensory signs on the contralateral limbs greater than hemiparesis. The thalamic hemorrhages that Fisher was able to diagnose clinically were large, and all were accompanied by blood in the cerebrospinal fluid.

Smaller hemorrhages in the thalamus were not recognized until the advent of MRI scanning. Chin-Sang Chung and colleagues in 1996 reviewed the findings among 175 patients with thalamic hemorrhages in various loci in the thalamus according to the distribution of the bleeding artery: tuberothalamic, thalamo-geniculate, thalamic-subthalamic, and posterior choroidal [27]. Midbrain and medullary hemorrhages were not separated from ischemic lesions in those sites until the advent of MRI.

NOTES AND REFERENCES

1. Sections and parts of this chapter have appeared in Caplan LR. *Posterior Circulation Disease: Clinical Findings, Diagnosis, and Management*. Boston: Blackwell Scientific, 1996; Caplan LR. *Vertebrobasilar Ischemia and Hemorrhage: Clinical Findings, Diagnosis, and Management of Posterior Circulation Disease*. Cambridge: Cambridge University Press, 2014; Caplan LR. History of vertebrobasilar territory stroke and TIA. In Kim JS (ed.), *Posterior Circulation Stroke*. Singapore: Springer, 2021, pp. 1–14.

2. Wepfer JJ. *Observationes anatomicae ex cadaveribus eorum, quos sustulit apoplexia, cum exercitatione de ejus loco affecto*. Schaffhausen: J. Caspari Suteri, 1658.

3. Wolf JK. *The Classical Brain Stem Syndromes*. Springfield, IL: Charles C. Thomas, 1971. The various brainstem syndromes are discussed in Chapter 10.

4. Wallenberg A. Acute bulbaraffection (Embolie der art. cerebellar post. inf.sinistr.?). *Arch. Psychiat. Nervenkr.* 1895;27:504–540. Wallenberg A. Anatomischer befund in einem als "acute bulbar affection (embolie der art. cerebellar post. inf. sinistra?)" beschreibenen falle. *Arch. Psychiat. Nervenkr.* 1901;34:923–959. Wallenberg A. Verschluss der arteria cerebelli inferior posterior sinistra. *Neurologische Zentralblatt* 1915;34:236–247. Wallenberg A. Verschluss der arteria cerebelli inferior posterior dextra (mit sektionbefund). *Deutsche Zeitschrift f Nervenheilk* 1922;73:189–212.

5. Duret H. Sur la distribution des arteres nouriclerres du bulb rachidien. *Arch. Physiol. Norm. Path.* 1873 5:97–113. Duret H. Reserches anatomiques sur la circulation de l'encephale. *Arch. Physiol. Norm. Pathol.* 1874;3:60–91, 316–353, 664–693, 919–957.

6. Stopford JSB. The arteries of the pons and medulla oblongata. *J. Anat. Physiol.* 1916;50:131–163, 255–280.

7. Caplan LR. Charles Foix, the first modern stroke neurologist. *Stroke* 1990;21:348–356. The career and contribution of Foix are the topic of Chapter 27.

8. Kubik C, Adams R. Occlusion of the basilar artery: A clinical and pathologic study. *Brain* 1946;69:73–121.

9. Hutchinson EC, Yates PO. The cervical portion of the vertebral artery, a clinicpathological study. *Brain* 1956;79:319–331. Yates PO, Hutchinson EC. Carotico-vertebral stenosis. *Lancet* 1957;1:2–8.

10. Fisher CM. Occlusion of the vertebral arteries. *Arch. Neurol.* 1970;22:13–19.

11. Reivich M, Holling E, Roberts B, Toole JF. Reversal of blood flow through the vertebral artery and its effect on cerebral circulation. *N. Engl. J. Med.* 1961;265:878–885.

12. Hennerici M, Klemm C, Rautenberg W. The subclavian steal phenomenon; a common vascular disorder with rare neurological deficits. *Neurology* 1988;88:669–673.

13. Millikan C, Siekert R. Studies in cerebrovascular disease. The syndrome of intermittent insufficiency of the basilar arterial system. *Mayo Clin. Proc.* 1955;30:61–68.

Bradshaw P, McQuaid P. The syndrome of vertebro-basilar insufficiency. *Quart. J. Med.* 1963;32:279–296. Williams D, Wilson TG. The diagnosis of major and minor syndromes of basilar insufficiency. *Brain* 1962;85:741–774.

14. Millikan C, Siekert R, Shick R. Studies in cerebrovascular disease: The use of anticoagulant drugs in the treatment of insufficiency or thrombosis within the basilar arterial system. *Mayo Clin. Proc.* 1955;30:116–126.

15. Chimowitz M, Lynn MJ, Howlett-Smith H, et al. for the Warfarin-Aspirin Symptomatic Intracranial Disease Trial investigators. Comparison of warfarin and aspirin for symptomatic Intracranial arterial stenosis. *N. Engl. J. Med.* 2005;352:1305–1316.

16. Denny-Brown D. Basilar artery syndromes. *Bull. N. Engl. Med. Center* 1953;15:53–60.

17. Caplan LR. *Vertebrobasilar Ischemia and Hemorrhage: Clinical Findings, Diagnosis, and Management of Posterior Circulation Disease.* Cambridge: Cambridge University Press, 2014.

18. Caplan LR, Chung C-S, Wityk RJ, et al. New England Medical Center posterior circulation stroke registry: I. Methods, data base, distribution of brain lesions, stroke mechanisms, and outcomes. *J. Clin. Neurol.* 2005;1:14–30. Caplan LR, Wityk RJ, Pazdera L, et al. New England Medical Center posterior circulation stroke registry: II. Vascular lesions. *J. Clin. Neurol.* 2005;1:31–49. Glass TA, Hennessey PM, Pazdera L, Chang H-M, Wityk RJ, DeWitt LD, Pessin MD, Caplan LR. Outcome at 30 days in the New England Medical Center Posterior Circulation Registry. *Arch. Neurol.* 2002;59(3):369–376. Searls DE, Pazdera L, Korbel E, Vysata O, Caplan LR. Symptoms and signs of posterior circulation ischemia in the New England Medical Center Posterior Circulation Registry. *Arch. Neurol.* 2012;69(3):346–351.

19. Cheyne J. *Cases of Apoplexy and Lethargy with Observations upon the Comatose Diseases.* London: J. Moyes printer, 1812.

20. Dana CL. Acute bulbar paralysis due to hemorrhage and softening of the pons and medulla with reports of cases and autopsies. *Med. Rec.* 1903;64:361–374.

21. Duret H. *Etudes experimentales et cliniques sur les traumatismes cerebraux.* Paris: V. Adrien Delahayes, 1878. Duret H. *Traumatismes craniocerebraux.* Paris: Librairie Felix Alcan, 1919.

22. Kornyey S. Rapidly fatal pontine hemorrhage: Clinical and anatomical report. *Arch. Neurol. Psychiatry* 1939;41:793–799.

23. Childs T. A case of apoplexy of the cerebellum. *Amer. Med. Month.* 1858;9:1–3.

24. Mitchell N, Angrist A. Spontaneous cerebellar hemorrhage: Report of fifteen cases. *Amer. J. Path.* 1942;18:935–953.

25. McKissock W, Richardson A, Walsh L. Spontaneous cerebellar hemorrhage. *Brain* 1960;83:1–9.

26. Fisher CM, Picard EH, Polak A, Dalal P, Ojemann R. Acute hypertensive cerebellar hemorrhage: Diagnosis and surgical treatment. *J. Nerv. Ment. Dis.* 1965;140:38–57.

27. Chung C-S, Caplan LR, Han W, Pessin MS, Lee K-H, Kim S-M. Thalamic haemorrhage. *Brain* 1996;119:1873–1886.

CHAPTER EIGHTEEN

ANEURYSMS AND SUBARACHNOID HEMORRHAGE

This chapter reviews the history of the diagnosis and evolution of knowledge about subarachnoid hemorrhage (SAH) and brain aneurysms. Chapter 57 discusses management.

As is often true, a main advance in the history of a topic often involves one single patient and one event. So it was in clarifying the relationship between bleeding into the space around the brain and aneurysms located at the base of the brain, a condition now well known as aneurysmal subarachnoid hemorrhage.

HARVEY CUSHING AND SIR CHARLES SYMONDS, 1920

The event occurred during the early days of September 1920 at the Peter Bent Brigham Hospital in Boston, Massachusetts. The three main characters were the neurosurgeon, Harvey Cushing; Charles Symonds, a young neurologist who came to the Brigham to study under Cushing; and the patient, BJH. Both Cushing and Symonds were destined to become giants in the fields of neurosurgery and neurology.

Harvey Cushing was born in Cleveland, Ohio, on April 8, 1869 [1]. Harvey's father was one of the third generation of physicians in the family. Harvey was educated at Yale where he played baseball, and then at Harvard Medical School. After a year as a house intern and surgeon at Massachusetts General Hospital, he received his surgical residency and training under the direction of pioneer surgeon William Halsted at the then fledgling Johns Hopkins Hospital in Baltimore, Maryland. After residency he traveled widely in Europe and gained valuable tutelage from some of the leading surgeons in Europe. He remained at Hopkins from 1896 until 1912 when he became surgeon-in-chief of the newly opened Peter Bent Brigham Hospital in Boston and professor of surgery at Harvard Medical School. At Hopkins, he began to specialize in operating on the brain and its contents. At that time, neurosurgery was not an independent specialty. In 1908 he authored a 259-page chapter in Keen's multivolume surgical textbook [2]. He emphasized the importance of designating neurosurgery as an important subspecialty. He is generally acknowledged as the father of modern neurosurgery. His time in Boston was interrupted by active surgical experience during World War I. Cushing served as the head of a surgical unit in a French military hospital outside Paris. By 1920 when the event occurred, Cushing had already written definitive textbooks on surgery for pituitary tumors and tumors of the acoustic nerve [3]. He had acquired a large neurosurgical practice with many referrals of patients with suspected brain tumors. Trainees and young surgeons traveled to Boston to learn from him.

Like Cushing, Charles ("Charlie") Symonds came from a medical family [4]. Symonds was born in London on April 11, 1890, to the Canadian-born Sir Charters Symonds, surgeon to Guy's Hospital. He matriculated at New College Oxford, graduating with a degree in physiology. He continued his medical training at Guy's Hospital on a scholarship. Like Cushing, Symonds had considerable experience during wartime. At the outbreak of World War I, Symonds left his medical studies and joined the British Army. He saw battlefield action, was wounded in September 1914, and was awarded the Military Medal. He then returned to his medical studies at Guy's Hospital, having resigned his military commission. Symonds completed his medical studies and was appointed to the National Hospital for Neurology and Neurosurgery at Queen Square London and to Guy's Hospital as assistant physician for nervous diseases. In 1920 he received a Radcliffe traveling fellowship, which he used to travel to the United States to study psychiatry under Adolf Meyer at the Johns Hopkins Hospital and neurosurgery with Harvey Cushing at the Peter Bent Brigham Hospital in Boston.

The patient, BJH, was a 52-year-old woman who was admitted to the Peter Bent Brigham Hospital on August 30, 1920. She was examined by Dr. Symonds, among others. Prior to her planned brain tumor surgery, Dr. Cushing reviewed her case with the staff. Symonds commented about that occasion: "We all stood in awe of Cushing, who was a hard taskmaster but demanded of himself the same standards he imposed on others. When I had suggested the diagnosis of intracranial aneurysm in a case in which he was about to operate, he was, to say the least skeptical" [4]. (The story that has been passed down is that Cushing actually said something rather demeaning to Symonds – something like, "Son, you will someday learn the difference between a tumor and an aneurysm.") Cushing performed a right subtemporal decompression on September 3 and found recently clotted blood that extended over the hemisphere. Uncontrollable hemorrhage developed during surgery. The patient died shortly thereafter and an autopsy was performed. Symonds comments in his memoir,

> The only time that Cushing could attend the post-mortem was on the following afternoon, on which most of us, and Cushing himself, had tickets for a great baseball match (at nearby Fenway Park). His edict was that the post-mortem be held at that time and we should be present and we were. When the aneurysm was disclosed he handed me the brain in the basin saying, "Symonds you made the correct diagnosis; either that was a fluke or there was reason in it. If so you will prove it. You will cease your ward duties as from now and spend all your time in the library. Anything you want translated I will arrange for." [4]

The report on intracranial aneurysms was written later but was not published until 1923, after Cushing had added his own addendum [5]. The report described five patients with aneurysmal subarachnoid hemorrhage, including the index case referred to above, and four other patients seen later in London. BJH, prior to her admission to the Brigham, had in 1919, "an illness causing her to take to her bed for 4 weeks which was diagnosed as influenza. With this was associated severe headache, pain in the back of the neck radiating down her back, and vomiting." There was also tinnitus and partial deafness in the right ear. Two weeks before her Brigham hospitalization, she developed severe right supraorbital pain, at first with vomiting, followed by drooping of the right eye. Examination by Symonds showed a right third nerve palsy and right eye papilledema. On the morning before surgery, she had a sudden severe worsening of her right orbital pain and lost consciousness for 20 minutes. After awakening she moaned with pain. That night she regained consciousness, recognized people, and talked freely. She later complained of severe headache radiating down into the back of her neck on the right side and again lost consciousness. Symonds reexamined her before surgery. She was comatose but made occasional purposeful movements of the right arm. The left limbs remained motionless and she now had a left Babinski response. The autopsy performed after the fateful surgery showed that the subdural and subarachnoid spaces at the base were found full of recently coagulated blood. This washed away easily disclosing a small saccular aneurysm about 8 mm in circumference at the junction of the right internal carotid artery and the posterior communicating artery (Figure 18.1). In the outer wall of this sac was a perforation the size of a pin head [5].

In his report with Cushing [5] and later in
more detailed publications [6], Symonds discussed the symptoms, signs, spinal fluid findings,   and   pathology   of   aneurysmal
subarachnoid hemorrhage. He noted: (1)
Often present are symptoms and signs due
to "mechanical pressure upon surrounding
structures – neighborhood signs. These
depend on the localization of the aneurysm."
Headache is often localized, as in BJH's right
temporal region. Pressure on nerves and/or
adjacent brain structures; in BJH a third nerve
paralysis. The third nerve exits from the midbrain and travels near the course of the posterior communicating artery. (2) "The almost
invariable occurrence from the sudden rupture of an artery, even if the subsequent
extravasation be small, of a brief initial loss
of consciousness." BJH had several episodes
of severe headache accompanied by loss of
consciousness. (3) Irritative effects. "In any
case of subarachnoid hemorrhage in which

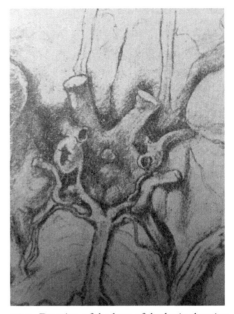

18.1 Drawing of the base of the brain showing
the aneurysm at the junction of the right internal
carotid and posterior communicating arteries.
Reprinted from Symonds C. Studies in
Neurology. London: Oxford University Press,
1970, p. 31, figure 1, with permission.

the extravasation is sufficiently extensive. The signs of meningitis – neck pain
and stiffness, pains in the back and limbs, and Kernig's sign may be expected."
BJH had several prodromal attacks of blood causing meningeal irritation. (4)
Findings "due to the disease which was the primary cause of the aneurysm."
Symonds discusses some cases in his reviews in which patients with bacterial
endocarditis had rupture of mycotic aneurysms. In those patients the presence
of symptoms and signs of endocarditis gave clues to the nature of attacks of
subarachnoid and intracerebral bleeding.

Symonds also reviewed the findings on lumbar puncture and examination
of the cerebrospinal fluid (CSF) [6]. Collection and analysis of the fluid
surrounding the brain was a relatively new technique when Symonds wrote
his reports. Heinrich Irenaeus Quinke, a professor of internal medicine in
Bern, Switzerland, is usually given credit for introducing lumbar puncture into
the armamentarium of medical diagnosis. His reports were published at the end
of the nineteenth and beginning of the twentieth century [7], about two
decades or so before Symonds's subarachnoid hemorrhage papers. Symonds
cited the work of Georges Froin (1874–1932), a French physician, who had
written a thesis about the spinal fluid findings in subarachnoid hemorrhage.
Froin described the gross and microscopic findings as well as the results of
spectroscopy on the fluid [8]. Symonds wrote [6]:

> Shortly after the onset of the hemorrhage, the fluid obtained by lumbar puncture appears on withdrawal to be mixed with blood, and is usually under increased pressure.... The distinctive macroscopic features of the cerebrospinal fluid are: 1) an even admixture of blood which is the same in a series of specimens collected at the same puncture; 2) absence of coagulum, and 3) orange, brown or yellow coloration of the fluid which is apparent when the red cells have been allowed to sink to the bottom of the tube.... The coloration of the supernatant fluid appears to be due to pigments derived from the red cells in process of destruction. The process of haemolysis is most active a few days after the initial effusion.... The rose yellow tint appears to coincide with the height of hemolysis in a large effusion and the spectroscope shows the oxyhaemoglobin or haemoglobin bands.

In his addendum to the initial report, Cushing remarked: "When rupture occurs and the true condition is recognized, whether there are surgical indications such as ligation of the internal carotid, further experience alone can tell" [5].

EARLIER REPORTS OF THE CLINICAL AND PATHOLOGICAL FINDING OF SUBARACHNOID HEMORRHAGE

The earliest description of the clinical findings is probably by Hippocrates, who wrote that "when persons in good health are suddenly seized with pains in the head and straightaway are laid down speechless and breathe with stertor, they die in seven days when fever comes on" [9]. In 1658, Johann Jacob Wepfer (1620–1695) had written a popular and detailed treatise on apoplexy [10]. Wepfer was the first to clearly show that hemorrhage into and around the brain was an important cause of apoplexy.

The next important description of subarachnoid hemorrhage was by Giovani Battista Morgagni (1682–1771), a renowned professor of anatomy at the University of Padua in Italy [11]. Morgagni opined that the extravasation of blood found in the cranium was from "an aneurysmal dilatation of the arteries and an enlargement of their delicate coats. The soft brain substance yielded to the impulse of blood causing apoplexy." Blood-filled cavities could rupture into the ventricles or onto the outer brain surface. Morgagni described five cases of subarachnoid hemorrhage and examples of intracranial aneurysms with and without SAH [11].

John Cheyne (1777–1836), a prominent Irish physician, wrote an influential treatise on apoplexy, which was published in 1812 [12]. One case described subarachnoid hemorrhage:

> Case XII. "A man of considerable literary attainments.... He was a man of inoffensive manners. Rather below the middle size, of a stout make,

with a short neck . . . and temperate in his habits. At 7 o'clock he entered the hall in perfect health and spirits. Soon after he rose to speak . . . but in a few minutes sat down. He complained of headache and sickness and retired to an anteroom where he vomited. His face was pale, there was a cold sweat on his forehead . . . he told me that soon after having begun to speak he felt a headache which rapidly increased to such severity as to give the idea that the sutures of the skull were about to be forced asunder." Later at home the same day "he complained of severe headache and sickness and slight coma had come on . . . it soon settled into complete insensibility until his death." The post-mortem dissection showed: "The surface of the brain appeared deluged with blood, which had insinuated itself between all its convolutions." [12]

Cheyne did not report finding an aneurysm in this patient. Figure 18.2 from Cheyne's monograph shows a brain with SAH at necropsy.

In 1828 John Abercrombie wrote of "primary apoplexy" in which "the apoplectic attack is a sudden deprivation of sense and motion, the patient falling down as in a profound sleep, the face being generally flushed, and the breathing stertorous. . . . In many cases the disease is speedily fatal, and we find on inspection, extensive extravasation of blood" [13]. Abercrombie wrote of the source of the bleeding in some cases: "from the rupture of small aneurysms in various parts of the cerebral vessels." He cites a case previously reported of a basilar artery aneurysm "as large as a small hen's egg": "A pound of blood had been discharged by the rupture of it" [13].

During the first half of the nineteenth century, physicians began to publish atlases illustrating human anatomy, clinical findings, and pathology. Richard Bright (1789–1858), an English physician and early pioneer in the research of kidney disease, was also very interested in apoplexy [14,15]. A subsection of his large atlas dealt with intracranial hemorrhage. Five cases are described in which "the effusion of blood has been found upon the surface of the brain." Bright gives detailed descriptions of the symptoms that characterize subarachnoid hemorrhage. In one of these cases, a 19-year-old man "while sitting on the

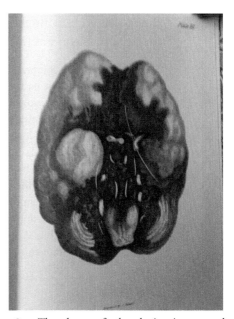

18.2 The base of the brain is covered extensively with a coagulum of blood owing to a rupture of the anterior artery of the cerebrum of the left side. From Cheyne J. *Cases of Apoplexy and Lethargy with Observations upon the Comatose Diseases.* London: J. Moyes printer, 1812. Reprinted in The Classics of Neurology and Neurosurgery Library, New York: Gryphon editions, 1986, plate III. Reprinted with permission.

chamber utensil suddenly exclaimed, 'Oh my head.'" Bright found blood on the surface of the brain and a ruptured, partially clotted middle cerebral artery aneurysm [14].

PRIOR REPORTS OF BRAIN ANEURYSMS

Morgagni wrote of "aneurysmal dilatation of cerebral vessels," but the first clear description of an aneurysm was probably by Francesco Biumi, an Italian physician, who in 1765 described a case of apoplexy in which, although there was no subarachnoid bleeding, an internal carotid aneurysmal sac was found in the cavernous sinus [16]. This was likely the first description of an unruptured aneurysm. In 1980, Gilbert Blane, a prominent British physician, published a detailed report that described bilateral carotid artery aneurysms [17]. The renowned surgeon John Hunter, a close colleague of Blane, performed the autopsy. After Bright's report [14] cited above, many physicians described finding aneurysms at necropsy, although few were found in patients who died of subarachnoid hemorrhage.

Sir William Withey Gull, a prominent Guy's Hospital physician and a colleague of William Bright, commented in 1859 on the scarcity of reports of intracranial aneurysms [18]:

> Aneurism of the cerebral vessels has been regarded as a disease of extreme rarity The apparent rarity, however, is doubtful . . . there is more reason to suspect it is only apparent and is due to careless inquiry. There are several reasons why intracranial aneurysm is likely to be overlooked. First of all, it has not been looked for.... When death occurs from rupture of the sac, recent coagula may so imbed and conceal it that unless strictly looked for it will not be found, for the sac is often small, and thin, and transparent, except at the point of rupture.... Unless a minute dissection be made, its true nature may not be discovered. Whenever young persons die with symptoms of ingravescent apoplexy, and after death large effusion of blood is found, especially if the effusion be over the surface of the brain in the meshes of the pia mater, the presence of an aneurysm is probable.

ANEURYSMAL SAH AFTER THE SYMONDS-CUSHING REPORT

Technological Advances: Angiography and CT Scanning

Symonds characterized the clinical findings in patients with aneurysmal sub-arachnoid hemorrhage but there were no available tests other than lumbar puncture that could substantiate bleeding and no investigations that could identify brain aneurysms. Further information and research had to wait for advances in technology. During the 1950s and 1960s arteriography of the arteries that supplied the brain became more feasible. Egas Moniz, in Portugal, introduced the technique of dye angiography into clinical medicine and neurology during the late 1920s [19]. Angiography initially involved a surgical cutdown on the artery to be studied. Contrast agents were potentially dangerous and filming was tedious and very inefficient. When I (LRC) was a stroke fellow during 1969–1970, angiography was performed by direct puncture of the carotid and vertebral arteries in the neck. The angiographer speared the artery against the bone, entered the lumen when the needle was pulled back toward the surface, and blood shot out under arterial pressure. The patient often looked up at the doctor anxiously. Injection was by hand and X-ray plates were hand pulled depending on the desired timing of the films. Only one plane could be filmed at a time. Each artery studied had to be pierced sequentially. The procedure was gruesome for the patient (and for the fellow) and was probably relatively dangerous. The movie *The Exorcist* (1973) featured a graphic depiction of a direct carotid stick.

An important advance in angiography was made when Sven Ivar Seldinger, in 1953, introduced angiography by catheterization of the femoral artery, allowing selective catheterization of all the vessels to be studied [20]. Selective catheter angiography become more widely used only decades later. During the 1970s, there were many changes and improvements in angiography performance: trained, experienced, full-time neuroradiologists began to perform the procedure; newer, safer dyes were developed and introduced; biplane filming techniques were perfected. These advances led to safer, more useful angiography. Digital subtraction angiography (DSA) was introduced in the 1980s as a method that used intravenous injection of contrast to image the arterial system. During the ensuing decades, the spatial resolution of DSA imaging improved. Further technical refinements included rotational angiography, 3D angiography, and flat panel detectors for imaging.

The introduction of computed tomography (CT) scanning into clinical practice in the 1970s further improved evaluation of patients with suspected SAH. Now physicians could see the locations and extent of bleeding into the subarachnoid space and the brain. These technical advances paved the way for research and data gathering in patients with brain aneurysms and in those suspected of having intracranial bleeding.

NATURAL HISTORY AND REBLEEDING

Once tools to diagnose patients with SAH and aneurysms became widely available, physicians began to collect data about natural history. Aneurysmal SAH was found to be a condition with very high mortality and long-term morbidity. Among 100 typical patients with SAH caused by ruptured aneurysms, about one third died before receiving medical attention; another one fifth died while in the hospital or remained incapacitated from the original hemorrhage; 17 patients who survived the initial hemorrhage deteriorated later, 8 patients recovered, and 9 patients were left with severe neurological deficits [21]. A delay often occurred in referring patients with SAH to neurological and neurosurgical centers for treatment.

Early observations and research led to attempts to predict prognosis by assigning grades of severity. The most commonly reported grading system was produced by neurologist and neurosurgeon William Hunt (a describer of the Tolosa-Hunt syndrome) and neurosurgeon Robert M. Hess, who worked together at Ohio State University. The grades were designed to predict the risk of surgery in patients with various grades of severity at the time of proposed surgery [22]. The grades they assigned (Hunt and Hess classification) were: grade 1: asymptomatic or minimal headache and slight neck stiffness; grade 2: moderate to severe headache, neck stiffness, no neurologic deficit except cranial nerve palsy; grade 3: drowsy, minimal neurologic deficit; grade 4: stuporous, moderate to severe hemiparesis, possibly early decerebrate rigidity and vegetative disturbances; and grade 5: deep coma, decerebrate rigidity, moribund [22]. These grades were in general used throughout the ensuing decades.

After the patient was admitted to the hospital, a major threat was rebleeding, recurrent aneurysmal rupture. The initial and subsequent bleeds were major causes of death in patients with aneurysmal SAH. In one study that had a 45 percent (36/80) mortality, 64 percent (23/36) of deaths were attributable to the initial SAH and 8 of the remaining 13 deaths were caused by recurrent hemorrhages [23]. The mortality rate in patients who rebled were as high as 50 percent [21,23]. Rebleeding was often heralded by the sudden onset of severe headache. Rebleeds tended to be both intraparenchymal and subarachnoid. Bleeding into the brain was more common than during the original aneurysm rupture. Signs included meningismus, focal neurological abnormalities associated with intraparenchymal hemorrhage, and often rapid development of coma. Among aneurysms that rebled, approximately 20 percent did so in the first two weeks, 30 percent by the end of the first month, and 40 percent by the end of six months. Beyond six months, re-rupture occurred at a rate of about 3 percent per year [21,22].

An early strategy used to prevent rebleeding was the administration of an antifibrinolytic agent, especially Amicar (aminocaproic acid). The rationale was that after the first bleed, a small clot filled the site of rupture. Fibrinolytic activity could theoretically lyse the thrombus capping the bleeding site and so lead to rebleeding. Although Amicar decreased the rate of rebleeding, it did not improve morbidity or mortality. Vasoconstriction, thrombophlebitis with pulmonary embolism, and hydrocephalus were more common in patients given antifibrinolytic agents [24].

Neurologists and neurosurgeons recognized that many patients, while recovering from the initial bleed, developed headache, decreased alertness, and sometimes focal neurological signs and did not have rebleeding. CT scans in these patients sometimes showed brain edema and localized areas of infarction but no new intracranial bleeding. When these patients had angiography, narrowing of intracranial arteries, as a result of vasoconstriction (vasospasm), was found. These patients often had unfavorable outcomes.

DELAYED CEREBRAL INFARCTION AND VASOCONSTRICTION

During the 1960s, British physician and pathologist M. R. Crompton wrote an MD thesis on the presence of brain infarcts found at necropsy in patients with aneurysmal SAH. That study was published in the journal *Brain* in 1964 [25]. Crompton noted that hypothalamic lesions were also often found at necropsy in patients who had ruptured aneurysm during life [26]. Although he speculated on the cause of the infarction, clinical studies before death were meager.

C. Miller Fisher, the first full-time neurological stroke specialist in the United States [27], and his colleagues at Massachusetts General Hospital were among the first to research brain infarction and vasoconstriction in patients with aneurysmal SAH. They observed that, often during the end of the first week after aneurysmal rupture, patients developed focal neurological deficits unrelated to rupture of an aneurysm. CT scans in these patients often showed a localized brain infarct. At autopsy brain infarcts were found. Fisher and his colleagues Glenn Roberson, a neuroradiologist, and Bob Ojemann, a neurosurgeon, called this condition delayed ischemic deficits (DID) (but in later years delayed cerebral infarction (DCI) was the more often used term) and studied the relationship of the ischemic lesions to constriction of intracranial arteries ("vasospasm") shown by angiography [28]. They reported in 1977 on the results of a study of 50 patients who had verified intracranial ruptured saccular aneurysms, among whom half developed a delayed ischemic deficit most often on the eighth day after the initial bleed. All of these patients had severe vasospasm shown by cerebral angiography. When vasospasm was absent, delayed infarction did not occur. With the aid of Phillip Kistler, Fisher and colleagues analyzed the relation of the amount and localization of blood to the development of vasospasm. They grouped patients according to the CT findings: Group 1: no detectable blood on CT; Group 2: diffuse blood that was not dense enough to represent a large, thick homogenous clot; Group 3: Dense collection of blood that represented a clot greater than 1 millimeter thick in the vertical plane or greater than 5 × 3 millimeters in longitudinal and transverse dimension in the horizontal plane; and Group 4: Intracerebral or intraventricular clots but with only diffuse blood or no blood in the basal cisterns [28,29]. The frequency of vasospasm increased with increasing grades in this scale. This method of grading blood on CT scans in patients with subarachnoid hemorrhage became widely used and was known as the "Fisher scale."

Two physicians merit mention for heavily contributing to research and knowledge about DCI and vasoconstriction, Nicholas Zervas and R. Loch McDonald. Each had a strong connection to the University of Chicago where Zervas attended medical school and McDonald was a professor of neurosurgery. Zervas was the Distinguished Higgins Professor of Neurosurgery at Harvard Medical School and was chair of neurosurgery, first at the Beth Israel Hospital then at Massachusetts General Hospital. Zervas was the longest serving chairman of the department of neurosurgery at Mass General. He was one of the first neurosurgery chairs to develop subspecialty neurosurgery groups in vascular disease, brain tumors, the spine, and other areas. McDonald spent much of his career as a professor of neurosurgery in Toronto, Canada.

Zervas and McDonald and colleagues investigated the necropsy findings in patients who had evidence of vasoconstriction during life. They found that patients who died from SAH who had vasoconstriction during less than three weeks after the initial hemorrhage showed necrosis of the media of cranial arteries, while patients who survived longer than three weeks showed marked concentric intimal thickening, subendothelial fibrosis, and medial atrophy [30]. The arterial adventitia showed an adherent clot with inflammatory cell infiltrates and degeneration of perivascular nerve terminals. The arterial media showed smooth muscle contraction with varying degrees of fibrosis and necrosis. The intima developed longitudinal furrows and endothelial cells were often desquamated or necrosed, and showed abnormalities of intercellular tight junctions [30]. Longer duration of vasoconstriction led to persistent morphological changes. The term "vasospasm" was incorrect since spasm conveyed the idea of temporary luminal contraction. Vasoconstriction was a more apt term.

The mechanism of vasoconstriction was also thoroughly investigated [31]. The peak timing for vasoconstriction was found to be between days 5 to 9 after the initial bleed. Most vasospasm resolved after the second week. Vasoconstriction was related to the release of substances into the CSF from the subarachnoid blood and the interaction of these substances with the arteries in the subarachnoid space. Erythrocytes and their subsequent hemolysis were shown to be necessary for vasospasm to develop. The most likely putative substance was oxyhemoglobin, which affects the function of platelet-derived growth factor, released from platelets adherent to the arterial wall; endothelial factors, especially endothelial-derived relaxing factor; and components of the coagulation cascade, especially thrombin, plasmin, and fibrinogen. These substances cause abnormal contraction or failure of relaxation of the arterial smooth muscle cells in the intracranial arteries bathed in blood [31].

Because calcium influx into vessel walls was a known mechanism of constriction of arterial lumens, doctors treating individuals at risk of developing vasoconstriction prescribed calcium channel–blocking drugs. These agents also were known to lower blood pressure. The most common agents used were nimodipine and nicardipine, rapid-acting calcium channel blockers.

The potential mechanisms of action of nimodipine, nicardipine, and other calcium channel blockers include a decrease in vasoconstriction, improved blood flow by dilation of collateral arteries, neuronal protection by decreasing entry of calcium into cells, and improvement of blood rheology. Therapeutic trials showed that nimodipine improved outcome and decreased the frequency of DCI [32]. A systematic review of 10 trials (including 2,756 patients) of calcium channel blockers in patients with SAH reported a 33 percent relative risk reduction in the frequency of ischemic neurological deficits and a 20 percent relative risk reduction in the development of infarcts on CT scans [33]. Administration of calcium channel–blocking agents sometimes caused hypotension and decreased renal function, especially when the drugs were given intravenously, so that blood pressure, urinary output, and renal function had to be carefully monitored. If vasoconstriction developed and did not respond to intravenous agents, endovascular angioplasty (mechanical dilatation of the arteries in spasm by balloons) and/or intraarterial infusions of vasodilators such as calcium channel blockers or papaverine were used, often successfully [34].

An important advance in the diagnosis and quantification of vasoconstriction occurred during the 1980s when transcranial Doppler (TCD) ultrasound began to be used to monitor SAH patients. One of the first clinical applications studied by Rune Aaslid (the developer of TCD) in collaboration with a group of Norwegian, Swiss, and German pioneers was in subarachnoid hemorrhage [35]. Blood in the subarachnoid space stimulated arteries at the base of the brain to constrict increasing blood flow velocities within these vessels. TCD could detect and quantitate the severity of this vasoconstriction. Increased blood-flow velocities measured by TCD correlated well with angiographically documented vasoconstriction [36]. In many medical centers TCD was used routinely to monitor SAH patients.

OTHER SEQUALAE AND COMPLICATIONS IN PATIENTS WITH ANEURYSMAL SAH

Many patients had poor outcomes unrelated to rebleeding and DCI. When patients with SAH were studied thoroughly in academic medical centers throughout the world other issues and problems were identified.

Hydrocephalus. CT scans often showed ventricular enlargement. Acute hydrocephalus was caused by alteration in normal CSF dynamics. CSF flow was blocked by blood in the cisterns around the brainstem and reabsorption was impaired when blood attached to pacchionian granulations. The syndrome was recognized clinically by worsening headache, lethargy, incontinence, and decreased spontaneity. Lumbar punctures with removal of CSF often sufficed to treat the ventricular enlargement. Temporary draining tubes or shunts were occasionally required to manage hydrocephalus [37].

Cardiopulmonary issues. Some patients with SAH had "waterfall T waves" on electrocardiograms, mimicking myocardial infarction. Further studies showed that these patients also had cardiac enzyme elevations mimicking myocardial infarction, regional left ventricular wall motion abnormalities, and cardiac arrhythmias [38]. Echocardiography often showed that the changes were explained by Takotsubo cardiomyopathy, a condition characterized by transient hypokinesis of the left ventricle often brought on by stress [39]. Acute pulmonary edema was also an occasional clinical finding [40].

Fluid, electrolyte, and endocrine abnormalities. Less common, but an important cause of neurological worsening, were fluid and electrolyte abnormalities. Slight sodium and potassium shifts without clinical consequence occurred often. In one eighth of patients, more severe abnormalities included diabetes insipidus, inappropriate secretion of antidiuretic hormone, and serious sodium and potassium shifts. In these patients, the serum sodium was often less than 130 mEq/liter and the potassium was greater than 5 mEq/liter. Hyponatremia was associated with a poor prognosis and was attributed to inappropriate secretion of antidiuretic hormone and elevated levels of plasma atrial natriuretic factor [41].

DEMOGRAPHY, EPIDEMIOLOGY, FAMILY, AND GENETIC INFORMATION ABOUT RUPTURED AND UNRUPTURED BRAIN ANEURYSMS

The Dutch, led by Jan van Gijn and Gabriel Rinkle, became leaders in developing useful data about brain aneurysms. The Netherlands is a small country. The leaders in stroke were trained together and continued to actively work together and to work avidly with the excellent primary care physicians in the Netherlands. Patients with suspected SAH were admitted to the neurology department and cared for jointly by both neurologists and neurosurgeons. Record keeping and following of patients were exemplary. Acute and long-term outcomes, familial incidence, and genetics were assiduously studied [42].

Studies showed that aneurysms were more common in women and that multiple aneurysms were present in about 14–24 percent of patients. In patients with multiple aneurysms, two were present in about three fourths, three in one eighth, and four or more in one twelfth. Saccular aneurysms were found to be more common in patients with polycystic kidney disease, coarctation of the aorta, fibromuscular dysplasia, pseudoxanthoma elasticum, and

Marfan's syndrome. About 7–20 percent of patients with a ruptured aneurysm had a first- or second-degree relative with an intracranial aneurysm. Among first-degree relatives of a patient who has had a ruptured intracranial aneurysm, the risk of having a ruptured intracranial aneurysm is approximately four times higher than in the general population. Dutch researchers suggested that late teenage and adult first-degree relatives in families where two or more first-degree relatives were shown to have a cerebral aneurysm should be screened with magnetic resonance angiography (MRA) or computed tomography angiography (CTA) for the presence of aneurysms [42].

Unruptured aneurysms are often found in the following: in patients who have had vascular studies for other indications; as additional aneurysms in patients with an aneurysmal rupture; in patients investigated because of a familial tendency; and in those studied because of a condition known to predispose to aneurysm formation, for example, polycystic kidney disease. Clinicians studied factors that might influence rupture of these previously unruptured aneurysms. Aneurysms ruptured at any time, but especially when blood pressure or blood flow were increased. Rupture often occurred during strenuous activity, such as weight lifting, exercise, coition, defecation, and heavy work, although many aneurysms leaked during relatively inactive periods and during sleep. Size, location, shape, and presence of daughter outpouchings were studied. Large aneurysms were more likely to rupture than smaller ones. In different autopsy series, the critical size for rupture has varied from 7 to 10 millimeters [43]. Aneurysms larger than 10 millimeters in diameter are more likely to rupture during follow-up than smaller aneurysms; however, many aneurysms that rupture are small. Hypertension and smoking are risk factors for the development of aneurysms and for their rupture. The highest risk is in women over 55 who have hypertension and smoke cigarettes [43].

NONANEURYSMAL SAH

Perimesencephalic Hemorrhages

In patients with aneurysmal SAH, the usual pattern of blood is located at the base of the brain and is widely disseminated in the sylvian fissures and subarachnoid spaces. Jan Van Gijn and colleagues noted that many patients with SAHs located predominantly in the perimesencephalic cisterns on CT scans had normal cerebral angiography [44]. Newer-generation CT scans and MRI showed that these hemorrhages were often centered around the prepontine cistern. Because these hemorrhages were concentrated around the brain stem, they are also referred to as pretruncal subarachnoid hemorrhages (truncus cerebri is another term for the brain stem), rather than perimesencephalic [45]. The clinical course in patients with pretruncal hemorrhage is different from aneurysmal SAH because few patients died, rebled acutely, or developed delayed cerebral infarction or hydrocephalus. The outcome is more benign than in patients with aneurysms shown by angiography [44].

Other Causes

Clinicians always recognized that trauma could cause blood in the subarachnoid region. This was common in neonates after traversing the birth canal. Bleeding disorders and hypertensive crises were also recognized as sources of SAH. MRI especially using susceptibility and T2$\star$ images began to show superficial bleeding in the subarachnoid space mainly in regions along the convexity of the brain. In older patients, the predominant cause of these local hemorrhages, often associated with superficial hemosiderosis, was cerebral amyloid angiopathy. In younger patients, the commonest cause was the reversible cerebral vasoconstriction syndrome, which also often began with a thunderclap headache mimicking aneurysmal SAH. Intracranial venous occlusions and dural fistulas were other rarer etiologies [46].

NOTES AND REFERENCES

1. Two detailed biographies describe the main life events and accomplishments of Harvey Cushing: Fulton J. *Harvey Cushing: A Biography – The Story of a Great Medical Pioneer.* Springfield, IL: Charles C. Thomas, 1946. Bliss M. *Harvey Cushing: A Life in Surgery.* New York: Oxford University Press, 2007.

2. Cushing H. Surgery of the head. In Keen WW (ed.), *Surgery: Its Principles and Practice.* Philadelphia: WB Saunders, 1911.

3. Cushing H. *Tumors of the Nervus Acusticus and the Syndrome of the Cerebellopontile Angle.* Philadelphia: WB Saunders, 1917. Cushing H. *The Pituitary Body and Its Disorders; Clinical States Produced by Disorders of the Hypophysis Cerebri. An Amplification of the Harvey Lecture for December, 1910.* Philadelphia: JB Lippincott, 1912.

4. Biographical information about Sir Charles Symonds was derived from the entry for Charles Symonds in Wikipedia. Available at https://en.wikipedia.org/wiki/Charles_Symonds. Shorvon S, Compston A. *Queen Square: A History of the Natil Hospital and Its Institute of Neurology.* Cambridge: Cambridge University Press, 2019, pp. 239–249. Symonds C. *Studies in Neurology: Autobiographical Introduction.* London: Oxford University Press, 1970, pp. 1–23.

5. Symonds C. Contributions to the clinical study of intracranial aneurysms, with Harvey Cushing. *Guy's Hospital Reports* 1923;73:139–158. The paper is reprinted in Symonds C. *Studies in Neurology.* London: Oxford University Press, 1970, pp. 27–47.

6. Symonds C. Spontaneous subarachnoid haemorrhage. *Quarterly Journal of Medicine* 1924;18:93–122. The paper is reprinted in Symonds C. *Studies in Neurology.* London: Oxford University Press, 1970, pp. 48–77, and Symonds CP. Spontaneous subarachnoid haemorrhage. *Proceedings of the Royal Society of Medicine* 1924;17(Neurology Section):39–52.

7. Quincke HI. *Verhandlungen des Congresses Innere Medizin.* Wiesbaden, 1891, 10:321–331. Quincke HI. *Die Technik der Lumbalpunktion.* Berlin, 1902.

8. Froin G. Les hémorrhagies sous-arachnoïdiennes et le méchanism de l'hématolyse en général. Thesis, Hôpitaux de Paris, 1904.

9. Hippocrates's work is described in Chapter 1 of this book. Clark E. Apoplexy in the Hippocratic writings. *Bulletin of the History of Medicine* 1963;37:301–314. Adams F. *Aphorisms of Hippocrates*. London: Dodo Press, 2009. Adams F. *Hippocrates: The Book of Prognostics*. London: Dodo Press, 2009.

10. Wepfer JJ. *Observationes anatomicae ex cadaveribus eorum, quos sustulit apoplexia, cum exercitatione de ejus loco affecto*. Schaffhausen: J. Caspari Suteri, 1658. Wepfer's contributions are described in Chapter 8.

11. Chapter 7 contains much more detail about Morgagni and his life, works, and influence. Morgagni GB. *The Seats and Causes of Diseases Investigated by Anatomy*. Trans. B. Alexander. London: Miller and Cadell, 1769.

12. Cheyne J. *Cases of Apoplexy and Lethargy with Observations upon the Comatose Diseases*. London: J. Moyes printer, 1812. Reprinted in The Classics of Neurology and Neurosurgery Library, Division of Gryphon editions, New York, 1986. Cheyne's work is discussed in Chapter 8.

13. Abercrombie J. *Pathological and Practical Researches on Diseases of the Brain and Spinal Cord*. Edinburgh: Waugh and Innes, 1828. Reprinted in The Classics of Neurology and Neurosurgery Library, Division of Gryphon editions, New York, 1993.

14. Bright R. *Reports of Medical Cases, Selected with a View of Illustrating the Symptoms and Cure of Diseases by a Reference to Morbid Anatomy. vol. II: Diseases of the Brain and Nervous System*. London: Longman, Rees, Orme, Brown, and Green, 1831. Bright and his work is described in more detail in Chapter 9.

15. Bright R. Cases illustrative of the effects produced when the arteries and brain are diseased. *Guy's Hospital Reports* 1836;1:9–16.

16. Biumi F. Observations anatomicae, scholiis ilustratae. Observatio V. In Sandifort E (ed.), *Thesaurus dissertationum*, vol. 3. Leyden: S et J Luchtmans, 1778, pp. 373–379.

17. Blane C. Case of aneurisms of the carotid arteries. *Trans. Soc. Improv. Med. Chir. Knowledge (London)* 1800;2.

18. The quote is from Gull WW. Cases of aneurism of the cerebral vessels. *Guy's Hospital Reports* 1859; 5:281–304. It is also reprinted in Symonds C. *Studies in Neurology*. London: Oxford University Press, 1970, pp. 27–47.

19. The topic of cerebral angiography is discussed in more detail in Chapter 25 and in Krayenbühl H. History of cerebral angiography and its development since Egaz Moniz. In *Egas Moniz Centenary: Scientific Reports*. Lisbon: Comissao Executiva das Comemoracoes do Centenario do Nascimento do Prof. Egas Moniz, 1977, pp. 63–74. Moniz E. L'encephalographie arterielle, son importance dans la localization des tumeurs cerebrales. *Rev. Neurol.* 1927;2 72–90. Moniz E. *L'angiographie cerebrale. Ses applications et resultats en anatomie, physiologie, et clinique*. Paris: Masson et Cie, 1931.

20. Seldinger SI. Catheter replacement of the needle in percutaneous arteriography. *Acta Radiol.* 1953;39:368–376.

21. Reviews of the natural history of aneurysmal SAH are found in Locksley HB. Report of the Cooperative Study of Intracranial Aneurysms and Subarachnoid Hemorrhage: Sec. V, part II. Natural history of subarachnoid hemorrhage, intracranial aneurysms, and arteriovenous malformation. *J. Neurosurg.* 1966;25:321–368. Weir B. *Aneurysms Affecting the Central Nervous System*. Baltimore, MD: Williams & Wilkins, 1987. Van Gign J, Kerr RS, Rinkel GJE. Subarachnoid haemorrhage. *Lancet* 2007;369:306–318. Jovin T, Caplan LR. Subarachnoid hemorrhage, aneurysms, and vascular malformations. In Caplan LR (ed.), *Caplan's Stroke*, 5th ed. Cambridge: Cambridge University Press, 2016, pp. 439–476.

22. Hunt WE, Meagher JN, Hess RM. Intracranial aneurysm: A nine-year study. *Ohio State Med. J.* 1966 Nov;62(11):1168–1171. Hunt WE, Hess RM. Surgical risk as related to time of intervention in the repair of intracranial aneurysms. *J. Neurosurg.* 1968 Jan;28 (1):14–20.

23. Broderick JP, Brott TG, Duldner JE, et al. Initial and recurrent bleeding are the major causes of death following subarachnoid hemorrhage. *Stroke* 1994;25:1342–1347. Suarez JI, Tarr RW, Selman WR. Aneurysmal subarachnoid hemorrhage. *N. Engl. J. Med.* 2006;354:387–396.

24. Mullan S, Dawley J. Antifibrinolytic therapy for intracranial aneurysms. *J. Neurosurg.* 1968 Jan;28(1):21–23. Kassell N, Torner D, Adams H. Antifibrinolytic therapy in the acute period following aneurysmal subarachnoid hemorrhage. *J. Neurosurg.* 1984;61:225–230.

25. Crompton MR. The pathogenesis of cerebral infarction following rupture of cerebral berry aneurysms. *Brain* 1964;87:491–510.

26. Crompton MR. Hypothalamic lesions following the rupture of cerebral berry aneurysms. *Brain* 1963;86:301–314.

27. Chapter 29 discusses Fisher's life and contributions to stroke. Fisher's life story is described in Caplan LR. *C. Miller Fisher: Stroke in the 20th* Century. New York: Oxford University Press, 2020.

28. Fisher CM, Roberson GH, Ojemann RG. Cerebral vasospasm with ruptured saccular aneurysm: The clinical manifestations. *Neurosurgery* 1977;1:245–248. Fisher CM, Kistler JP, Davis JM. Relation of cerebral vasospasm to subarachnoid hemorrhage visualized by computerized tomographic scanning. *Neurosurgery* 1980;6(1):1–9.

29. Kistler JP, Crowell RM, Davis KR, Heros R, Ojemann RG, Zervas NT, Fisher CM. The relation of cerebral vasospasm to the extent and location of subarachnoid blood visualized by CT scan: A prospective study. *Neurology* 1983;33:424–437.

30. Conway LW, McDonald LW. Structural changes of the intradural arteries following subarachnoid hemorrhage. *J. Neurosurg.* 1972;37:715–723. Hughes JT, Schianchi PM. Cerebral artery spasm: A histological study at necropsy of the blood vessels in cases of subarachnoid hemorrhage. *J. Neurosurg.* 1978;48:515–525. Wellum GR, Peterson JW, Zervas NT. The relevance of in vivo smooth muscle experiments to cerebral vasospasm. *Stroke* 1985;16:573–581.

31. Heros RC, Zervas NT, Varsos V. Cerebral vasospasm after subarachnoid hemorrhage: An update. *Ann. Neurol.* 1983;14:599–608. Heros RC, Zervas NT, Varsos V. Cerebral vasospasm after subarachnoid hemorrhage: An update. *Ann. Neurol.* 1983;14:599–608. Macdonald RL, Weir BKA. A review of hemoglobin and the pathogenesis of cerebral vasospasm. *Stroke* 1991;22:971–982. Macdonald RL. Cerebral vasospasm. In Welch KMA, Caplan LR, Reis DJ, et al. (eds.), *Primer on Cerebrovascular Diseases*. San Diego, CA: Academic, 1997, pp. 490–497.

32. Pickard JD, Murray GD, Illingworth R, et al. Effect of oral nimodipine in cerebral infarction and outcome after subarachnoid hemorrhage: British aneurysm nimodipine trial. *BMJ* 1981;298:636–642. Allen GS. Cerebral arterial spasm: A controlled trial of nimodipine in subarachnoid hemorrhage patients – The Nimodipine Cerebral Arterial Spasm Study Group. *Stroke* 1983;14:122.

33. Feigin VL, Rinkel GJE, Algra A, et al. Calcium antagonists in patients with aneurysmal subarachnoid hemorrhage: A systematic review. *Neurology* 1998;50:876–883.

34. Higashida RT, Halbach VV, Cahan LD, et al. Transluminal angioplasty for treatment of intracranial arterial vasospasm. *J. Neurosurg.* 1989;71:648–653. Hoh BL, Ogilvy CS.

Endovascular treatment of cerebral vasospasm: Transluminal balloon angioplasty, intra-arterial papaverine, and intra-arterial nicardipine. *Neurosurg. Clin. N. Am.* 2005;16:501–516.

35. Chapter 34 discusses the history of ultrasound and of transcranial Doppler imaging. Aaslid R (ed.). *Transcranial Doppler Sonography*. Wien: Springer-Verlag, 1986.

36. Sloan MA, Haley EC, Kassell NF, et al. Sensitivity and specificity of transcranial Doppler ultrasonography in the diagnosis of vasospasm following subarachnoid hemorrhage. *Neurology* 1989;391:1514–1518. Sekhar L, Wechsler L, Yonas H, et al. Value of transcranial Doppler examination in the diagnosis of cerebral vasospasm after subarachnoid hemorrhage. *Neurosurgery* 1988;22:813–821. Davis SM, Andrews JT, Lichtenstein M, et al. Correlations between cerebral arterial velocities, blood flow, and delayed ischemia after subarachnoid hemorrhage. *Stroke* 1992;23:492–497.

37. Graff-Radford NR, Torner J, Adams HP, Kassell NF. Factors associated with hydrocephalus after subarachnoid hemorrhage. *Arch. Neurol.* 1989;46:744–752.

38. Caplan LR, Hurst JW. Cardiac and cardiovascular findings in patients with nervous system diseases. In Caplan LR, Hurst JW, Chimowitz MI (eds.), *Clin. Neurocardiol.* New York: Marcel Dekker, 1999, pp. 298–312.

39. Lee VH, Connolly HM, Fulgham JR, Manno EM, Brown RD Jr, Wijdicks EF. Takotsubo cardiomyopathy in aneurismal subarachnoid hemorrhage: An underappreciated ventricular dysfunction. *J. Neurosurg.* 2006;105:264–270.

40. Ciongoli AK, Poser CM. Pulmonary edema secondary to subarachnoid hemorrhage. *Neurology* 1972;22:867–870. Weir BK. Pulmonary edema following fatal aneurysmal rupture. *J. Neurosurg.* 1978;49:502–507.

41. Takaku A, Shindo K, Tanaki S, et al. Fluid and electrolyte disturbances in patients with intracranial aneurysms. *Surg. Neurol.* 1979;11:349–356. Diringer MN, Lim JS, Kirsch JR, Hawley DF. Suprasellar and intraventricular blood predict elevated plasma atrial natriuretic factor in subarachnoid hemorrhage. *Stroke* 1991;22:572–581. Wijdicks EFM, Ropper AH, Hunnicutt EJ, et al. Atrial natriuretic factor and salt wasting after aneurysmal subarachnoid hemorrhage. *Stroke* 1991;22:1519–1524.

42. Van Gijn J, Kerr RS, Rinkel GJE. Subarachnoid haemorrhage. *Lancet* 2007;369:306–318. Bromberg JE, Rinkel GJ, Algra A, et al. Familial subarachnoid hemorrhage: Distinctive features and patterns of inheritance. *Ann. Neurol.* 1995;38:929–934. Raaymakers TW, Rinkel GJ, Ramos LM. Initial and follow-up screening for aneurysms in families with familial subarachnoid hemorrhage. *Neurology* 1998;51:1125–1130. Ruigrok YM, Rinkel GJE. Genetics of intracranial aneurysms. *Stroke* 2008;39:1049–1055. Zuurbier CCM, Greving JP, Rinkel GJE, Ruigrok YM. Higher risk of intracranial aneurysms and subarachnoid hemorrhage in siblings of families with intracranial aneurysms. *Euro. Stroke J.* 2020;5;73–77.

43. Rinkel GJE, Djibuti M, Algra A, van Gijn J. Prevalence and risk of rupture of intracranial aneurysms: A systematic review. *Stroke* 1998;29:251–256. The International Study of Unruptured Intracranial Aneurysms Investigators. Unruptured intracranial aneurysms: Risk of rupture and risks of surgical intervention. *N. Engl. J. Med.* 1998;339:1725–1733. Vlak MH, Rinkel GJE, Greebe P, Algra A. Independent risk factors for intracranial aneurysms and their joint effect: A case-control study. *Stroke* 2013;44:984–987.

44. Van Gijn J, van Dongen KJ, Vermeulan M, et al. Perimesencephalic hemorrhage: A nonaneurysmal and benign form of subarachnoid hemorrhage. *Neurology* 1985;35:483–487. Rinkel GJ, Wijdicks E, Vermeulen M, et al. The clinical course of

perimesencephalic nonaneurysmal subarachnoid hemorrhage. *Ann. Neurol.* 1991;29:463–468.

45. Schievink WI, Wijdicks EFM. Pretruncal subarachnoid hemorrhage: An anatomically correct description of the perimesencephalic subarachnoid hemorrhage. *Stroke* 1997;28:2572.

46. Kumar S, Goddeau RP, Selim MH, Thomas A, Schlaug G, Alhazzani A, Searls DE, Caplan LR. Atraumatic convexal subarachnoid hemorrhage: Clinical presentation, imaging patterns, and etiologies. *Neurology* 2010;74:893–899.

CHAPTER NINETEEN

INTRACEREBRAL HEMORRHAGE

VERY EARLY RECOGNITION

Apoplexy is a historical term (*apo*, from or outside, and *pléttô*, to strike) that was defined as the abrupt, more or less complete suspension of brain activity [1]. In the epic poems of Homer that are the foundational works of ancient Greek literature, sudden death is a sign of divine wrath, by the arrows of Apollo for men, and those of Artemis for women. These arrows are often referred to as "soft," rapid death, rather than long suffering. They are considered to be a favor of the gods [2]. During the seventh and eighth centuries BCE, observers recognized the existence of sudden ailments, often fatal, that developed in the absence of any apparent injury and occurred in healthy individuals. In the "Treatise on Diseases II and III," Hippocrates used "apoplexy" as a clinical term that described instances in which the patient is "staggered," with sudden headache and loss of vision, movement, and consciousness [3]. He attributed the condition to an excess of impurities in the brain, by an influx of phlegm or black bile in the blood. Erasistratus, one of the first physicians to conduct recorded dissections during the second century BCE, rejected this humoral theory; he attributed apoplexy to a sudden abundance of blood in the brain [4].

The term "apoplexy" was used to describe acute stroke syndromes including both brain ischemia and brain hemorrhage. In 1761, Morgagni dissected brains at necropsy and distinguished "serous apoplexy" from "blood apoplexy" [5]. While "bloody" (hemorrhagic) stroke was recognized during the eighteenth and nineteenth centuries, the term "apoplexy" was often used as a synonym for brain hemorrhage. Hemorrhages both intracerebral and subarachnoid were well described, and nearly all writers recognized "sanguinous apoplexies." The designation "serous apoplexies" was applied when no gross bleeding was found at necropsy. Some writers believed that even these cases were somehow related to bleeding and that congestion and blood were absorbed before necropsy.

NINETEENTH- AND EARLY TWENTIETH-CENTURY INTEREST IN THE LOCATIONS AND CAUSES OF BRAIN HEMORRHAGE

During the latter years of the nineteenth century, interest turned to the nature and causes of brain hemorrhage. In 1873, John Liddell, a surgeon and anatomist, included a section on cerebral hemorrhage in his treatise on brain diseases [6]. Liddell's description of the important gross pathological features of brain hematomas is applicable even today:

> Size of the clot varies from that of a hemp-seed to that of the fist. If the extravasation occurs in the vicinity of a ventricle, it often breaks through the walls of the latter, and flows therein. Extravasations forming near the surface of the brain not infrequently break through the cortical substance and escape into the subarachnoid space. Usually there is only one hemorrhagic effusion in the whole brain, occasionally several. The most frequent seat of these effusions is the corpus striatum, the thalamus opticus, and the large medullary masses of the cerebral hemispheres; less frequently, they occur in the cortical substance of the cerebrum, the cerebellum, and in the pons varioli. [6]

Charles Bouchard (1837–1915), a young physician and researcher working in the laboratory of the French neurologist Jean-Martin Charcot, sought the origin of brain hemorrhages. Charcot and Bouchard found tiny aneurysms within large intracerebral hematomas in three of 84 patients with fatal strokes [7]. They also found small lesions that resembled tiny globules of grain along many penetrating arteries. These so-called miliary aneurysms were described and liberally illustrated. Bouchard later published his ideas and findings in a monograph on brain hemorrhage [7]. Bouchard was also one of the first to posit that arterial hypertension might be an important cause of brain hemorrhages. He reviewed the evidence that left ventricular hypertrophy and "a state of rigidity of the main arterial trunks or some obstacles to the flow of blood" were common in patients with intracerebral hemorrhage (ICH) [7]. Johann Wepfer, in 1658, had alluded to a predisposition for apoplexy in those "whose faces and hands are livid" [8]. John Cheyne in 1812 noted vascular congestion, an "excitement of the arteries of the brain" in his treatise [9]. One of Cheyne's patients had severe headache, attributed by the author to possible hypertension, before his fatal pontine hemorrhage. Recall that sphygmomanometers were not introduced into clinical medicine until the early twentieth century so that earlier physicians had no way to clinically quantify blood pressure.

Physicians during this period also began to show interest in and to document the clinical findings in patients found to have brain hemorrhages at necropsy. In 1903, Charles Dana, then professor of neurology at Cornell University in New York, reviewed prior reports and his own personal experience, and summarized the clinical aspects of pontine hemorrhages and infarcts [10]. Among 2,288 hematomas found at necropsy, 205 (9%) were pontine. Dana described the prototypic case:

> Some prodromal headache and malaise for a few days ... then he falls suddenly as if by a lightning stroke, into a coma, usually very profound. There are twitching of the face or of the limbs or both ... the pupils are contracted to a pinpoint ... there is convergent strabismus or conjugate deviation of the eyes. The limbs are at first stiff but tone may be reduced later and the reflexes increased. The patient cannot be aroused but can be made to vomit ... the patient dies in 6 to 20 hours usually with paralysis of respiration. [10]

English-speaking physicians and students who sought information about stroke and other neurological diseases during the first quarter of the twentieth century consulted the popular textbook of neurology by Sir William Gowers [11] and the textbook of medicine written by Sir William Osler [12]. Gowers began his coverage of intracerebral hemorrhage by discussing etiology: "Hemorrhage is always due to rupture of a vessel" [11]. Gowers noted that the vessel ruptured was nearly always an artery and that rupture was caused by an injury or "internal causes." Gowers cited hypertension as a predisposing cause with additional "exciting causes" superimposed at the time of the bleeding. Gowers wrote, "When the wall of an artery is weakened, it yields before the blood pressure and becomes bulged" [11]. Gowers and Osler both described the common locations of spontaneous hemorrhages: the putamen, thalamus, lobar white matter, cerebellum, and pons.

THE TWENTIETH CENTURY AND HYPERTENSIVE ICH

Introduction of the sphygmomanometer into every day medical practice during the first quarter of the twentieth century led to realization of the importance of accelerated and severe hypertension in causing ICH [13]. Unfortunately, recognition of hypertension did not lead to effective treatment. Effective treatment of hypertension did not occur until the last quarter of the twentieth century. The report on one patient emphasized the importance of hypertension and the gradual, inexorable development of the symptoms and signs in hypertensive ICH [14].

The patient was sent to the hospital by his physician because of "malignant hypertension." While his history was being taken, the patient became weak and dizzy. He said that he had noted that his hands became numb and tingled just before he left the admitting area while his heart was examined. He was extremely restless and apprehensive while his history was taken. He complained of inability to hear, difficulty in swallowing, and dyspnea. The patient was placed on the examining table, and his blood pressure was found to be 245 systolic, 170 diastolic. Under the eyes of several examiners, a complete bilateral sixth nerve palsy developed, both pupils dilated, and the corneal reflexes disappeared. The patient was still able to talk, but speech became slurred. He appeared almost completely deaf. His left leg became paretic, and rapid clonic movements were observed. Babinski's sign was present bilaterally. Within an hour, the patient became comatose and his blood pressure had risen to 280/170 mmHg. He soon died of a large pontine hemorrhage. Kornyey commented that this rapidly progressive chain of events was most unpleasant to witness and produced a depressing effect on nurses and physicians [14].

One of C. Miller Fisher's main early projects involved exploring the mechanisms that led blood vessels to rupture, giving rise to brain hemorrhages. He also focused on clinical presentations of ICH [15]. At a March 1959 meeting at the Texas Medical Center in Houston, Fisher presented a description of his own series of 134 brains that contained ICH, examined during 3.5 years [16]. He emphasized that ICH in hypertensive patients occurred mainly at four sites: basal ganglia, thalamus, pons, and cerebellum. These were the same sites where most lacunar infarcts were found. There was likely a common pathological mechanism underlying the two different stroke types, hypertensive penetrating artery disease. Before Fisher's research, ICH was considered a uniformly fatal condition diagnosed only at necropsy. Most patients who had a large hemorrhage died in his series, but Fisher also described ICH patients who survived the event with some degree of neurological deficit. A slit-like cavity was found at the prior hemorrhage site in these patients.

Combining meticulously performed serial clinical exams and pathological studies, Fisher contributed greatly to ICH clinicopathological correlations. Before his time, different theories for the mechanism of acute ICH were posited, including rupture of a small aneurysm or an arteriosclerotic vessel wall without aneurysm formation, simultaneous bleeding from many small vessels, and rupture of a vessel due to the loss of support of surrounding tissue. Fisher published his "Pathological Observations in Hypertensive Cerebral Hemorrhage" in 1971 [17]. He performed meticulous sequential thin section pathological examinations of a large pontine hemorrhage and two small putaminal hemorrhages. One of the most striking observations was the finding

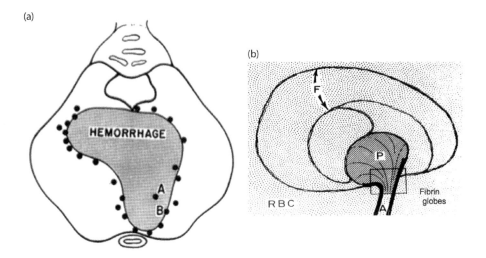

19.1. Miller Fisher's drawings of a necropsy specimen of a patient who died of a pontine hemorrhage. (a) Along the circumference of the hemorrhage dots mark the presence of fibrin globes that represented recently ruptured capillaries. (b) View of the fibrin globes that represent enlarged capillaries or arterioles; platelets are in the center and fibrin on the periphery. From Fisher CM. Pathological observations in hypertensive cerebral hemorrhages. *J. Neuropathol. and Exp. Neurol.* 1971;30:536–550. With permission.

of many (namely, 24) small ruptured arteries around the circumference of the large pontine hemorrhage (Figure 19.1). Fibrin globes, meshes of platelets encircled by a thin layer of fibrin, protruded from ruptured sites and clearly marked vessels that had bled into the pons. He also identified large "fibrin globes" in both of the smaller putaminal hemorrhages and suggested that these fibrin globes represented the primary bleeding sites. The arterial defect took many forms and the artery appeared to have completely parted in 19 instances, while in five only a segment of the arterial circumference was involved. There was no arterial or periarterial infiltration of cells that might represent a chronic inflammatory or reactive process. No aneurysmal formation or arterial dissection was identified [17].

Fisher posited a theory to explain growth of ICH. He interpreted the circumferential bleeding sites as evidence that hematomas developed gradually with pressure effects beginning and maximal at the center of the hematoma. This led to secondary pressure damage sequentially to vessels on the periphery of the expanding hematoma. Hypertension caused a penetrating artery to rupture. Often this occurred when the hypertension first developed. Hemorrhages would begin small. Pressure in the center due to the high pressure within the leaking artery exerted force on arterioles and capillaries at the periphery, causing them in turn to bleed. The hematoma grew on its outer circumference much like a snowball rolling downhill. This process of growth of the hematoma would stop if and when the hematoma drained onto the brain or ventricular surface and, in so doing, partially decompressed itself. Alternatively, tissue pressure and intracranial pressure external to the hematoma would increase until pressures inside and outside the hematoma equalized. Fisher recognized that anticoagulants increased the risk of ICH and that anticoagulant-related ICHs were larger and had even worse clinical outcomes.

At the same Houston meeting in 1959, Fisher described the usual clinical findings in patients with hematomas located in the basal ganglia, thalamus, and pons. He and his colleagues had previously clarified the clinical findings in patients with cerebellar hemorrhages, emphasizing oculomotor abnormalities and gait as early findings [18,19]. These clinical and pathological findings were in patients who had large fatal hemorrhages or large lesions that shed blood into the cerebrospinal fluid, allowing diagnosis during life.

Other neuropathologists sought the nature of the vascular lesions that led to hypertensive ICH. Cole and Yates examined the brains of 100 hypertensive patients and 100 normotensive controls [20]. All 13 patients with ICH had microaneurysms and were hypertensive. Among 63 patients with microaneurysms, 46 patients had hypertension recognized during life. Among 21 hypertensive patients younger than 50 years, only two patients had microaneurysms, while the brains of 71 percent of hypertensive patients in the 65- to 69-year-old age range had microaneurysms [20].

Rosenblum analyzed the morphology of microaneurysms and their parent vessels [21]. Some arteries had early aneurysmal dilatations, whereas others had sclerosed aneurysms with flask-shaped collections of collagen joined to a small artery by a narrow neck. Microaneurysms were often surrounded by hemosiderin-laden macrophages, indicating prior leakage. The lesions were most common in penetrating arteries that supplied the basal ganglia, thalamus, pons, and cerebellum, and arteries supplying the gray-white matter cortical junctions of the hemispheres. The same arteries that bore microaneurysms also contained foci of lipohyalinosis and fibrinoid degeneration.

Angiographic observations and examination of surgical specimens of patients who had acute ICH in Japan showed that penetrating arteries broke, but often not in relation to microaneurysms [22]. Sudden increase in blood pressure was shown to cause ICH in relation to drug use, especially cocaine and amphetamines [23]; pheochromocytoma-related hypertensive surge; exposure to extreme cold weather [24]; dental procedures [25]; and stimulation of the fifth cranial nerve [26]. More important than these unusual circumstances were events of everyday life that abruptly raised blood pressure. Kinnier Wilson in his textbook of neurology that was very popular during the first three quarters of the twentieth century was aware of this concept. He wrote that "emotional experience, joy, anger, fear, or apprehension may disturb the action of the heart, trivial though the incident may be – an address at a public meeting, trouble with a cook, and so on" [27]. Hypertensive ICH could arise from degenerative changes in penetrating arteries and arterioles but also could develop in previously normal vessels subjected to sudden severe rises in systemic blood pressure.

CT, MRI, AND DEVELOPMENTS DURING THE LAST QUARTER OF THE TWENTIETH CENTURY AND BEYOND

When CT became available in the mid- to late 1970s, studies of patients with acute ICHs using sequential CT scans showed that hematomas often expanded dramatically over hours. Some of these observations occurred when IV thrombolytic agent was given soon after the onset of neurological symptoms. Investigators assessed some patients before CT scans, sometimes revealing ICH rather than ischemic stroke as the presenting event. This led to the discovery of early hematoma growth between the baseline CT and later ones, at times performed because of neurological deterioration observed after hospital presentation. Tom Brott and Joe Broderick and colleagues from the University of Cincinnati confirmed the fact that ICHs grew over hours using serial CTs scans in the 1990s [28]. Additional observations established the dynamic course of the early stages of ICH with growth of lesions for hours [29]. Hematoma expansion became a therapeutic target in subsequent clinical trials based on its close correlation with early neurological deterioration and poor clinical outcome.

CT and later MRI made it possible to diagnose small hemorrhages. Often these were in very localized portions of the basal ganglia (caudate nucleus, putamen, anterior limb of the internal capsule, posterior limb), in the various arterial supply zones of the arteries to the thalamus, and in regions within the pontine base, and lateral and medial tegmentum. Small hemorrhages in the cerebral lobes, midbrain, and medulla were now recognized. Some of these arose in cavernous malformations, lesions that were most often not seen on CT scans. The clinical findings in these patients was the focus of many reports and reviews. MRI scans also began to show blood within the cerebral sulci along the brain convexities and evidence of old meningeal bleeding (hemosiderosis) and tiny hemorrhages dubbed microbleeds.

CEREBRAL AMYLOID ANGIOPATHY

Vascular deposition of amyloid beta proteins (Aβ) was first described by Gustav Oppenheim in 1909 as degeneration of capillary walls presumably from the same substance (amyloid) that caused pericapillary necrosis in autopsied brains of individuals with "senile" dementia [30]. The first report that focused on vascular amyloid pathology was published in 1938 [31]. Later observations showed that amyloid deposition could be limited to the vascular media without involvement of adjacent parenchymal tissues [32].

Kurt Jellinger, a prominent professor of neurology and neuropathology at the Medical University of Vienna, first called attention to brain hemorrhages in patients with amyloid-laden arteries and arterioles [33]. The first study of a large series of patients showing an association between amyloid within vessels and lobar intracerebral hemorrhage as well as multiple asymptomatic cortical petechial hemorrhages in autopsies was published in 1979 [34]. The term "cerebral amyloid angiopathy" (CAA) was coined for this process. The Aβ peptide became recognized as the principal component of amyloid deposits in the brain parenchyma and superficial cerebral vasculature of patients with Alzheimer disease as well as CAA; the shared 4-kDa subunit indicated a common origin.

Steve Greenberg became a driving force in expanding knowledge about CAA. He completed his undergraduate studies at Harvard in 1981, majoring in biochemistry. He then obtained MD and PhD degrees from Columbia University. He had a medicine internship at Pennsylvania Hospital followed by a neurology residency at Massachusetts General Hospital in Boston. He then trained in basic science research at the Brigham and Women's Hospital, working on the mechanisms underlying Alzheimer disease. Greenberg was also active clinically. He recognized that patients with CAA presented with unexpected symptoms. In a 1993 article, Greenberg and colleagues described "the clinical spectrum of cerebral amyloid angiopathy: presentations without lobar hemorrhage" [35]. Further studies showed that patients with CAA had a variety of clinical manifestations, including transient focal neurological episodes, cognitive impairment, and gait disturbances, as well as the focal neurologic deficits and death and disability resulting from ICH. The introduction of MRI methods that could detect cerebral microbleeds and convexal and meningeal bleeding greatly facilitated clinical diagnosis. Greenberg and his MGH colleagues developed and validated clinico-radiological criteria for the diagnosis of CAA in living patients [36].

NOTES AND REFERENCES

1. Chapter 8 discusses writings about apoplexy in detail.

2. Grmek MD. *Les maladies à l'aube de la civilisation occidentale*. Paris: Payot, 1994.

3. Poirier J, Derouesné C. *Apoplexy and Stroke*. Cambridge: Cambridge University Press, 1993.

4. Corvisier JN. *Santé et société en Grèce ancienne*. Paris: Economica, 1985

5. Morgagni G. *De sedibus et causis morborum per anatomen indagates* (The seats and causes of diseases investigated by anatomy). London: Millar and T. Cadell, 1769. Morgani's life and contributions is the topic of Chapter 7.

6. Lidell JA. *A Treatise on Apoplexy, Cerebral Hemorrhage, Cerebral Embolism, Cerebral Gout, Cerebral Rheumatism, and Epidemic Cerebrospinal Meningitis*. New York: William Wood and Co., 1873. Reprinted as part of the Classics of Neurology and Neurosurgery Library. Birmingham, AL: Gryphon Editions, 1990, quote on p. 128.

7. Charcot JM, Bouchard C. Nouvelle recherches sur la pathogenie de l'hemorrhagie cerebrale. *Arch. Physiol. Norm. Pathol.* 1868;1:110–127, 634–665, 725–734. Bouchard C. *A Study of Some Points in the Pathology of Cerebral Hemorrhage.* London: Simpkin, Marshall and Co., 1872.

8. Wepfer JJ. *Observationes anatomicae ex cadaveribus eorum, quos sustulit apoplexia, cum exercitatione de ejus loco affect.* Schaffhausen: J. Caspari Suteri, 1658.

9. Cheyne J. *Cases of Apoplexy and Lethargy with Observations upon the Comatose Diseases.* London: J. Moyes printer, 1812.

10. Dana CL. Acute bulbar paralysis due to hemorrhage and softening of the pons and medulla with reports of cases and autopsies. *Med. Rec.* 1903;64:361–374.

11. Gowers WR. *A Manual of Diseases of the Nervous System.* London: J. and A. Churchill, 1893.

12. Osler W. *The Principles and Practice of Medicine,* 5th ed. New York: D. Appleton and Co., 1903, pp. 997–1008.

13. The story of the introduction of the sphygmomanometer into medical practice is discussed in Chapter 49.

14. Kornyey S. Rapidly fatal pontile hemorrhage: Clinical and anatomic report. *Arch. Neurol. Psychiatry* 1939;41:793–799.

15. The career and contributions including those related to ICH are covered in Chapter 29 and in Caplan LR. *C. Miller Fisher: Stroke in the 20th Century.* New York: Oxford University Press, 2020.

16. Fisher CM. Pathology and pathogenesis of intracerebral hemorrhage in pathogenesis and treatment of cerebrovascular disease. In Fields W (ed.), *Proceedings of the Annual Meeting of the Houston Neurological Society.* Springfield, IL: Charles C. Thomas, 1961, pp. 295–317.

17. Fisher CM. Pathological observations in hypertensive cerebral hemorrhages. *J. Neuropathol. Exp. Neurol.* 1971;30:536–550.

18. Fisher CM. Clinical syndromes in cerebral hemorrhage in pathogenesis and treatment of cerebrovascular disease. In Fields W (ed.), *Proceedings of the Annual Meeting of the Houston Neurological Society.* Springfield, IL: Charles C. Thomas, 1961, pp. 318–342.

19. Fisher CM, Picard EH, Polak A, Dalal P, Ojemann RG. Acute hypertensive cerebellar hemorrhage: Diagnosis and surgical treatment. *J. Nerv. Ment. Dis.* 1965;140:38–57.

20. Cole F, Yates P. Intracerebral microaneurysms and small cerebrovascular lesions. *Brain* 1967;90:759–768.

21. Rosenblum WI. Miliary aneurysms and "fibrinoid" degeneration of cerebral blood vessels. *Hum. Pathol.* 1977;8:133–139.

22. Mizukami M, Araki G, Mihara H, Tomita T, Fuginaga R. Arteriographically visualized extravasation in hypertensive intracerebral hemorrhage; report of seven cases. *Stroke* 1972; 3: 527–537. Takebayashi S, Kaneko M. Electron microscopic studies of ruptured arteries in hypertensive intracerebral hemorrhage. *Stroke* 1983;14:28–36.

23. Caplan LR. Drugs. In Kase CS, Caplan LR (eds.), *Intracerebral Hemorrhage.* Boston: Butterworth-Heinemann, 1994, pp. 201–220.

24. Caplan LR, Neely S, Gorelick PB. Cold-related intracerebral hemorrhage. *Arch. Neurol.* 1984;41:227.

25. Barbas N, Caplan LR, Baquis G, et al. Dental chair intracerebral hemorrhage. *Neurology* 1987;37:511–512. Cawley CM, Rigamonti D, Trommer B. Dental chair apoplexy. *South. Med. J.* 1991;84:907–909.

26. Haines S, Maroon J, Janetta P. Supratentorial intracerebral hemorrhage following posterior fossa surgery. *J. Neurosurg.* 1978;49:881–886. Sweet WH, Poletti CE,

Roberts JT. Dangerous rises in blood pressure upon heating of trigeminal rootlets: Increased bleeding times in patients with trigeminal neuralgia. *Neurosurgery* 1985;17:843–844.

27. Wilson SAK, Bruce AN. *Neurology*, 2nd ed. London: Butterworth, 1955, pp. 1367–1383.

28. Broderick JP, Brott TG, Tomsick T, Barsan W, Spilker J. Ultra-early evaluation of intracerebral hemorrhage. *J. Neurosurg.* 1990; 72: 195–199.

29. Kazui S, Naritomi H, Yamamoto H, Sawada T, Yamaguchi T. Enlargement of spontaneous intracerebral hemorrhage: Incidence and time course. *Stroke* 1996;27:1783–1787. Brott T, Broderick J, Kothari R, et al. Early hemorrhage growth in patients with intracerebral hemorrhage. *Stroke* 1997;28:1–5.

30. Oppenheim, G. Uber "drusige Nekrosen" in der Großhirnrinde. *Neurol. Centralbl.* 1909;28:410–413.

31. Scholz, W. Studien zur pathologie der hirngefabe II: Die drusige entartung der hirnarterienundcapillaren. *Z. gesamte Neurol. Psychiatr.* 1938;162:694–715.

32. Pantelakis S. A particular type of senile angiopathy of the central nervous system: Congophilic angiopathy, topography and frequency. *Monatsschr. Psychiatr. Neurol.* 1954;128:219–256.

33. Jellinger K. Cerebral hemorrhage in amyloid angiopathy. *Ann. Neurol.* 1977;1:604. Jellinger K. Cerebrovascular amyloidosis with cerebral hemorrhage. *J. Neurol.* 1977;214:195–206.

34. Okazaki H, Reagan TJ, Campbell RJ. Clinicopathologic studies of primary cerebral amyloid angiopathy. *Mayo Clin. Proc.* 1979;54(1):22–31.

35. Greenberg SM, Vonsattel JP, Stakes JW, Gruber M, Finklestein SP. The clinical spectrum of cerebral amyloid angiopathy: Presentations without lobar hemorrhage. *Neurology* 1993;43(10):2073–2079.

36. Knudsen K, Rosand AJ, Karluk D, Greenberg SM. Clinical diagnosis of cerebral amyloid angiopathy: Validation of the Boston criteria. *Neurology* 2001;56(4):537–539.

CHAPTER TWENTY

VASCULAR MALFORMATIONS

ARTERIOVENOUS MALFORMATIONS

Before the advent of modern brain and vascular imaging, recognition of vascular malformations was only at necropsy or surgery. William Hunter, the brother of the surgeon John Hunter, is often credited for the first description of an arteriovenous communication [1]. In 1757 Hunter reported two patients who had acquired systemic arteriovenous fistulas as a result of overexuberant phlebotomies. He heard a loud hissing murmur and a strong tremulous thrill in the arm at the location of the vascular communication. The brachial artery was much enlarged and large tortuous venous sacs visibly pulsated. Hunter was able to reduce the size of the veins and eliminate the murmur and thrill by pressing on a local spot that he recognized to be the point of the arteriovenous communication. He suggested the word "anastamosis" for this union [1].

In 1863 Rudolph Virchow described the pathology of a number of different types of intracranial vascular malformations [2]. He noted the presence of arteriovenous and capillary types of malformations in the brains at necropsy. Virchow was convinced that some of the lesions, which he called "angiomas," were of congenital origin and were not new growths.

S.O. Steinheil authored the first detailed clinical report of a brain arteriovenous malformation in 1895 [3]. Harvey Cushing with Percival Bailey [4], and Walter Dandy [5] in 1928, reported series of patients with intracranial vascular malformations treated surgically. The treatments consisted of decompressive craniotomies, and partial coagulation or occlusion of parts of the blood supply but not direct excisions. Bailey was a neuropathologist who worked with Cushing in classifying brain tumors and other brain lesions [6].

Walter Dandy was born in Missouri in 1886, the son of British and Irish immigrants. After matriculating at the University of Missouri, he graduated from Johns Hopkins Medical School in 1910 at the age of 24, and became the sixth appointee to the Hunterian Laboratory of Experimental Medicine under Harvey Cushing in 1910. He joined the Johns Hopkins Hospital surgical house staff for one year as Cushing's assistant resident (1911–1912). Dandy completed his general surgery residency at the Johns Hopkins Hospital under William S. Halsted in 1918 [7]. He then had a long and distinguished career at the University of Missouri and pioneered ventriculography and other neurosurgical procedures. He and Cushing did not get along and became rivals during their entire later careers.

Dandy described eight patients with arteriovenous malformations (AVMs) and reviewed the prior literature [5]. Dandy separated patients with direct arteriovenous fistulas from those in whom a "network of vessels – a so-called angioma – is interposed between an artery and one or several veins. A capillary bed between the artery and vein is lacking in both types; the arterial blood, therefore, passes directly into the veins". One patient had a large scalp, dural, and brain malformation visible externally. All patients except the man with the externally visible pulsatile lesion were thought preoperatively to have brain tumors. The diagnosis of vascular malformation was made only at surgical exploration [5].

Dandy's patient with a posterior circulation AVM is among the first such cases recognized and studied during life [5]. At age 33 an otherwise healthy man developed a staggering gait. He began to swerve and veer to the left. Diplopia, headaches, and slurred speech followed and gradually worsened. He then became drowsy. Examination showed gait ataxia, dysarthria, nystagmus, falling to the left, and "choked discs." A cerebellar exploration was performed. When the cerebellum was exposed, "six large tortuous veins stood out ... about equally on both sides. They converged to two large trunks." Further exploration showed a very large venous structure and a greatly enlarged artery. Dandy noted that convulsions were common and often were the presenting clinical problem in AVM patients. In other patients there was a gradually progressive loss of function. Symptoms could begin in childhood or middle life. Dandy estimated that about 40 percent of patients had hemorrhages and that bleeding was the major cause of death in these patients.

By 1930 there were only 30 reported cases of brain arteriovenous malformations [8]. As was the situation in arterial aneurysms, the advent of angiography by Egas Moniz in Portugal greatly facilitated recognition of AVMs during life [9]. During the 1950s there were three reports of intracranial

AVMs diagnosed mostly by angiography [10]. Among the total of 369 patients in these three large series, 138 (37%) had hemorrhaged. In 1966, George Perret and Hiro Nishioka reported the results of the Cooperative Study of Intracranial Aneurysms and Subarachnoid Hemorrhage on the 500-plus cases of vascular malformation reported to them [11]. In the cooperative study aneurysms were 6.5 times more common than vascular malformations (mostly AVMs). Among the patients with vascular malformations, 307 presented with subarachnoid bleeding and 146 had not had recognized hemorrhages. These studies antedated CT scanning. Diagnosis was primarily made by the clinical findings, lumbar puncture, and cerebral angiography. The availability of brain and vascular imaging using CT and MRI led to more diagnoses of AVMs as well as to better separation of the different types of intracranial vascular malformations.

Beginning in the 1960s, McCormick and colleagues made major contributions in defining the pathology, frequency, and distribution of brain vascular malformations and in their classifications. William F. McCormick received his undergraduate education at the University of Chattanooga, and then a master of science degree and an MD from the University of Tennessee. He served as a clinical professor of pathology at the University of Texas Medical Branch in Galveston, Texas [12].

McCormick divided malformations into AVMs, dural arteriovenous fistulas, cavernous angiomas, and developmental venous anomalies [13]. Vascular malformations usually arose from the failure of normal development of embryonic vascular networks. Some malformations such as some arteriovenous fistulas, especially dural arteriovenous malformations and some cavernous angiomas, were acquired during life.

McCormick noted that AVMs contained arteries, arteriolized veins, and draining veins. The size of the component vessels varied greatly but the largest vessels were always venous. Sometimes the arterial supply was small and "cryptic." No recognizable normal capillary bed was present and abnormal gliotic parenchyma usually was found between the component vessels. Thrombosis and inflammation were often found within AVMs. Arteriograms usually were able to show shunting directly from the arteries to the venous components of the malformations.

CAVERNOUS MALFORMATIONS (CAVERNOMAS)

McCormick noted that some lesions were composed entirely of capillaries. They had no prominent arterial input or abnormal venous drainage. Cavernous angiomas consisted of a relatively compact mass of sinusoidal vessels close together without intervening brain parenchyma. These lesions were usually encapsulated. Hyalinization and thickening of the component vessels, especially on the periphery of the angiomas, was very common. These angiomas were not visualized well if at all on angiography because they had no direct arterial input. CT missed cavernomas that had not hemorrhaged. These lesions were usually readily visible on MRI scans as well-circumscribed, well-defined lesions, with a central core of mixed heterogeneous signal intensity surrounded by a rim of signal void. The heterogeneous center was attributable to blood and blood metabolites in various stages of evolution, and the dark rim was hemosiderin.

Cavernous malformations were found to occur in a sporadic, nonhereditary form, in patients with single isolated lesions, and often in a familial form in patients with multiple lesions. In the familial form, which occurred most often in Hispanic people, the number of lesions increased with age [14]. Mutations in the Krev interaction trapped 1 (KRIT1) gene have been identified as underlying the familial form of cerebral cavernous malformations. The KRIT1 protein, the product of the KRIT1 gene, was found in vascular endothelium, astrocytes, and pyramidal cells in adult brains [15].

Once it became possible to image cavernomas using MRI, their prognosis became important to study. Kelly Flemming and her Mayo Clinic colleagues identified 292 patients who harbored cavernomas [16]. Seventy-four patients presented with hemorrhage, 108 with symptoms not related to hemorrhage (seizures or focal deficits), and 110 were asymptomatic. Patients who presented initially with hemorrhage were at higher risk for future hemorrhage, and hemorrhage risk decreased with time. Men and those with multiple cavernomas had a higher risk than women and those with single lesions [16].

DEVELOPMENTAL VENOUS ANOMALIES AND OTHER VENOUS LESIONS

Before McCormick's pathology studies, others had noted that lesions consisting only of venous structures were occasionally the source of bleeding into the brain [17]. These lesions were called "venous hamartomas" and "venous angiomas." On angiography only prominent draining veins were visualized. McCormick recognized that these lesions represented an abnormality of development of venous drainage and preferred to designate them as developmental venous anomalies (DVAs). Because some veins were absent or underdeveloped, accessory and anomalous venous structures developed to aid drainage of blood from areas within the brain. The anomaly consisted of a collection of dilated medullary veins that converged and drained into an enlarged transcortical or subependymal collector vein. One or more large central draining veins were usually conspicuous and could be dilated into a venous varix or varices. The walls of the veins can become thick and hyalinized. These lesions were the commonest type of vascular malformation found in the brain by MRI or at necropsy. DVAs were often associated with cavernous angiomas [18]. McCormick also described telangiectasias, small lesions in which the component capillaries were separated from each other by normal brain parenchyma. They appeared as small, pink, spongy areas most often in the pons. He also noted that some brains contained venous varices, dilated draining veins without an important parenchymal component.

DURAL ARTERIOVENOUS FISTULAS

Dural AVFs (DAVFs) were characterized by abnormal arteriovenous shunting within the leaflets of the dura mater usually within or near the walls of a dural venous sinus. Dural AVMs represented from 10 to 15 percent of all arteriovenous malformations. C. W. Kerber and T. H. Newton showed during the early 1970s that some arteriovenous shunts were often normally present within the dura mater [19]. The major meningeal arteries lay on the outer, periosteal surface of the dura and fed into a rich anastamotic layer of vessels. These arteries and their branches gave rise to vessels that penetrated into the dura toward the pial surface. Arteriovenous shunts were present within the midportion of the dural leaves. Angiographically visible DAVFs exaggerated and enlarged the normal situation. DAVFs could have drainage limited only into dural sinuses or there might be prominent drainage into the cortical and deep veinous systems. DAVFs that had prominent cortical venous drainage had a much higher incidence of bleeding than those without [20].

The cause of most of the complications and the symptoms and signs in patients with DAVFs was attributable to venous hypertension. Previous occlusion of a dural sinus was an important cause of DAVMs [21]. Thrombosis or stenosis within the draining dural sinus often caused enlargement of the DAVFs and augmented venous hypertension [20].

NOTES AND REFERENCES

1. Hunter W. Further observations upon a particular species of aneurysm. *Observ. Inquiries* 1762;2:390–414.
2. Virchow R. *Die krankhaften Geschwulste*. Berlin: Aug. Hirschwald, 1863, vol. 3, pp. 456–461. Rudolph Virchow's career and contributions are discussed in Chapter 13.
3. Steinheil SO. Ueber einen Fall von varix aneurysmaticus im bereit der gehirngefoesse. Inaugural dissertation, Wurzburg, 1895.
4. Cushing H, Bailey P. *Tumors Arising from the Blood-Vessels of the Brain. Angiomatous Malformations and Hemangioblastomas*. Springfield, IL: Charles C. Thomas, 1928. Harvey Cushing is introduced in Chapter 18 on aneurysms and subarachnoid hemorrhages.
5. Dandy WE. Arteriovenous aneurysm of the brain. *Arch. Surg.* 1928;17:190–243.
6. Bucy, Paul C. *Percival Bailey 1892–1973*. Washington, DC: National Academy of Sciences, 1989.

7. Walter Dandy. Wikipedia. Available at https://en.wikipedia.org/wiki/Walter_Dandy. Marmaduke, ME. *Walter Dandy: The Personal Side of a Premier Neurosurgeon.* Philadelphia: Lippincott Williams and Wilkins, 2002. Fox, WL. *Dandy of Johns Hopkins.* Baltimore, MD: Williams and Wilkins, 1984.

8. Pool JL. Arteriovenous malformations of the brain. In Vinken PJ, Bruyn GW (eds.) *Handbook of Clinical Neurology, vol. 12, part II: Vascular Diseases of the Nervous System.* Amsterdam: North-Holland, 1972, pp. 227–266.

9. Moniz and his role in the introduction of cerebral angiography into clinical medicine are discussed in Chapter 31.

10. Paterson JH, McKissock W. A clinical survey of intracranial angiomas with special reference to their mode of progression and surgical treatment: A report of 110 cases. *Brain* 1956;79:233–266. Olivecrona H, Ladenheim J. *Congenital Arteriovenous Aneurysms of the Carotid and Vertebral Systems.* Berlin: Springer, 1957. Tonnis W, Schieffer W, Walter W. Signs and symptoms of supratentorial arteriovenous aneurysms. *J. Neurosurg.* 1958;15:471–480.

11. Perret G, Nishioka H. Report on the Cooperative Study of Intracranial Aneurysms and Subarachnoid Hemorrhage. Section VI. Arteriovenous malformations. An analysis of 545 cases of cranio-cerebral arteriovenous malformations and fistulae reported to the Cooperative Study. *J. Neurosurg.* 1966;25:467–490.

12. William F. McCormick, MD. Marquis Who's Who Top Doctors. Available at https://marquistopdoctors.com/2019/07/01/william-f-mccormick/.

13. McCormick WF. The pathology of vascular ("arteriovenous") malformations. *J. Neurosurg.* 1966;24:807–816. McCormick WF. Pathology of vascular malformations of the brain. In Wilson CB, Stein BM (eds.), *Intracranial Arteriovenous Malformations: Current Neurosurgical Practice.* Baltimore, MD: Williams and Wilkins, 1984. McCormick WF, Boulter TR. Vascular malformations ("angiomas") of the dura mater. *J. Neurosurg.* 1966:309–311. McCormick WF. The pathology of angiomas. In Fein JM, Flamm ES (eds.), *Cerebrovascular Surgery*, vol. 4. New York: Springer-Verlag, 1985, pp. 1073–1095.

14. Rigamonti D, Hadley M, Drayer B, et al. Cerebral cavernous malformations: Incidence and familial occurrence. *N. Engl. J. Med.* 1988;319:343–347. Metellus P, Kharkar S, Lin D, et al. Cavernous angiomas and developmental venous anomalies. In Caplan LR (ed.), *Uncommon Causes*, 2nd ed. Cambridge: Cambridge University Press, 2008, pp. 189–219.

15. Labauge P, Denier C, Bergametti F, Tournier-Lasserve E. Genetics of cavernous angiomas. *Lancet Neurol.* 2007;6(3):237–244.

16. Flemming KD, Link MJ, Christianson TJH, Brown RD Jr. Prospective hemorrhage risk of intracerebral cavernous malformations. *Neurology* 2012;78(9):632–636.

17. Truwit C. Venous angiomas of the brain: History, significance, and imaging findings. *Am. J. Radiol.* 1992;159:1299–1307. Crawford JV, Russell DS. Cryptic arteriovenous and venous hamartomas of the brain. *J. Neurol. Neurosurg. Psychiatry* 1956;19(1):1–11. Wolf PA, Rosman NP, New PFJ. Multiple small cryptic venous angiomas of the brain mimicking cerebral metastases: A clinical, pathological, and angiographic study. *Neurology* 1967;17:491–501.

18. Wilms G, Bleus E, Demaerel P, et al. Simultaneous occurrence of developmental venous anomalies and cavernous angiomas. *AJNR Am. J. Neuroradiol.* 1994;15:1247–1254. Abe T, Singer RJ, Marks MP, et al. Coexistence of occult vascular malformations and developmental venous anomalies in the central nervous system: MR evaluation. *AJNR Am. J. Neuroradiol.* 1998;19:51–57.

19. Kerber CW, Newton TH. The macro and microvasculature of the dura mater. *Neuroradiology* 1973;6:175–179.

20. Castaigne P, Bories J, Brunet P, et al. Les fistules arterio-veineuse meningees pures a drainage veineux cortical. *Rev. Neurol.* 1976;132:169–181. Dion J. Dural arteriovenous malformations: Definition, classification, and diagnostic imaging. In Awad IA, Barrow DL (eds.), *Dural Arteriovenous Malformations*. Park Ridge, IL: American Association of Neurological Surgeons, 1993, pp. 1–19.

21. Houser OW, Campbell JK, Campbell RJ. Arteriovenous malformation affecting the transverse dural venous sinus: An acquired lesion. *Mayo Clin. Proc.* 1979;54:651–661.

CHAPTER TWENTY ONE

CEREBRAL VENOUS THROMBOSIS

La pathologie veineuse de l' encéphale occupe une place restreinte dans les traités et dans l'esprit des neurologistes. (Venous pathology of the brain occupies a limited place in treatises and in the minds of neurologists.) [1]

In 1949, Raymond Garcin and Maurice Pestel began their monograph on cerebral vein and dural sinus thrombosis (CVDST) with this sentence cited above that acknowledged that cerebral venous disease was underreported and seldom considered by neurologists [1]. Marie Mathieu Jean Raymond Garcin (1897–1971) was one of the outstanding figures in neurology in France and internationally during the twentieth century. Born in 1897 in the Caribbean island of Martinique, he traveled at age 18 to Paris to study medicine. He was a medical intern in 1923, Médecin des Hôpitaux in 1930, and Professeur agrégé à la Faculté de Médecine in 1939. His early career as a consultant and teacher was associated with the Hospice Debrousse, the Hôpital Saint-Antoine, and l'Hôtel-Dieu. His major contributions were made during his long stay at the Salpêtrière where in 1948 he was officially nominated Médecin. His monograph with Pestel was based primarily on autopsy material. The authors recognized CVDST as an important but rare cause of death.

During recent decades, CVDST started to be more often on the differential diagnosis for several neurological clinical presentations. Cerebral venous thrombosis is now a constant presence in *l'espirit* of neurologists.

THE FIRST PATIENTS

The first detailed description of CVDST is attributed to M. F. Ribes, a French physician, who in 1825 described a 45-year-old man who developed severe headache and epilepsy and died six months later after a month of delirium. Autopsy showed thrombosis of the superior sagittal sinus and the left lateral sinus, as well as subdural effusion and brain metastases [2].

Three years later, John Abercrombie, physician to King George IV, described the first case associated with the postpartum period. A 24-year-old woman had severe headache after the delivery of her second child. A sense of uneasiness in her head and numb feelings in her occiput and neck developed and were followed by sudden weakness and numbness of her right hand, loss of speech, and twisting of her mouth. Frequent seizures were followed by coma and death. At necropsy, the sagittal sinus was occluded and the draining veins were distended and turgid. The brain showed softening and hemorrhage [3]. At the end of the nineteenth century, Heinrich Irenaeus Quinke, the Swiss clinician given credit for originating lumbar puncture, described patients who had headache, visual symptoms, papilledema, and evidence of raised intracranial pressure who often recovered and did not have brain tumors. At necropsy, one of Quinke's patients had occlusion of both transverse sinuses and the vein of Galen [4].

INSIGHTS FROM DIFFERENT SPECIALTIES

CVDST started to be described in specific settings such as pediatrics, obstetrics, ophthalmology, and otorhinolaryngology. One of the most interesting legacies about this condition was first reported in newborns and children. Victor Hutinel, in 1877, dedicated a large part of his thesis to the study of the newborn's venous conditions. He considered that athrepsia, dehydration, malnutrition, and cardiovascular asthenia favored the development of thrombosis. He suggested that the supine position was a predisposing factor for occlusion of cerebral veins and dural sinuses. The signs of the condition could be nonspecific during the first year of life [5]. After the first year of age, infections were the main cause of thrombosis. Hutinel noted that the brain lesions were initially congestive and edematous, and later acquired the appearance of hemorrhagic softening. The diagnosis was established at postmortem examinations.

Another group of patients in whom the frequency of CVDST was soon described was that of pregnant and puerperal women. In 1905, R. von Hösslin, a German neurologist, described several instances occurring during the postpartum period [6]. Von Hösslin published a review of paralysis during pregnancy and dedicated special attention to those arising from thrombosis of cerebral vessels, especially veins and dural sinuses. Paresis and focal or generalized seizures were important in diagnosis. The spontaneous regression of the symptoms was very suggestive of venous pathology [6]. During the 1940s, J. Purdon Martin and H. L. Sheehan described the symptoms of puerperal thrombophlebitis and noted occasional spontaneous cures, the late occurrence of seizures, and incomplete recovery from hemiparesis [7]. Ross Stansfield, a British obstetrician and gynecologist and a pioneer in the use of heparin in the treatment of CVDST, wrote in 1942: "The introduction of heparin gives us an effective weapon to treat what has invariably been a fatal complication of the puerperium" [8].

Ophthalmologists were also well aware of this condition from the beginning of the twentieth century. Infections of the face were the most common source of cavernous sinus thrombosis that led to cranial nerve involvement (cranial nerves III, IV, V, and VI), fullness of retinal veins, proptosis, and papilledema. Infection of the cavernous sinus was considered to be due to an infected thrombus extending backward from an infected area in the face or paranasal sinuses [9]. Until the advent of antibiotics, the mortality was very high.

CVDST was also familiar to otolaryngologists occurring in association with ear and sinus infections. The infectious component usually dominated the clinical picture, often with meningitis or brain abscesses. In 1924, Fraser published a report about lateral sinus thrombosis after acute or chronic otitis. Diagnosis was confirmed by surgical exploration, and septic sinus thrombosis was more common in acute than in chronic cases of middle ear infection [10]. A few years later, Sir Charles Symonds described the syndrome of intracranial hypertension in relation to middle ear infections, under the name of "otitic hydrocephalus" [11]. This syndrome had a spontaneous cure in most cases. Symonds posited that the cause of the increased intracranial pressure could be failure of absorption of cerebrospinal fluid as the result of clot blocking the arachnoid villi. The appearance of focal signs or seizures was explained by extension of thrombosis to cortical veins [11].

Independent of the setting where the patients were seen, most of them had a poor prognosis, and the diagnosis was typically made at autopsy. Over time, the collection of isolated cases clarified aspects such as the clinical presentation, etiology, and prognosis. Later the development of auxiliary exams made it possible to diagnose CVDST during life.

IMPROVING THE DIAGNOSIS OF CVDST: BROADENING OF THE CLINICAL SPECTRUM

In these early years, CVDST diagnosis was made by autopsy. Knowledge about the clinical presentation and prognosis were based on the worst cases. Most of them occurred in the setting of infections, hence the designation of "cerebral thrombophlebitis." Less severe cases were seldom described as having spontaneous neurological recovery, although the diagnosis was mostly presumptive in such patients. Publication of case series and reviews was essential to disseminate knowledge about this condition.

The first comprehensive review of the subject was carried out by Louis Tonnellé in 1829 [12]. Tonnellé grouped his cases into those due to changes in the circulating blood and those with changes in the walls of the sinus. He was aware of the tendency of the left lateral sinus to be narrower than the right. Jean Cruveilhier included a chapter on inflammation of the dural sinuses in his popular pathologic anatomy atlas [13]. Tonnellé and Cruveilhier noted that dural sinus thrombosis was common in children, especially those with fever and infections, and that dural sinus thrombosis also tended to develop during the puerperium and in older, ill individuals, so-called senile cases. In 1861, T. von Dusch reviewed 57 cases of CVDST from the literature [14]. He separated CVDST into groups, according to the site of beginning of the thrombosis (dural sinuses or cerebral veins) and the underlying circumstances (septic or aseptic). In 1883, James Ross reinforced the varied spectrum of presentations – apathy, depression, headache, nausea, and vomiting – that could be followed by coma, strabismus, trismus and contractures affecting any limbs, and paresis limited to the facial or ocular muscles, hemiparesis, or bilateral paresis [15].

During the early years of the twentieth century, several case series, autopsy studies, and monographs were published. These reports characterized CVDST as a rare and severe condition characterized by headache, papilledema, seizures, focal deficits, coma, and death, and large or multiple hemorrhagic infarcts at necropsy. In 1949, Raymond Garcin and Maurice Pestel summarized the early literature regarding the clinical diagnosis and therapeutics of CVDST [1]. In 1967, R. M. Kalbag, a neurosurgeon, and A. L. Woolf, a neuropathologist, wrote a monograph on the topic of cerebral venous thrombosis. These physicians reviewed the history of recognition of this disorder, ideas about pathogenesis, and past contributions [16]. The increased use of neurosurgery contributed to the report of a few patients in whom the diagnosis of cerebral thrombophlebitis was established during the course of craniotomy. The diagnosis was occasionally possible in life, through the visualization of a thrombosed cerebral vein during surgical exploration. It started to become clear that the prognosis was not always fatal and that some patients could recover from the condition.

Cerebral Angiography: CVDST, Not So Lethal!

Dural sinus venography was introduced and shown to contribute to the diagnosis of intracranial thrombosis during life [17]. This technique was difficult and had risks. An important advance in the history of cerebral venous diseases was the introduction of cerebral phlebography by António Egas Moniz

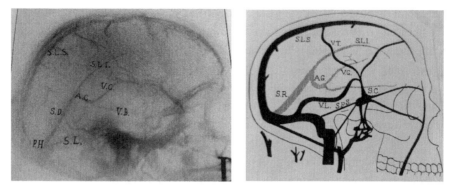

21.1. Cerebral phlebographie and scheme made from phlebograms by Egas Moniz. Published in Bumke O, Foerster O. *Handbuch der Neurologie. Ergänzungsserie ll. Die cerebrale Arteriographie und Phlebographie von Egas Moniz.* Berlin: Verlag von Julius Springer, 1940. S.L.S., superior sagittal sinus; S.L., lateral sinus; P.H., torcular herophili; S.D, straight sinus; S.L.I., inferior sagittal sinus; A.G., Galen ampoule; V.G., Galen vein; V.B., basal vein of Rosenthal; V.T., Trolard vein; V.L., Labbé vein; S.P.S., superior petrousus sinus; S.C., cavernous sinus.

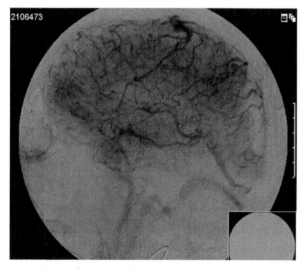

21.2. Cerebral angiography showing extensive thrombosis of superior sagittal sinus and prominent collateral veins.

[18]. The career and contributions of Egas Moniz are described in Chapter 31. Egas Moniz opened a new era for the study of cerebral venous pathology. Figure 21.1 shows one of Egas Moniz's diagrams of the cranial venous structures. Several signs found on cerebral angiography supported the diagnosis of venous or dural sinus occlusion: direct signals (e.g., interruption of filling of venous sinuses or veins) and indirect signals (e.g., delay in filling or emptying of veins, dilation of collateral veins with a tortuous "corkscrew" appearance). (Figure 21.2 shows an angiogram from a patient with occlusion of the superior sagittal sinus.)

During the 1950s and 1960s, several case series were published with the diagnosis based not only on autopsy or surgery but also on angiography. Hugo Krayenbühl, a Swiss neurosurgeon, reported a series of 92 patients and showed that the diagnosis of cerebral venous thrombosis could be made at the onset of symptoms by cerebral angiography. Forty percent of the patients had an infectious cause. The most frequent symptoms were headaches, seizures, paresis, somnolence, or coma. The mortality was high (38%), but, remarkably, only three of the survived patients were "more or less disabled," and a "mild residual epilepsy" was observed in three patients [19]. In the years that followed, evidence accumulated and confirmed that the disease was not as rare nor as severe as suggested by older reports.

Computed Tomography: CVDST, Not So Rare nor So Severe!

The next progress in the history of CVDST was the advent of computed tomography (CT) during the late 1970s. Direct signs of venous or dural sinus thrombosis and their frequency were described: the cord sign, a hyperdense thrombosed vein visualized on unenhanced CT scans; the dense triangle sign, a spontaneously hyperdense superior sagittal sinus; the empty delta sign, non-filling of the superior sagittal sinus after contrast injection. Besides these direct signs, many indirect and nonspecific signs of CVDST were described: general or localized brain edema, small ventricles, nonhemorrhagic venous infarcts seen as focal hypodensity, hemorrhagic infarcts seen as isolated or multifocal hematomas, contrast enhancement of the falx cerebri and tentorium.

Although not pathognomonic, with low sensitivity and specificity, the presence of these direct and indirect signs made it possible to suspect CVDST in some clinical settings. Physicians gradually became more familiar with CT findings that could be caused by venous thrombosis and more aware of the condition. Still considered necessary was the performance of conventional angiography to confirm the diagnosis.

During the last two decades of the twentieth century several retrospective series illustrated a wider clinical spectrum of presentation and prognosis. Bousser and colleagues published a series of 38 patients with angiographically proven CVDST confirming that the disease was not as rare or severe as previously thought [20]. Marie-Germaine Bousser graduated from Paris-Sorbonne University in neuropsychiatry in 1972. She then trained at the Pitié-Salpêtrière Hospital. She spent a year at the National Hospital for Neurology and Neurosurgery, Queen Square, in London, working closely with the neurovascular team, particularly with Ralph Ross Russell, with whom she later wrote a monograph on CVDST [20]. She returned to Paris and became a professor of neurology at the Pitié-Salpêtrière Hospital in 1981, one of the very first women professors within the Paris University medical system. She later was appointed head of neurology at the Saint-Antoine Hospital in Paris in 1989. In 1997 she moved to Lariboisière hospital where she became head of the neurology department and professor of neurology at the Saint Louis Lariboisière faculty.

In Bousser's series, clinical symptoms and modes of onset were very variable, rendering the clinical diagnosis sometimes difficult [20]. Most CT findings were nonspecific; angiography remained the best diagnostic tool to confirm the diagnosis. Only four patients died (10.5%), which suggested a more benign outcome than classically described. Anticoagulants were already used in most patients, and seemed to be safe [20]. This was the first of many publications of Bousser's Paris group. The sample of patients in Paris was steadily enlarged, and understanding of clinical presentation, diagnosis, etiology, and prognosis was increasingly consolidated. Although the prognosis was much more favorable than previously accepted, the unpredictable course was considered to be a distinctive feature of this condition.

Published series of patients from different parts of Europe, typically with a retrospective design, confirmed a benign clinical profile and prognosis compared with older reports. Case fatality ranged between 5.5 and 30 percent. The prognosis for recovery among survivors was much better than in patients with arterial thrombosis. The incidence of sequelae such as seizures, optic atrophy, and focal neurological deficits affected usually less than 25 percent of patients. The first prospective study by Karl Max Einhäupl, the director of the department of neurology at the very large Charité hospital in Berlin, contained 71 CVDST patients [21]. Einhäupl and colleagues performed the first clinical trial that evaluated the efficacy of heparin in CVDST [22].

Experience with CVDST began to be reported outside Europe. In India, cerebral venous thrombosis occurring in the puerperium was suggested to be much more frequent than in Western countries. K. Srinavasan published a study of 135 patients with cerebrovascular diseases in the puerperium, showing that cerebral venous thrombosis was common compared to arterial thrombosis [23]. The illness usually occurred within the first two weeks after delivery, with multifocal seizures, stupor or coma, regressing focal signs, and, at times, "pseudotumor cerebri." Contrary to previous reports, mortality was less than 20 percent, and patients who survived had minimal physical disability. Carlos Cantu and Fernando Barinagarrementeria published a large series of 113 Mexican patients [24]. They compared 67 cases associated with pregnancy or the puerperium with 46 cases unrelated to obstetric causes. Pregnant or puerperal women had a more acute onset and had better outcomes than patients with other causes (good outcome in 80% vs. 58%; mortality rate of 9% vs. 33%) [24]. These series and others from India and Mexico uncovered many associations and postulates about mechanisms in relationship to pregnancy and the postpartum period. Women tended to develop CVDST during the first three weeks after delivery, but venous thromboses also developed at any time during pregnancy. Postpartum cerebral venous thrombosis was more common in patients who had venous thromboses outside the nervous system during previous pregnancies (pelvic or lower extremity phlebothrombosis and pulmonary embolism). Puerperal intracranial venous thrombosis was also most often found in multiparous women, women from lower socioeconomic strata who had less prenatal care, and after deliveries at home. Explanations for the frequency of intracranial venous thrombosis in pregnancy and the puerperium included poverty, vegetarian and vitamin-deficient food intake, depletion of vitamin and protein stores by multiple pregnancies, and anemia. These factors may lead to hypercoagulability. Other series of patients with CVDST showed a relatively frequent occurrence in women who took oral contraceptives containing female hormones. In Saudi Arabia, a review of 40 patients showed that almost half had a clinical picture of "pseudotumor cerebri"; Behçet's disease was the cause in 25 percent, and infection was no longer an important cause [25].

Magnetic Resonance Imaging and CT venography: CVDST, Mostly Benign, but Unpredictable

From the early 1990s, magnetic resonance imaging (MRI) became the method of choice to diagnose CVDST. MRI was noninvasive and enabled visualization of the brain and confirmation of the thrombosis by visualizing the thrombus itself. Venous MRI examinations added complementary information by showing the lack of visualization of venous flow in thrombosed structures. A variety of MR signs was described, related to the evolution of the thrombus. Specific MRI sequences, such as T2* or susceptibility weighted imaging (SWI), further enabled the diagnosis of cortical vein thrombosis in patients who had been difficult to diagnose even with the use of cerebral angiography. CT venography also emerged as an alternative to MR venography or intraarterial angiography by showing filling defects, sinus wall enhancement, and increased collateral venous drainage. The more widespread use of MRI and CT venography allowed easier and earlier diagnosis of CVDST. Most series reported after their introduction typically used one of these techniques to diagnose CVDST.

During the late 1990s and early twenty-first century, studies focused on the clinical presentation and on the description of the short and long-term prognosis. Alain Ameri and Marie-Germaine Bousser, among a series of 110 CVDST patients, noted a reduced frequency of focal deficits, seizures, and disorders of consciousness compared to older descriptions [20]. The mode of onset was categorized as acute (less than 48 hours; 28% patients), subacute (more than 48 hours but less than 30 days; 42% of patients) and chronic (more than 30 days; 30% of patients). Clinical presentation was separated into four groups: isolated intracranial hypertension, focal cerebral signs, cavernous sinus syndrome, and unusual presentations. Isolated intracranial hypertension was shown to be a common occurrence (40%). Prognosis was better than previously shown: 77 percent of patients made a complete recovery, 17 percent had sequelae, and less than 6 percent died [20]. In a prospective study of 77 patients, Maurice Preter et al. showed that CVDST had a good long-term prognosis, with death or dependency occurring in about 20 percent of patients [26]. The frequency of long-standing epilepsy was low, but subsequent thrombotic episodes occurred in 20 percent of patients [26].

In addition to conditions traditionally associated with CVDST (e.g., heart disease, cachexia or marasmus, local or generalized infections, pregnancy or puerperium), other conditions were added as precipitating or predisposing to CVDST: malignancies, bowel inflammatory diseases, Behçet's, connective tissue diseases, essential thrombocythemia, polycythemia, sickle cell disease, paroxysmal nocturnal hemoglobinuria, coagulation defects (e.g., antithrombin III, protein S or C deficiency, factor V, and prothrombin gene mutation), oral contraceptives and other prothrombotic drugs, head trauma, lumbar puncture, and jugular vein catheters [20]. CVDST was increasingly diagnosed in young women, mainly related to pregnancy and the puerperium in developing countries, and with oral contraceptives in developed countries; the incidence of septic CVDST became less frequent, even in developing countries.

CONSORTIUMS DEVELOPED IN SEVERAL REGIONS TO STUDY CVDST

Several hospitals were assembled in the Netherlands to study cerebral venous thrombosis. In 1995, a retrospective study reported 62 patients admitted to the neurological wards of nine Dutch teaching hospitals, from 1970 to 1990. Three months after the diagnosis, 10 patients (16%) were seriously disabled and 11 patients (18%) had died. Coma and hemiparesis at the time of diagnosis were associated with a poor outcome [27]. A prospective study of 59 patients included in a therapeutic trial evaluating the efficacy of heparin ensued by the Cerebral Venous Sinus Thrombosis Study Group (14 centers from the Netherlands and two UK centers) [27]. They concluded that the overall prognosis of CVDST was good (only 17% of patients had poor outcome), and coma and intracerebral hemorrhage were independent predictors for poor outcome [27].

Sharing the concept of the benefit of network research on infrequent conditions, José Ferro, the chair and professor of neurology at the Santa Maria Hospital in Lisbon, launched a mixed retrospective and prospective study in Portugal [28]. The study reported results among 142 patients studied between 1980 to 1998 from 20 Portuguese hospitals. Nine (6%) patients died, and only six (4%) were dependent at discharge. This study suggested that it was possible to identify patients with a potentially poor prognosis. Central nervous system infection, encephalopathy on admission, and hemorrhage on CT/MRI done on admission were predictors of death or dependency [28]. The long-term functional prognosis of patients with CVDST was good, with complete recovery in most patients. This collaborative study suggested a moderate risk of further thrombotic events (5%) and seizures (10%) [28].

Gabrielle deVeber, from the Hospital for Sick Kids in Toronto, Canada, led the formation of the Canadian Pediatric Ischemic Stroke Registry [29]. This registry was initiated in 1992 at 16 pediatric tertiary care centers. During the first six years of the registry, 160 children with CVDST were included. DeVeber et al. showed that CVDST affected mostly neonates. Clinical presentation was different from adult patients; 58 percent of the children had seizures, 76 percent had diffuse neurologic signs, and 42 percent had focal neurologic signs. Risk factors were also different in children, and most often included head and neck disorders (29%), acute systemic illnesses (54%), chronic systemic diseases (36%), and prothrombotic states (41%). Venous infarcts occurred in 41 percent of the children. About half of the patients received antithrombotic treatment. Neurologic deficits were present in 38 percent of the children, and 8 percent died. Predictors of poor outcomes were seizures at presentation and venous infarcts [30].

Worldwide, at the end of the twentieth and the beginning of the twenty-first century, venous thrombosis had become a well-known condition, easily diagnosed, its causes investigated and patients treated with anticoagulation in most instances. Although the prognosis was better than previously thought, it was still considered unpredictable. It was not possible to anticipate which patients would worsen or have a poor outcome. Data on long-term prognosis was scarce and inconclusive. Prospective studies, based on single-center or single-country studies, had given contradictory results: death at the end of the follow-up varied between 0 and 39 percent, and death or dependency varied between 8.8 and 44.4 percent.

THE ISCVT: A NEW ERA, CLARIFYING THE PROGNOSIS

The previous experiences of collecting cases by a network of centers led to the organization of the International Study on Cerebral Vein and Dural Sinus Thrombosis (ISCVT). The Steering Committee was composed of José Ferro, Jan Stam, Marie-Germaine Bousser, Fernando Barinagarrementeria, and Karl Einhäupl. By assembling a large sample of patients from different world sites, the objective was to perform a study with high internal and external validities.

The ISCVT aimed to acquire reliable evidence on clinical presentation, risk factors, outcome, and prognostic factors.

Between 1998 and 2001, 624 patients older than 15 years were included in this multinational (21 countries) and multicenter (89 centers) observational prospective study. Due to the participation of many different sites, data on the clinical presentations of ISCVT was more representative of the condition. This study confirmed the variability of the condition. The mode of onset was more often acute (37.2%) or subacute (55.5%), and less frequently chronic. Headache was by far the most frequent symptom (88.8%), followed by seizures (39.3%) and paresis (37.2%), while stupor or coma occurred only in 13.9 percent of patients. About 23 percent of patients presented with isolated intracranial hypertension, and this subgroup of patients had an excellent prognosis. More than 60 percent of patients had any type of brain lesion on CT or MR; 18 percent had bilateral lesions, and about 40 percent of patients had hemorrhagic lesions. Thrombophilia, either genetic or acquired, and oral contraceptives were the most common risk factors. Many patients (43.6%) had more than one known risk factor, and no recognized risk factor was identified in 12.5 percent of patients [31].

The prognosis was better than reported in previous studies. Less than 5 percent of patients died during the acute phase. Death was mainly caused by transtentorial herniation, which could be due to a unilateral focal mass effect or to diffuse edema and multiple parenchymal lesions [32]. At the last follow-up (median 16 months), almost 80 percent of patients made a complete recovery, and 13 percent had a poor outcome (death or dependency). Multivariate analysis identified the following independent predictors for an unfavorable outcome: male sex, age above 37 years, coma, mental status disorder, intracranial hemorrhage, thrombosis of the deep cerebral venous system, central nervous system infection, and cancer [31]. Using the ISCVT data, Ferro and colleagues derived a prognosis risk score (the CVT risk score) and further validated it in two samples. This score had a good estimated overall rate of correct classifications in both validation samples, but its specificity was low. The score could be helpful in identifying high-risk CDSVT patients [33]. ISCVT also provided data concerning complications during follow-up. Severe headache (14.1%) and seizures (10.6%) were frequent complaints, while recurrent CVDST (2.2%) and other thrombotic events (4.3%) were not common, and severe visual loss was rare (0.6%) [33].

This large collaborative prospective study collected a large amount of data, allowing analyses of CVDST in specific subgroups of patients, for example, elderly women and those with particular types of brain lesions, for example, intracerebral hemorrhage and non-hemorrhagic lesions. The ISCVT also studied the risk of seizures in CVDST and the frequency of venous thromboembolic events during follow-up. In a case-control study, Patricia Canhão and colleagues showed that steroids in the acute phase were not useful and were detrimental in patients without parenchymal cerebral lesions [34]. After these results, the use of steroids was discouraged in patients with cerebral venous thrombosis.

ISCVT marked a new era in the study of CVDST. Since the publication of the first paper in 2004, a plethora of studies arose from different parts of the world and validated their main results. ISCVT identified patients at risk of poor prognosis, and this information was critical to select patients for aggressive therapies such as endovascular therapy. Understanding the causes of death led to the evaluation of the effect of therapies such as decompressive craniectomy. ISCVT also identified areas of uncertainty to clarify in future studies, such as the safety of future pregnancy and the risk of epilepsy.

Besides all the data revealed by ISCVT, one of the important legacies of this international study was to confirm that it was possible to study an infrequent condition by building networks of interested clinicians and researchers. Other collaboratives became operant: the European Collaborative Paediatric Database on Cerebral Venous Thrombosis [35], the Biorepository to Establish the Aetiology of Sinovenous Thrombosis (BEAST Consortium) [36], the VENOST study of 1,144 patients with CVDST [37], the Asian study of cerebral venous thrombosis [38], and the International CVT Consortium. The data derived will continue to broaden the knowledge of this condition, which is not so rare, mostly benign, and still presenting us with much to learn.

NOTES AND REFERENCES

1. Garcin R, Pestel M. *Thrombophlébites cérébrales*. Paris: Masson et Cie, 1949.

2. Ribes MF. Des recherches faites sur la phlébite. *Revue Médicale Française et Etrangère et Journal de Clinique de l'Hôtel-Dieu et de la Charité de Paris* 1825;3:5–41.

3. Abercrombie J. *Pathological and Practical Researches on Diseases of the Brain and the Spinal Cord*. Edinburgh, 1828.

4. Quinke H. Ueber meningitis serosa und verwandte Zustände. *Dtsch. Z. Nervenheilk.* 1896;9:149–168.

5. Hutinel VH. *Contribution à l'étude des troubles de la circulation veineuse chez l'enfant et en particulier chez le nouveau-né*. V. Adrien Delahaye et Cie, 1877.

6. Von Hösslin R. Die Schwangerschaftlähmungen der Mutter. *Arch. für Psychiatrie* 1904;38:779; 1905;40:445 (cited in Garcin R, Pestel M. *Thrombophlébites cérébrales*. Paris: Masson et Cie, 1949).

7. Purdon Martin J, Sheehan HL. Primary thrombosis of cerebral veins (following childbirth). *BMJ* 1941 Mar 8:349–353.

8. Stansfield FR. Puerperal cerebral thrombophlebitis treated by heparin. *BMJ* 1942 April 4;1(4239):436–438.

9. Eagleton WP. *Cavernous Sinus Thrombophlebitis, and Allied Septic and Traumatic Lesions of the Basal Venous Sinuses*. New York: Macmillan, 1926.

10. Fraser JS. Septic otitic thrombosis of the cranial blood sinuses and jugular bulb. *Edinb. Med. J.* 1924 Apr;31(4):T75–T89. PMID: 29647779; PMCID: PMC5305757.

11. Symonds CP. Otitic hydrocephalus. *Brain* 1931;54, part I:55–72. Symonds CP. Hydrocephalic and focal cerebral symptoms in relation to thrombophlebitis of the dural sinus and cerebral vein. *Brain* 1937;60:531–550. Symonds CP. Intracranial thrombophlebitis. Otolaryngology lecture delivered at the Royal College of Surgeons of England on April 3, 1952, pp. 347–356.

12. Tonnellé ML. Mémoire sur les maladies des sinus veineux de la dure-mère. *J. hebd. Méd.* 1829;5:337–403.

13. Cruveilhier J. *Anatomie pathologique du corps humain: Descriptions avec figures lithographiées et caloriées des diverses alterations morbides dont le corps humain est susceptible.* Paris: JB Bailliere, 1835–1842.

14. Von Dusch T. *On Thrombosis of the Cerebral Sinus.* London: New Sydenham Society, 1861.

15. Ross J. *A Treatise on the Diseases of the Nervous System*, 2nd ed., vol. 2. London, 1883, pp. 385–390.

16. Kalbag RM, Woolf AL. *Cerebral Venous Thrombosis*, vol. 1. London: Oxford University Press, 1967.

17. Ray BS, Dunbar HS, Dotter CT. Dural sinus venography as an aid to diagnosis in intracranial disease. *J. Neurosurg.* 1951;8(1):23–37.

18. Moniz E, Lima A. Phlébographie cérébrale. Essai de détermination de la vitesse du sang dans les capillaires du cerveau chez l'homme. Comptes rendus des séances de la Société de biologie. Société de biologie de Lisbonne. Séance du 29 Janvier 1932, t CIX, p. 1037. Moniz E. Phlébographie cérébral. In Masson et Cie (eds.), *L'angiographie cérébrale. Ses applications et résultats en anatomie, physiologie et clinique.* Paris, 1934.

19. Krayenbühl HA. Cerebral venous thrombosis; diagnostic value of cerebral angiography. *Schweiz. Arch. Neurol. Psychiat.* 1954;74:261–287. Krayenbühl HA. Cerebral venous and sinus thrombosis. *Neurologia medico-chirurgica* 1968;10:1–24.

20. Bousser MG, Chiras J, Bories J, Castaigne P. Cerebral venous thrombosis: A review of 38 cases. *Stroke* 1985;16:199–213. Ameri A, Bousser MG. Cerebral venous thrombosis. *Neurologic Clinics* 1992;10(1):87–111. Bousser M-G, Ross Russell R. *Cerebral Venous Thrombosis.* London: Saunders, 1997.

21. Einhäupl KM, Villringer A, Haberl RL, et al. Clinical spectrum of sinus venous thrombosis. In Einhäupl K, Kempski O, Baethmann A (eds.), *Cerebral Sinus Thrombosis.* Boston: Springer, 1990, pp. 149–155.

22. Einhäupl KM, Villringer A, Mehraein S, et al. Heparin treatment in sinus venous thrombosis. *Lancet* 1991;338:597–600.

23. Srinivasan K. Cerebral venous and arterial thrombosis in pregnancy and puerperium. A study of 135 patients. *Angiology* 1983 Nov;34(11):731–746.

24. Cantu C, Barinagarrementeria F. Cerebral venous thrombosis associated with pregnancy and puerperium. Review of 67 cases. *Stroke* 1993;24(12):1880–1884.

25. Daif A, Awada A, Al-Rajeh S, et al. Cerebral venous thrombosis in adults: A study of 40 cases from Saudi Arabia. *Stroke* 1995;26(7):1193–1195.

26. Preter M, Tzourio C, Ameri A, Bousser MG. Long-term prognosis in cerebral venous thrombosis: follow-up of 77 patients. *Stroke* 1996;27(2):243–246.

27. de Bruijn SF, de Haan RJ, Stam J. Clinical features and prognostic factors of cerebral venous sinus thrombosis in a prospective series of 59 patients. For the Cerebral Venous Sinus Thrombosis Study Group. *J. Neurol. Neurosurg. Psychiatry* 2001;70(1):105–108. de

Bruijn SF, Stam J, CVST Study Group. Randomized, placebo-controlled trial of anticoagulant treatment with low-molecular-weight heparin for cerebral sinus thrombosis. *Stroke* 1999;30:484–488.

28. Ferro JM, Correia M, Pontes C, Baptista MV, Pita F. Cerebral vein and dural sinus thrombosis in Portugal: 1980–1998. *Cerebrovascular Diseases* 2001;11(3):177–182. Ferro JM, Lopes MG, Rosas MJ, Ferro MA, Fontes J. Long-term prognosis of cerebral vein and dural sinus thrombosis. *Cerebrovasc. Dis.* 2002;13(4):272–278.

29. The career and contributions of Gabrielle deVeber are discussed in detail in Chapter 40.

30. deVeber G, Andrew M, Adams C, et al., Canadian Pediatric Ischemic Stroke Study Group. Cerebral sinovenous thrombosis in children. *N. Engl. J. Med.* 2001 Aug 9;345 (6):417–423.

31. Ferro JM, Canhão P, Stam J, Bousser MG, Barinagarrementeria F, ISCVT Investigators. Prognosis of cerebral vein and dural sinus thrombosis: Results of the International Study on Cerebral Vein and Dural Sinus Thrombosis (ISCVT). *Stroke* 2004;35:664–670.

32. Canhão P, Ferro JM, Lindgren AG, Bousser, MG, Stam J, Barinagarrementeria F, ISCVT Investigators. Causes and predictors of death in cerebral venous thrombosis. *Stroke* 2005;36:1720–1725.

33. Ferro JM, Bacelar-Nicolau H, Rodrigues T, et al. Risk score to predict the outcome of patients with cerebral vein and dural sinus thrombosis. *Cerebrovasc. Dis.* 2009;28 (1):39–44.

34. Canhão P, Cortesão A, Cabral M, et al. Are steroids useful to treat cerebral venous thrombosis? *Stroke* 2008;39(1):105–110.

35. Kenet G, Kirkham F, Niederstadt T, et al. Risk factors for recurrent venous thromboembolism in the European collaborative paediatric database on cerebral venous thrombosis: A multicentre cohort study. *Lancet Neurol.* 2007 Jul 1;6(7):595–603.

36. Cotlarciuc I, Marjot T, Khan MS, et al. Towards the genetic basis of cerebral venous thrombosis – The BEAST Consortium: A study protocol. *BMJ Open* 2016 Nov 1;6(11).

37. Duman T, Uluduz D, Midi I, et al. A multicenter study of 1144 patients with cerebral venous thrombosis: The VENOST study. *J. Stroke Cerebrovasc. Dis.* 2017;26 (8):1848–1857.

38. Wasay M, Kaul S, Menon B, et al. Asian study of cerebral venous thrombosis. *J. Stroke Cerebrovasc. Dis.* 2019;28(10):104247.

CHAPTER TWENTY TWO

ARTERIAL DISSECTIONS, FIBROMUSCULAR DYSPLASIA, MOYAMOYA DISEASE, AND REVERSIBLE CEREBRAL VASOCONSTRICTION SYNDROME

During the second half of the twentieth century and first quarter of the twenty-first, new cerebrovascular syndromes were identified. The advent of modern brain and vascular imaging allowed identification of previously unrecognized or underrecognized conditions. Once the diagnosis could be made clinically, further experience allowed recognition of the frequency, demography, clinical findings, and course of the conditions and paved the way for treatment. Four representative entities have been chosen that illustrate discovery and evolution during this time.

ARTERIAL DISSECTIONS

Dissection of the aorta was described by Giovanni Morgagni in the seventeenth century. A detailed postmortem description of cardiac tamponade resulting from aortic dissection in King George II was published by his personal physician more than 250 years ago [1,2]. During the first half of the twentieth century, aortic dissection became a well-recognized and important entity to diagnose. The first large series was described by T. Shennan, who reported the findings in 302 patients with aortic dissection, including 77 of his own, among whom only six were accurately diagnosed during life [3]. A review of 505 patients seen at the Massachusetts General Hospital was published in 1958 [4]. Frederick Moersch and George Sayre in 1950 reviewed the Mayo Clinic experience with aortic dissections and emphasized the neurological findings [5]. Surprisingly, dissections involving other major arteries – coronary, cervico-cranial, renal, and gastrointestinal – took much longer to be recognized and diagnosed by general physicians.

In 1972, C. Miller Fisher and his surgical colleagues Robert Ojemann and Charles Rich reported the eleventh published case of dissection of the internal carotid artery (ICA) in the neck, and reviewed the previously described cases [6]. As has often been the case, a single patient experience led the authors to identify a relatively new entity. The patient was a 41-year-old man who had had several attacks of decreased vision in the left eye and then developed aphasia and right hemiparesis. He had been thrown from a boat months before. His cerebral angiogram was unusual. It showed an irregular narrowing of the ICA extending from approximately 1 centimeter beyond the carotid bifurcation to the base of the skull. The surgical specimen showed regions of dilatation and narrowing due to dissection of the arterial wall. The authors emphasized the angiographic appearance of a long narrow column of contrast, which they dubbed "the string sign." They had not seen a similar picture in patients with occlusive disease due to atheroma. Miller Fisher commented on this finding in his memoirs:

> It was largely a chance observation that contributed to the opening of the field of dissection of the carotid and cerebral arteries. Dr. Robert Ojemann and I had described the pathological findings in a patient with carotid obstruction whom he had operated on by removing the blocked segment. The diagnosis of dissection was established. Only 10 cases of carotid dissection had been previously described in the literature and almost all had been fatal. Our patient's angiogram had shown a thin column of dye in the carotid where the lumen was compromised by blood dissecting in the wall of the artery. Three of the cases in the literature had a somewhat similar appearance. The narrow column of dye was termed "the string sign" and tentatively it was suggested that it might be a sign of dissection. Not long afterwards there was admitted to the hospital another stroke patient with the string sign on angiography.... After the introduction of the "string sign" as a diagnostic clue, it was not long before we were consulted concerning numerous cases far and wide. The "string sign" was extended to dissection in other arteries, middle cerebral, vertebral, and posterior cerebral and the ranks of obscure strokes underwent further shrinkage. [6,7]

Further research and experience clarified the nature of arterial dissections, a term used for a mechanically or traumatically induced tear within the wall of an artery. The tear causes bleeding within the arterial wall that can spread (dissect) within the media along the longitudinal course of the artery. The pressure within the wall can break through the inner lining of the wall, the endothelium (intimal flap), and introduce into the lumen a fresh blood clot and chemical substances such as tissue factor contained within the wall.

That blood clot and the swollen wall can obstruct the artery and become the source of blood clot that embolizes into intracranial branches, causing brain ischemia and infarction. Dissection in the plane between the media and adventitia can cause aneurysmal outpouching of the artery.

During the 1970s and 1980s standard catheter cerebral angiography identified the angiographic features of carotid artery dissection. Abnormalities usually began more than 2 centimeters distal to the origin of the ICA. Often a gradually tapering segment ended in occlusion. Localized aneurysmal sacs or outpouchings were shown along or both proximal and distal to a narrowed, normal, or unusually dilatated portion of the artery. String signs and intimal flaps were common. Similar angiographic abnormalities allowed recognition of dissections within the extracranial cervical vertebral arteries (ECVAs) [8]. Arterial dissections became diagnosable through angiography. When magnetic resonance angiography (MRA), computed tomography angiography (CTA), and ultrasound became widely available, more knowledge accrued about the vascular imaging features. Further experience allowed recognition of the causes, locations, and clinical symptoms and signs in patients with cervical artery dissections [9]. By the later years of the twentieth century, arterial dissection had become a relatively common and important diagnosis.

Most cervical arterial dissections involved some trauma, stretch, or mechanical stress. The vulnerable portions of the arteries were those that were readily movable and not anchored.. The ICAs were anchored at the bifurcation and the skull base. The pharyngeal portions were mobile. The ECVAs were anchored at their origin from the subclavian arteries and by the cervical vertebrae. The portion between the origins before penetration into bone, and the distal portion after exit from the cervical vertebrae before skull entry, were mobile. These mobile regions of the carotid and vertebral arteries were spared by atherosclerosis. Trauma could be trivial, for example, twisting the neck to avoid a falling tree branch, lunging for a ball, or turning the neck abruptly while backing up a car or skiing, or neck movement during chiropractic manipulation [9,10]. Congenital or acquired abnormalities of the connective tissue elements in the media and/or elastica of the arteries, and edema of the arterial wall, could promote dissection. Marfan's syndrome, cystic medial necrosis, fibromuscular dysplasia (FMD), Ehlers–Danlos type 4 syndrome, Loeys–Dietz syndrome, osteogenesis imperfecta type 1, and migraine were found more often than expected in patients with arterial dissections [9].

The most common and characteristic feature in patients with ICA dissections was pain. Ipsilateral throbbing headache and sharp pain locally in the neck, jaw, pharynx, or face distinguished dissections from ordinary atherosclerotic occlusion of the artery in which pain was rare. Sympathetic fibers traveling along the wall of the ICA can be perturbed, leading to an ipsilateral partial Horner's syndrome characterized by ptosis and miosis. Facial sweat function was preserved because sympathetic innervation of the sweat glands traveled along the external carotid artery. Transient ischemic attacks (TIAs) were common and involved the ipsilateral eye and/or brain. The spells often occurred in rapid succession over hours or a few days. Visual scintillations and bright sparkles resembling migraine were often reported even in non-migraineurs. Some patients heard a pulsatile noise in the head or ipsilateral ear. TIAs were attributable to luminal compromise with distal hypoperfusion, but most patients with severe strokes had evidence of embolization of clot to the middle cerebral artery (MCA) from thrombus at the site of the dissection. When the ICA dissection extended to the carotid siphon, ischemic optic neuropathy sometimes occurred. Strokes usually occurred soon after the ICA dissection but could ensue during the days and weeks after the event. Patients with medial-adventitial dissections often presented with compression or ische-mia of the lower cranial nerves; weakness of the pharynx, palate, tongue, and trapezius were found.

Some patients with vertebral artery neck dissections had only neck pain and did not develop neurologic symptoms or signs. TIAs most often include dizziness, diplopia, veering, staggering, and dysarthria. TIAs were less common in vertebral artery dissections than ICA dissections. Infarcts usually were accompanied by signs that began suddenly. The most common patterns of ischemic brain damage were cerebellar infarction in posterior inferior cerebel-lar artery (PICA) distribution and lateral medullary infarction. Some dissections extended intracranially. Infarcts were invariably explained by fresh thrombus within the intracranial vertebral artery and its branches Sometimes, emboli reached the superior cerebellar arteries (SCAs), basilar artery, or posterior cerebral arteries (PCAs). ECVA dissections could also cause cervical root pain. Aneurysmal dilatation of the ECVA adjacent to nerve roots led to radicular distribution pain and motor, sensory, and reflex abnormalities. Occasionally, spinal cord infarction resulted because of hypoperfusion in the supply zones of ECVA branches that supplied the cervical spinal cord [9].

Once considered rare, intracranial arterial dissections began to be recognized by vascular imaging features similar to those found in cervical artery dissections. High-resolution CT and MRI imaging of intracranial arteries became useful in identifying those features

Intracranial dissections resulted in brain infarction, subarachnoid bleeding, and mass effects [11]. When the dissections were between the media and the intima, luminal narrowing and local hypoperfusion usually occurred and led to infarction in the regions of supply. Ischemia attributed to intracranial dissec-tions was considered in the past to always be devastating or fatal, but modern technology has led to increased recognition of patients who have only minor symptoms and signs. When dissections developed between the media and the adventitia, aneurysms and tears through the adventitia caused subarachnoid hemorrhage (SAH), which could be repeated. At times, dissecting aneurysms presented as space-taking lesions that compressed adjacent cranial nerves or brain parenchyma. Intracranial dissections have been most often detected in patients of Asian origin. In the anterior circulation, the supraclinoid ICA and main stem of the MCA were most often involved [11,12]. In the posterior circulation, the intracranial vertebral arteries (ICVAs) and basilar artery were most often affected [11,13]. The posterior cerebral arteries were occasionally involved [14].

FIBROMUSCULAR DYSPLASIA

Renal artery fibromuscular dysplasia (FMD) was first described in 1938 as a cause of arterial hypertension in a patient with unilateral kidney disease who had an intraluminal mass of smooth muscle [15]. Lawrence McCormack and colleagues described the renal artery pathology of FMD 20 years later [16]. For many years fibromuscular disease was assumed to be limited to the renal arteries. A. J. Paslubinskas and H. R. Ripley were the first to report the angiographic appearance of FMD in extrarenal arteries in a patient who had involvement of the celiac artery and an angiographic lesion in an internal carotid artery [17]. Knowledge soon accrued about the common locations of FMD and their angiographic and clinical features. Burton Sandok, the chair of neurology at the Mayo Clinic and founder and later dean of the Mayo Clinic Medical School, deserves credit for bringing FMD to the attention of neurologists [18]. During the past decades, the United States Registry for Fibromuscular Dysplasia has yielded important information about the demography, locations, clinical findings, diagnosis, and treatment of FMD [19].

As in arterial dissection, the appearance of vessels at angiography identified the condition. The most common finding was alternating zones of widening and narrowing of the arterial lumen on angiograms – a "string of beads" appearance. Dilatations in the artery are wider than the normal lumen and are separated from each other by sharply localized regions of vasoconstriction. Some patients with typical "string of beads" lesions also have localized regions of tubular constriction and diverticulum-like aneurysmal dilatations. Hypertrophy of fibrous tissues in the adventitia or intima cause segmental areas of tubular stenosis, which can appear as shelves, ridges, or webs in arteries. Occasionally, patients have had band-like shelves or diaphragms within greatly enlarged carotid bulbs in the neck that sometimes contain thrombi.

FMD occurs predominantly in Caucasian women, mostly in their fourth to sixth decades of life. In the US Registry, 92 percent of patients were female [15,19]. Fibromuscular dysplasia is a nonatheromatous multifocal condition that can affect almost any systemic or brain-supplying artery but has special predilection for some arterial sites. It tends to involve medium-sized muscular arteries, especially renal, splanchnic, and cervicocranial arteries. In the US Registry cohort of more than 400 patients, nearly 80 percent had renal artery involvement and almost 75 percent had carotid artery FMD lesions [19]. The vertebral artery was the third most common site. FMD was most often localized to the portions of the extracranial vertebral and carotid arteries adjacent to the second cervical vertebra. FMD can occasionally involve the cavernous carotid arteries and the arteries of the circle of Willis.

FMD affects primarily the connective tissue elements of the arteries. Any or all of the three arterial walls can be involved. The most common form affects the media. Constricting bands composed of fibrous dysplastic tissue and proliferating smooth-muscle cells in the media alternate with areas of luminal dilatation related to medial thinning and disruption of the elastic membrane. An adventitial form is characterized by narrowing of the vascular lumen by fibrous tissue hypertrophy surrounding an artery. An intimal form is character-ized by an increase in the fibrous components of the intima, producing concentric narrowing of the arterial lumen.

Hypertension related to renal arterial FMD can lead to brain infarcts and hemorrhages. Patients with FMD often have intracranial arterial aneurysms. The involvement of the nuchal carotid and vertebral arteries renders these sites vulnerable to dissections.

In some patients with transient or persistent brain ischemia, FMD of an artery appropriate to explain the brain imaging and clinical findings was the only vascular abnormality found. The lumen may not appear severely com-promised in these patients. The mechanism of the distal ischemia in this circumstance is uncertain. Functional changes in vessel contraction (vasocon-striction) could lead to distal hypoperfusion. Altered blood flow with stasis could lead to thrombus formation and distal intraarterial embolism. A striking observation in series of patients with cervico-cranial fibromuscular dysplasia is the relative benignity of the condition [15]. Even in those who present with strokes, further vascular episodes are unusual and much less frequent than in patients with atherosclerotic vascular lesions.

MOYAMOYA SYNDROME AND DISEASE

The first patient with a new condition, later recognized as Moyamoya disease, was presented at an annual meeting of the Japanese Neurosurgical Society in 1955 [20]. This 29-year-old man had had visual dysfunction and seizures since age 10 and had become functionally blind. Carotid angiography showed occlusion of the internal carotid arteries intracranially. A biopsy of an extracra-nial external carotid artery branch showed proliferative changes in the media and adventitia of the artery [20]. Subsequent similar cases studied by angiog-raphy showed a net of blood vessels that developed at the base of the brain to provide collateral circulation in response to the progressive occlusive process. These vessels formed large, prominent, anastomosing channels, basal telangiectasias, that on angiograms resembled a "cloud of smoke." These arteries were especially prominent because of the sparsity of MCA sylvian branches. The appearance of these basal telangiectasias led Japanese clinicians to use the non-medical term "Moyamoya," which colloquially means something is hazy, vague or indescribable, like "a puff of smoke drifting in the air."

Jiro Suzuki, professor of neurosurgery at the Tohoku University in Sendai, Japan, launched intensive research on this entity during more than two decades before his sudden death from a brain glioma [21]. Six generations of his family before him had been physicians. He described the angiographic stages of the condition, shown in Figure 22.1. He and his Sendai colleagues were among the first to attempt surgical treatment of the condition in children [22].

In classical Moyamoya disease, the intracranial carotid arteries undergo progressive tapering and progressive occlusion at their intracranial bifurcations (the so-called T-portion of the ICAs). Basal penetrating branches of the ICAs,

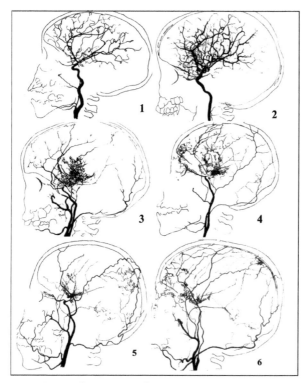

22.1. Stages of Moyamoya after Suzuki: (1) Narrowing of the intracranial ICA; (2) start of basal Moyamoya; (3) intensification of the Moyamoya, middle cerebral artery and anterior cerebral artery diminished; (4) minimization of Moyamoya, posterior cerebral artery disappearing; (5) reduction of Moyamoya, all major internal carotid artery branches lost; (6) supply only by external carotid artery and collaterals from vertebrobasilar system. From Suzuki J, Kodama N. Moyamoya disease – A review. *Stroke* 1983;14:105–109, with permission.

ACAs, and MCAs enlarge to provide collateral circulation. The deep lenticulostriate branches enlarge and form a basal telangiectasia, from which the term "Moyamoya" arose. Although initially described in Japan, the condition occurs worldwide.

Once the angiographic features were recognized, experience in Asia and elsewhere led to characterization of the demography, clinical features, prognosis, and effect of various therapeutic maneuvers. Childhood-onset Moyamoya disease was found to be much more common in girls and women than in boys and men. Clinically, the condition had a bimodal distribution, presenting most often in very young children and adolescents and in adults in their third to fifth decades of life. Children usually presented with transient episodes of hemiparesis, abnormal movements, or other focal neurologic signs often precipitated by physical exercise or hyperventilation. Others had sudden-onset deficits, such as hemiplegia, or the gradual development of intellectual deterioration. Headaches and seizures were common. Adults, in contrast, usually presented with brain hemorrhages, most often in the thalamus, basal ganglia, and deep white matter. These hemorrhages were attributable to degenerative changes (aneurysmal dilatation and thinning) in the anastomotic basal vessels that were overburdened and could not accommodate the volume of blood needed for perfusion. Some hemorrhages were subarachnoid and intraventricular.

Necropsy studies, although few, showed severe vascular occlusive abnormalities characterized by endothelial hyperplasia and fibrosis, with intimal thickening and abnormalities of the internal elastic lamina [23]. The intracerebral perforating arteries show microaneurysm formation, lipohyalinosis, focal fibrin deposition, and thinning of the elastic laminas and arterial walls. The vessels did not show inflammatory abnormalities.

Although classified as a disease, Moyamoya is probably better considered a syndrome defined by a characteristic angiographic appearance. Moyamoya vascular abnormalities have been found in a variety of conditions that cause intimal changes leading to fibrosis and luminal narrowing. Known conditions that cause Moyamoya-like changes are sickle cell disease, neurofibromatosis, Takayasu's disease, Down syndrome, atherosclerosis, and fibromuscular dysplasia. Similar findings were found in young women, especially those who smoke cigarettes and take oral contraceptives.

A variety of different surgical revascularization procedures have been used. These usually involve anastomosing the superficial temporal artery to the MCA, placing the superficial temporal and middle meningeal arteries adjacent to the pia, or placing vascularized connective tissue elements and muscle on the surface of the pia matter [24]. The surgical revascularization created is often called synangiosis. More recently, making a number of burr holes and opening the arachnoid membranes has been performed [25].

A strong association has been established between Moyamoya disease and polymorphisms of the RING finger 213 (*RNF213*) gene on chromosopme17q25-ter [26]. About one third of patients who have the p. R4810K polymorphism of *RNF213* gene develop Moyamoya disease. The RING finger gene has been found predominantly in Asians and is much less common in those of European descent [27].

REVERSIBLE CEREBRAL VASOCONSTRICTION SYNDROME

Marie Fleming, a neurologist at St. Elizabeth's Medical Center in Boston, presented two patients who had headaches and abnormal cerebral angiograms at a 1987 Boston Stroke Society meeting. After the meeting, Miller Fisher and his Massachusetts General Hospital (MGH) colleagues, including Greg Call, a stroke fellow at the time, collected similar cases and published a report in the journal *Stroke* [28]. The condition that they described was characterized by persistent headache and transient, fully reversible vasoconstriction and dilatation prominently involving arteries around the circle of Willis. The condition was referred to as the "Call-Fleming" syndrome [29].

Aneesh Singhal dubbed the condition reversible cerebral vasoconstriction syndrome (RCVS). He and his MGH colleagues studied large number of patients with this syndrome, analyzed the features that separated RCVS from vasculitis (a much less common condition), and elaborated on the clinical symptoms and signs, precipitating conditions, imaging characteristics, and prognosis [30]. Clinicians and investigators in Paris at Lariboisière Hospital, led by Anne Ducros and Marie-Germaine Bouser, professor of neurology at Paris Diderot University, later clarified the clinical and imaging characteristics of this entity [31]. By the end of the first quarter of the twenty-first century, the entity had become well known, although treatment was debated.

RCVS was found to most often affect young women, especially during the puerperium, but it also occurred at menopause and at all ages. When it occurred after childbirth, the syndrome had been referred to as postpartum angiopathy [32]. Many of the patients have had a history of migraine. The use of serotonin reuptake inhibitors prescribed for depression and use of cannabis, especially when smoked in a binge, could provoke the syndrome [30].

Vasoconstriction involved many large, medium, and small-sized brain-supplying arteries. Neck arteries were also involved and could show areas of dissection [30,31]. The onset was often with a severe headache likened to a thunderclap. The clinical findings included severe persistent but fluctuating headache, decreased alertness, seizures, and changing multifocal neurologic signs. Brain edema and death occasionally occurred. In many cases the headaches gradually subsided after weeks or a few months even without treatment.

Brain imaging could show focal subarachnoid blood on the surface of the brain and in adjacent sulci and small regions of abnormality on FLAIR-MRI imaging representing brain ischemia. Angiography showed sausage-shaped focal regions of vasodilatation and multifocal regions of vascular narrowing. Transcranial Doppler (TCD) ultrasound could show increased blood flow velocities indicative of vasoconstriction even before angiographic abnormalities were identified. The initial vascular imaging studies (CTA, MRA, and even digital cerebral angiography) were often normal and only became abnormal after a few days or a week.

Management was debated. Many patients recovered without treatment. Corticosteroid treatment was not effective and might be harmful. Some clinicians favored calcium-channel inhibitor treatment.

NOTES AND REFERENCES

1. Caplan LR, Biller J. *Uncommon Causes of Stroke*, 3rd ed. Cambridge: Cambridge University Press, 2017.

2. Nicholls F. 1761. Observations concerning the body of His Late Majesty. *Philos. Trans. Royal Soc. Lond.* 1761;52:265–275.

3. Shennan T. *Dissecting Aneurysms*, Medical Research Council, Special Report Series 193. London: His Majesty's Stationery Office, 1934.

4. Hirst AE Jr, Johns VJ, Kime SW. 1958. Dissecting aneurysm of the aorta: A review of 505 cases. *Medicine* 1958;37:217–279.

5. Moersch FP, Sayre GP. 1950. Neurologic manifestations associated with dissecting aneurysm of the aorta. *JAMA* 1950;144:1141–1148.

6. Ojemann RG, Fisher CM, Rich JC. Spontaneous dissecting aneurysms of the internal carotid artery. *Stroke* 1972;3:434–440.

7. Fisher CM. *Memoirs of a Neurologist*, vol. 1. Rutland, VT: Sharp & Co. Printers, 2006, p. 157. Caplan LR. *C. Miller Fisher: Stroke in the 20th Century*. Oxford: Oxford University Press, 2020, pp. 201–212.

8. Caplan LR, Zarins CK, Hemmati M. Spontaneous dissection of the extracranial vertebral arteries. *Stroke* 1985;16:1030–1038. Bradac G, Kaernbach A, Bolk-Weischedel D, Finck G. Spontaneous dissecting aneurysm of cervical cerebral arteries. *Neuroradiology* 1981;21:149–154. Goldstein S. Dissecting hematoma of the cervical vertebral artery. *J. Neurosurg.* 1982;56:451–454.

9. Caplan LR: Dissections of brain-supplying arteries. *Nat. Clin. Pract. Neurol.* 2008;4:34–42. Debette S, Leys D. Cervical-artery dissections: Predisposing factors, diagnosis, and outcome. *Lancet Neurol.* 2009;8:668–678. Schievink WI. Spontaneous dissection of the carotid and vertebral arteries. *N. Engl. J. Med.* 2001;344:898–906.

10. Biller J, Sacco RL, Albuquerque FC, Demaerschalk BM, Fayad P, et al. Cervical arterial dissections and association with cervical manipulative therapy: A statement for healthcare professionals from the American Heart Association/American Stroke Association. *Stroke* 2014;45:3155–3174.

11. Arnold M, Sturznegger M. Cervicocephalic arterial dissections. In Biller J, Caplan LR (eds.), *Uncommon Causes of Stroke*. Cambridge: Cambridge University Press, 2018, pp. 509–533.

12. Chaves C, Estol C, Esnaola MM, et al. Spontaneous intracranial internal carotid artery dissection. *Arch. Neurol.* 2002;59:977–981.

13. Caplan LR, Baquis G, Pessin MS, et al. Dissection of the intracranial vertebral artery. *Neurology* 1988;38:868–879. Hosoya T, Adachi M, Yamaguchi K, et al. Clinical and neuroradiological features of intracranial vertebrobasilar artery dissection. *Stroke* 1999;30:1083–1090.

14. Caplan LR, Estol CJ, Massaro AR. Dissection of the posterior cerebral arteries. *Arch. Neurol.* 2005;62:1138–1143.

15. Caplan LR. Fibromuscular dysplasia in uncommon causes of stroke. In Biller J, Caplan LR (eds.), *Uncommon Causes of Stroke*. Cambridge: Cambridge University Press, 2018, pp. 575–580. Sandok BA. Fibromuscular dysplasia of the cephalic arterial system. In Toole JF (ed.), *Handbook of Clinical Neurology*, vol. 11. Amsterdam: Elsevier Science Publishers, 1989, pp. 283–292. Slovut DP, Olin JW. Fibromuscular dysplasia. *N. Engl. J. Med.* 2004;350:1862–1871.

16. McCormack LJ, Hazard JB, Poutasse EF. Obstructive lesions of the renal artery associated with remediable hypertension. *Amer. J. Pathol.* 1958;34:582.

17. Palubinskas AJ, Ripley HR. Fibromuscular hyperplasia in extrarenal arteries. *Radiology* 1964;82:451–455.

18. Sandok BA. Fibromuscular dysplasia of the internal carotid artery. In Barnett HJM (ed.), *Neurologic Clinics*, vol. 1. Philadelphia: Saunders, 1983, 17–26. Sandok BA. Fibromuscular dysplasia of the cephalic arterial system. In Toole JF (ed.), *Handbook of Clinical Neurology*, vol. 11. Amsterdam: Elsevier Science Publishers, 1989, pp. 283–292.

19. Olin JW, Froehlich J, Gu X, et al. The United States Registry for Fibromuscular Dysplasia: Results in the first 447 patients. *Circulation* 2012;125:3182–3190.

20. Yonekawa Y, Handa H, Okuno T. Moyamoya disease: Diagnosis, treatment, and recent achievement. In Barnett HJM, Mohr JP, Stein B, Yatsu FM (eds.), *Stroke: Pathophysiology, Diagnosis, and Management*, vol. 2. New York: Churchill-Livingstone, 1986, pp. 805–829.

21. Suzuki J, Kowada M, Asahi M, Takaku A. A study on disease showing singular cerebral-angiographical findings which seem to be new collateral circulation. Proceedings of the 22nd Meeting of the Japan Society, 1963. Suzuki J, Takaku A, Asahi M. The disease showing the abnormal vascular network at the base of the brain, particularly found in Japan. *Brain Nerve (Tokyo)* 1966;18:897–908. Suzuki J, Takaku A. Cerebral vascular "Moyamoya" disease: A disease showing abnormal net-like vessels in base of brain. *Arch. Neurol.* 1969; 20: 288–299. Suzuki J, Kodama N. Moyamoya Disease: A review. *Stroke* 1983;14:105–109. Suzuki J. *Moyamoya Disease*. Berlin: Springer-Verlag, 1986.

22. Suzuki, J, Takaku A, Kodama N, et al. An attempt to treat cerebrovascular Moyamoya disease in children. *Child Brain* 1975;1:193–206.

23. Bruno A, Adams HOP, Bilbe J, et al. Cerebral infarction due to Moyamoya disease in young adults. *Stroke* 1988;19:826–833.

24. Matsushima T, Inoue TK, Suzuki SO, Inoue T, Ikezaki K, Fukui M, et al. Surgical techniques and the results of a fronto-temporo-parietal combined indirect bypass procedure for children with Moyamoya disease: A comparison with the results of encephalo-duro arterio-synangiosis alone. *Clin. Neurol. Neurosurg.* 1997;99:123–127. Scott RM, Smith ER. Moyamoya disease and Moyamoya syndrome. *N. Engl. J. Med.* 2009;360:1226–1237.

25. Sainte-Rose C, Oliveira R, Puget S, Beni-Adani L, Boddaert N, Thorne J, et al. Multiple burr hole surgery for the treatment of Moyamoya disease in children. *J. Neurosurg.* 2006;105:437–443.

26. Kamada F, Aoki Y, Narisawa A, et al. A genome-wide association study identifies *RNF213* as the first Moyamoya disease gene. *J. Hum. Genet.* 2011;56(1):34–40.

27. Raso A, Biassoni R, Mascelli S, et al. Moyamoya vasculopathy shows a genetic mutational gradient decreasing from East to West. *J. Neurosurg. Sci.* 2020;64 (2):165–172.

28. Call GK, Fleming MC, Sealfon S, Levine H, Kistler JP, Fisher CM. Reversible cerebral segmental vasoconstriction. *Stroke* 1988;19(9):1159–1170.

29. Dodick DW. Reversible segmental cerebral vasoconstriction (Call-Fleming syndrome): The role of calcium antagonists. *Cephalalgia* 2003;23(3):163–165.

30. Singhal AB. Cerebral vasoconstriction without subarachnoid blood: Associated conditions, clinical and neuroimaging characteristics. *Ann. Neurol.* 2002;52 (3S):59–60. Singhal AB, Caviness VS, Begleiter AF, Mark EJ, Rordorf G, Koroshetz WJ. Cerebral vasoconstriction and stroke after use of serotonergic drugs. *Neurology* 2002;58(1):130–133. Singhal AB, Koroshetz WJ, Caplan LR. Reversible cerebral vasoconstriction syndromes. In Caplan LR (ed.), *Uncommon Causes of Stroke.* Cambridge: Cambridge University Press, 2008, pp. 505–514. Singhal AB, Hajj-Ali RA, Topcuoglu MA, et al. Reversible cerebral vasoconstriction syndromes: Analysis of 139 cases. *Arch. Neurol.* 2011;68(8):1005–1012.

31. Ducros A, Boukobza M, Porcher R, Sarov M, Valade D, Bousser MG. The clinical and radiological spectrum of reversible cerebral vasoconstriction syndrome: A prospective series of 67 patients. *Brain* 2007;130(12):3091–3101. Ducros A. Reversible cerebral vasoconstriction syndrome. *Lancet Neurol.* 2012;11:906–917.

32. Bogousslavsky J, Despland PA, Regli F, Dubuis PY. Postpartum cerebral angiopathy: Reversible vasoconstriction assessed by transcranial Doppler ultrasound. *Eur. Neurol.* 1989;29:102–105.

CHAPTER TWENTY THREE

BLOOD DISORDERS

EARLY STUDIES

Marcello Malpighi (1628–1694), an Italian physiologist and physician, is credited with introducing the microscope into medicine. He was probably the first to study blood clotting. He examined both thrombi in the heart and in vitro blood clots using a light microscope and found that their structures were similar. He described red blood cells for the first time and noted the appearance of a meshwork of fibrous texture that later was labeled "fibrin" [1].

The next advance was by Johannes Peter Müller (1801–1858), a German physiologist and comparative anatomist. He became professor of physiology in Bonn in 1830. In 1833, he went to the University of Berlin, where he filled the chair of anatomy and physiology until his death. Müller was very interested in nerve function, both cranial and spinal. He maintained that all stimuli acting on the nerves had the same effect, whether they were mechanical chemical, thermal, or galvano-electric. His physiological research identified fibrin, the substance in the blood that led to clotting [2]. In 1856, Müller entrusted the lectures on pathological anatomy at Berlin to his brilliant student Rudolf Ludwig Karl Virchow.

While it is now evident that blood disorders and conditions that promote hypercoagulability play an important role in the pathogenesis of stroke, this concept was not understood until the mid-nineteenth century when Virchow (1821–1902) studied mechanisms of ischemia and described the phenomena he called "thrombosis" and "embolism" [3,4]. Virchow studied medicine at the Friedrich-Wilhelms-Institut in Berlin and began his professional career at the Charité Hospital, which to this day is one of Europe's largest university teaching hospital and research institutions. He was one of the first physicians to examine disease at the cellular level. He proposed that pathology originated not in a tissue or an organ but rather in individual cells or groups of cells, thereby launching the field of cellular pathology [5].

Virchow studied venous thromboembolism (VTE) extensively and opined that the thrombus did not originate locally in the pulmonary artery, but rather dislodged and traveled from a distant source ("embolus"). He stated:

> In contrast to that kind of obliterating clot we find another kind. Here there is either no essential change in the vessel wall and its surroundings, or this is ostensibly secondary. I feel perfectly justified in claiming that these clots never originated in the local circulation but that they are torn off at a distance and carried along in the blood stream as far as they can go. [6,7]

Virchow was able to confirm this hypothesis and described a set of factors that promote thrombosis, which became known as Virchow's Triad. These include intravascular vessel wall (endothelial) damage, stasis of flow, and blood coagulation. He studied the blood and, in 1847, identified a slowly clottable substance that he called *fibrinogen*. While Virchow's triad was originally described in venous disease, its concepts also apply to arterial thromboembolism and ischemic stroke. Virchow and his extensive contributions are the topic of Chapter 13.

Alexander Schmidt (1831–1894), a German physiologist born in Estonia, studied extensively the process of coagulation of the blood and showed that the transformation of fibrinogen into fibrin was the result of an enzymatic process. He named the hypothetical enzyme *thrombin* and called its precursor *prothrombin* [8].

CLINICAL KNOWLEDGE OF BLOOD COAGULATION

Virchow and Schmidt had discovered the final pathway in which blood coagulated. Thrombin catalyzed the reaction of fibrinogen to fibrin and a clot formed. Clots blocked arteries and led to organ ischemia and infarction.

It took many decades, and many clinicians and investigators, to clarify the intricate process of blood coagulation. Platelets circulated within the blood and repaired breeches in vessels caused, for example, by trauma. An excess of platelets could lead to increased clotting; a deficiency of platelets could lead to bleeding. As Virchow had proposed, blood vessels and tissue could release a factor or factors that increased the tendency for blood to clot. This pathway was later labeled the "extrinsic pathway" because it did not begin with factors within the blood, but rather by the release of *tissue factor* under conditions of injury or inflammation. Investigators also found that various proteins present within the plasma were necessary for clot formation. This pathway of coagulation was labeled the "intrinsic pathway." These two pathways come together with the conversion of prothrombin to thrombin. Several individuals were instrumental in discovering key components of blood clotting.

Giulio Bizzozero (1846–1901) was a physician who pioneered the study of histology. He graduated from the University of Pavia in 1866 at the age of 20. He then traveled and worked with Rudolf Virchow in Berlin. In 1867, he was appointed the chief of general pathology and histology at the University of Pavia. In 1881, he described platelets as a third element in blood after erythrocytes and leukocytes. He called them *petit plaques*, *plaquettes*, or *Blutplättchen*. He showed their role in clotting through aggregation that led to the formation of clumps admixed with thread-like strands of fibrin [9].

Paul Oskar Morawitz (1879–1936) was a German physician and physiologist whose most important work was the study of blood coagulation [10]. After completing his medical studies in Leipzig in 1901, he completed his army service and became a physician's assistant in Tübingen. In 1905, while at the University of Tübingen, Morawitz coined the term "thrombokinase" to describe the clot-promoting protein in tissue [11.] He suggested that platelets were the principal source. He recognized four necessary and sufficient components for blood coagulation: thrombokinase (later referred to as tissue factor), calcium, prothrombin, and fibrinogen. In 1907, he completed his thesis on blood coagulation and was appointed chief physician at the University Clinic in Freiburg. He then became director of medical inpatients in Greifswald and later worked as a physician in Würzburg and Leipzig. He was also a pioneer in blood transfusion.

Armand James Quick (1894–1978) was an American researcher and clinician [12,13]. His work was important in calling attention to the intrinsic pathway of coagulation. As a boy, he contracted tuberculosis of the cervical spine, leaving him with restricted neck motion. In 1920, he earned his PhD in organic chemistry at the University of Illinois. He then worked at the Philadelphia General Hospital and the University of Pennsylvania, before beginning his medical studies. He obtained his MD in 1928 at Cornell. In 1935, he was offered an assistant professorship at Marquette's medical school, where he later became chairman of biochemistry, a position he held until retirement. He was the initiator of the *prothrombin time* test still in use today. In researching this test, he showed that blood clotted in the test tube without platelets and that this depended on various blood protein substances [14]. In his later years, Quick studied the effects of aspirin on hemostasis. He showed that aspirin could prolong the skin bleeding time. He was also an exacting clinician and could take hours to extract a detailed clinical history.

The biochemical factors in the blood that are active in the process of coagulation were mostly discovered during the first half of the twentieth century. The use of roman numerals rather than eponyms or systematic names was agreed upon during annual conferences. Prothrombin became known as factor II. The best known was factor VIII, originally termed anti-hemophilic globulin because of its role in hemophilia. Each of factors V, VII, X, XI, and XII was shown to have a role in the intrinsic pathway of the coagulation cascade.

INHERITED THROMBOPHILIAS

When young patients with deep vein thrombosis and pulmonary embolism or with brain infarcts were investigated, it began to be recognized that some of these thrombotic events occurred due to an increased tendency for blood clotting. Normal hemostasis depended on a delicate balance between pro-thrombotic and antithrombotic processes mediated by cellular components, soluble plasma proteins, and endothelium-derived factors [15]. Thrombosis was a result of an imbalance between the prothrombotic and anticoagulant activities of the vascular milieu and plasma in favor of thrombosis.

Individuals with an increased tendency to thrombosis were defined as having thrombophilia, either acquired or inherited. Acquired or secondary thrombophilias were found to occur in the presence of antiphospholipid antibodies or in the setting of malignancy, myeloproliferative diseases, hyper-viscosity syndromes, nephrotic syndrome, paroxysmal nocturnal hemoglobi-nuria, trauma, prolonged immobilization, or pregnancy/puerperium [16]. Inherited or primary thrombophilias were found to be due to genetic defects directly or indirectly involved with hemostasis. Clinically, inherited thrombo-philia was characterized by thrombotic events that occurred early in life, typically before 45 years of age, thrombosis at unusual sites (retinal veins, intraabdominal veins, upper limbs, or central nervous system), and a family history of thromboembolic events in 30–50 percent of patients.

FACTOR V LEIDEN

Before 1993, the diagnosis of a hereditary coagulation disorder could be established in only about 5–15 percent of individuals. The major disorders known at the time were deficiencies of antithrombin III, protein C, or protein S. These naturally occurring plasma proteins had anticoagulant activity. Activated *protein C* and *protein S* were found to inhibit the action of factors Va and factor VIIIa. A deficiency of any of these factors weighted the balance of hemostasis toward excess clotting.

In 1993, Dahlbäck and his Swedish colleagues identified a coagulation abnormality that was found to be highly prevalent among patients with venous thrombosis [17]. The initial patient described had developed multiple episodes of deep vein thrombosis, the first in his leg at age 19. Several family members also had developed unexplained thrombotic events. The patient and his family were investigated, and the authors observed that the addition of exogenous activated protein C (APC) to their plasma did not result in the expected prolongation of clotting time seen in controls, a phenomenon they called "APC resistance." Subsequent studies identified this phenotype in 20–50 percent of patients with deep vein thrombosis and pulmonary embolism. It became recognized as a novel mechanism underlying the development of thromboembolic disease.

A year later, Rogier M. Bertina and his Dutch colleagues identified that APC resistance was present in over 95 percent of cases, the result of a G to A point mutation in the coagulation factor V gene that rendered the mutant factor V resistant to proteolytic inactivation, thereby leading to augmented generation of thrombin [18]. This point mutation was described and investigated at the University of Leiden in the Netherlands, and has been referred to since as factor V Leiden (FVL). Factor V Leiden was found to be the most common genetic defect involved in the etiology of venous thrombosis. The increased risk of deep vein thrombosis, pulmonary embolism, and cerebral venous thrombosis associated with FVL was confirmed in a number of studies [19]. Factor V Leiden was found to be highly prevalent among Caucasians with carrier frequencies in the population ranging from 1 to 15 percent worldwide. The Dutch investigators found that heterozygosity for FVL increased the risk of VTE between three- and eight-fold [20], while homozygosity was associated with a 50- to 100-fold increase in risk [21].

PROTHROMBIN GENE MUTATION

Prothrombin (factor II) had been identified as a vitamin K–dependent zymogen produced by the liver. Its activated form, thrombin, catalyzed the conversion of fibrinogen into fibrin. In 1996, Swibertus Poort, Rogier Bertina, and their Dutch colleagues identified a G to A substitution at nucleotide 20210 in the 3'-untranslated region of the prothrombin gene associated with elevated plasma prothrombin levels and an increased risk of VTE [22]. Carriers of the 20210A allele were found to have an almost three-fold increase in the risk of venous thrombosis. Studies later established prothrombin 20210A as the second most prevalent inherited thrombophilia, leading to a two- to five-fold increase in risk of VTE [23].

HYPERHOMOCYSTEINEMIA

A correlation between homocysteine and atherothrombosis was first suggested by Kilmer McCully [24]. He reported autopsy evidence of extensive arterial thrombosis and atherosclerosis in two children with homocystinuria and proposed that elevated plasma homocysteine levels could cause atherosclerotic vascular disease. Homocystinuria had been described seven years before McCully's study in a search among individuals with intellectual disabilities [25]. Hyperhomocysteinemia became a well-established independent risk factor for atherosclerosis and atherothrombosis. Although severe hyperhomocysteinemia was found to be rare, abundant epidemiologic evidence showed that even slight hyperhomocysteinemia, which occurs in approximately 5–7 percent of the general population, was an independent risk factor for atherosclerosis in the coronary, cerebral, and peripheral vasculature [26].

The normal plasma homocysteine concentration was found to vary between 5 and 15 μmol/L in the fasting state. Hyperhomocysteinemia could be classified into moderate (15–30 μmol/L), intermediate (>30–100 μmol/L), and severe (>100 μmol/L) based on fasting plasma levels of the amino acid. Elevations in plasma homocysteine could be attributed to a wide range of conditions, the most important of which were determined to be genetic defects in the enzymes involved in homocysteine metabolism and by nutritional deficiencies in vitamin cofactors.

Homocystinuria and severe hyperhomocysteinemia were found to be caused by inborn errors of metabolism resulting in marked elevations of plasma and urine homocysteine concentrations. Cystathionine β-synthase deficiency was identified as the most common genetic cause of severe hyperhomocysteinemia. The homozygous form of this autosomal recessive disorder, congenital homocystinuria, had a frequency of approximately 1 in 250,000 in the general population and can be associated with plasma homocysteine concentrations of up to 400 μmol/L during fasting, leading to severe pathological effects [27]. The clinical manifestations included premature, severe atherosclerosis, venous thromboembolism, intellectual disability, ectopic lenses, and skeletal deformities. Atherothrombotic complications developed at a young age, and about half of untreated patients had a thromboembolic event before age 30. Heterozygotes typically had much less marked hyperhomocysteinemia, with plasma homocysteine concentrations in the range of 20–40 μmol/L. Patients with mild hyperhomocysteinemia had none of the clinical signs of severe hyperhomocysteinemia or homocystinuria, and were typically asymptomatic until the third or fourth decade of life when premature coronary artery disease or stroke could develop, as well as recurrent arterial and venous thrombosis.

In 1988, Kang and his colleagues in the genetics section of the department of pediatrics at Rush Medical College reported a thermolabile variant of methylenetetrahydrofolate reductase (MTHFR), an enzyme involved in homocysteine metabolism [28]. This variant had less than 50 percent specific activity at $37°C$ compared to the normal enzyme. They determined that this thermolability was caused by a C677T point mutation in the coding region of the MTHFR gene, which led to a single amino acid substitution in a potential folate binding site. The thermolabile variant of MTHFR was inherited as an autosomal recessive trait and caused slight to moderate hyperhomocysteinemia. The frequency of homozygosity was found to lie between 5 and 15 percent among populations of Caucasian, Middle Eastern, and Japanese origin and below 1.5 percent among African Americans.

In addition to genetic abnormalities in enzymes of the homocysteine metabolic pathways, nutritional deficiencies in the vitamin cofactors (folate, vitamin B_{12}, and vitamin B_6) required for homocysteine metabolism were found to lead to hyperhomocysteinemia. Serum homocysteine levels were elevated in more than 95% of individuals with nutritional deficiencies of the essential cofactor vitamin B_{12} or the cosubstrate folate, and levels of homocysteine could range from two- to three-fold over control to greater than 400 μmol/L. Selhub and colleagues suggested that low plasma concentrations of one or more B vitamins were contributing factors in approximately two thirds of all cases of hyperhomocysteinemia [29].

ANTIPHOSPHOLIPID ANTIBODIES AND ANTIPHOSPHOLIPID SYNDROME

The term *antiphospholipid antibodies* (aPL) refers to a heterogeneous group of antibodies to phospholipid-binding proteins. The discovery of aPL would not have been possible without the creation of a test for syphilis by Wasserman in 1906 in which cardiolipin was extracted from bovine tissue and used as an antigen [30]. The first description of aPL was reported in 1951 when "unusual circulating anticoagulants" were described [31]. The name "lupus anticoagulant" (LA) was applied, although it was a misnomer since the antibody was associated with increased coagulability, not bleeding. Lupus anticoagulant was found to be a phospholipid antibody that interfered with the formation of the prothrombin activator. In 1952, the earliest association with lupus erythematosus was reported [32]. In 1989, antiphospholipid syndrome (APS) was formally described as a syndrome in which the lupus anticoagulant (LA) was associated with fetal loss, thrombosis, or thrombocytopenia [33].

Although laboratory recognition had occurred for the LA and anticardiolipin antibodies (aCL), it was not until 1990 that a cofactor was identified as beta-2 glycoprotein, which allowed for the binding of anticardiolipin to cardiolipin on ELISA testing, expanding the ability to test for these antibodies [34]. Laboratory technology evolved to allow for increased precision in recognizing the syndrome. Case series began to convey a more complete picture of the various components of the syndrome. The Sapporo criteria were published in 1999, followed by the revised Sydney criteria in 2006 [35].

Primary APS was distinguished from secondary APS, which occurred in patients with systemic lupus erythematosus. The most common clinical presentation of primary APS was found to be venous thromboembolism, most often manifested as deep vein thrombosis (DVT) or pulmonary embolism. For those who had a first event, elevated aCL served as a predictor of recurrence and mortality. Many neurologic clinical presentations were associated with APS, including cerebrovascular disease, headache, seizures, movement disorders, multiple sclerosis–like syndrome, transverse myelitis, and migraine. By far the most common presentation was brain ischemia – transient ischemic attack and stroke – described in up to 30 percent of initial presentations. In patients with a neurologic presentation of APS, elevated aCL were found in 70 percent of cases; LA positivity was found in 20 percent; and anti-beta-2 glycoprotein antibodies were found in 10 percent [36]. Patients with a neurologic manifestation of APS had an increased risk of morbidity and mortality compared to those with other presentations.

Strokes in patients with APS were found to be attributable to hypercoagulability or embolism arising from non-bacterial endocarditic lesions. The cardiac lesions were identical to those in Libman-Sacks endocarditis and involved the valves and the endothelium of the heart. The mechanism of increased coagulability and valvular changes was posited to relate to immune-mediated endothelial and valve-surface injuries [37]. Angiography in patients with APS showed a high frequency of intracranial occlusive disease, atypical extracranial occlusive arterial disease, and venous and dural sinus occlusions [38].

The Antiphospholipid Antibodies and Stroke Study (APASS) found that positivity for both LA and aCL, but not anticardiolipin alone, predicted a higher risk of recurrence in patients with a first ischemic stroke [39]. Patients who were "triple positive" – meaning positive for LA, IgG or IgM anticardiolipin, and anti-beta-2 glycoprotein – were at the highest risk for recurrent vascular events. The RATIO study showed that in a younger female population, the presence of LA was a major risk factor for arterial events such as myocardial infarction and stroke in the presence of oral contraceptive use and smoking [40].

A devastating form of APS became recognized as the catastrophic antiphospholipid syndrome (CAPS), first described in 1992 [41]. This syndrome described acute disseminated, often microvascular thrombosis involving multiple organs. This presentation was found in less than 1 percent of APS patients, but it conferred a high mortality rate. A European study noted that 62 percent of CAPS patients had a neurologic presentation, which ultimately led to mortality in 13 percent of patients [42].

BRAIN HEMORRHAGE DUE TO BLEEDING DISORDERS

Hereditary and acquired platelet and coagulation factor disorders are important causes of bleeding in the body. Bleeding is usually into the skin, gums, and internal organs but less often into the brain or its coverings. Iatrogenic causes, such as prescription of anticoagulants and antiplatelet agents, and thrombolysis are much more frequent causes of intracranial bleeding than inherited coagulopathies or platelet disorders. Thrombocytopenia and hemophilia were found to be very rare causes of major intracranial hemorrhages. The causes of intracerebral hemorrhage are discussed in Chapter 19.

NOTES AND REFERENCES

1. Malpighi, Marcello. *De polypo cordis*. Bologna, 1666.
2. Müller, Johannes. *Handbuch der Physiologie des Menschen*. 4 editions. Coblenz: J. Hölscher, 1835–1840.
3. Safavi-Abbasi S, Reis C, Talley MC, et al. Rudolf Ludwig Karl Virchow: Pathologist, physician, anthropologist, and politician. Implications of his work for the understanding of cerebrovascular pathology and stroke. *Neurosurg. Focus* 2006 Jun 15;20(6):E1.
4. Dickson BC. Venous thrombosis: On the history of Virchow's Triad. *University of Toronto Medical Journal* 2004;166–171.
5. Virchow, Rudolf. *Die Cellularpathologie in ihrer Begründung auf physiologische und pathologische Gewebelehre*. Berlin: A. Hirschwald, 1858.
6. Virchow, Rudolf. Über die akute Entzündung der Arterien. *Arch. Path. Anat. Physiol.* 1847;1:272–378.
7. Schiller F. Concepts of stroke before and after Virchow. *Med. Hist.* 1970;14:115–131.
8. Schmidt A. Neue Untersuchungen ueber die asserstoffesgerinnung. *Pflügers Archiv für die gesamte Physiologie* 1872;6:413–538.
9. Ribatti, D, Crivellato, E. Giulio Bizzozero and the discovery of platelets. *Leukemia Research* 2007;31(10):1339–1341.
10. Boulton F. A hundred years of cascading – Started by Paul Morawitz (1879–1936), a pioneer of haemostasis and of transfusion. *Transfus. Med.* 2006;16(1):1–10.
11. Morawitz P. Die Chemie der Blutgerinnung. *Ergebnisse der Physiologie* 1905;4:307–423.
12. Dirckx JH. Armand J. Quick: Pioneer and prophet of coagulation research. *Ann. Intern. Med.* 1980;92(4):553–558.
13. Ebel EM. *The Quick Tests: The Life and Work of Dr. Armand J. Quick*. Blacksburg, VA: Pocahontas Press, 1995.
14. Quick AJ. The development and use of the prothrombin tests. *Circulation* 1959;19 (1):92–96.
15. Rosenberg RD, Aird WC. Vascular-bed-specific hemostasis and hypercoagulable states. *N. Engl. J. Med.* 1999;340(20):1555–1564.
16. Bauer KA. Inherited and acquired hypercoagulable states. In Loscalzo J, Schafer AK (eds.), *Thrombosis and Hemorrhage*, 2nd ed. Baltimore, MD: Williams & Wilkins, 1998, pp. 863–900.
17. Dahlbäck B, Carlsson M, Svensson PJ. Familial thrombophilia due to a previously unrecognized mechanism characterized by poor anticoagulant response to activated

protein C: Prediction of a cofactor to activated protein C. *Proc. Natl. Acad. Sci. USA* 1993;90:1004–1008.

18. Bertina RM, Koeleman BP, Koster T, et al. Mutation in blood coagulation factor V associated with resistance to activated protein C. *Nature* 1994;369(6475):64–67.

19. Voorberg J, Roelse J, Koopman R, et al. Association of idiopathic venous thromboembolism with single point-mutation at Arg506 of factor V. *Lancet* 1994;343 (8912):1535–1536. Vandenbroucke JP, Bertina RM, Holmes ZR, et al. Factor V Leiden and fatal pulmonary embolism. *Thromb. Haemost.* 1998;79(3):511–516. Lüdemann P, Nabavi DG, Junker R, et al. Factor V Leiden mutation is a risk factor for cerebral venous thrombosis: A case-control study of 55 patients. *Stroke* 1998;29 (12):2507–2510.

20. Koster MDT, Vandenbrouke JPV, Rosendaal FR, de Ronde H, Bertina RM. Venous thrombosis due to poor anticoagulant response to activated protein C: Leiden Thrombophilia Study. *Lancet* 1993;342:1503–1506.

21. Rosendaal FR, Koster T, Vandenbroucke JP, Reitsma PH. High risk of thrombosis in patients homozygous for factor V Leiden (activated protein C resistance). *Blood* 1995;85 (6):1504–1508.

22. Poort SR, Rosendaal FR, Reitsma PH, Bertina RM. A common genetic variation in the 3′-untranslated region of the prothrombin gene is associated with elevated plasma prothrombin levels and an increase in venous thrombosis. *Blood* 1996;88 (10):3698–3703.

23. Leroyer C, Mercier B, Oger E, et al. Prevalence of 20210 A allele of the prothrombin gene in venous thromboembolism patients. *Thromb. Haemost.* 1998;80(1):49–51.

24. McCully KS. Vascular pathology of homocysteinemia: Implications for the pathogenesis of arteriosclerosis. *Am. J. Pathol.* 1969;56(1):111–128.

25. Carson NAJ, Neill DW. Metabolic abnormalities detected in a survey of mentally backward individuals in Northern Ireland. *Arch. Dis. Child* 1962;37:505–513.

26. Clarke R, Daly L, Robinson K, et al. Hyperhomocysteinemia: An independent risk factor for vascular disease. *N. Engl. J. Med.* 1991;324(17):1149–1155. Kang SS, Wong PW, Malinow MR. Hyperhomocyst(e)inemia as a risk factor for occlusive vascular disease. *Ann. Rev. Nutr.* 1992;12:279–298.

27. Mudd SH, Skovby F, Levy HL, et al. The natural history of homocystinuria due to cystathionine beta-synthase deficiency. *Am. J. Hum. Genet.* 1985;37:1–31.

28. Kang SS, Zhou J, Wong PW, Kowalisyn J, Strokosch G. Intermediate homocysteinemia: A thermolabile variant of methylenetetrahydrofolate reductase. *Am. J. Hum. Genet.* 1988;43(4):414–421.

29. Selhub J, Jacques PF, Wilson PW, Rush D, Rosenberg IH. Vitamin status and intake as primary determinants of homocysteinemia in an elderly population. *JAMA* 1993;270 (22):2693–2698.

30. Svenungsson E, Antovic A. The antiphospholipid syndrome – often overlooked cause of vascular occlusions? *J. Intern. Med.* 2020;7(4):349–372.

31. Mueller JF, Ratnoff O, Heinle RW. Observations on the characteristics of an unusual circulating anticoagulant. *J. Lab. Clin. Med.* 1951;8(2):254–261.

32. Conley CL, Hartmann RC. A hemorrhagic disorder caused by circulating anticoagulant in patients with disseminated lupus erythematosus. *J. Lab. Clin. Invest.* 1952;31:621–622. Bowie EJ, Thompson JH Jr, Pascuzzi CA, Owen CA Jr. Thrombosis in systemic erythematosus despite circulating anticoagulants. *J. Clin. Invest.* 1963;62:416–430.

33. Hughes GR, Asherson RA, Khamashta MA. Antiphospholipid syndrome: Linking many specialties. *Ann. Rheum. Dis.* 1989;48:355–356.

34. de Groot PG, Meijers JCM. β(2)-Glycoprotein I: Evolution, structure and function. *J. Thromb. Haemost.* 2011;9(7):1275–1284.

35. Wilson WA, Gharavi AE, Koike T, et al. International consensus statement on preliminary classification criteria for definite antiphospholipid syndrome: Report of an international workshop. *Arthritis Rheum.* 1999;42:1309–1311. Miyakis S, Lockshin MD, Atsumi T, Branch DW, et al. International consensus statement on an update of the classification criteria for definite antiphospholipid syndrome (APS). *J. Thromb. Haemost.* 2006 Feb;4(2):295–306.

36. Levine JS, Ware Branch D, Rauch J. The antiphospholipid syndrome. *N. Engl. J. Med.* 2002;346(10):752–763.

37. Ziporen L, Goldberg I, Arad M, et al. Libman-Sacks endocarditis in the antiphospholipid syndrome: Immunopathologic findings in deformed heart valves. *Lupus* 1996;5(3):196–205.

38. Provenzale JM, Barboriak DP, Allen NB, Ortel TL. Antiphospholipid antibodies: Findings at arteriography. *AJNR Am. J. Neuroradiol.* 1998;19:611–616.

39. Levine SR, Brey RL, Tilley BC, Thompson JL, et al. Antiphospholipid antibodies and subsequent thrombo-occlusive events in patients with ischemic stroke. *JAMA* 2004;291:576–584.

40. Urbanus RT, Siegerink B, Roest M, Rosendaal FR, et al. Antiphospholipid antibodies and risk of myocardial infarction and ischemic stroke in young women in the RATIO study: A case control study. *Lancet Neurol.* 2009;8:998–1005.

41. Asherton RA. The catastrophic antiphospholipid syndrome. *J. Rheumatol.* 1992;19:508–512.

42. Bucciarelli S, Espinosa G, Cervera R. The CAPS Registry: Morbidity and mortality of the catastrophic antiphospholipid syndrome. *Lupus* 2009;18(10):905–912.

CHAPTER TWENTY FOUR

STROKE GENETICS

A BRIEF HISTORY OF THE EVOLUTION OF GENETICS

The earliest recorded beliefs about heredity were provided by ancient Greeks who observed that animals gave birth to other animals of the same species and that children tended to resemble their parents. They deduced the "particulate theory" from this observation, suggesting that some information from body parts of each parent passed directly into the corresponding body parts of their offspring. Aristotle (384–322 BCE) posited that the father provided a miniature organism and the mother provided the necessary conditions for its growth. He refuted the notion of a simple, direct transfer of body parts from parent to offspring by observing that animals and humans who had been mutilated or lost body parts did not confer these losses to their offspring. Aristotle described a process he called *epigenesist*, in which the offspring was gradually generated from an undifferentiated mass by the addition of parts [1].

Aristotle's theory relied on macroscopic observations rather than microscopy. At the end of the seventeenth century, British scientist Robert Hooke put a cork under a microscope and observed that it was composed of miniature rectangles. He called them "cells," referring to the private chambers of monks in monasteries. He inferred that everything both living and nonliving was composed of cells. Later, French scientist René Dutrochet revised Hooke's theory through a microscopic study in 1824, concluding that only plant and animal tissues were composed of cells [1].

In 1858, British naturalist Charles Darwin and Alfred Russel Wallace presented the ground-breaking new theory of evolution through natural selection, the idea that members of a population who are better adapted to their environment will be the ones most likely to survive and pass their traits on to the next generation. Darwin published his theory in *On the Origin of Species by Means of Natural Selection*. His work was not viewed favorably, especially by religious leaders, who believed it refuted the biblical story of how life on Earth began. Even in the twenty-first century, the dispute over creationism and evolution continues [1,2].

The connection between cytology and inheritance was revealed by studies of cellular components, processes, and functions. The nineteenth-century German biologist August Weissmann studied medicine, biology, and zoology and contributed to genetics. He proposed the evolutionary theory known as the germplasm theory of heredity. He asserted that the genetic code of each organism was contained in its germ cells. He also suggested that the amount of genetic material in the gametes was reduced by one half by a reduction division now known as miosis. He refuted the claims that physical characteristics acquired through environmental exposure were passed from generation to generation by cutting the tails of several consecutive generations of mice and observing that none of their offspring was born tailless [1,3].

Gregor Mendel (1822–1884) was born into a peasant family in the Czech Republic. He spent much of his youth working in his family's orchards and gardens. Mendel is regarded as the "Father of Genetics." He devised the laws of heredity, which were published in his 1865 paper titled "Versuche über Pflanzenhybriden" (Experiments on Plant Hybridization). Mendel's contributions were not acknowledged during his lifetime. Not until the early twentieth century, nearly 40 years after he published his findings, did the scientific community resurrect Mendel's work and affirm the importance of his ideas [4].

In 1902, Sir Archibald E. Garrod, a British physician and chemist, applied Mendel's principles and identified the first disease attributable to genetic causes, which he called, "inborn errors of metabolism." The disease was alkaptonuria, a condition in which an abnormal buildup of homogentisic acid or alkapton accumulates. Mendel's work was translated from German to English by the British geneticist William Bateson, who coined the term *genetics* in 1905, along with other descriptive terms used in modern genetics [1]. The scope of Mendel's laws of heredity was expanded from individuals to populations by British mathematician Godfrey Harold Hardy and German geneticist Wilhelm Weinberg. In 1908, they independently devised a mathematical formula known as the Hardy-Weinberg equilibrium to quantify genetic variations in any given population [5].

In the early twentieth century, American geneticist Thomas Hunt Morgan researched genetic variations in fruit flies at Columbia University's famous "Fly

Room" and confirmed theories derived from Mendel's pea experiments. Morgan and his team explored sex chromosomes and sex-linked inheritance after they learned that all white-eyed flies were male. Morgan was awarded the Nobel Prize in Physiology or Medicine in 1933 for his work on the chromosomal theory of inheritance [6]. Fifty years later, in 1983 American geneticist Barbara McClintock was awarded the Nobel Prize in Physiology or Medicine for her discovery of the existence of jumping genes, mobile transposons that can move between different positions on a chromosome [7].

British biologist Fredrick Griffith discovered a transforming principle that could transfer the ability to cause fatal pneumonia from one strain of *Streptococcus pneumoniae* to another. Griffith assumed that transforming factor was a protein. In 1944 Canadian microbiologist Oswald Theodore Avery, American scientist Maclyn McCarty, and Colin Munro Macleod discovered that the transforming factor was DNA and not a protein [8]. Austrian biochemist Erwin Chargaff discovered that DNA contained equivalent amounts of adenine, thymine, cytosine, and guanine. This suggested that DNA underwent base-pairing. British biochemist Rosalind Elsie Franklin (1920–1958) and British biophysicist Maurice Wilkins discovered a repeating sequence of molecules that appeared like DNA through an experimental technique called X-ray crystallography. The collective efforts of Chargaff, Franklin, and Wilkins helped biologist James D. Watson and biophysicist Francis Crick to discover the structure of DNA: a double helix. Wilkins, Watson, and Crick won the Nobel Prize in Physiology or Medicine in 1961. Franklin did not qualify for this honor since she had died four years earlier [1,9]. The semi-conservative nature of DNA replication was discovered by American geneticist Franklin W. Stahl and American biochemist Matthew Stanley Meselson in 1958 [10].

In 1966, DNA was found to be present not only in chromosomes but also in mitochondria. The first single gene was isolated in 1969. In 1972 the American biochemist Paul Berg developed a technique to splice DNA fragments from different organisms and created the first recombinant DNA. In 1980 Berg was awarded the Nobel Prize in Chemistry for his achievement. The first genetically engineered drug, a type of human insulin grown in genetically modified bacteria, was marketed by the Eli Lilly pharmaceutical company [1,11].

The polymerase chain reaction (PCR) was invented in 1985. This technique, which amplified DNA, enabled geneticists, medical researchers, and forensic specialists to analyze and manipulate DNA from very small samples. PCR was described as the "genetic equivalent of the printing press," with the potential to revolutionize genetics in the same way that the printing press had revolutionized mass communications [1].

In 1990, the first gene therapy was administered to a four-year-old girl who had inherited an immunodeficiency disorder, adenine deaminase deficiency. In 1996, the British embryologist Ian Wilmut and his colleagues at the Roslin

Institute in Scotland successfully cloned the first adult mammal that was able to reproduce [1].

The term *genetics* refers to the study of a single gene at a time, and *genomics* is the study of all genetic information contained in a cell. The Human Genome Project (HGP) set as one of its goals to determine the entire nucleotide sequence of the more than 3 billion bases of DNA contained in the nucleus of a human cell. Beginning in 1987, automated sequencing, which enabled researchers to decode millions, as opposed to thousands, of letters of genetic code per day, was a pivotal technological advance for the HGP. American geneticist Francis S. Collins was appointed the director of the project and helped oversee sequencing of an entire human chromosome for the first time. The human genome was published in 2001. It estimated that humans had between 30,000 and 35,000 genes. In October 2004, the human gene count estimates were revised downward to between 20,000 and 25,000. During 2005 and 2006, sequencing of more than 10 human chromosomes was completed, including the human X chromosome [1,12].

In 2006 Roger D. Kornberg, a physician and American structural biologist at Stanford University, was awarded the Nobel Prize in Chemistry for determining the intricate way in which information in the DNA of a gene was copied to provide instructions for building and running a living cell [1,13].

The Nobel Prize in Chemistry in 2020 was awarded to Emmanuelle Charpentier and Jennifer Doudna for developing a way to edit genes [14]. They used CRISPR (clustered regularly interspaced short palindromic repeats), a family of DNA sequences found in the genomes of prokaryotic organisms such as bacteria and archaea. Cas9 (CRISPR-associated protein 9) is an enzyme that uses CRISPR sequences as a guide to recognize and cleave specific strands of DNA. Cas9 enzymes together with CRISPR sequences form the basis of a technology known as CRISPR-Cas9 that can be used to edit genes within organisms. This editing process has a potentially wide variety of applications, including basic biological research, development of biotechnological products, and treatment of disease.

KEY DEVELOPMENTS IN THE FIELD OF STROKE GENETICS

Stroke genetic information and strategies gradually evolved during the last years of the twentieth century and beyond. Targets for understanding the hereditary and genetic influences of conditions of clinical interest included (1) molecular genetic variations affecting risk of monogenic stroke syndromes; (2) molecular genetic variations affecting risk of common stroke syndromes; (3) genetics of conditions associated with stroke risk, for example, white matter hyperintensities, atrial fibrillation, hypercholesterolemia, and hypertension; (4) hereditary causes of familial aggregation of stroke; (5) epigenetic impact on protein expression during acute brain injury; (6) genetic influence on stroke recovery; and (7) pharmacogenetics [15].

Genetic variants predisposing to stroke were found to act at various levels, for example, by increasing the risk of and susceptibility to "conventional" stroke risk factors such as hypertension and diabetes; by influencing specific mechanisms underlying stroke, such as the occurrence and progression of atherosclerosis and lipohyalinosis; by predisposing to arterial thrombosis or bleeding; and by modifying tolerance to brain ischemia or more largely brain injury [16].

The most popular research techniques that clinicians and geneticists began to use became candidate gene studies and genome-wide association studies (GWAS). The candidate gene approach to conducting genetic association studies focused on associations between genetic variation within prespecified genes of interest and phenotypes and disease states. This approach was limited by reliance on existing knowledge about the known or theoretical biology of disease. Results of candidate gene studies in stroke have been disappointing and the genomic analysis of stroke shifted more to GWAS [17].

The development of accurate and high-throughput technologies, using microarrays, to perform genotype analysis across the entire genome of a study subject led to GWAS. GWAS consists of genotyping a very large number of genetic variants across the genome and testing their association with a phenotype without any prior hypothesis or underlying biology. This approach led to identifying a very large number of genetic associations with various traits and diseases that were convincingly replicated in independent samples, mostly near previously unsuspected genes, providing new hypotheses on the underlying biology. For stroke, most genome-wide significant associations were identified for ischemic or hemorrhagic subtypes, suggesting that the genetic contributions to stroke risk are largely subtype-specific. Some risk loci for all ischemic strokes have also been reported. An elaborate analysis of shared genetic variation also showed a high genetic correlation between the large-artery atherosclerosis and small artery disease subtypes of ischemic stroke. These discoveries required large collaborative efforts made possible through the creation of international consortia.

International Stroke Genetics Consortium

The International Stroke Genetics Consortium (ISGC) was founded in April 2007 by Jonathan Rosand, a professor of neurology at Harvard, an endowed chair in neurology at Massachusetts General Hospital (MGH), and an associate member of the Broad Institute. He convened the founding members – 16 investigators from Europe and North America – at the Broad Institute in Cambridge, Massachusetts. He then served as chair of the ISGC from

2007 through 2010 and the inaugural chair of the ISGC steering committee when it was created in 2011. His laboratory continued to support the ISGC convener. He was the senior author of the ISGC's first GWAS of hemorrhagic stroke and the landmark NINDS-SiGN GWAS of ischemic stroke. Rosand launched the ISGC's Cerebrovascular Disease Knowledge Portal. His research group at the MGH Center for Genomic Medicine and Broad Institute served as a training ground for many investigators who later developed internationally distinguished research programs of their own [18].

The ISGC has been at the forefront of genetic discovery to understand the stroke mechanisms. Formed with the principle that collaboration and coordinated effort would produce the highest quality of results in the most efficient manner, the ISGC has developed other major stroke collaborations, including the METASTROKE consortium and the SiGN consortium, and partnered with the CHARGE consortium. The ISGC grew substantially encompassing over 250 members from six continents, spanning more than 50 countries. There have been multiple publications from the data derived from the ISGC. The first ISGC workshop was held in London in July 2007. Since then, the ISGC has held its international workshop every six months [19].

DISCOVERIES WITHIN MONOGENIC STROKE CONDITIONS

During the last quarter of the twentieth century, major advances were made in studying monogenic conditions (disorders controlled by single genes). Discovery of the gene often led to interrogation of the gene products and the pathology and pathophysiology of the conditions.

CADASIL

In 1976, a 50-year-old man arrived at the University of Paris for treatment of a minor stroke. He had no vascular risk factors. His CT scan showed multiple subcortical infarcts and white matter abnormalities, tracing stroke to the small, rather than large arteries of the brain. The presence of these lesions was confirmed 10 years later by magnetic resonance imaging (MRI) that had by then become available. The absence of known risk factors made the cause unclear. The patient's doctors settled on a diagnosis of Binswanger's disease [20].

Marie-Germaine Bousser was the assistant neurologist assigned to the case. She had graduated from the Paris-Sorbonne University in neuropsychiatry in 1972. She then trained at the Pitié-Salpêtrière Hospital. She spent a year at the National Hospital for Neurology and Neurosurgery, Queen Square, in London, working closely with the neurovascular team. She returned to Paris and became professor of neurology at the Pitié-Salpêtrière Hospital in 1981, one of the first woman professors within the Paris University medical system. She later was appointed chair of neurology at the Saint-Antoine Hospital in Paris in 1989. In 1997 she moved to Lariboisière hospital where she became head of the neurology department and professor of neurology at the Saint Louis Lariboisière faculty.

Bousser was not convinced of the diagnosis. In order to keep an eye on the patient, she enrolled him in one of the first aspirin stroke prevention clinical trials. The patient was followed regularly until his death 20 years later after he progressively developed gait and balance difficulties and dementia. In parallel, this gave an opportunity to see the patient's two children, both in their thirties. They had already had minor strokes and there were small deep infarcts and white matter abnormalities on MRI as observed in their father. The hypothesis of a family-related condition became possible [20].

Armed with these three cases of unusual, familial stroke, Bousser caught the attention of Tournier-Lasserve, a fellow neurologist with a growing interest in genetics research. Élisabeth Tournier-Lasserve was born in 1954. She trained in medicine and neurology at the Pitié-Salpêtrière Hospital in Paris. After obtaining a doctorate in medicine in 1984, she worked at the Pitié-Salpêtrière Hospital for two years and trained at the National Institutes of Health in the United States. In 1989, she joined the Institut national de la santé et de la recherche médicale (INSERM), the French National Institute of Health and Medical Research. She became director of research at the Necker-Enfants Malades Hospital and, in 1999, formed the INSERM genetics of vascular diseases unit at the Molecular Genetics Laboratory at Lariboisière Hospital where Bousser worked. She became the head of the Molecular Genetics Laboratory, which provided a diagnostic service for hereditary neurovascular diseases for all French hospitals.

Bousser and Tournier-Lasserve collaborated and began their research in 1990. They planned to investigate the relatives of the first three initial cases through detailed clinical evaluation, an MRI examination, and a blood sample for DNA extraction. Owing to the willingness of the whole family, which allowed 57 adult members to be evaluated, they confirmed that the disease was an autosomal dominant condition affecting cerebral small arteries and capillaries. The main clinical manifestations were reported. White matter signal abnormalities were found in some individuals in the absence of symptoms. In the wall of small arteries, swollen myocytes were found surrounded by collagen, elastin, and a compact and granular electron-dense material they called granular osmiophilic material (GOM) deposits, which emerged as a specific pathological feature of CADASIL. The data was first presented as "recurrent strokes in a family with diffuse white matter and muscular lipidosis – a new mitochondrial cytopathy?," then as "autosomal dominant syndrome with stroke-like episodes and leukoencephalopathy," and later as "autosomal dominant leukoencephalopathy and subcortical ischaemic strokes" [20].

In 1993, the data obtained from this family study allowed the gene locus of the disease to be assigned to chromosome 19q12, which was confirmed immediately in a second French family. Because of the confusion raised by different names, the label "cerebral autosomal dominant arteriopathy with subcortical infarcts and leukoencephalopathy" (CADASIL) was given by Bousser to designate the condition [20].

Bousser and Tournier-Lasserve expanded their research and recruited 32 additional French families with CADASIL to participate and collaborated with two other young neurologists. Tournier-Lasserve welcomed Anne Joutel, who had recently completed a residency with Bousser, into her lab to shift into the basic sciences to identify the mutation. Hugues Chabriat, who had also trained with Bousser, became the group's expert on the clinical aspects of CADASIL, honing the criteria for identifying the disorder using MRI [20].

Joutel and Tournier-Lasserve subsequently identified the responsible gene as *NOTCH3*, a gene that had previously only been studied in fruit flies. Before identification of the gene, many patients with CADASIL were misdiagnosed as having multiple sclerosis. CADASIL was found to be the most common inherited cerebral small artery disease. *NOTCH3* encodes a cell-surface receptor involved in vascular smooth muscle cell survival and vascular remodeling. The underlying vascular lesion is a non-arteriosclerotic amyloid-negative angiopathy involving small arteries and capillaries. The most common manifestation of the condition is recurrent lacunar strokes occurring at a mean age of 49 years. The second most common manifestation was progressive cognitive impairment. The first symptom was usually an attack of migraine with aura. Patients also developed various psychiatric disturbances such as mood disturbances and severe depression. MRI abnormalities appear before the onset of clinical symptoms at a mean age of 30 years [21].

The discovery of CADASIL opened the door to the discovery of several other genes involved in monogenic cerebral small vessel diseases. CADASIL became recognized as one of the best models for exploring the mechanisms and pathophysiology of migraine with aura, stroke, and cognitive decline in ischemic small vessel disease.

In 2019, the Brain Prize crowned the discovery of CADASIL in the 1990s and research efforts on this archetypal small vessel disease of the brain over 40 years.

CARASIL

Probably the first recorded encounter with a patient with cerebral autosomal recessive arteriopathy with subcortical infarcts and leukoencephalopathy

(CARASIL) was reported by Seiji Nemoto in 1960, when a 30-year-old man was admitted to Tohoku University's department of neuropsychiatry. The patient died 18 months later following frequent seizures after cerebral angiography. An autopsy was performed. Nemoto described the clinical and pathological features of that patient and of two similar brothers of another family in 1966. In 1965, Maeda and colleagues presented a preliminary description of the autopsy findings in one of those brothers at a clinicopathological conference at which the first case was discussed. In 1976, Maeda and coworkers, including Nemoto, reported the clinical and pathological findings of the two brothers, born of consanguineous parents, using the term "familial unusual encephalopathy of Binswanger's type without hypertension." These three patients had dementia, pyramidal and extrapyramidal symptoms, and pseudobulbar palsy accompanied by severe lumbago (acute middle to lower back pain) and premature baldness. The condition started in the third decade, with steady progression leading to death within nine years [22].

In the period between 1965 and 1976, two other groups reported clinical and autopsy findings of similar but sporadic cases of young men. In 1985, Toshio Fukutake and his group reported a family of three brothers with strikingly similar clinical features and cerebral diffuse white matter disease on CT scans, and proposed a new systemic syndrome termed "familial juvenile encephalopathy (Binswanger type) with alopecia and lumbago." Based on their clinical and pathological/neuroradiologic criteria, approximately 50 patients were reported almost exclusively from Japan. In 2009, Hara et al. applied linkage analysis and fine mapping in five consanguineous families with CARASIL and identified homozygous mutations in the *HTRA1* gene on chromosome 10q25. *HTRA1* encoded a serine protease thought to repress signaling by transforming growth factor-beta (TGF-beta) family members [21]. The term "CARASIL" was proposed by Bowler and Hachinski based on the disorder's recessive inheritance and resemblance to CADASIL [23].

RETINAL VASCULOPATHY AND CEREBRAL LEUKODYSTROPHY

Cerebral retinal vasculopathy was first reported in 1985 at Washington University School of Medicine in St. Louis, Missouri. A patient presented with visual loss, and examination showed a microvascular abnormality involving the macula. On learning that three relatives had a progressive neurologic disease attributed to a "brain tumor," a collaborative effort was undertaken to evaluate this family. The characteristic ophthalmic findings were found in 10 family members and were suspected in eight additional family members spanning four generations. An autosomal dominant pattern was recognized [24].

Hereditary endotheliopathy with retinopathy, nephropathy, and stroke (HERNS) was reported in 1991 at UCLA and hereditary vascular retinopathy

(HRV) in 1998 at Leiden University, Netherlands. Retinal vasculopathy and cerebral leukodystrophy (RVCL) is a group of inherited small vessel diseases. HERNS was found to be due to mutations in the *TREX1* gene on chromosome 3p21.1–21.3. The disease was localized to chromosome 3 in 2001 and the specific genetic defect *TREX1* was discovered in 2007 [25]. All types of RVCL are characterized by progressive loss of vision secondary to retinal vasculopathy and variable neurological findings. Visual loss, stroke, and dementia began in middle age, and death occurred in most families 5–10 years later.

COLLAGEN 4A1 (COL4A1) SYNDROME

Douglas Gould and colleagues were able to identify mutations in *COL4A1* gene in mice and in human families that led to porencephaly in children and hemorrhage and small-vessel disease related infarcts in adults [26]. The gene was further identified on chromosome 13q34. The genetic defect led to basement membrane vascular defects. COL4A1 related disorders were found to cover a spectrum of overlapping phenotypes characterized by cerebral small vessel disease of varying severity and associated with eye abnormalities and systemic findings mainly in kidney and muscles. Clinical expression varied even within the same family. Cerebrovascular manifestations included perinatal intracerebral hemorrhage and porencephaly, adult or childhood-onset intracranial hemorrhage (in all locations), and, less often, lacunar ischemic strokes [16,27].

SICKLE CELL DISEASE

The first description of sickle cell disease was given by James Herrick, a cardiologist practicing in Chicago. The patient was a 20-year-old dental student from the island of Grenada in the Caribbean. He developed what is now called acute chest syndrome and was admitted to the Presbyterian Hospital in Chicago where he was monitored by an intern, Ernest Irons, and his attending physician Dr. Herrick. In 1910 Irons saw "peculiar elongated and sickle-shaped" cells in the patient's blood. The second case, published only three months later, was a 25-year-old woman who had been observed for some years in the wards of the Medical College of Virginia. The third case reported was a 21-year-old woman with a characteristic blood film. The fresh blood film obtained from the father of this patient was normal, but when the blood preparation was sealed and observed days later, there were similarly abnormal red cells. The authors inferred that sickling might be an inherited phenomenon. The fourth case, a 21-year-old man, reported from Johns Hopkins Hospital, was the first in which the term "sickle cell anemia" was used. Memphis physician Lemuel Diggs first introduced the distinction between sickle cell disease and trait in 1933 [28].

In November 1949, Linus Carl Pauling, Harvey Itano, S. J. Singer, and Ibert Wells published "Sickle Cell Anaemia, a Molecular Disease" in the journal *Science*. It was the first proof of a human disease being caused by an abnormal protein. Sickle cell anemia became the first disease understood at the molecular level. Using electrophoresis, they showed that individuals with sickle cell disease had a modified form of hemoglobin in their red blood cells and that individuals with sickle cell trait had both the normal and abnormal forms of hemoglobin. This was the first demonstration causally linking an abnormal protein to a disease and also the first demonstration that Mendelian inheritance determined the specific physical properties of proteins, not simply their presence or absence – the dawn of molecular genetics [29].

In 1956, Vernon Ingram determined that the change in the hemoglobin molecule in sickle cell disease and trait was the substitution of the glutamic acid in position 6 of the beta chain of the normal protein by valine. Ingram used electrophoresis and chromatography to show that the amino acid sequence of normal human and sickle cell anemia hemoglobins differed due to a single substituted amino acid residue. This was the first time a researcher showed that a single amino acid exchange in a protein could cause a disease or a condition. As a result, Vernon Ingram is sometimes referred to as "The Father of Molecular Medicine" [30].

FABRY DISEASE

The first descriptions of Fabry disease were made in 1898 by two physicians working independently. William Anderson and Johannes Fabry described patients with "angiokeratoma corporis diffusum," red-purple maculopapular skin lesions now recognized as a characteristic feature of the condition. William Anderson, who trained at St. Thomas' Hospital in London, first saw his patient in 1897 and described the dermatological findings without commenting on the cause. Johannes Fabry, who studied dermatology at the University of Bonn, also saw his first patient in 1897. The patient was 13 years old at the time and four years previously had developed cutaneous eruptions in the hollow of his left knee that spread to the left thigh and trunk. Fabry suggested that the disease might represent a form of nevus or developmental defect. Although the condition is now commonly known as Fabry disease, it is also referred to as Anderson-Fabry disease in recognition of the original descriptions. In 1952, it was recognized that the disorder is due to abnormal storage of lipids. In 1960s, the inheritance pattern was established as being X-linked, and the molecular defect responsible for causing the accumulation of glycolipids was identified. In 1965, Ken Hashimoto published his classic paper on the electron microscopic findings in Fabry disease. The first specific treatment of the disease was approved in 2001 [31].

Fabry disease was identified as an X-linked lysosomal storage disorder, caused by lysosomal accumulation of neutral glycosphingolipids, primarily globotriaosylceramide, due to deficiency of the enzyme α–galactosiade A. Progressive accumulation of substrate is associated with a wide range of disease signs and symptoms, including renal failure, cardiovascular dysfunction, neuropathy, stroke, and angiokeratomas. Fabry disease leads to ischemic stroke due to both small artery occlusion and large artery vasculopathy with a predominance in the vertebrobasilar circulation. The pathophysiology of cerebrovascular events in Fabry disease is complex and incompletely understood, resulting from a combination of abnormalities in blood vessel walls, altered blood components, and altered blood flow. Some patients develop dolichoectasia of the basilar and vertebral arteries. Strokes can also be cardioembolic, resulting from arrhythmia caused by cardiomyopathy [16,31].

MELAS

Mitochondrial abnormalities were long suspected of leading to strokes amid a host of other systemic abnormalities. One of the first mitochondrial disorders to be studied in depth was mitochondrial myopathy, encephalopathy, lactic acidosis and stroke-like episodes (MELAS), a progressive neurodegenerative disorder characterized by acute neurological episodes resembling brain ischemia associated with hyperlactatemia and mitochondrial myopathy. The acronym MELAS was proposed by Pavlakis et al. in 1984 [32]. They reported two patients and reviewed nine other cases with similar presentations. They differentiated MELAS from two other clinical disorders known to be associated with mitochondrial myopathy and brain disease: Kearns–Sayre syndrome and the myoclonus epilepsy ragged red fiber syndrome. They suggested that MELAS was transmitted by maternal inheritance and that the ragged red fibers were due to an abnormality of the electron transport system [32].

MELAS was found to be the most prevalent inherited mitochondrial disorder. The most common initial symptoms were seizures, recurrent headaches, anorexia, recurrent vomiting, and myopathy with exercise intolerance or proximal limb weakness. Additional features included short stature, hearing loss and visual impairment, migraine, abdominal pain, obstipation, cognitive defects, and cardiomyopathy [16]. Stroke-like episodes were the clinical disease hallmark. They were usually characterized by aphasia, cortical blindness, hemianopia, or hemiparesis, which were at least partially reversible. The term "stroke-like episodes" was coined to stress the nonischemic, metabolic origin of these events.

INHERITED DISORDERS OF CONNECTIVE TISSUE

Conditions that affect the body's connective tissues often have prominent cerebrovascular abnormalities. Inherited disorders of connective tissue are monogenic diseases that affect structure and function. While these disorders are transmitted within families according to a Mendelian inheritance pattern, de novo mutations are common and many patients do not have a family history of the disease. Most neurologic manifestations are cerebrovascular, due to alterations in the vascular connective tissue. Other neurologic manifestations are mostly secondary to osteoarticular complications [33].

Ischemic stroke is a classic complication of vascular Ehlers-Danlos syndrome (type IV), homocystinuria, and arterial tortuosity syndrome and may occasionally be seen in Marfan syndrome and pseudoxanthoma elasticum with distinct underlying mechanisms for each condition. Vascular Ehlers-Danlos syndrome can also lead to cervical artery dissection, carotid-cavernous fistula, intracranial dissections, and aneurysms potentially causing subarachnoid or intracerebral hemorrhage and arterial rupture.

FAMILIAL CEREBRAL AMYLOID ANGIOPATHY

Vascular β-amyloid deposition in the central nervous system was first described by Gustav Oppenheim in 1909. Oppenheim found foci of necrosis in the brain parenchyma adjacent to hyalinized capillary walls in six of 14 brains of autopsied individuals with senile dementia and the pathological changes of Alzheimer disease. In 1938, Scholz published the first article that focused solely on cerebral vascular abnormalities now recognized as cerebral amyloid angiopathy (CAA). Stefanos Pantelakis observed in 1954 that CAA was limited to vascular media without adjacent parenchymal involvement. He described many of the hallmark pathological features of CAA. Okazaki and colleagues published a seminal article in 1979, clarifying the relationship between CAA and lobar intracerebral hemorrhage (ICH). They identified 23 consecutive cases of moderate to severe CAA from autopsies at Mayo Clinic. A history of lobar, multiple hemorrhages was very common in these patients [34].

CAA mostly occurred in a sporadic form in the elderly, while rare familial forms occurred in younger patients (often younger than 55 years) and generally led to more severe clinical manifestations. One form of familial CAA, associated with intracerebral hemorrhage, was identified as hereditary cerebral hemorrhage with amyloidosis (HCHWA). HCHWA was comprised of various subtypes that all had an autosomal dominant pattern of inheritance but were caused by different types of mutation: in the *APP* gene chromosome 21q21.2 for most (Dutch, Italian, Flemish, Iowa, Piedmont types), and in the *CST3* gene on chromosome 20p11.2 (encoding cystatin C) for another (Icelandic type). The accumulating peptide was Aβ for the first five types and ACys for the Icelandic type. Typically, patients presented with hemorrhagic stroke and/or dementia. Transient neurologic symptoms and seizures also occurred [16,34].

NOTES AND REFERENCES

1. Wexler B. *Genetics and Genetic Engineering*. Detriot, MI: Thomson/Gale Group, 2005.
2. Charles Darwin: Theory, Book & Quotes. Biography.com. Available at www.biography.com/scientist/charles-darwin.
3. August Weismann. Wikipedia. Available at https://en.wikipedia.org/w/index.php?title=August_Weismann&oldid=1017702452.
4. Gregor Mendel. Biography.com. Available at www.biography.com/scientist/gregor-mendel.
5. Edwards AWF. G. H. Hardy (1908) and Hardy-Weinberg equilibrium. *Genetics* 2008;179(3):1143–1150.
6. Miko I. Thomas Hunt Morgan and sex linkage. *Nature Education* 2008;1(1):143. Available at www.nature.com/scitable/topicpage/thomas-hunt-morgan-and-sex-linkage-452.
7. The Nobel Prize in Physiology or Medicine, 1983. NobelPrize.org. Available at www.nobelprize.org/prizes/medicine/1983/mcclintock/facts/.
8. Griffith's experiment. Wikipedia. Available at https://en.wikipedia.org/w/index.php?title=Griffith%27s_experiment&oldid=1035936961.
9. The Discovery of the Double Helix, 1951–1953. National Library of Medicine. Profiles in Science: Francis Crick. Available at https://profiles.nlm.nih.gov/spotlight/sc/feature/doublehelix.
10. The Meselson-Stahl Experiment (1957–1958), by Matthew Meselson and Franklin Stahl. The Embryo Project Encyclopedia. Available at https://embryo.asu.edu/pages/meselson-stahl-experiment-1957-1958-matthew-meselson-and-franklin-stahl.
11. Paul Berg. Wikipedia. Available at https://en.wikipedia.org/w/index.php?title=Paul_Berg&oldid=1008152020.
12. The Human Genome Project. Genome.gov. Available at www.genome.gov/human-genome-project.
13. Roger D. Kornberg. NobelPrize.org. Available at www.nobelprize.org/prizes/chemistry/2006/kornberg/biographical/.
14. CRISPR. Wikipedia. Available at https://en.wikipedia.org/w/index.php?title=CRISPR&oldid=1037242001. Nobel Prize in Chemistry 2020. NobelPrize.org. Available at www.nobelprize.org/prizes/chemistry/2020/press-release/. Isaacson W. *The Code Breaker*. New York: Simon & Schuster, 2021.
15. Lindgren A. Stroke genetics: A review and update. *J. Stroke* 2014 Sep;16(3):114–123.
16. Debette S, Caplan L. Genetics of stroke. In Caplan L (ed.), *Caplan's Stroke: A Clinical Approach*, 5th ed. Cambridge: Cambridge University Press, 2016, pp. 129–144.
17. Candidate gene. Wikipedia. Available at https://en.wikipedia.org/w/index.php?title=Candidate_gene&oldid=1026115546.
18. Jonathan Rosand, MD. International Stroke Genetics Consortium. Available at www.strokegenetics.org/node/372.
19. What is the ISGC? International Stroke Genetics Consortium. Available at www.strokegenetics.org/what_is_isgc. Raffeld MR, Debette S, Woo D. International Stroke Genetics Consortium Update. *Stroke*. 2016 Apr 1;47(4):1144–1145.
20. Chabriat H, Joutel A, Tournier-Lasserve E, Bousser MG. CADASIL: Yesterday, today, tomorrow. *Eur. J. Neurol.* 2020;27(8):1588–1595. The Discovery of CADASIL. BrainFacts.org. Available at www.brainfacts.org/Diseases-and-Disorders/Injury/2019/The-Discovery-of-CADASIL-040319.

21. Chabriat H, Joutel A, Dichgans M, Tournier-Lasserve E, Bousser M-G. CADASIL. *Lancet Neurol.* 2009;8(7):643–653.

22. Fukutake T. Cerebral autosomal recessive arteriopathy with subcortical infarcts and leukoencephalopathy (CARASIL): From discovery to gene identification. *J. Stroke Cerebrovasc. Dis.* 2011;20(2):85–93.

23. Bowler JV, Hachinski V.Progress in the genetics of cerebrovascular disease: Inherited subcortical arteriopathies. *Stroke* 1994;25(8):1696–1698.

24. Grand MG, Kaine J, Fulling K, Atkinson J, Dowton SB, Farber M, et al. Cerebroretinal vasculopathy: A new hereditary syndrome. *Ophthalmology* 1988;95 (5):649–659.

25. Autosomal dominant retinal vasculopathy with cerebral leukodystrophy. Wikipedia. Available at https://en.wikipedia.org/w/index.php?title=Autosomal_dominant_ret inal_vasculopathy_with_cerebral_leukodystrophy&oldid=989941105.

26. Gould DB, Phalan FC, Breedveld GJ, et al. Mutations in Col4a1 cause perinatal cerebral hemorrhage and porencephaly. *Science* 2005;308:1167–1171. Gould DB, Phalan FC, van Mil SE, et al. Role of COL4A1 in small-vessel disease and hemor-rhagic stroke. *N. Engl. J. Med.* 2006;354:1489–1496.

27. Lanfranconi S, Markus HS. COL4A1 mutations as a monogenic cause of cerebral small vessel disease: A systematic review. *Stroke* 2010;41(8):e513–e518.

28. Sickle cell disease. Wikipedia. Available at https://en.wikipedia.org/wiki/Sickle_cell_ disease. Serjeant GR. One hundred years of sickle cell disease. *British Journal of Haematology* 2010 Dec;151(5):425–429. https://onlinelibrary.wiley.com/doi/10.1111/j .1365-2141.2010.08419.x.

29 Linus Pauling. Wikipedia. Available at https://en.wikipedia.org/wiki/Linus_ Pauling#Biological_molecules.

30. Vernon Ingram. Wikipedia. Available at https://en.wikipedia.org/w/index.php?title= Vernon_Ingram&oldid=1038204705.

31. Mehta A, Beck M, Linhart A, Sunder-Plassmann G, Widmer U. History of lysosomal storage diseases: An overview. In Mehta A, Beck M, Sunder-Plassmann G (eds.), *Fabry Disease: Perspectives from 5 Years of FOS.* Oxford: Oxford PharmaGenesis, 2006. Available at www.ncbi.nlm.nih.gov/books/NBK11615/. Fabry disease. Wikipedia. Available at https://en.wikipedia.org/w/index.php?title=Fabry_disease&oldid= 1037635440.

32. Pavlakis SG, Phillips PC, DiMauro S, De Vivo DC, Rowland LP. Mitochondrial myopathy, encephalopathy, lactic acidosis, and strokelike episodes: A distinctive clin-ical syndrome. *Ann. Neurol.* 1984;16(4):481–488.

33. Debette S, Germain DP. Neurologic manifestations of inherited disorders of connect-ive tissue. *Handb. Clin. Neurol.* 2014;119:565–576.

34. Cerebral amyloid angiopathy is also discussed in Chapter 19 on intracerebral cemor-rhages. See also Biffi A, Greenberg SM. Cerebral amyloid angiopathy: A systematic review. *J. Clin. Neurol.* 2011;7(1):1–9.

CHAPTER TWENTY FIVE

EYE VASCULAR DISEASE

EARLY BACKGROUND AND OPHTHALMOSCOPY

Physicians of the nineteenth century were aware that some patients developed sudden or persistent loss of vision, but they did not connect the disorder with stroke. In 1835 in a book on eye diseases, Richard Middlemore used the term "periodical amaurosis" to describe attacks of temporary visual loss [1]. Later, amaurosis fugax (from the Greek *amaurosis*, meaning dark, and the Latin *fugax*, meaning fleeting) was a common term used for transient loss of vision in one or both eyes.

In 1851, renowned scientist Hermann von Helmholtz invented the ophthalmoscope, which revolutionized the methods of assessing and examining the eyes [2]. In 1915, Francis Welch and William Allyn made the world's first hand-held direct illuminating ophthalmoscope, the precursor to the device now used by clinicians worldwide. This refinement of von Helmholtz's invention enabled ophthalmoscopy to become one of the most ubiquitous medical screening techniques. The company Welch Allyn started as a result of this invention [2].

SIR WILLIAM GOWERS

One of his generation's leading neurologists, Sir William Gowers (1845–1915) authored a book on medical ophthalmology in 1879 [3]. Gowers had a very unusual personal history [4]. He was born above his father's ladies' bootmaker shop. By the time he was 11 his father and all three of his siblings had died, and his mother had left, leaving the boy to live with relatives in Oxford where he attended Christ Church school. He tried farming, but this was not a success. On a visit to his paternal grandmother, his aunt introduced him to the local doctor and suggested that he become a medical apprentice, which he did during the next three years. He matriculated at the University of London, achieving an outstanding record. Gowers applied successfully for the newly created position of medical registrar at the National Hospital for the Paralyzed and Epileptic at Queen Square London, a position he held from 1870 to 1872. He was then promoted to assistant physician at Queen Square and spent the rest of his career at the hospital, retiring in 1910. Gowers produced most of his major works, including the two-volume *Manual of Diseases of the Nervous System* and his ophthalmology text, during the years between 1870 and 1890. A master of diagnosis, his clinical teaching at Queen Square earned him an international reputation. Gowers maintained copious case notes. He wrote about his diagnostic strategy [5]:

> Whenever you find yourself in the presence of a case that is not at once and completely familiar to you in all its details, forget for the time all your types and all your names. Deal with the case as one that has never been seen before, and work it out as a new problem. Observe each symptom and consider its significance, then put all the symptoms together and consider their meaning.

Gowers was appointed professor of clinical medicine University College London in 1887. He was a self-taught artist and skilled etcher, an accomplishment he enjoyed both as a hobby and in his work. William Gowers was knighted in 1897. He emphasized the use of the ophthalmoscope in medical diagnosis. His medical ophthalmology monograph contained descriptions of many personally studied cases, and the ophthalmic findings and pathological studies were heavily illustrated with Gowers's own drawings. Gowers described the appearance of the retina and the fundic vessels in cases of embolism to the central retinal artery and its branches. He attributed these instances to rheumatic heart disease and atheroma of the aorta. He described the resultant monocular visual field abnormalities that resulted. One patient described in detail was case 47, a 30 year-old man with severe rheumatic heart disease who suddenly lost consciousness and was aphasic and right hemiplegic. His ophthalmological exam showed that he had embolized to his eye as well as his brain. Figure 25.1a and b shows Gowers's drawing of the necropsy findings in the ophthalmic artery and the appearance of the optic fundus in this case. He opined that retinal vascular changes could occur in patients with carotid artery disease but he did not cite any observations or cases of his own.

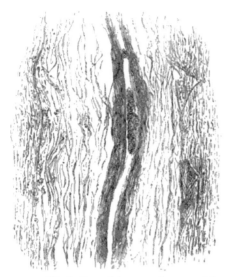

25.1A. "Embolism of the central artery of the retina (case 47). Longitudinal section through the artery, one-eight of an inch (3mm) behind the eyeball. On each side the nerve fibers are indicated and between these and the vessel is much loose connective tissue. Within the contracted vessel is an oval granular mass (thrombus), and in front of this a small round body (x300)." From [3].

C. MILLER FISHER AND ROBERT HOLLENHORST

It was not until the early 1960s, that two giants in their respective clinical specialties – C. Miller Fisher in neurology and Robert Hollenhorst in ophthalmology – noted that transient visual loss was an important precursor to stroke and that findings found by examining the eyes and ocular fundus could be important in the diagnosis of cerebrovascular disease. When Miller Fisher was a junior staff neurologist in Montreal, he encountered several patients with attacks of monocular visual loss that preceded the development of strokes characterized by hemiplegia [6]. These patients' histories stimulated Fisher to review the anatomy of the blood vessels that supply the eye and the brain. The transient blindness could best be explained by a lack of blood flow to the eye. The eye was supplied by blood through the ophthalmic artery, the very first branch of the internal carotid artery (ICA) originating just after the artery entered the cranium. There were no branches of the ICA between the neck and the ophthalmic artery. The ICA then gave off branches that supplied the cerebral hemispheres on the same side. So Fisher concluded that the most likely explanation for the patients symptoms was an obstruction of blood flow in the ICA. This could lead to a lack of blood flow to the eye and ischemic damage to the same side of the brain, causing paralysis of the contralateral limbs. The blockage in the carotid artery might be a clot that could break off and land in its branches (the anterior and middle cerebral arteries) in the head. The presence and location of a carotid artery lesion as the cause of the strokes in his patients was speculative and unproven. It was a hypothesis that floated in his mind and thoughts. Questions abounded in his mind. How often did warning attacks occur before strokes? In patients with blindness or visual loss, how did they describe the change in vision? He read to determine if others had observed and written of transient attacks that preceded strokes. He was also curious about disease of the carotid artery. Were there previous writings about carotid artery disease?

The first patient he had seen who had had transient right visual loss and later left hemiplegia developed colon cancer and died on June 16, 1950. Fisher obtained permission for a postmortem examination. At 11 pm on a Sunday night, after visiting hours, the funeral director and Fisher performed a limited autopsy that included examination of the right carotid artery in the neck. When Fisher cut down on the artery and found that it was totally occluded, he felt a wave of emotion. The hypothesis of a young, inexperienced, clinically naïve individual that the responsible lesion must be in that carotid artery in the neck had proven to be correct.

Fisher then focused intently in the pathology laboratory at Montreal General Hospital, during his clinical encounters at hospitals, and in medical libraries on transient loss of vision in one eye, on warnings before strokes, and on carotid artery disease. He collected clinical information from patients and pathological data from his autopsies. In 1951 he presented a report at a meeting of the American Neurological Association entitled "Transient Monocular Blindness Associated with Hemiplegia" [7]. In the presentation, he described seven patients in whom paralysis on one side of the body was preceded by attacks of temporary loss of vision involving the opposite eye. Fisher wrote two more detailed reports concerning occlusion of the internal carotid artery [8]. In 1952 Fisher presented his research on carotid artery disease at a meeting of physicians and surgeons in his native Canada [9]. He also authored a 36-page report in an ophthalmology journal that included a history of writings concerning transient loss of vision in an eye [10]. Fisher must have spent months in the library reviewing the 150 prior literature reports of transient visual symptoms localizable to one eye, many written in French and German. This historical review consumed a full 18 pages of text.

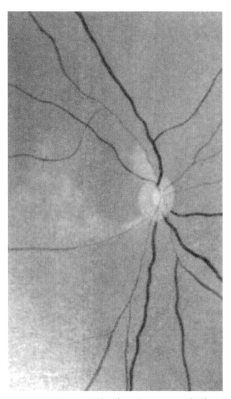

25.1B. "Case 47. The drawing was made about a fortnight after the occurrence of the embolism. The disc is clear and pale (not quite pale enough in the figure), the peripheral part almost, but not quite so clear as the central cup. Its edges are sharp. The veins have a normal size and course.... The arteries are filiform on the disc and for some distance beyond. Some remain, as far as can be seen, narrow (even to the periphery of the retina); others become wider at a distance from the disc, which varies in the case of different branches. From the upper part of the disc a white opacity extends a short distance on to the retina. A similar but narrower white area extends from the lower part of the disc, being evidently situated behind the level of an artery, and it gradually widens and becomes less intense, and is continuous with a mottled opacity which occupies the region of the macula, and is the remains of a large white area which at first occupied this region. A branch of an artery which courses across the upper part of this area is evidently dilated, and the minute branches which come from it are abnormally distinct." From [3].

Years later, after moving to Boston and Massachusetts General Hospital, he published his personal observations of the retina through an ophthalmoscope in a patient who developed blindness in one eye while hospitalized [11]. The patient was a pharmacist who had had many prior attacks of partial or total blindness in the left eye. He was sitting in a chair reading when early one morning during a period of one minute, his vision failed in all fields of the left eye except the upper temporal quadrant. Vision remained unchanged when Fisher examined him 20 minutes after the onset of the attack. The visual loss lasted one hour. Fisher noted a whitish platelet embolus that blocked a main retinal branch artery. The embolus moved during Fisher's examination of the eye. He included within his report his own drawings (Figure 25.2) and descriptions of the retinal arteries that changed as he watched. This showed the importance of careful observation of a single patient and the usefulness of looking in the eyes of individuals suspected of having carotid artery disease.

Robert Hollenhorst (1913–2008) was born in Minnesota and spent his entire medical career at the Mayo Clinic in Rochester, Minnesota. He held many leadership positions in the field of American ophthalmology. In 1961 he described what came to be known as Hollenhorst crystals or plaques [12]:

> Bright, orange-colored plaques were found at bifurcations of the retinal arterioles in 27 of 235 patients with occlusive disease within the carotid arterial system and in 4 of 93 patients with occlusive disease of the vertebral-basilar arterial system. Some of these plaques later disappeared from the retina, some remained stationary, and still others were observed to move distally. In 6 of 35 patients with recent carotid endarterectomy, new plaques appeared during or shortly after the operation. An occasional plaque caused occlusion of the arteriole. These plaques apparently consist of embolic material from atheromatous lesions in the aorta or carotid arteries. The finding of such plaques on routine ophthalmoscopy constitutes an important sign of atherosclerosis. [12]

Hollenhorst and Fisher drew attention to the carotid artery as a source of embolism to the eye, and they and their colleagues made major contributions to the importance, prevalence, diagnosis, and treatment of carotid artery disease [13].

RALPH ROSS RUSSELL

During the beginning of the second half of the twentieth century, one of the most important contributors to knowledge about vascular disease of the eye and to cerebral vascular disease in general was Ralph William Ross Russell. He was born in 1928 in Edinburgh, Scotland, and obtained his medical education at Cambridge and later Oxford Universities. He spent his early career in

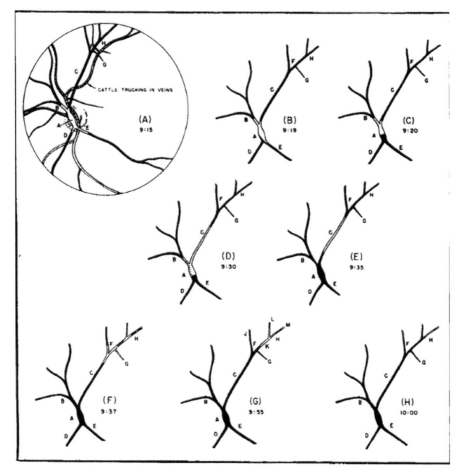

25.2. Fisher's drawings of the blood vessels of the left eye in a patient with transient left eye blindness. From Fisher CM. Observations of the fundus oculi in transient monocular blindness. *Neurology* 1959;9:333–347, with permission.

Oxford where he was stimulated by Sir George Pickering to study hypertension and cerebral vascular disease. He spent a year in Boston with Professor Derek Denny-Brown concentrating on neuropathology. He spent the great part of his clinical career in London where he was a consultant neurologist at St. Thomas' Hospital, Moorfields Eye Hospital, and the National Hospital Queen Square.

At Moorfields, he had extensive experience with vascular disease of the eye. He was one of the first to write about the fundic changes in amaurosis and retinal infarcts and their accompanying visual field changes and to describe the various types of retinal emboli and their sources [14]. Ross Russell also published widely on other aspects of cerebral vascular disease, including the nature of microaneurysms and on venous and arterial diseases [15].

Jean-Claude Gautier, a neurologist at the Pitiè-Salpêtrière Hospital in Paris, and Shirley Wray, a neuro-ophthalmologist at the Massachusetts General

Hospital in Boston, were also prominent contributors to knowledge about vascular disease of the eye. By the beginning of the final quarter of the twentieth century the types, nature, sources, and prognosis of retinal emboli were well known. The most frequent emboli were cholesterol crystals (Hollenhorst plaques) [16]. These are actually white but often appear yellow-orange because the red blood column shows through behind thin crystals. They are 2–3 μm thick and 10–250 μm in diameter. They usually do not obstruct flow in branch arteries and arterioles and often disappear quickly from the retina. Platelet-fibrin emboli are long and white-gray in color and often progress slowly through retinal vessels. Fragments may drift off from their distal regions. This was the embolic type Fisher documented passing through the retina in his 1959 report and illustrated in Figure 24.2 [11]. Calcific emboli are chalky white. They often block blood flow in the recipient vessel. Most often they arise from calcium in aortic valves [16]. Talc, silicone, and other foreign injected materials are also occasionally seen in the retinal vessels [16,17].

CHRONIC EYE ISCHEMIA

Occlusion of the internal carotid artery occasionally caused chronic hypoper-fusion of the structures of the eye. In 1963 Thomas Reed Hedges Jr. and Robert Hollenhorst with his Mayo Clinic colleague Thomas Kearns described the ophthalmoscopic and clinical findings in patients with chronic ophthalmic hypoperfusion caused by carotid artery occlusion [18]. They dubbed the condition "venous-stasis retinopathy." Hedges established and ran the section of ophthalmology at Pennsylvania Hospital for over 30 years and was professor of ophthalmology at the University of Pennsylvania. Hedges performed research on pressure effects on the optic nerve and blood flow to the eye. Sohan Singh Hayreh of the University of Iowa was also a major contributor to knowledge about the anatomy of blood flow to the eye and conditions that effect the vascular supply of the eye [19].

The earliest changes of venous stasis retinopathy consist of microaneurysms and small dot-and-blot retinal hemorrhages and nerve fiber layer splinter hemorrhages [18,19]. These findings are most prominent beginning at the vascular arcades and extend throughout the mid-periphery of the fundus. More severe ischemia produces dilatation and darkening of the retinal veins, often with marked irregularity of caliber of the major retinal veins. The optic disc may be slightly swollen. Severe chronic ischemia may cause pallor or a gray cast to the macula due to retinal edema similar to that seen in central retinal artery occlusion [18,19].

Clinicians reported other eye signs that sometimes accompanied carotid artery occlusion and dissection. Some patients had Horner's syndrome, attrib-utable to perturbation of the sympathetic nerve fibers that coursed along the artery. Irregularity of the iris with red speckling (rubreosis iridis) and dilatation and irregularity of the pupil were sometimes noted [20]. Tony Furlan and his then Mayo Clinic colleagues reported a syndrome of temporary monocular visual loss in patients with carotid artery occlusion when they were exposed to bright light [21]. The light increased metabolism of the retina; the proximal arterial occlusion prevented the needed augmentation of flow, a kind of retinal claudication.

RETINAL VASCULAR SPASM

Jaqueline Winterkorn deserves the most credit for bringing monocular vasospastic visual loss to the attention of the medical community. Jacqueline Marjorie Schuker Winterkorn was born and raised in Queens, New York [22]. After graduating from Barnard College, her first career was as a laboratory neuroscientist. She received her PhD in neurobiology from Cornell and taught neuroanatomy while researching the neurobiology of the visual system. She later earned her MD from Cornell University Medical College and completed a residency in ophthalmology at Mount Sinai Medical School – Beth Israel Hospital and a fellowship in neuro-ophthalmology at Columbia University Medical School – Harkness Eye Institute. She practiced neuro-ophthalmology on Long Island for many years. During the later years of her life, Winterkorn remained active and productive in patient care and teaching despite Parkinson's disease with severe treatment-related dyskinesias.

In a series of reports Winterkorn and her colleagues described the clinical symptoms, findings on examination of the ocular fundus, precipitants, and treatment of retinal vascular spasm [23]. John Selhorst (chair of neurology at St. Louis University and a neuro-ophthalmologist) and colleagues reported their observations of the fundus oculi during the same year as the initial Winterkorn report [24]. Although often called "retinal migraine," Winterkorn et al. noted that vasospasm also occurred in other conditions that provoked vasoconstriction.

During the subsequent years, the clinical features of retinal vascular spasm became clarified. The vision changes attributable to retinal vascular spasm were monocular, as opposed to the binocular vision changes that occurred in migraine with aura affecting the striate region of the brain. Some patients described an awareness of the eye or an unpleasant ocular sensation before the visual loss developed. Patients most often described blurring or graying or a "blackout" or whiteout" of their vision, usually of the entire visual field in that eye. Sometimes the visual loss was partial, sectoral, or altitudinal. Attacks were usually brief, most often lasting less than five minutes, but occasionally they lasted up to 30 minutes, rarely hours. Attacks were often repeated and could recur many times in some patients. Sometimes repeated attacks occurred during a 24-hour period. Attacks often involved the same eye in most if not all episodes. The most common ophthalmoscopic finding was constriction of both arteries and veins. The narrowing could be focal or diffuse. At times segmentation of blood in a thin and slowly moving column of blood and pallor of the macula or optic disc was visible. A relative afferent pupillary reflex abnormality could be found during an attack. As the attack cleared, slow flow in venules with rouleux formation could be seen.

Conditions known to cause systemic vasoconstriction such as cocaine and amphetamine use, hypercalcemia, pheochromocytoma, eclampsia, and hypereosinophilic syndrome can also stimulate retinal vasoconstriction. When precipitants were not present and the episodes were repeated in young individuals, the diagnosis of retinal migraine can be applied. The diagnosis of retinal migraine should be reserved for patients with repeated brief visual loss in one eye, who have a history of headaches, and who show vasoconsriction on fundoscopy and have none of the known precipitants of systemic vasoconstriction. Treatments have not been systematically studied, but calcium channel blockers have been the preferred treatment.

ISCHEMIC OPTIC NEUROPATHY, AND GIANT-CELL ARTERITIS AND THE EYE

During the last quarter of the twentieth century, ophthalmologists and neuro-ophthalmologists began to define the syndrome of ischemic optic neuropathy. Sohan Singh Hayreh of the University of Iowa was among the earliest observers to report the clinical findings in this condition [25]. In contradistinction to retinal ischemia, the visual findings were related to ischemia of the optic nerve. The nerve was supplied mostly by ciliary branches of the ophthalmic artery rather than by the central retinal artery. Once the distinction between retinal and optic nerve ischemia and infarction became clear, observations during the next decades clarified the causes, clinical syndrome, and ophthalmoscopic findings in ischemic optic neuropathy. Arteritic (giant-cell arteritis) and non-arteritic causes were separated because they dictated the urgency and nature of treatment [26].

Sir Jonathan Hutchinson is usually assigned credit for first calling attention to inflammation of the superficial temporal arteries on the face, a condition later dubbed *temporal arteritis*, and later referred to as *giant cell arteritis* because of the pathology of the involved vessels. Hutchinson (1828–1913) was clearly a man for all seasons, a leader in many medical fields: surgery, ophthalmology, venereology, neurology, and pathology [27]. He was president of the Hunterian Society in 1869 and 1870, professor of surgery and pathology at the Royal College of Surgeons from 1877 to 1882, president of the Pathological Society (1879–1880), of the Ophthalmological Society (1883), of the Neurological Society (1887), of the Medical Society (1890), and of the Royal Medical and Chirurgical Society from 1894 to 1896. In 1889, he was president of the Royal College of Surgeons. He published more than 1,200 medical articles and also produced the quarterly *Archives of Surgery* from 1890 to 1900, being its only contributor.

In 1890 he wrote:

> The subject was an old man, the father of a well-remembered beadle at the London Hospital College 30 years ago. I was asked to see him because he had red "streaks on his head" which were painful and prevented his wearing a hat. The "red streaks" proved to be the temporal arteries which were inflamed and swollen. Pulsation could be feebly detected in the affected vessel, but it finally ceased. The redness then subsided and the vessels were left impervious cords. [28]

Bayard Taylor Horton (1895–1980), a Mayo Clinic physician, described the entity in more detail [29]. Horton received his MD degree in 1922 from the University of Virginia and then interned at the University of Virginia Hospital. He was professor of biology at Emory and Henry College in Emory, Virginia, from 1923 to 1925. In 1925, Horton began his fellowship in medicine at the Mayo Graduate School of Medicine. He became a member of the Mayo staff in 1929. In 1940, he was appointed head of the Section of Clinical Investigation at the clinic. In 1932, Horton and colleagues reported two patients whose temporal artery biopsies showed arteritis. In 1937, these workers summarized information from seven patients who had systemic symptoms, headache, fever, anemia, and jaw claudication. Temporal artery biopsies showed granulomatous inflammation with giant cells. The authors considered this a new vasculitis, calling it "temporal arteritis" [30]. It soon became clear that this form of arterial inflammation was an important cause of sudden blindness in one or both eyes. Once one eye was involved, the other was at risk, so that urgent diagnosis and treatment of temporal arteritis was mandated.

Experience was gained during the years of the twentieth century about both arteritic and nonarteritic ischemic optic nerve damage [26]. Temporal arteritis-related ischemic optic neuropathy developed in elderly individuals often after weeks of fatigue and headache. There may have been prodromal temporary visual loss. Blindness developed suddenly. Markers of systemic inflammation were present; the temporal and other superficial facial and posterior auricular vessels were firm, tender, and often painless in regions; and biopsy of the temporal arteries showed a giant cell arteritis. Nonarteritic ischemic optic neuropathy often was noticed on awakening in those patients who had a history of hypertension and/or diabetes. Visual field defects were often altitudinal. There could be a small optic cup on ophthalmoscopy [26].

NOTES AND REFERENCES

1. Middlemore R. *A Treatise the Diseases of the Eye and Its Appendages*. London: Longmans & Co., 1835, p. 303. Cited in Fisher CM. Transient monocular blindness associated with hemiplegia. *AMA Arch. Ophthalmol.* 1952;47:167–203.

2. Friedenwald H. The history of the invention and of the development of the ophthalmoscope. *JAMA* 1902;38;549–552.

3. Gowers W. *A Manual and Atlas of Medical Ophthalmoscopy*. London: Churchill, 1879.

4. William Gowers (neurologist). Wikipedia. Available at https://en.wikipedia.org/wiki/William_Gowers_(neurologist). Shorvon S, Compston A. *Queen Square: A History of the National Hospital and Its Institute of Neurology*. Cambridge: Cambridge University Press, 2019, pp. 145–155. Gowers's textbook of neurology is discussed in Chapter 14.

5. Gowers WR. General principles of the diagnosis of the diseases of the nervous system. *Lancet* 1892;139:403–405; also cited in Shorvon S, Compston A. *Queen Square: A History of the National Hospital and Its Institute of Neurology*. Cambridge: Cambridge University Press, 2019, p. 148.

6. C. Miller Fisher is the subject of Chapter 29. The history of his observations and research on visual loss and stroke and carotid artery disease is contained in Caplan LR. *C. Miller Fisher: Stroke in the 20th Century*. New York: Oxford University Press, 2020.

7. Fisher CM. Transient monocular blindness associated with hemiplegia. *Trans. Am. Neurol. Assoc.* 1951;76:154–158.

8. Fisher CM: Occlusion of the internal carotid artery. *Am. Med. Assoc. Arch. Neurol. Psych.* 1951;65:346–377. Fisher CM. Occlusion of the carotid arteries: Further experiences. *Am. Med. Assoc. Arch. Neurol. Psych.* 1954;72:187–204.

9. Fisher CM. Disease of carotid arteries: A clinico-pathological correlation. In Report of the Annual Meeting and Proceedings of the Royal College of Physicians and Surgeons of Canada. October 3–4, 1952, pp. 60–67.

10. Fisher CM. Transient monocular blindness associated with hemiplegia. *AMA Arch. Ophthalmol.* 1952;47:167–203.

11. Fisher CM. Observations of the fundus oculi in transient monocular blindness. *Neurology* 1959;9:333–347.

12. Hollenhorst RW. Significance of bright plaques in the retinal arterioles. *JAMA* 1961;178:23–29. The history of the recognition and description of retinal emboli is reviewed in Graff-Radford J, Boes CJ, Brown RD. History of Hollenhorst plaques. *Stroke* 2015:46:e82–e84.

13 Carotid artery disease and its history are discussed in detail in Chapters 15, 29, 54, and 55.

14. Ross Russell RW. Observations on the retinal blood vessels in monocular blindness. *Lancet* 1961;2:1422–1428. Ross Russell RW. Atheromatous retinal embolism. *Lancet* 1963;2;1354–1356. Ross Russell RW. The source of retinal emboli. *Lancet* 1968;292:789–792.

15. Ross Russell RW. Observations on intracranial aneurysms. *Brain* 1963;86:425–442. Ross Russell WR. *Cerebral Arterial Disease*. Edinburgh: Churchill Livingstone, 1976. Bousser MG, Ross Russell R. *Cerebral Venous Thrombosis*, vol 1. London: WB Saunders, 1997.

16. Gautier J-C. Clinical presentation and differential diagnosis of amaurosis fugax. In Bernstein EF (ed.), *Amaurosis Fugax*. New York: Springer-Verlag, 1988, pp. 24–42.

17. Atlee WE. Talc and cornstarch emboli in the eyes of drug abusers. *JAMA* 1972;219:49–51. Caplan L, Banks G, Thomas C. Central nervous system complications of addiction to "T's and Blues." *Neurology* 1982;32:623–628.

18. Hedges TR. Ophthalmoscopic findings in internal carotid artery occlusion. *Am. J. Ophthalmol.* 1963;55:1007–1012. Kearnes TP, Hollenhorst RW. Venous-stasis retinopathy of occlusive disease of the carotid artery. *Mayo Clin. Proceed.* 1963;38:304–312.

19. Hayreh SS. Chronic ocular ischemic syndrome in internal carotid artery occlusive disease. In Bernstein EF (ed.), *Amaurosis Fugax*. New York: Springer-Verlag, 1988, pp. 135–158. Carter JE. Chronic ocular ischemia and carotid vascular disease. In Bernstein EF (ed.), *Amaurosis Fugax*. New York: Springer-Verlag, 1988, pp. 118–134.

20. Fisher CM. Dilated pupil in carotid occlusion. *Trans. Am. Neurol. Assoc.* 1966;91:230–231.

21. Furlan AJ, Whisnant JP, Kearns TP. Unilateral visual loss in bright light: An unusual symptom of carotid artery occlusive disease. *Arch. Neurol.* 1979;36: 675–676.

22. Jacqueline Winterkorn. Legacy.com. Available at www.legacy.com/us/obituaries/newmilfordspectrum/name/jacqueline-winterkorn-obituary?pid=175295971.

23. Winterkorn JM, Teman AJ. Recurrent attacks of amaurosis fugax treated with calcium channel blockers. *Ann. Neurol.* 1991;30:423–425. Winterkorn JM, Kupersmith M, Wirtschafter JD, Forman S. Treatment of vasospastic amaurosis fugax with calcium channel blockers. *N. Engl. J. Med.* 1993;329:396–398.

24. Burger SK, Saul RF, Selhorst JB, Thurston SE. Transient monocular blindness caused by vasospasm. *N. Engl. J. Med.* 1991;325:870–873.

25. Hayreh SS. Anterior ischemic optic neuropathy. 1. Terminology and pathogenesis. *Br. J. Ophthalmol.* 1974;58:955–963.

26. Glaser J. The ischemic optic neuropathies. In Levin L, Iessell S (eds.), *Principles and Practices of Ophthalmology, vol. 5: Neuroophthalmology*, 2nd ed. Philadelphia: WB Saunders, 2000.

27. Jonathan Hutchinson. Wikipedia. Available at https://en.wikipedia.org/wiki/Jonathan_Hutchinson.

28. Hutchinson, J. Diseases of the arteries. *Arch. Surg.* 1890;1:323–333. Cited in Ross RT. From the Archives of Surgery: Sir Jonathan Hutchinson's (1829–1913) modern description of symmetrical temporal arteritis. *J. Neurol. Neurosurg. Psychiatry* 1988;51(9):1192.

29. Capobianco DJ, Swanson JW. Historical vignette: Neurological contributions of Bayard T. Horton. *Mayo Clin. Proceed.* 1998;73(9):912–915.

30. Horton BT, Magath TB, Brown GE. An undescribed form of arteritis of the temporal vessels. *Proc. Staff Meet. Mayo Clin.* 1932;7:700–701. Horton BT, Magath TB, Brown GE. Arteritis of the temporal vessels: Previously undescribed form. *Arch. Int. Med.* 1934;53:400–409. Horton BT, Magath TB. Arteritis of the temporal vessels: Report of 7 cases. *Proc. Staff Meet. Mayo Clin.* 1937;12:548–553.

CHAPTER TWENTY SIX

SPINAL CORD VASCULAR DISEASE

The first recorded instance of spinal cord infarction was by Sir Astley Cooper [1]. In 1825 Cooper ligated the abdominal aorta of a patient who, soon after, developed loss of feeling in his lower limbs and incontinence of urine. The patient died after several days and a postmortem was carried out but not of the spinal cord.

Astley Cooper was born at Brooke, Norfolk, on August 23, 1768 [1]. His father was a clergyman and his mother authored several novels. At the age of sixteen he was sent to London and placed under Henry Cline, a surgeon at St. Thomas' Hospital. Cooper studied anatomy and attended the lectures of John Hunter. In 1789 he was appointed demonstrator of anatomy at St. Thomas', and in 1800 he was appointed surgeon at Guy's Hospital where he spent his entire career. In 1820, he was made a baron. He was appointed sergeant surgeon to George IV in 1828. He served as president of the Royal College of Surgeons in 1827 and again in 1836. He died on February 12, 1841, in London. A statue of Cooper was erected in St. Paul's Cathedral. Sir Astley's greatest contribution was in vascular surgery. He was the first to demonstrate experimentally the effects of bilateral ligation of the carotid arteries in dogs and to propose treatment of aneurysms by ligation of the vessel. In 1805 he published an account of his attempt to tie the common carotid artery for treating an aneurysm. A patient with a leaking iliac artery aneurysm was treated in 1817 by Cooper as an emergency during the night by lamplight at the patient's bedside without anesthesia.

The next important contribution related to vascular spinal cord injury was by Henry Charlton Bastian [2]. He entered University College, London, in 1856, and graduated in 1863. He served as assistant curator of the University College Museum. He lectured in pathology at St. Mary's Hospital, and in 1867 was appointed professor of pathology and assistant physician at the University College Hospital London where he worked most of his life. He successively became professor of clinical medicine and physician to the National Hospital for the Paralyzed and Epileptic at Queen Square. He developed a strong reputation as a neurological diagnostician and intellectual and was one of the pioneers of scientific neurology. He was described as "a quiet and reserved man considered one of the most intellectual physicians of the day although reluctant to lecture or teach on ward rounds" [3]. Bastian described several patients with "acute myelitis" that resulted in softening of the spinal cord [4]. He wrote a report in *The Lancet* in 1910 that was mostly an essay that debunked the prevalent idea of the time that spinal cord infarcts were due to inflammatory causes. He also reviewed the prior literature [5].

> There seems little room for doubt that the common "softenings" met with in the spinal cord are in all essential respects similar to the common "softenings" met with in the brain. It is now generally acknowledged that these latter softenings are due to vascular occlusions (embolism and thrombosis), cutting off the blood-supply from the affected region of the brain, and thereby leading to degenerative processes in the sites supplied by the occluded vessels.

> There is absolutely no reason for supposing that inflammation should be more common in the spinal cord than in the brain, nor that the process which causes the great majority of softenings of the brain (simple vascular occlusions) should not be capable of producing analogous results in the spinal cord. Yet works on medicine at the present day and for some time would have us believe that while the common softenings of the brain are results of non-inflammatory degenerations, those of the spinal cord are due to inflammation. [5]

Another important early description of spinal cord infarction was by William Gibson Spiller (1863–1940). At the time he was professor of neurology at the University of Pennsylvania. Spiller had made the rounds during four years in Europe, studying internal medicine and neurology with Hermann Oppenheim, Ludwig Edinger, William Gowers, and Jules Dejerine [6]. He became an expert in neuroanatomy and neuropathology. In 1909 he described a patient who at autopsy had an occlusion of the anterior spinal artery that Spiller attributed to syphilis [7]. The spinal cord infarct extended from C4 to T3. Spiller described the clinical findings in detail. During the early years of the twentieth century it became fashionable to attribute rapid onset paraplegia to syphilis. M. F. Chung described 24 Chinese patients that he opined developed spinal cord infarction attributable to syphilis [8].

During the later years of the nineteenth century, Albert Adamkiewicz, Henryk Kadyi, and others studied the blood supply of the spinal cord [9]. One reason for the dearth of information about spinal cord vascular disease was the rarity of postmortem studies. Erichson wrote in a monograph in 1875 on spinal cord concussion, that the spinal cord was probably the structure that was least frequently examined in the death house because of the technical difficulty of preparation [10]. He knew of only one published postmortem of the spinal cord, a case of delayed gradual paraparesis after a railway collision. Erichson wrote about "spinal anemia" as did other authors but without any necropsy studies [10]. William Blackwood, a neuropathologist at the National Hospital Queen Square, affirmed in 1958 that no examples of arterial softening of the cord were encountered at the National Hospital, Queen Square, in 3,737 postmortem examinations from 1909 to 1958 [11].

THE AORTA AND SPINAL CORD ISCHEMIA

Astley Cooper had drawn attention to ligation of the aorta as a cause of spinal cord infarction in 1825 [1]. Authors of medical and neurological texts mentioned the aorta when they wrote of "spinal anemia" but provided little or no detail and no actual case descriptions. Byrom Bramwell, a Scotch pathologist and surgeon, authored the treatise *Diseases of the Spinal Cord*, published first in 1881 [12]. He discussed extramedullary and intramedullary spinal hemorrhages in some detail, but only one paragraph in the entire text concerned "anemic paraplegia." Bramwell wrote: "Paraplegia sometimes results from the sudden stoppage of the blood supply to the lower end of the cord, an accident which occurs in the course of some abdominal aneurysms in consequence of detachment of the clot or obstruction of the abdominal aorta" [12]. Charles Dana in his text on nervous diseases wrote about spinal hemorrhage, both meningeal and into the cord substance, which he attributed mostly to syphilitic small aneurysms [13]. He commented that little was known about spinal anemia. "An aortic obstruction which cuts off the circulation of blood from the spinal cord will produce a spinal anemia and when this is severe the functions of the cord are nearly abolished" [13]. William Osler in his textbook of medicine noted that "there were some very interesting facts with reference to the profound anemia of the cord which follows ligature of the aorta." In experiments made in Welch's lab by Herter, it was found that within a few moments after the application of the ligature to the aorta paraplegia came on" [14].

Early writings including the classic Spiller report [7] often posited that spinal cord infarctions were likely attributable to occlusions (usually thought to be syphilitic) of the anterior spinal artery. Recall that, similarly, brain infarcts were attributed to middle cerebral artery (MCA) occlusions before Fisher and others showed that the occlusive process was most often in the larger carotid artery in the neck, not the MCA [15]. Because of the paucity of necropsy examination of the spinal cord and its supplying vasculature, there were virtually no documented cases of cord infarction caused by occlusion of the anterior spinal artery.

Jean Lapresle (1921–2000) was one of the first neurological clinicians to make important observations about spinal cord vascular disease [16]. He also wrote about spinal cord tumors and angiomas. Lapresle studied at the Faculté de Médecine de Paris, graduating in 1950. He then trained in the United States in neuropathology with Harry Zimmerman at the Montefiore Hospital in New York. Lapresle followed the academic route from student to "interne des Hôpitaux" to "chef de clinique" to chairman. He trained in neurology with Guillain, Alajouanine, Garcin, Lhermitte, and André-Thomas. Lapresle was appointed head of the department of neurology at Bicêtre in 1970. Lapresle was first and foremost a neurologist. He organized the Sixth International Congress of Neuropathology in Paris in 1970. He was president of the French Neurological Society in 1986.

In 1962, Gruner and Lapresle collected 21 anatomically verified cases of arteriosclerotic vascular disease of the spinal cord, examined at necropsy at the Salpêtrière Hospital in Paris or in Strasbourg [17]. None showed thrombosis of the anterior spinal artery. Atheroma of the aorta was noted in eight, an aortic aneurysm in two, and an aortic embolus in one. Nineteen of the spinal cords showed complete softening. Among these, 12 were in the anterior three quarters of the cord, that is, in anterior spinal artery territory [17].

More information about the role of the aorta in spinal cord ischemia came after reviews of the complications of aortic dissection and surgery on aortic aneurysms, aortic dissections, and coarctation of the aorta. In 1966, Hugh Garland and colleagues reviewed the prior literature concerning spinal cord infarction and reported six new cases, four studied at necropsy [18]. Among the autopsied cases were a 62-year-old man who became paraplegic after surgery on an aortic aneurysm and an 18-year-old lad who developed paraplegia shortly after an aortic dissection [18]. During the first half of the twentieth century, aortic dissection became a well-recognized and important entity to diagnose [19]. Mayo Clinic physicians reviewed the neurological complications of aortic dissection and found two instances of spinal cord infarction among 26 patients [20]. In a larger review of aortic dissections, Albert Hirst et al. noted that 27 of 505 patients who had dissection of the aorta became paraplegic due to spinal cord infarction [21].

A large surgical series of aortic surgery concluded in 1978 [22]:

> As regards postoperative cord complications, they occurred only in cases of aneurysm, were 10 times more common in ruptured than in unruptured aneurysms, and the neurological loss usually was complete flaccid paraplegia with high mortality and rare partial or complete recovery.... The cause of postoperative spinal cord damage was ischemia resulting from the interruption of a critical radicular artery at the lower thoracic or high lumbar vertebral levels in the presence of anomalously located greater radicular or infrarenal radicular arteries. High aortic clamping and hypotension increased the probability of this occurrence, which essentially was unpredictable and, therefore, unavoidable. [22]

When surgeons began to treat abdominal aortic aneurysms and aortic dissections using endovascular rather than open surgery, the frequency of spinal cord infarction was not significantly reduced when compared to open repair [23].

Patients with coarctation of the aorta can also develop spinal cord ischemia and infarction [24]. Spinal cord infarction is very rare without surgery. More common is paraplegia after primary repair of aortic coarctation and even more frequent after secondary repair of recoarctation.

HYPOTENSION AND AORTIC BORDER ZONES

Occasionally, patients recover from coma without obvious cerebral damage but instead have paraplegia related to hypoxic-ischemic damage to the spinal cord. The most vulnerable spinal regions are the upper and lower thoracic and lumbar spinal cord segments. The cervical cord was rarely involved, so that the arms were normal despite severe weakness of the lower limbs [25]. Studies of the spinal cord at necropsy in patients who had cardiac arrest or severe hypotension confirmed the frequency of necrosis of neurons mostly in the anterior and posterior horns of the gray matter of the lumbosacral spinal cord [26].

Klaus Joachim Zülch, director of the Max Planck Institute for Brain research in Köln, Germany, and his colleagues posited the presence of border-zone regions of the spinal cord that received the least blood supply from the aorta and so were vulnerable to infarction [27]. Zülch had previously described cerebral border zones and used these observations to postulate spinal locations for circulatory vulnerability [28]. The most vulnerable region was posited to be in the rostral thoracic spinal cord at T3–T4, a region that was located between the cervical supply from the vertebral arteries and the caudal supply from the aorta. Areas within the spinal cord were also considered most vulnerable. Figure 26.1 depicts these regions.

ARTERIOVENOUS FISTULA
AND MALFORMATIONS

Dural arteriovenous fistulas are now known to be one of the most frequent, most important, and most remediable of the causes of spinal cord infarction, especially in men. One of the earliest pioneers in bringing attention to these lesions was Giovanni Di Chiro (1926–1997), a neuror-adiologist at the National Institutes of Health in the United States [29].

Di Chiro was born in Vinchiaturo, Italy. His father was a professor of Greek and Latin. Di Chiro studied medicine at the University of Naples, graduating in 1949. He originally intended to work as a cardi-ologist in Switzerland, but changed his mind and traveled to Sweden instead. While on the train to Stockholm he met a radiologist who convinced him to pursue a career in radiology. He did his radiology residency in multiple Swedish hospitals affiliated with the Karolinska University from 1949 to 1953. He then traveled to Boston where he began working at the Boston City Hospital on a Fulbright Fellowship. In October 1957, he

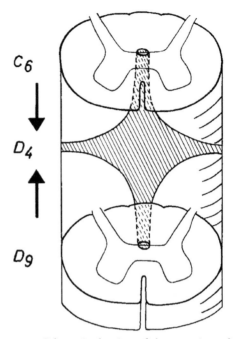

26.1. Schematic drawing of the extension of a spinal infarct. In the "critical segment," it will be the largest and may cover the whole segment. Above and below, there is a reduction in size, so that the form is "biconcal." From Zülch KJ, Kurth-Schumacher R. The pathogenesis of "intermittent spinovascular insufficiency" ("spinal claudication of Dejerine") and other vascular syndromes of the spinal cord. *Vasc. Surg.* 1970;4 (2):116–136, with permission.

began working at the National Institute of Neurological Diseases and Blindness as a visiting scientist, and in January 1958, he established what became known as its neuroimaging branch. After years of leg pain, in May 1958, he underwent exploratory surgery to remove a spinal cord ependymoma. He bled postopera-tively, and two days after surgery he became paraplegic, and remained so for the rest of his life. At that time, he was 32 years old, an immigrant for only five months, a father of three children under the age of 3 three, and unable to stand or walk. Giovanni's adjustment to this catastrophic change in his life was an inspiration to all who worked with and knew him. He embarked on a brilliant career as an investigator, teacher, editor, and spokesperson for neuroradiology [29]. One of his important contributions was in the field of spinal cord arterio-graphy where he, with John Doppman and Ayub Ommaya, studied the radio-graphic appearances of spinal malformations and their interventional obliteration by embolization [30]. Despite his paraplegia, Di Chiro served as the head of neuroimaging branch of the NIH from its founding until his death in 1997.

When advanced spinal imaging became available, it became possible to diagnose spinal dural arteriovenous fistulas often before spinal catheter angiography. The fistulas were most often localized in the thoracic region. The most frequent clinical presentation was of progressive neurologic worsening, often with acute deteriorations and occasionally with spinal TIAs.

The most frequent symptoms included radicular pain, abnormal gait, sensory abnormalities in the lower extremities and/or perineum, and lower extremity weakness. Most patients by the time a diagnosis was made had important symptoms and signs that indicated dysfunction of sacral cord segments: loss of sensation in the perineum, and abnormalities of micturition, defecation, and sexual function.

Michael Aminoff was among the first individuals to clarify the pathogenesis of spinal cord infarction that developed in patients with spinal dural arteriovenous fistulas. He was born and educated in England, graduating from University College London in 1962 [31]. He trained in neurology and neurophysiology at the National Hospital (Queen Square) in London. In 1974, while working in the United Kingdom, Aminoff and his colleagues (Robin Barnard, a neuropathologist at Maida Vale Hospital in London, and Valentine Logue, a pioneering British neurosurgeon) described the pathophysiology of spinal vascular malformations and their clinical features [32]. Aminoff then moved to the United States in 1976 and had a long and fruitful career as professor of neurology at the University of California at San Francisco. Aminoff and colleagues attributed the spinal cord infarction to a rise in venous pressure in the draining veins caused by the arteriovenous fistula. In order to adequately nourish the cord, the arterial supply pressure had to exceed the venous pressure, which was often not possible because of the low pressure within the small arteries and arterioles that fed spinal cord segments. Aminoff also authored a monograph on spinal angiomas [33]. Later neurosurgeons, including Roberto Heros at the University of Miami and David Piepgras at the Mayo Clinic in Rochester, Minnesota, gained considerable experience and became leaders in the surgical management of these spinal arteriovenous fistulas.

OTHER LESS COMMON CAUSES OF SPINAL CORD INFARCTION

During much of the twentieth century, spinal cord–related clinical care and research was performed by physiatrists and physical therapists who cared for patients with traumatic spinal cord damage often at special spinal cord rehabilitation facilities. Few neurologists specialized in spinal cord disease other than those focused on multiple sclerosis. One neurologist who collated information about spinal cord infarction was Richard Satran [34]. He came to Rochester in 1962 as one of three neurologists who practiced general neurology at the University of Rochester Medical Center, even before the neurology department was established. Other authors described the usual anatomical locations and patterns and accompanying clinical symptoms related to spinal cord infarction [35]. Figure 26.2 depicts the various patterns of spinal cord infarction.

More recently, other etiologies of spinal cord vascular disease have been reported. Since the early 1980s, pathologists and clinicians have become aware that cartilaginous material from intervertebral disks somehow invades the spinal arteries and veins and causes spinal cord strokes [36]. Most reported cases are cervical and involve young women. Some patients have been pregnant, puerperal, or on oral contraceptives. Minor trauma, sudden neck motion, or lifting was often an immediate precipitant. The first symptoms were usually pain in the neck or upper back or radicular pain. Then, a rapidly progressive, sometimes asymmetric, spinal cord syndrome with quadriparesis developed [36].

Infarction and inflammation of the spinal cord meninges can spread to the spinal arteries, causing acute spinal cord infarction. The phenomenon is similar to Heubner's arteritis found in the brain in the presence of tuberculosis, syphilis, and fungal infections. Lyme borreliosis occasionally causes spinal cord infarcts. Schistosomiasis, especially caused by *Schistosoma mansoni*, is well known to affect the spinal cord. This parasite reaches the spinal cord through the blood vessel supply and can cause spinal cord infarction or granulomatous inflammation, most often involving the conus medullaris and the cauda equina [37].

Chronic adhesive arachnoiditis from any cause, especially meningeal infection, can cause scarring and obliteration of spinal penetrating arteries and ischemic necrosis of the central portion of the spinal cord [38]. The clinical findings are similar to syringomyelia, except that any level of the spinal cord may be involved. Spinal cord

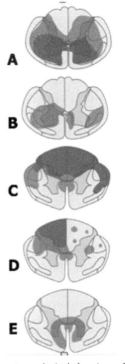

26.2. Artists' drawing of patterns of spinal cord infarction. From *Caplan's Stroke: A Clinical Approach*, 5th ed. Cambridge: Cambridge University Press, 2016, and based on Novy J, Carruzzo A, Maeder P, Bogousslavsky J. Spinal cord ischemia: Clinical and imaging patterns, pathogenesis, and outcomes in 27 patients. *Arch. Neurol.* 2006;63:1113–1120.

A. Bilateral, predominantly anterior. These patients have bilateral motor and spinothalamic type sensory deficits. Posterior column sensory functions are spared.

B. Unilateral, predominantly anterior. These patients have a hemiparesis below the lesion and a contralateral spinothalamic tract sensory loss: a Brown-Sequard syndrome.

C. Bilateral, predominantly posterior. These patients have a posterior column type of sensory loss below the lesion with variably severe bilateral pyramidal tract signs.

D. Unilateral, mostly posterior. These patients have ipsilateral hemiparesis and posterior column sensory loss.

E. Central. Bilateral pain and temperature loss with spared posterior column and motor functions, similar to a syrinx.

infarcts are occasionally explained by varicella-zoster virus infection. Rare patients with systemic vasculitis develop spinal cord as well as brain infarcts. Spinal cord ischemia has also been reported after injection of heroin and inhalation of cocaine [39].

An unusual and perplexing syndrome of spinal cord infarction was discovered and analyzed in Hawaii and entitled surfer's myelopathy [40]. In one study, 19 patients, 14 male, aged 15–46 years, had the sudden onset of low back pain while surfing. This was followed by bilateral leg numbness and paralysis progressing over 10–60 minutes. All were novice surfers; 17 of 19 surfed for the first time. All patients had MRI evidence of spinal cord infarction that extended from the lower thoracic spinal cord to the conus medullaris. A subsequent series reported another 23 Hawaiian cases [41]. The condition is opined to be caused by hyperextension of the back leading to perturbation of the vascular supply of the lower spinal cord.

Bleeding in and around the spinal cord has also been recognized but rarely. Cavernomas can be found in the spinal cord, especially in patients with multiple cavernomas on a genetic basis. Angiomas can cause intramedullary and extramedullary hemorrhaging. Spinal ependymomas often present with bleeding into the spinal cord [36].

NOTES AND REFERENCES

1. Brock RC. *The Life and Work of Astley Cooper.* Edinburgh: E&S Livingstone, 1952. Astley Cooper. Wikipedia. Available at https://en.wikipedia.org/wiki/Astley_Cooper. Silver JR. History of infarction of the spinal cord. *J. Hist. Neurosci.* 2003;12:2:144–153.
2. Pearce JMS. Henry Charlton Bastian (1837–1915): Neglected neurologist and scientist. *Eur. Neurol.* 2010;63:73–78.
3. Shorvon S, Compston A. *Queen Square: A History of the National Hospital and its Institute of Neurology.* Cambridge: Cambridge University Press, 2019, p. 107.
4. Bastian HC. Special diseases of the spinal cord. In Quain R (ed.), *A Dictionary of Medicine: By Various Writers.* London: Longmans, Green & Co., 1882, pp. 1479–1483.
5. Bastian HC. Thrombotic softening of the spinal cord: A case of so-called "acute myelitis." *Lancet* 1910;2:1531–1534.
6. McHenry LC. *Garrison's History of Neurology.* Springfield, IL: Charles C. Thomas, 1969, pp. 331–332.
7. Spiller WG. Thrombosis of the cervical anterior median spinal artery. *J. Nerv. Ment. Dis.* 1909;36:601–613.
8. Chung M-F. A study of thirty-four cases of rapidly developing syphilitic paraplegia. *Arch. Derm. Syphilol.* 1926;14(2):111–121.
9. The works of Adamkiewitz and colleagues is described in Chapter 12 on vascular anatomy.
10. Erichsen, John E. *On Concussion of the Spine.* London: Longmans, Green and Co., 1875.
11. Blackwood, W. Discussion on vascular disease of the spinal cord. *Proc. R. Soc. Med.* 1958;51:543.

12. Bramwell B. *Diseases of the Spinal Cord*, 2nd ed. New York: William Wood and Co., 1884.

13. Dana CL. *Textbook of Nervous Diseases*, 4th ed. New York: William Wood and Co., 1897.

14. Osler W. *The Principles and Practice of Medicine*, 5th ed. New York: D. Appleton and Co., 1903.

15. The topic of carotid artery disease is discussed in Chapters 15, 29, 54, and 55.

16. Duckett, S, Said G. Jean Lapresle, MD (1921–2000). *Neurology* May 2001 May;56(9):1167. Bousser MG. Éloge de Jean Lapresle, Société médicale des hôpitaux de Paris, 4 mai 2001. Vie Professionelle. *La Lettre du Neurologue* 2002 Feb;6(2).

17. Gruner J, Lapresle J. Étude anatomo-pathologique des médullopathies d'origine vasculaire. *Rev. Neurol.* 1962;107:592–631.

18. Garland H, Greenberg J, Harriman DGF. Infarction of the spinal cord. *Brain* 1966;89:645–662.

19. The history about recognition of aortic dissection is discussed briefly in Chapter 22.

20. Moersch FP, Sayre GP. Neurologic manifestations associated with dissecting aneurysm of the aorta. *JAMA* 1950;144:1141–1148.

21. Hirst AE Jr, Johns VJ, Kime SW. Dissecting aneurysm of the aorta: A review of 505 cases. *Medicine* 1958;37:217–279.

22. Szilagyi DE, Hageman JH, Smith RF, et al. Spinal cord damage in surgery of the abdominal aorta. *Surgery* 1978;83(1):38–56.

23. Hamdy A, Ramadan ME, El Sayad HF, et al. Spinal cord injury after thoracic endovascular aortic aneurysm repair. *Can. J. Anaesth.* 2017;64(12):1218–1235.

24. Brewer LA, Fosburg RG, Mulder GA, Verska JJ. Spinal cord complications following surgery for coarctation of the aorta: A study of 66 cases. *J. Thoracic Cardiovasc. Surgery* 1972;64(3):368–381. Selioutski O, Bhatt A, Kelly AG. Acute paraplegia in a patient with repaired coarctation of the aorta. *Neurol. Clin. Practice* 2017;7(2): e16–e18.

25. Caronna J, Finkelstein S. Neurologic syndromes after cardiac arrest. *Stroke* 1978;9:517–520. Silver JR, Buxton PH. Spinal stroke. *Brain* 1974;97:539–550.

26. Azzarelli B, Roessmann U. Diffuse "anoxic" myelopathy. *Neurology* 1977;27:1049–1052. Duggal N, Lach B. Selective vulnerability of the lumbosacral spinal cord after cardiac arrest and hypotension. *Stroke* 2002;33:116–121.

27. Zülch KJ, Kurth-Schumacher R. The pathogenesis of "intermittent spinovascular insufficiency" ("spinal claudication of Dejerine") and other vascular syndromes of the spinal cord. *Vasc. Surg.* 1970;4(2):116–136.

28. Zulch K. On the circulatory disturbances in the borderline zones of the cerebral and spinal vessels. In Greenfield JG, Russell D (eds.), *Proceedings of the Second International Congress on Neuropathology*, vol. 8. Amsterdam: Excerpta Medica, 1955, pp. 894–895. Zülch KJ, Behrend RCH. The pathogenesis and topography of anoxia, hypoxia, and ischemia of the brain in man. In Meyer JS, Gastaut H. *Cerebral Anoxia and Electroencephalogram*. Springfield, IL: Charles C. Thomas, 1961, p. 144.

29. Huckman M. Memorial: Giovanni Di Chiro (1926–1997). *Am. J. Neuroradiol.* 1998;19:1007–1010.

30. DiChiro G, Doppman JL, Ommaya AK. Radiology of spinal cord arteriovenous malformations. *Prog. Neurol. Surg.* 1971;4:329–354. Doppman JL, Di Chiro G, Ommaya AK. Obliteration of spinal cord arteriovenous malformation by percutaneous embolisation. *Lancet* 1968;1:477. Ommaya A, Di Chiro G, Doppman J. Ligation

of arterial supply in the treatment of spinal cord arteriovenous malformations. *J. Neurosurg.* 1969;30:679–692.

31. Michael Jeffrey Animoff. Wikipedia. Available at https://en.wikipedia.org/wiki/ Michael_Jeffrey_Aminoff.

32. Aminoff MJ, Logue V. Clinical features of spinal vascular malformations. *Brain* 1974; 97:197–210. Aminoff MJ, Barnard RO, Logue V. The pathophysiology of spinal vascular malformations. *J. Neurol. Sci.* 1974;23:255–263.

33. Aminoff MJ. *Spinal Angiomas.* Oxford: Blackwell, 1976.

34. Satran R. Spinal cord infarction. Current concepts of cerebrovascular disease. *Stroke* 1987;22:13–17.

35. Novy J, Carruzzo A, Maeder P, Bogousslavsky J. Spinal cord ischemia: Clinical and imaging patterns, pathogenesis, and outcomes in 27 patients. *Arch. Neurol.* 2006;63:1113–1120.

36. Caplan LR, Massaro A. Spinal cord vascular disease. In Caplan LR (ed.), *Caplan's Stroke*, 5th ed. Cambridge: Cambridge University Press, 2016, pp. 534–543. Caplan LR, McKee A. Case records of the Massachusetts General Hospital: Case 5-1991. *N. Engl. J. Med.* 1991;324:322–332. Srigley JR, Lambert CD, Bilbao JM, Pritzker KP. Spinal cord infarction secondary to intervertebral disc embolism. *Ann. Neurol.* 1981;9:296–301.

37. Haribhai HC, Bhigjee AI, Bill PL, et al. Spinal cord schistosomiasis: A clinical, laboratory and radiological study, with a note on therapeutic aspects. *Brain* 1991;114:709–726.

38. Caplan LR, Noronha A, Amico L. Syringomyelia and arachnoiditis. *J. Neurol. Neurosurg. Psychiatry* 1990;53:106–113.

39. Brust JCM. Stroke and substance abuse. In Caplan LR (ed.), *Uncommon Causes of Stroke*, 2nd ed. Cambridge: Cambridge University Press, 2008, pp. 365–370.

40. Chang CW, Donovan DJ, Liem LK, et al. Surfers' myelopathy: A case series of 19 novice surfers with nontraumatic myelopathy. *Neurology* 2012;79(22):2171–2176.

41. Nakamoto BK, Siu AM, Hashiba KA, Sinclair BT, Baker BJ, Gerber MS, McMurtray AM, Pearce AM, Pearce JW. Surfer's myelopathy: A radiologic study of 23 cases. *Am. J. Neurorad.* 2013;34(12):2393–2398.

SOME KEY PHYSICIANS

CHAPTER TWENTY SEVEN

CHARLES FOIX

Charles Foix was born in 1882 in Salies-de-Bearn, a small village in southern France where his father was a physician. Foix traveled from the provinces to Paris to study medicine and spent his entire medical career within the hospital systems of Paris at the Hotel-Dieu, Necker, Bicétre, and Salpêtrière [1–5].

As a medical student, he was allowed to serve a shortened time in the military service, which he completed in 1902 in an infantry regiment. He continued to serve as a physician in the reserve army and became a major aide of second-class reserve (*médecin aide-major de 2e classe de reserve*) in 1912. Passing the Paris entrance exam (*internat*) in 1905, he became a student of the neurologists Édouard Brissaud, Jean Sicard, and Pierre Marie. He then passed the very competitive examination for the position of an intern (*interne hôpitaux*) in France in 1906. This was an appointment in the Paris hospital system of one to four years with duties similar to those of resident doctors in the United States. In order to get a university teaching position (*agrégé*), he passed another competitive examination and presented a thesis (*these d'Agrégation*). During his fourth year of training he won the Gold Medal Competition, a coveted and prestigious award. He worked in pathology and neuropathology with his mentor Pierre Marie and became head of Marie's laboratory at the Salpêtrière in 1912 [6].

Then came World War I. Foix fought in France and on the Eastern Front. In addition to his pathology laboratory work, Foix had just been named hospital physician when war broke out. During August 1914, he was mobilized for ambulance duty. In January 1915, he was assigned to the Parisian military government while he was recovering from a bout of typhoid fever [7].

He came in contact with the militarized neurology departments of the Parisian hospitals, particularly that of his teacher Pierre Marie (le Grand Pére), whose contributions to neurology and cerebrovascular disease are discussed in Chapter 17. Foix worked on wartime aphasias resulting from lesions in the left cerebral hemisphere. With the help of Ivan Bertrand, Foix and Pierre Marie established a schematic cerebral map that allowed better anatomical-clinical correlations. They made detailed descriptions of the different types of aphasia resulting from lesions of the supramarginal gyrus and the angular gyrus. Foix was assigned to the Eastern Army Hospital in Salonika, which mostly treated patients with infectious diseases, especially malaria.. In April 1917, he was assigned to an ambulance unit that covered the Veria Pass area in Greece. In September 1917, the death of his friend Henry Salin from illness was especially painful for Foix. In September 1918, he was assigned to Zeitenlik Hospital No. 2, the Salonika neurology center [7]. He remained there until February 1919, taking advantage of the time by giving free rein to his passion for writing poetry. He wrote the *Trilogy of Dionysus* in Salonika, a mythological long poem in January 1919 [8].

After returning to Paris he was named hospital physician in 1919 and joined the faculty in 1923. As an associate professor he succeeded Clovis Vincent at the Hôpital Ivry-sur-Seine in 1924 where his reputation began to attract many foreign visitors. He performed many of his cerebrovascular studies there.

Of medium height with a mobile expression and dancing eyes, Foix let his hair grow in ringlets over the left side of his head and would sweep the unruly locks away from his face when bending over a patient. Figure 27.1 shows Foix early in his career. His voice was warm, vibrant, and captivating, and his demeanor was aristocratic. He was described as gentle and kind, characteristics that endeared him to friends and students. He had a brisk walk, staccato speech, and responded quickly, and to the point [5]. For someone who was not a native Parisian in a city that often did not welcome outsiders from small villages, he was very popular with students and junior and senior faculty alike; his teaching conferences were well attended. He was a compulsive and effective diagnostician with few peers. Roussy, a long-term colleague, wrote: "In his hospital ward when he examined a patient, how many times would he forget the time and not leave the consultation room until the diagnosis had been made or the sign searched for was detected" [3].

Foix's initial research studies were in general medicine. He studied and reported the leukocyte-activating powers of body fluids and hemolysis. He was a student and disciple of Pierre Marie, "from whom he learned a strict method of observation and a strong scientific discipline" [3]. His first neurologic papers were with Marie and concerned abnormalities of motor and reflex function such as medullary automatisms and synkineses, flexor spinal reflexes, and synkinetic movements in hemiplegics [9,10]. The anatomy, functions, and diseases of the extrapyramidal system were lifelong interests of his and led to publication of a book with Nicolesco on the basal ganglia and subopticmesencephalic region [11]. Foix also wrote extensively on higher cortical function abnormalities, especially aphasia and apraxia, and on cerebellar degenerations and syndromes. Two of his best-known nonvascular contributions were recognition with Sicard of albuminocytologic dissociation in the cerebrospinal fluid in patients with spinal cord compression [12] and description of the syndrome of subacute necrotizing myelitis (Foix-Alajouanine syndrome) [13].

His major contributions were in the field of cerebrovascular disease. Hillemand, one of his major collaborators, cited an initial single

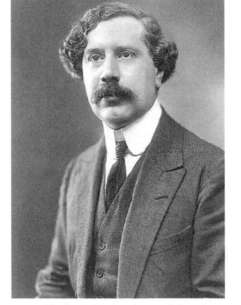

27.1. Charles Foix after the war (photo from a private collection). From Walusinski O, Tatu L, Bogousslavsky J. French neurologists during World War l. In Tatu L, Bogousslavsky J (eds.), *War Neurology*. Basel: Karger, 2016, vol. 38, pp. 107–118.

observation as the stimulus for Foix's cerebrovascular studies [14]. In the neuropathology laboratory, he noted the frequent coexistence of thalamic infarction and softening of the inferior parts of the occipital and temporal lobes. At that time the thalamic syndrome was well known, having been described a decade previously by Joseph Jules Dejerine and Gustave Roussy [15]. Those authors made no comment on the vascular supply or the vascular lesions involved. Foix was intrigued by the coincidence of thalamic and cerebral hemisphere lesions and, meticulously dissecting the arterial supply, found that the calcarine cortex was not irrigated by the middle cerebral artery (MCA) but that the posterior cerebral artery (PCA) supplied the visual cortex, the splenium of the corpus callosum, and the inferior temporal lobe, as well as the thalamus. Now, Foix understood the association. All the lesions were due to obliteration of the same arterial vessel, and the thalamic syndrome fell into the framework of a more extensive vascular syndrome, that of the PCA [16]. Hillemand commented that "from that point an unexplored avenue opened up before him – the study of the extensive vascular syndromes ... which would fill the most fruitful years of his career" [14].

Foix's major focus was on the anatomy and supply of the major brain-supplying arteries, the distribution of softenings (ramollissements), and the

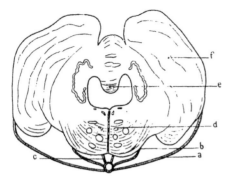

27.2. Schema of brainstem blood supply: (a) long circumferential artery, (b) short circumferential artery, (c) paramedian artery, (d) pons (protuberance), (e) cerebellar vermis, (f) lateral lobe of the cerebellum. From Foix C, Hillemand P. Les artères de l'axe encephalique jusqu'au diencephale inclusivement. *Rev. Neurol. (Paris)* 1925;41:705–739, p. 709.

clinical signs and phenomenology found in patients with variously located lesions. His tools were primarily anatomic, pathologic, and clinical, and he worked hard and long in his anatomico-pathologic laboratory at the Salpêtrière, at the bedside, and in the outpatient clinic. Foix recognized that previous treatises on anatomy often gave incomplete and erroneous descriptions of the brain vascular supply and that the figure legends and writings did not always agree with the illustrations. The vascular and brain anatomy had to be reviewed and studied from the very beginning. For months Foix meticulously dissected the intracranial arteries and their branches, subjecting both dye and opaque injections to X-rays [14]. First, he analyzed the distribution of brainstem arteries with their three systems of paramedian and short and long circumferential arteries (Figure 27.2), and then he found this same general schematic arrangement in the major cerebral arteries, the anterior cerebral artery (ACA), the MCA, and the PCA.

Foix's published reports were detailed and very systematic, and most followed a uniform system and schema. First came a description of the anatomy of the arteries being considered and their deep and superficial branches, then a description of the anatomic regions and nuclear structures supplied by each branch, and then an analysis of the distribution of softenings and their accompanying neurological signs. Foix paid little attention to the pace of illness, the accompanying risk factors, or the mechanism of infarction, and until the very end he gave little attention to the vascular pathology. His papers were well illustrated with diagrams that he drew himself and with pictures of gross and stained pathologic specimens. During Foix's time, duplication was common and accepted, and many of his diagrams and verbatim descriptions appeared in multiple publications on the same topic. He rarely mentioned in his vascular papers the number of patients or specimens studied or quantified the relative frequency of various findings and signs.

Foix's first important cerebrovascular report concerned the syndrome of the PCA and was written with Masson [16]. The paper began with descriptions and drawings of the branching of the PCA and the brain regions supplied by its branches. The major components of the clinical findings (hemianopsia, hemisensory loss, and alexia) in patients with complete PCA-territory infarcts were described. Descriptions of partial syndromes followed: an "anterior syndrome affecting the proximal PCA and cerebral peduncle with cerebellar findings and sensory loss, a thalamic syndrome, and a posterior syndrome affecting the occipital lobe with hemianopia and alexia the major findings" [16]. Abundant photographs of gross pathologic specimens illustrated the verbal descriptions. Foix later wrote an article with Hillemand on the role of the splenium of the corpus callosum in alexia without agraphia [17], a posterior cerebral hemisphere syndrome that was described and explained by one of his mentors, Jules Dejerine [18]. Dejerine and his contributions to cerebrovascular disease are discussed in Chapter 10.

Foix and his colleagues studied both the rostral and the caudal intracranial portions of the posterior circulation concurrently and during the next two years he and his colleagues Hillemand and Schalit published reports on the blood supply of the pons [19,20], the thalamic syndromes, [21] the lateral medullary syndrome [22], and a major work on arteries of the brainstem, including the diencephalon [23]. The paper on the thalamic syndromes contained detailed schematic drawings of the blood supply and the thalamic nuclei and regions supplied; the remainder of the paper analyzed the clinical findings in patients with infarcts in selected thalamic regions [21]. In the report that reviewed the arterial supply of the brainstem, Foix and Hillemand included detailed drawings of the blood supply; even the angulation of the arteries was illustrated. The authors successively reviewed the arterial supply of the pons, medulla, midbrain, and diencephalon and the clinical syndromes at each level [23]. The syndromes of the pontine arteries were characterized as follows: syndrome of the paramedian territory – the clinical "table" is very simple, the illness presents as a banal hemiplegia; syndrome of a short circumferential artery cerebellar signs on the side of the lesion and abnormalities of pyramidal and sensory function on the opposite side; softenings of the pontine tegmentum were "numerous and particularly complex" [20,23].

The reports by Foix and his colleagues on the major anterior circulation arteries (ACA [24], MCA, [25], and anterior choroidal artery (AChA) [26]) were equally detailed and complete. These studies were also published from 1925 to 1927, concurrent with the posterior circulation reports. Foix and his colleagues must have studied the two circulations at the same time, extensively examining each pathologic specimen and each patient irrespective of the location of infarction. Using the same schematic outline used in the posterior circulation papers, in discussing the anterior circulation arteries, Foix and Hillemand first noted the normal distribution of the artery and its branches and the brain regions supplied by each branch (Figure 27.3) and then described the clinical findings in each partial syndrome. The three most common presentations of ACA-territory infarction were enumerated as: (1) a simple crural monoplegia, (2) a hemiplegia with major crural predominance, and (3) a crural monoplegia (or hemiplegia with crural predominance) and a unilateral left ideomotor apraxia [24].

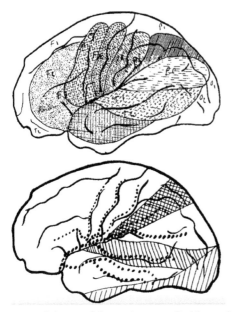

27.3. Schema of the territory supplied by each sylvian branch. F1, F2, and F3 refer to frontal gyri; P, parietal gyri; T, temporal gyri; O, occipital gyri. Territories (hatched) of supply (from superior to inferior) in the bottom figure are posterior parietal, superior temporal, and posterior temporal. From Foix C, Levy M. Les ramollissements sylviens. *Rev. Neurol. (Paris)* 1927;43:1–51, pp. 26 and 33.

Foix's analyses of the MCA syndromes were perhaps the most detailed of all his vascular studies. With Lévy, Foix described the normal usual MCA anatomy, the deep and superficial territories of the MCA, and its branches and the accompanying clinical syndromes [25].

The report on the anterior choroidal artery (AchA) syndrome was very brief and was delivered to the French Society of Ophthalmology [26]. This paper is difficult to find, but it may be the most often cited of Foix's works, probably because of the dearth of reports of AchA infarction in the succeeding five decades. This report gives a misleading interpretation of the clinical findings in AchA infarction, citing the invariable coexistence of hemiplegia, hemianesthesia, and hemianopsia and the absence of prominent cortical function abnormalities [26]. We now know that contralateral visual, sensory, and motor loss of function are uncommon after occlusion of the AchA, that only rarely are all three deficits present together, and that cortical function abnormalities are common, at least transiently. With his young ophthalmological colleague Suzanne Schiff-Wertheimer, Foix described the various vascular territorial lesions that could give rise to a hemianopia (Figure 27.4) [27].

Foix and colleagues reports contained no discussion of the pathology within the arteries. They emphasized only the distribution of the softenings and the accompanying clinical signs. Several weeks before his death, Foix, Hillemand, and Lévy-Valensi delivered a report at a meeting of the Medical Society of the Hospitals of Paris on a study of vascular pathology in arteries supplying regions of brain softening. An abstract of this report was published in the *Revue Neurologique* [28], but a full report never appeared. In an abstract of the report, Foix and colleagues described an analysis of 56 cases of brain softening. Some patients had hemorrhagic infarcts. Among these cases, the artery supplying the infarct was totally occluded in 12 and subtotally occluded in 14, but in 30 cases the arteries were essentially open or had relatively unimportant stenosis. The authors stepped beyond their colleagues of the era in speculating on possible explanations for the frequent lack of arterial occlusion. Four possibilities were cited: (1) occlusion followed softening and would have developed later; (2) embolism with passage of material by the time of autopsy; (3) insufficiency ("l'insuffisance cardio-artérielle"), that is, more proximally located circulatory failure; and (4) vasospasm ("spasme artérielle"). With these last two suggestions Foix was decades ahead of his time.

Foix died in 1927 at the age of 45. His terminal illness was acute and accompanied by abdominal pain and fever. He died quickly after surgery, never recovering postoperatively. I (LRC) found no diagnosis proffered, but appendicitis with rupture and peritonitis is most likely. The hospital and its geriatric unit and university where he worked is now named Hôpital Charles Foix at Ivry in the Val-de-Marne suburb south of the river Seine.

The major legacy of Foix was his methodology: meticu-

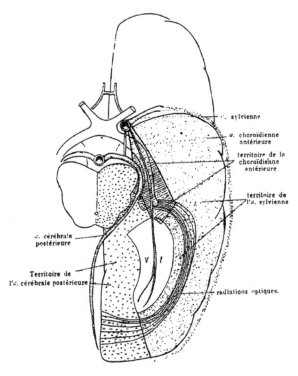

27.4. Drawing of one cerebral hemisphere, the midbrain and the optic chiasm. The arteries and their territories are labeled: middle cerebral artery (MCA) (*sylvienne*); anterior choroidal artery (AchA) (*choroidienne antérieure*); posterior cerebral artery (PCA) (*cérébrale postérieure*). From Foix C, Schiff-Wertheimer S. Revue d'oto-neuro-oculistique. In Schiff-Wertheimer S (ed.), *Les syndromes hémianopsiques dans le ramollissement cerebral*. Paris: Gaston Doin et Cie, 1926, pp. 561–584.

lous anatomic and pathologic examination of blood vessels and brain lesions, detailed clinical descriptions, and correlation of anatomy, pathology, and clinical signs. The pathology laboratory at the Salpêtrière was dedicated to Charles Foix. Foix was the first stroke neurologist, and, in fact, he really has no competition for this designation. During the half century since his untimely death, many clinicians and pathologists have followed his methodology. Some examples in France and Europe include Raymond Escourolle, Paul Castaigne, Jean-Claude C. Gautier, Jean-Jacques Hauw, Julien Bogousslovsky, Marie-Germaine Bousser, Pierre Amarenco, and Ralph Ross-Russell; while in the United States, C. Miller Fisher, Raymond Adams, John Moosy, Jay P. Mohr, Louis Caplan, Carlos Kase, Michael Pessin, J. Phillip Kistler, L. Dana DeWitt, Cathy Helgason, Dan Hier, Larry Wechsler, and Joseph Masdeu have followed the methodology of Foix. More recently, clinico-radiologic and radiologic-pathologic correlations have partially replaced and enriched our knowledge, but these have been gained by the same systematic approach.

There are many parallels between the careers of the first cerebrovascular specialist, Charles Foix, and the second specialist, C. Miller Fisher. Both spent years in the military during world wars; both were dedicated pathologists who worked during their entire careers in the pathology laboratory and in the clinic; both were very meticulous observers who worked long hours; both had a keen interest in neurological phenomenology and descriptions of neurological signs and deficits; and both made major contributions to general neurology. Foix contributed to knowledge of aphasia, basal ganglia disorders, and spinal cord conditions, while Fisher contributed to knowledge about hydrocephalus, memory, migraine, and many other topics. Both were dedicated superb teachers and role models. Each described syndromes that are eponymously named after them: Foix-Alajuanine syndrome, a vascular myelopathy [13]; the Foix-Chavany-Marie syndrome of mutism and facio-lingual dysfunction due to lesions of the operculum [29]; and the Miller Fisher variant of the Guillain-Barré syndrome [30].

NOTES AND REFERENCES

1. Caplan LR. Charles Foix: The first modern stroke neurologist. *Stroke* 1990;21:348–356.
2. Caplan LR. Charles Foix (1882–1927). *J. Neurology* 2010;257:1941–1942.
3. Roussy G. Charles Foix (1882–1927). *Rev. Neurol. (Paris)* 1927;43:44–446.
4. Lévy-Valensi. Charles Foix 1882–1927. *Sem. Hop. Paris* 1927;3:185–189.
5. Freeman W. Charles Foix. In Haymaker W (ed.), *The Founders of Neurology.* Springfield, IL: Charles C. Thomas, 1953, pp. 286–289.
6. Seilhean D. Neuropathology in Pitie-Salpetriere hospital: Past, present, and prospect. *Neuropathology* 2020;40:3–13.
7. Walusinski O, Tatu L, Bogousslavsky J. French neurologists during World War I. In Tatu L, Bogousslavsky J (eds.), *War Neurology.* Basel: Karger, 2016, vol. 38, pp. 107–118.
8. Vinchon J. L'oeuvre poetique de Charles Foix. *Aesculape* 1927;17:241–251.
9. Guillain G. L'oeuvre neurologique de Charles Foix. In *Études neurologiques.* Paris: Masson et Cie, 1933, ser. 5, pp. 439–458.
10. Boucher M. Charles Foix, sa vie, son œuvre. In *Conférences Lyonnaises d'Histoire de la Neurologie et de la Psychiatrie.* Lyon: Oberval, 1982.
11. Foix C, Nicolesco J. *Les noyaux gris centraux et la region mesencephalo-sous-optique.* Paris: Masson et Cie, 1925.
12. Sicard JA, Foix C. L'albumino reaction du liquide cephalorachidien; dissociation albumino-cytologique au cours des compressions rachidiennes. *Presse Med.* 1912;20:1013–1014.
13. Foix C, Alajournine T. La myelite necrotique subaigue. *Rev. Neurol. (Paris)* 1926;42:1–42.

14. Hillemand P. Charles Foix (1882–1927) anatomical studies. *Ann. Anat. Pathol. (Paris)* 1927;4:530–532.

15. Dejerine J, Roussy G. Le syndrome thalamique. *Rev. Neurol. (Paris)* 1906;14:521–532.

16. Foix C, Masson A. Le syndrome de l'artère cerebrale posterieure. *Presse Med.* 1923;31:361–365.

17. Foix C, Hillemand P. Role vraisemblable du splenium dans la pathogenie de l'alexie pure par lesion de la cerebrale posterieure. *Bull. Mem. Soc. Med. Hopitaux Paris* 1925;49:393–395.

18. Dejerine J. Contribution à l'étude anatomo-pathologique et clinique des différentes variétés de cécité verbal. *C. R. Soc. Biol. (Paris)* 1892;4:61–90.

19. Foix C, Hillemand P. Irrigation de la protuberance. *C. R. Soc. Biol. (Paris)* 1925;92:35–36.

20. Foix C, Hillemand P. Contribution a l'etude des ramollissements protuberantiels. *Rev. Med.* 1926;43:287–305.

21. Foix C, Hillemand P. Les syndromes de la region thalamique. *Presse Med.* 1925;33:113–117.

22. Foix C, Hillemand P, Schalit I. Sur le syndrome lateral du bulbe et l'irrigation du bulbe superieur. *Rev. Neurol. (Paris)* 1925;41:160–179.

23. Foix C, Hillemand P. Les artères de l'axe encephalique jusqu'au diencephale inclusivement. *Rev. Neurol. (Paris)* 1925;41:705–739.

24. Foix C, Hillemand P. Les syndromes de l'artère cerebrale anterieure. *Encephale* 1925;20:209–232.

25. Foix C, Levy M. Les ramollissements sylviens. *Rev. Neurol. (Paris)* 1927;43:1–51.

26. Foix C, Chavany H, Hillemand P, Schiff-Wertheimer M. Obliteration de l'artère choroidienne anterieure: Ramollissement de son territoire cerebral. Hemiplegie, hemianesthesie et hemianopsie. *Bull. Soc. Ophtalmol. Fr.* 1925;27:221–223.

27. Foix C, Schiff-Wertheimer S. Revue d'oto-neuro-oculistique. In Schiff-Wertheimer S (ed.), *Les syndromes hémianopsiques dans le ramollissement cérébral.* Paris: Gaston Doin et Cie, 1926, pp. 561–584.

28. Foix C, Hillemand P, Ley J. Relativement au ramollissement cerebral a sa frequence et a son siege, et a l'importance relative des obliterations artèrielles, completes ou incompletes dans sa pathogenie. *Rev. Neurol. (Paris)* 1927;43:217–218.

29. Foix C, Chavany J-A, Marie J. Diplégie facio-linguomastcatrice d'origine cortico sous-corticale sans paralysie du membres (contribution a l'étude de la localization des centres de la face du membre supérieur). *Rev. Neurologique* 1926;33:214–219.

30. Fisher CM. An unusual variant of acute idiopathic polyneuritis (syndrome of opthalmoplegia, ataxia, and areflexia). *N. Engl. J. Med.* 1956;255:57–65.

CHAPTER TWENTY EIGHT

HOUSTON MERRITT AND CHARLES ARING

By the end of the first third of the twentieth century, much progress had been made in neuropathology, in recognizing the necropsy findings in patients with brain and subarachnoid hemorrhages and brain infarctions. The anatomy and distribution of the arteries that supplied the brain had been extensively studied and published (see Chapters 12 and 23). The clinical neurological symptoms and signs in patients with various localized brain lesions had been studied and discussed in published literature (see Chapters 10, 11, 14, and 23). Neurosurgeons had begun to attempt to drain brain hemorrhages. But stroke continued to be of little interest to most general physicians and neurologists. There were no doctors who called themselves stroke specialists.

In that milieu two young neurologists working in a city hospital in Boston wrote an important report published in an internal medicine journal that attempted to awaken interest in the clinical diagnosis of stroke [1].

The report began: "The purpose of this study is to present an analysis of 245 cases of lesions of the cerebral vessels in which the diagnosis was proved at necropsy in order to determine the significant findings in the history and examination that will aid in the differential diagnosis between cerebral hemorrhage and cerebral thrombosis" [1].

Charles Aring and Houston Merritt noted that most strokes were labeled as cerebral hemorrhage but that few physicians attempted to differentiate hemorrhage from infarction despite differences in the symptoms, the signs, and the prognosis of these conditions:

Treatment or the possible alleviation of any cerebral lesion demands accurate knowledge of the nature and location of that lesion. It seems, therefore, that the hope of occasionally relieving the previously almost totally fatal cerebral hemorrhage will force the members of the medical profession to learn not only to localize but to determine more accurately the nature of the process in patients with cerebral vascular lesions. The need of a series of proved cases of cerebral vascular lesions is indisputable and has been repeatedly noted in the literature. [1]

Each of the authors was in his early years of neurology training at the time of the report, what would now be referred to as neurology residency. Each had a long distinguished career as a neurology department chair and held a key leadership position in medical and neurological societies. Each wrote widely in his later career about a variety of topics. Each was a general neurologist. Curiously, neither showed any special interest in stroke after their training, although Aring authored a later report on stroke diagnosis in 1964 [2].

Charles D. Aring was born on June 24, 1904, in Dent Ohio. By age five both of his parents had died and he had been partially crippled by poliomyelitis [3]. At age seven he entered a German Protestant orphanage in Cincinnati and stayed there until age 15. He worked his way through undergraduate studies and the University of Cincinnati Medical School, graduating in 1929. After a year and a half as a receiving physician and neuropsychiatry resident at Cincinnati General Hospital, he had a two-and-a-half-year fellowship in neurology and neuropathology at the Boston City Hospital. The Harvard Neurological Unit at the hospital was recognized as the premier academic neurological center in the United States at that time. It was there that he met Houston Merritt and performed the studies cited in the report.

Hiram Houston Merritt was born in Wilmington, North Carolina, on January 12, 1902. He attended Wilmington High School, graduating with high honors at age 16. He attended the University of North Carolina and Vanderbilt University, attaining an undergraduate degree in three years. He graduated from Johns Hopkins Medical School at age 24 and then served a medical internship at Yale. In 1928 he moved to the Boston City Hospital for training in neurology. Merritt remained at Boston as a staff physician. He rose to the rank of professor of neurology at Harvard University and remained there until 1944 when he went to New York to chair the department of neurology at Columbia University. He had a very distinguished career in neurology. A prominent lecture presented at the annual American Academy of Neurology meeting carries his name. At Boston he was best known for his part in introducing Dilantin into medicine as a treatment for epilepsy and for his studies of neurosyphilis [4,5].

The Aring and Merritt review of 245 cases included 106 examples of cerebral hemorrhage, 106 cases of cerebral thrombosis, and 23 cases of cerebral embolism. At that time there was no effective treatment of hypertension, so that intracerebral hemorrhage was a common occurrence in hypertensive individuals and a frequent cause of death. The distinction between thrombosis (customarily used to refer to a local in situ blockage of a vessel) and embolism (blockage of a vessel by a particle arising proximally) was difficult, and, in fact, the term "thromboembolism" was often used. Thrombi could develop in an artery, break off, and embolize distally, so that thrombosis and embolism often coexisted. At the time of this report, the only accepted sources of embolism were rheumatic heart disease, infective endocarditis, and recent myocardial infarction. Arterial sources of embolism were not referred to under the rubric of embolism. Since all of the patients died and had autopsies, only large hemorrhages and infarcts were studied.

The results began with demography. Most patients were between 50 and 80 years old. There were more men than women. More strokes occurred in winter. No particular time of day was prevalent. Few strokes occurred during vigorous activity or emotional stress. A history of previous "cerebral vascular injury" was obtained in 14 cases of cerebral hemorrhage, in 19 patients with cerebral thrombosis, and in six patients who had cerebral embolism. The authors sought instances of prodromal symptoms noted in the hospital charts. Headache was common in the days before cerebral hemorrhage. Only 8 of 106 patients with "cerebral thrombosis" had preceding warnings:

> In one patient there had been repeated and numerous attacks of tingling and numbness in the right and the left side of the face and the left extremities for five days before the onset of left hemiplegia. During these attacks speech was incomprehensible, and the left arm and leg would become rigid and then flaccid, with increased tendon reflexes and an extensor plantar response. Between attacks the patient could use the left arm and leg, and the plantar response was normal. A softening of the right half of the pons was observed at autopsy. [1]

The onset and course of illness were analyzed. Figure 28.1 is a table from their report showing the frequency of headache, vomiting, coma, and seizures, at onset and later in the hospital. Progression of signs was much commoner in patients who had cerebral hemorrhage. Progression occurred in 18.7 percent of the 112 hemorrhage cases in which this point was recorded, compared with 2 percent of the cases of cerebral thrombosis. In only one case was progression (of one day's duration) noted in patients with cerebral embolism. Survival was shorter in those who died of hemorrhage.

TABLE 3.—*Incidence of Headache, Vomiting, Convulsion and Coma at the Onset of Cerebral Vascular Lesions*

	Headache		Vomiting		Convulsion		Coma	
	At Onset	In Hospital	At Onset	In Hospital	At Onset	In Hospital	At Onset	On Admission
Cerebral hemorrhage..	26	13	19	14	8	11	35	79
Cerebral thrombosis...	3	2	3	2	2	6	16	39
Cerebral embolism.....	6	4	4	2	2	1	5	9

28.1. A table from the original report.

Blood and urine tests did not differentiate between stroke subtypes. High spinal fluid pressures were more common in patients with hemorrhage. The spinal fluid was grossly bloody in three quarters of the hemorrhage patients who had lumbar punctures, in one patient with cerebral thrombosis, and in two patients who had embolic strokes. Atherosclerosis was a constant finding in the thrombosis cases and was rare in those with hemorrhage. Kidney infarcts were common in cases of embolism. The authors concluded rather confidently:

> The differential diagnosis between cerebral hemorrhage and thrombosis can usually be made during life. A carefully taken history of the onset and progress is of paramount importance. A thorough analysis of the history, together with the results of the physical and neurological examinations and of the examination of the cerebrospinal fluid should make the differentiation possible in nearly 100% of the cases. [1]

Thirty years later Aring wrote: "Dealing since with many stroke patients, and sharing the experience with successive groups of medical students and house officers, has led naturally to some formulations. A cross section of our ongoing experience is presented, with the hope that a crisp summary may be useful for those not in the thick (one might say the thicket!) of vascular neurology" [2].

There were very important limitations of the Aring and Merritt study. It included only fatal cases. It was retrospective; the history was taken from the medical charts and often information was not recorded. The authors recognized that the frequency of stroke subtypes was skewed by the need for autopsy. They prospectively collected 407 stroke cases and, using their own diagnosis rules, found that 82 percent were thrombotic, 15 percent hemorrhagic, and only 3 percent embolic.

This was the first stroke clinico-pathologic series. It served as a model for later clinico-pathologic and clinico-radiologic studies. When Jay Mohr and I (LRC) prospectively collected cases for the Harvard Cooperative Stroke registry a full 40 years after the original study, we used the data items of Aring and Merritt's study as a guide.

NOTES AND REFERENCES

1. Aring CD, Merritt HH. Differential diagnosis between cerebral hemorrhage and cerebral thrombosis: A clinical and pathological study of 245 cases. *Arch. Intern. Med. (Chic).* 1935;56(3):435–456. doi:10.1001/archinte.1935.00170010023002.

2. Aring CD. Differential diagnosis of cerebrovascular stroke. *Arch. Intern. Med.* 1964 113:195–199.

3. Trufant S, Asbury A. Charles D. Aring (1904–1998). *Annals of Neurology* 1998;44;710.

4. Rowland LP. H. Houston Merritt (1902–1979). *Neurology* 1979;29:277–279.

5. Rowland LP. *The Legacy of Tracy J. Putnam and H. Houston Merritt: Modern Neurology in the United States.* New York: Oxford University Press, 2009.

CHAPTER TWENTY NINE

C. MILLER FISHER

Charles Miller Fisher was born on December 5, 1913. Like his older sister and older brother and the five other siblings who followed, Miller (as he liked to be called) was delivered at home. His parents lived in a simple frame house in Waterloo, in the southern part of Ontario, Canada. When Miller was 11, his mother died during childbirth while giving birth to the tenth child, who also died. He was raised by his father and a succession of stepmothers. As a young boy, he was often referred to as "Doctor." He was an average student in school, spending much of his time with sports and outdoor activities. During high school, a respected teacher criticized a report that he submitted, admonishing him that he could do much better. This criticism stimulated him, and during his last two years in high school, Miller "turned up the burners" and began to study more assiduously. He read avidly. By graduation he was recognized as "the scholar in the class." He was awarded a scholarship to the University of Toronto in recognition of his performance during high school [1].

Fisher matriculated at the University of Toronto. He chose the "biology and medicine" pathway, which exposed him to four years of general studies at one of the arts colleges affiliated with the University of Toronto. The curriculum included religion, philosophy, English literature, French or German, psychology, physics, and mathematics. The arts and science courses were intermingled with standard preclinical medical classes in anatomy, pathology, and physiology. The medical school curriculum followed during the next four years. He was stimulated most by the courses and experiments in physics. Fisher was critical of the clinical teaching. There were no full-time physicians, and instruction was unsystematic and haphazard. Special effort was neither encouraged nor welcomed. After graduation he was awarded a coveted internship at the Henry Ford Hospital in Detroit, Michigan. There he met and worked with his lifetime friend and colleague Bill Fields, another physician who dedicated his professional career to stroke.

Because Fisher was a Canadian citizen, his stay in Detroit at Henry Ford Hospital was limited by statute to one year. In 1939, Fisher enlisted in the Canadian military and married Doris Stiefelmeyer. Canada followed Great Britain into the war. While awaiting mobilization, he was invited to join the medical house staff at the Royal Victoria Hospital in Montreal. His time was divided between the general medicine and diabetic wards at the Royal Vic, the Alexandria Hospital for Infectious Diseases where diphtheria was a major problem, and a tuberculosis sanitarium. Kenneth Evelyn, a mentor, and his experience on the diabetic ward became important influences on Fisher, so much so that he planned to specialize in metabolic conditions when he returned from military service. The emphasis on metrics – carefully studying and quantifying variables – appealed to him and later became an important characteristic during his career.

He entered the Royal Canadian Navy as a surgeon lieutenant, and after some postings, he was a ship's doctor aboard the *Voltaire* headed across the ocean toward Sierra Leone. On the third day out, on April 4, 1941, disaster unexpectedly struck and the ship was sunk by a German warship. Fisher spent about 10 hours in the ocean and then was rescued by a German ship. He was eventually taken to a prisoner of war camp at Stalag X-B, near Sandbostel in northern Germany, where he spent the next three and a half years. He served as a doctor for the sick bay. During his time in the POW camp, Fisher occupied himself with learning German and reading literature and science. When the camp was liberated in 1944, he returned to Canada, determined to work earnestly and to make up for lost time in his career.

Having been away from medical practice for nearly five years, Fisher began retraining in medicine in Montreal. The six-month refresher course at the Royal Victoria Hospital included a six-week rotation on the neurology service at the Montreal Neurological Institute (MNI). As would be true during his career, a single patient provided a turning point. Fisher examined a high-ranking US Army officer admitted to the MNI to treat focal epileptic seizures. The seizures began by the patient hearing the beating of tom-tom drums. Fisher "sleuthed" in the medical library and reviewed the brain anatomy related to hearing. The next day on rounds, Fisher presented the case to Wilder Penfield, the head of the institute, a world-renowned neurosurgeon and a very charismatic individual. After the presentation, Penfield asked Fisher what he thought was going on. Fisher replied that the patient most likely had a tumor that involved hearing cerebral cortex near Heschl's gyrus in the temporal lobe. Surgical exploration confirmed Fisher's guess. This experience and others impressed Penfield with Fisher's thoroughness and willingness to explore the literature and to think about his patients.

Penfield offered Fisher the post of acting neurology registrar while another physician was away on sabbatical leave. This gave Fisher an opportunity to continue to participate in the neurology ward and clinical services at the MNI, the Royal Victoria Hospital, and the Queen Mary Veterans Hospital. During the next three years, Fisher showed proclivities that were to characterize his modus operandi later. He was dedicated to learning by extracting the maximum from each patient encounter. He also liberally used the library facilities to seek and review past reports. He often took nighttime and weekend duty in the emergency department of the MNI. He began to gain experience with neurological conditions and developed an interest in headache and hypertension. He found the academic environment in Montreal very stimulating.

In 1948, Wilder Penfield met with Fisher and suggested that he should go elsewhere to get post-graduate training and broadening in the United Kingdom or United States. Roy Swank, who recently had been recruited to the MNI, convinced Fisher that the best place to obtain further training was the Harvard Neurological Unit at Boston City Hospital (BCH). Fisher said that the major reason he decided on Boston rather than other sites was the presence of Derek Denny-Brown and Raymond Adams. He became convinced that these two were among the very few neurologists who "knew everything" [1].

The experience at BCH proved to be career- and life-changing for Fisher. The vigorous academic milieu and the work ethic on the neurological unit were a new experience for him. There he contacted individuals who would prove to be role models, mentors, and colleagues during much of his later career. In his memoirs, Fisher wrote: "There was an air of hustle and bustle, vigor, enthusiasm, excitement and cockiness. It was medicine in depth, painstaking, penetrating, inquiring, competing" [2]. "Every case, every inquiry, was the occasion for a penetrating yet wide-ranging account into every facet of a problem. In some areas Dr. Denny-Brown was superior and in many areas it was Dr. Adams" [3].

He learned pathology staining and other techniques under Adams, his mentor and chief of neuropathology at BCH. Later, when Fisher reflected on his career, he opined that the discoveries that he found on one, particular day during this training determined his entire future career in medicine and neurology. That afternoon he dissected three brains that had hemorrhagic infarctions. In each he found that the arteries that supplied the infarcts were not obstructed, indicating that an embolus had temporarily blocked the arteries and had moved distally. Reperfusion had incited bleeding into the tissues. Each of the patients had atrial fibrillation diagnosed during life. These cases raised many unanswered questions about brain embolism that he sought to answer during the subsequent years.

After the fellowship year in Boston, he returned to Montreal. Arrangements were made for Fisher to set up a neuropathology laboratory at the Montreal General Hospital dedicated to the study of strokes. William Osler, a Canadian like Fisher, had created the pathology department at Montreal General Hospital (1876–1884) and performed more than 800 autopsies while in Montreal. Fisher's clinical work involved attending rounds at the Montreal General and Royal Victoria Hospitals and consulting on patients at the Queen Mary Veterans Hospital and Ste. Anne's Hospital, which primarily served veterans of the Canadian Forces and specialized in long-term and geriatric care.

Again, it was a single patient encounter that stimulated Fisher into new avenues of inquiry. He wrote in his memoirs: "Hardly had my family and I settled back in Montreal when in the clinic at Queen Mary Veterans Hospital I examined an unfortunate veteran who had suffered a rather severe left hemiplegia two and a half years before" [4]. This disabled man who had preserved intellect but severe paralysis of his left limbs told Fisher that during the weeks before the stroke he had had several attacks of temporary blindness in one eye. While Fisher was writing his consultation note, the veteran remarked, "Isn't it funny, I went blind in the wrong eye. I am paralyzed on the left side and I went blind in the right eye" [4]. One week later another veteran told Fisher a similar story. Before he had his stroke, he was in his favorite tavern when he went blind in one eye. These two patients' histories stimulated Fisher to review the anatomy of the blood vessels that supplied the brain. The transient blindness could best be explained by a lack of blood flow to the eye. The eye is supplied by blood through the ophthalmic artery, the first branch of the internal carotid artery. The stories told by these two veterans raised the question in Fisher's mind of how often patients who had a stroke had temporary minor episodes that preceded the stroke and provided a warning that strokes might develop. He began to assiduously question stroke patients as to whether they had had any temporary neurological dysfunctions before their strokes. He also asked about transient visual symptoms. Fisher extracted detailed histories from stroke patients and their spouses and visitors. Always a stickler for details, the questions abounded in his mind. How often did warning attacks occur? What was their nature? How long before the stroke? How many attacks? How long did each warning attack last? Were the symptoms the same in each attack or did they vary? How did patients describe changes in vision? He also read to determine if others had observed and written of transient attacks preceding strokes. He was also curious about disease of the carotid artery. Were there previous writings about carotid artery disease?

The first patient who had described transient visual loss and stroke developed colon cancer and died on June 16, 1950. Fisher obtained permission for an autopsy. At 11 pm on a Sunday night, after visiting hours, the funeral director and Fisher performed a limited autopsy that included examination of the right carotid artery in the neck. Postmortem removal of the carotid arteries in the neck was usually forbidden at that time by undertakers, who depended on these vessels for embalming the head. Despite this custom and dictum, that particular funeral director was fully cooperative and went out of his way to help Fisher obtain the information needed. Fisher said that when he cut down on the artery and found that it was totally occluded, he felt a wave of emotion. The hypothesis of a young, inexperienced, clinically naïve individual that the responsible lesion must be in that carotid artery in the neck had proven to be correct. Figure 29.1 shows a drawing Fisher made of an occluded carotid artery at necropsy.

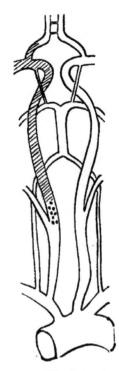

29.1. Fisher's drawing of the findings in the blood vessels of the neck in one patient. The firm blood clot originated at the origin of the internal carotid artery (shown by black dots on the left of the figure) and extended all the way into the carotid artery branches within the cranium (cross lines).

Fisher devised a method of removing the arteries in the neck, including the carotid bifurcation, by placing a red rubber catheter in the external carotid arteries so that morticians could perfuse the face with fixative. He and his hospital dieners collected a large number of specimens of the neck and intracranial arteries taken at necropsy. He continued to assiduously collect clinical information mostly from veterans who had strokes. The clinical and pathological data were the substance of several influential presentations at international meetings and reports on carotid artery disease [5–7] and on transient visual symptoms [8,9]. Fisher showed that occlusive disease of the internal carotid artery was common, as were transient ischemic attacks (a term he originated). He speculated that one day surgeons might be able to operate on the carotid artery after transient attacks and in doing so prevent strokes (the topic of carotid artery surgery is discussed in Chapter 54).

In the neuropathology laboratory at the Montreal General Hospital, Fisher continued to work on small deep infarcts (lacunes) and on brain embolism, topics he had begun studying with Raymond Adams in Boston during his fellowship. Another major project was to define the usual locations and severities of atherosclerotic plaques and narrowings found in the arteries in the neck and head that supplied the brain. He collected 1,100 pairs of carotid arteries collected at autopsies. The removal often extended to the aorta, and all of the arterial branches were dissected and preserved in formalin. The arteries within the cranium were also analyzed and preserved. In 1954, a group of international researchers came to Montreal to witness progress there. Fisher laid out his specimens on tables in the pathology laboratory. His exhibit was the last stop on the research tour. The researchers told him that this was the best thing they had seen in Canada. He was justifiably very proud and was determined to complete his work on disease of these brain-supplying arteries. Shortly thereafter he was talking with Edward Mills, the chief of the department of medicine at Montreal General Hospital, who was one of the highest-ranking and most influential physicians at McGill University at that time. Mills was a practical physician who had little or no interest in research. He asked Fisher: "Why are you studying these stroke patients? They are already paralyzed. All that carotid work is a bunch of crap" [1].

About a month after the harsh remarks of Mills, which portended a difficult future for him in Montreal, Fisher received a call from Raymond Adams urging him to come to Boston to join the neurology service at the Massachusetts General Hospital (MGH). Fisher was determined to pursue a career centered on stroke, and he knew that he could not accomplish his goals in Montreal. He had great respect for Adams, and the opportunity to help create a new department and a stroke service was a great attraction for him. While in Montreal, Fisher had become a productive researcher. His work on carotid artery disease and temporary episodes of eye and brain ischemia had gained him widespread recognition.

Fisher, his wife Doris, and their three children came to Boston and settled in a northern suburb, Winchester. Doris took major control of the household and parenting. Elizabeth later became a lawyer, and Hugh and Peter became physicians. After beginning work at the MGH in 1954, Fisher devoted his career and the great majority of every waking day to the study of neurology and stroke, both in the pathology laboratory and in patients. He created the first stroke training program. In his memoirs he reflected on his thoughts at the time that he began his efforts:

> How does one go about a practical useful study in a broad and nebulous field where the goals are difficult to discern? It was decided to methodically consult on stroke patients throughout the hospital to determine if promising avenues of approach would not open up. One or two or three neurological Fellows at a time joined me in the project and we called it the Stroke Service. [10]

Fisher worked at the hospital long and hard in his pathology laboratory and in the clinic. He arrived during the morning and left near midnight each day except Sunday, working only "half day" then. He was a methodical observer, trying to approach each pathology specimen and each patient without preconceived notions. He was unconcerned about time. His goal was to make the absolute most out of each encounter. "The patient is the clinical laboratory." He would spend many hours examining a clinical sign. Patients knew that he would take as much time as needed and they would willingly wait hours to be seen. He took copious notes in little books that he carried. He collected symptoms, signs, and observations in manila folders, waiting until enough data was collected before fully analyzing and trying to understand its meaning and significance. When he had clarified in his own mind the nature and meaning of his observations, he authored a detailed, carefully worded report.

Below are listed are some of the major contributions that he made in stroke and cerebrovascular disease.

1. **Decreased level of consciousness, stupor, and coma**. Soon after arriving at MGH, Fisher turned his attention to patients who came to the hospital unconscious or nearly so or became unconscious after entry into the hospital. The potential causes were many; stroke was a frequent etiology. Stuporous or frankly comatose patients could not give an account of their symptoms, and there were no imaging tests that could localize the lesions within the brain. Localization depended on the clinical signs obtained at the bedside. Fisher and his stroke fellows set out to examine consecutive patients who had stupor or coma. They noticed the spontaneous presence and absence of movements and activities such as coughing, sneezing, swallowing, tongue protrusion, lip licking, sighing, and yawning. The patterns of breathing were important. The eyes were examined in detail. Pupil size, position within the iris, and response to light and painful stimuli were categorized. Fisher and his colleagues noted the position of the eyes at rest and tested eye movements to each side and up and down when various stimuli were given. The position of the arms and legs at rest and their response to passive movement and to painful stimuli were studied. Fisher published a long and very detailed monograph on examination of the patient with reduced consciousness [11], and he and his colleagues authored a number of reports on eye signs and their localization [12].

2. **Small deep infarct (lacunes)**. While in Montreal, Fisher began to follow up on the work of Pierre Marie and colleagues (discussed in Chapter 16) on lacunar infarcts. At MGH, he began to systematically examine serial sections of brain specimens. One brain might yield 1,000 or more thinly cut sections. Among 1,042 brains studied at autopsy, 114 (11%) had lacunar infarcts, often multiple [13]. The commonest locations were deep within the brain: the internal capsule, basal ganglia, thalamus, and pons, the same locations as hypertensive intracerebral bleeds. Recent infarcts represented small regions of brain softening. Older lesions were cavities ranging from one to 17 millimeters in size. Often, strands of fibrillary connective tissue traversed the cavities. He studied the small penetrating arteries and arterioles that supplied these small deep infarcts and found segmental occlusions within them [14]. He

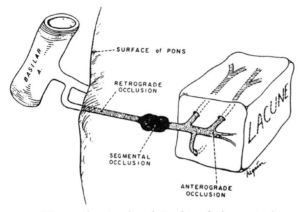

29.2. Diagram showing the relationship of a lacune in the pons to the causative penetrating artery vascular lesion. The artery beyond the region of arterial disorganization is thrombosed (anterograde occlusion) and thrombus has also formed in a retrograde manner extending toward the parent basilar artery. From Fisher CM. The arterial lesion underlying lacunes. *Acta Neuropathologica* 1969;12:1–15.

dubbed the pathology "segmental arterial disorganization" and also applied the term "lipohyalinosis," indicating that fatty material (lipid) was included and that the wall took on a glassy (hyaline) appearance. Lipid material and connective tissue called fibrinoid thickened the wall of the small arteries, causing encroachment on the vascular lumen. Figure 29.2 shows a drawing of the lesion in an artery leading to a lacune.

Later, Fisher and Caplan described another vascular lesion that caused small deep infarcts [15]. The initial designation for this alternate pathology was "basilar branch infarcts" since the pathology was found in studying branches of the basilar artery. This pathology also involved branches of the main arteries supplying the cerebral hemispheres and was labeled "intracranial branch atheromatous disease" [16]. In the clinic during many decades he reported and analyzed the different syndromes that were found in patients with these lacunar infarcts [17].

3. **Hemorrhages outside and inside the brain**. Fisher was one of the first to clarify the pathology and clinical findings in patients with intracerebral hemorrhages [18]. The first major presentation of his findings concerning hemorrhage was in 1959 at a meeting at the Texas Medical Center that was organized by William Fields, his colleague during medical internship in Detroit and also a stroke pioneer. Fisher had examined 134 brains that contained brain hemorrhages during a period of three and a half years. Most hemorrhages in patients with hypertension occurred at four sites: basal ganglia, thalamus, pons, and cerebellum. He described the usual clinical course and findings in these patients. Later, he and his colleagues were the first to clarify the clinical findings in patients with cerebellar hemorrhages [19].

Studying hematomas in serial section, he noted that small globoid caps were situated around the circumference of the hematomas [20]. These caps represented bleeding capillaries or small arterioles. He interpreted the circumferential bleeding sites as evidence that hematomas developed gradually with pressure effects beginning and maximal at the center of the hematomas and causing secondary pressure damage sequentially to small vessels on the periphery of the expanding hematoma. Hypertension would cause a penetrating artery to rupture. Often this occurred when the hypertension first developed or worsened. Hemorrhages would begin small. Pressure in the center due to the high pressure within the leaking artery exerted force on vessels at the periphery, causing them, in turn, to bleed. The hematoma grew on its outer circumference much like a snowball rolling downhill. This process of growth of the hematoma would stop if and when the hematoma drained onto the brain or ventricular surface, partially decompressing itself. Alternatively, tissue pressure and intracranial pressure external to the hematoma would increase until pressures inside and outside the hematoma equalized. The clinical course of patients with brain hematomas corresponded to what was expected from gradual enlargement of the lesions.

When computed tomography (CT) became available in the 1970s, Fisher and his colleagues turned their attention to aneurysmal subarachnoid hemorrhage. They recognized that blood within the subarachnoid space stimulated vasoconstriction. They studied the frequency and clinical findings in patients with vasoconstriction and delayed brain ischemia and the relationship of the clinical features to the location and extent of blood found on CT scans [21].

4. **The distribution and severity of cervico-cranial atherosclerosis and carotid and subclavian artery disease**. While in Montreal, Fisher had accumulated necropsy specimens of the neck and cranial arteries. In Boston, he collaborated with cardiologists and a pathologist in describing the usual locations of atherosclerotic plaques within the brain-supplying arteries. The carotid bifurcations extending into the internal carotid arteries, the carotid siphon, the first centimeters of the middle cerebral arteries, the subclavian arteries extending into the vertebral artery origins, the intracranial vertebral arteries, and the basilar arteries were the most frequent sites [22]. Fisher and Robert Ojemann, a neurosurgeon, described the pathological findings and their correlation with clinical findings in patients whose surgical specimens were serially analyzed after carotid artery surgery [23]. Fisher coined the term and described the phenomenology of the subclavian steal syndrome [24].

5. **Cervical artery dissections**. Fisher and his surgical colleague Robert Ojemann were among the very first to call attention to dissection of arteries in the neck and head that supplied the brain [25]. At the time of their reports (the 1970s) arterial dissection was known to occur in the aorta but was not often

considered as involving systemic arteries in the neck, head, abdomen, and coronary circulations.

6. **Published diagrams of the clinical symptoms and signs in patients with lesions attributable to brain ischemia related to the various obstructed cervico-cranial arteries**. One of Fisher's major contributions to the care of patients with cerebrovascular disease and strokes was his lengthy descriptions and diagrams of the symptoms and signs in patients with occlusive cerebrovascular disease that appeared in textbooks of internal medicine and neurology. The first major presentation of this material was in a chapter included in a volume of the proceedings of a March 1959 meeting at the Texas Medical Center organized by Bill Fields [26]. The drawings and much of the text that Fisher presented at this meeting were later incorporated into chapters in very popular, widely read medical textbooks, for example, in successive editions of Harrison's textbook of Internal Medicine and Victor and Adams's textbook of neurology. Figure 29.3 is a diagram showing the pons and its syndromes.

7. **Atrial fibrillation as a cause of brain embolism**. While a neuropathology fellow during 1949, the first three cases of brain embolism studied by Fisher all had atrial fibrillation. Fisher remained interested in this topic during his long career at MGH [27]. While performing postmortem examinations in Boston in his neuropathology laboratory, he was impressed by the frequency of atrial fibrillation in patients whose brains showed embolic infarcts. In Montreal, he had shown that studies of serial sections of the left atrial appendage in patients who had had embolic brain infarcts invariably exhibited mural thrombi within the interstices of the trabeculae carnae of the appendage. In 1972 he sent a letter to the editor urging consideration of anticoagulation in patients with atrial fibrillation before they had a stroke [28]. He was the first to make this suggestion: "In our cerebrovascular studies, we have been struck by the number of patients in atrial fibrillation who have a severe stroke as the first manifestation of embolism. All patients with chronic atrial fibrillation should be considered for prophylactic anticoagulant therapy . . . to avoid a fate worse than death" [28].

Fisher organized a study along with his stroke fellows and cardiology colleagues to formally study the heart and other organs at autopsy to clarify the role of atrial fibrillation in causing brain embolism. The results showed that atrial fibrillation was important not only in patients with mitral valve disease but also in patients without cardiac valve disease [29].

8. **Migraine and brain ischemia; separation from occlusive cerebrovascular disease**. Fisher had a lifelong interest in headache and migraine. He carefully studied, noted, and reported the common sites of headache in patients with various vascular lesions [30]. He analyzed auras in migraineurs and contrasted these visual symptoms with those found in visual loss due to

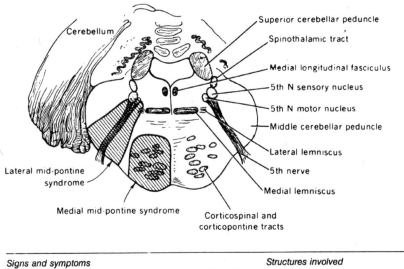

29.3. The clinical findings in patients with brainstem infarcts located in the pons. From Fisher CM. Clinical syndromes in cerebral arterial occlusion. In Fields W (ed.), *Proceedings of the Annual Meeting of the Houston Neurological Society*. Springfield, IL: Charles C. Thomas, 1961, pp. 151–181. N = nerve.

Signs and symptoms	Structures involved
1. Medial midpontine syndrome (paramedian branch of midbasilar artery)	
a. On side of lesion	
(1) Ataxia of limbs and gait (more prominent in bilateral involvement)	Middle cerebellar peduncle
b. On side opposite lesion	
(1) Paralysis of face, arm, and leg	Corticobulbar and corticospinal tract
(2) Deviation of eyes	
(3) Variably impaired touch and proprioception when lesion extends posteriorly. Usually the syndrome is purely motor.	Medial lemniscus
2. Lateral midpontine syndrome (short circumferential artery)	
a. On side of lesion	
(1) Ataxia of limbs	Middle cerebellar peduncle
(2) Paralysis of muscles of mastication	Motor fibers or nucleus of fifth nerve
(3) Impaired sensation over side of face	Sensory fibers or nucleus of fifth nerve

carotid artery disease [31] and to posterior cerebral artery territory infarctions. He called attention to the common occurrence of late-life migraine accompaniments that mimicked transient ischemic attacks [32]. Fisher noted that migraine could occasionally cause brain infarction [33].

9. **Neuro–ophthalmological signs and syndromes in stroke patients**. During his early studies of comatose patients during the 1950s and 1960s, Fisher became aware of the importance of eye movements and visual function in localizing brain lesions [12]. The human brain is all about looking and seeing. He authored many reports of new and important "eye signs." He correlated

the size of the pupils with vascular lesions that affected various parts of the brainstem. The pupils were often very small, pinpoint, in lesions of the pons. Using a bright light and a magnifying lens, the very small pupils could be shown to react to light stimulation. The pupils could be widely dilated or mid-position and the shape could become oval in patients with midbrain lesions [34,35]. The pupil could be dilated and unreactive on the side of a carotid artery occlusion, the mechanism being ischemia to the iris of the eye [36].

Some patients closed one eye repeatedly without being aware that they were doing so, a sign that Fisher dubbed "unwitting closure of one eye" [34]. This was a subtle indication that the patient was seeing double.

He analyzed unusual situations in which one or both eyes failed to move normally and was the first to describe the "one-and-a-half syndrome" [34]. In this condition, both eyes failed to move on gaze to one side. On gaze to the other side, only one eye moved. If gaze to each side was counted as one, the patient had only half gaze to one side, so that one and a half gaze was lost. This finding was diagnostic of a lesion in the upper, medial portion of the pons. In some patients, there was abnormal spontaneous movements of one or both eyes. Intermittent, rhythmic, up and down movement of the eyes, vertical nystagmus, indicated a lower brainstem localization [34]. He was the first to describe a different type of abnormal vertical motion of the eyes found in unresponsive patients. "In a typical case, the eyeballs intermittently dip briskly downwards through an arc of a few millimeters and then return to the primary position in a kind of bobbing action" [37]. Ocular bobbing indicated a hemorrhage or infarct in the pons. Fisher reported that ocular nerve palsies could occur in patients with temporal arteritis and other forms of arterial inflammation [38].

Fisher, like Charles Foix, throughout his career practiced general neurology in addition to his stroke work. Fisher made many contributions to understanding brain functions and to clinical neurology. These important contributions included transient and persistent memory dysfunction, hydrocephalus, cognitive and behavioral abnormalities, and decreased and increased behavior (abulia, impersistence, intermittent interruption of behavior, and agitated hyperactivity). He is also remembered for a syndrome that carries his name: the Miller Fisher variant of the Guillain-Barré syndrome [39]. Although he officially retired in 1980, he continued to work at MGH, in his laboratory and in the clinic, and to write and teach until 2007.

He was 98 years old when he died. He had been a witness to remarkable changes during his near century of life. Much of the change in the care of patients with stroke and cerebrovascular disease could be directly attributable to his research, his writings, and his teachings and to the physicians he had mentored lovingly during his long and fruitful career.

NOTES AND REFERENCES

1. The biographical information in this chapter is from Caplan LR. *C. Miller Fisher: Stroke in the 20th Century*. New York: Oxford University Press, 2020.

2. Fisher CM. *Memoirs of a Neurologist*. Rutland, VT: Sharp, 2006, vol. 1, p. 47.

3. Fisher CM. *Memoirs of a Neurologist*. Rutland, VT: Sharp, 2006, vol. 1, p. 49.

4. Fisher CM. *Memoirs of a Neurologist*. Rutland, VT: Sharp, 2006, vol. 1, p. 53.

5. Fisher CM. Occlusion of the internal carotid artery. *American Medical Association Archives of Neurology and Psychiatry* 1951;65:346–377.

6. Fisher CM. Disease of carotid arteries: A clinico-pathological correlation. In *Report of the Annual Meeting and Proceedings of the Royal College of Physicians and Surgeons of Canada. October 3–4, 1952*, pp. 60–67.

7. Fisher CM. Occlusion of the carotid arteries: Further experiences. *American Medical Association Archives of Neurology and Psychiatry* 1954;72:187–204.

8. Fisher CM. Transient monocular blindness associated with hemiplegia. *Transactions of the American Neurological Association* 1951;76:154–158.

9. Fisher CM. Transient monocular blindness associated with hemiplegia. *AMA Archives of Ophthalmology* 1952;47:167–203.

10. Fisher CM. *Memoirs of a Neurologist*. Rutland, VT: Sharp, 2006, vol. 1, p. 132.

11. Fisher CM. The neurological examination of the comatose patient. *Acta Neurologica Scandinavica* 1969;49(suppl 6):4–57.

12. Abnormalities of the pupil and eye movements are described in Fisher CM. Oval pupils. *Archives of Neurology* 1980;37:502–503. Fisher CM. Some neuro-ophthalmologic observations. *Journal of Neurology, Neurosurgery, and Psychiatry* 1967;30:383–392. Fisher CM Ocular bobbing. *Archives of Neurology* 1964;11:543–546. Fisher CM. Dilated pupil in carotid occlusion. *Transactions of the American Neurological Association* 1966;91:230–231. Fisher CM. Ocular flutter. *Journal of Clinical Neuroophthalmology* 1990;10:155–156.

13. Fisher CM. Lacunes, small deep cerebral infarcts. *Neurology* 1965;15:774–784.

14. Fisher CM. The vascular lesion in lacunae. *Transactions of the American Neurological Association* 1965;90:243–245. Fisher CM. The arterial lesions underlying lacunes. *Acta Neuropathologica* 1969;12:1–15.

15. Fisher CM, Caplan LR. Basilar artery branch occlusion: A cause of pontine infarction. *Neurology* 1971;21:900–905. Fisher CM. Bilateral occlusion of basilar artery branches. *Journal of Neurology Neurosurgery and Psychiatry* 1977;40:1182–1189.

16. Caplan LR. Intracranial branch atheromatous disease: A neglected, understudied and underused concept. *Neurology* 1989;39:1246–1250.

17. Clinical syndromes were reported in Fisher CM. Pure motor hemiplegia of vascular origin. *Archives of Neurology* 1965;13:30–44. Fisher CM. Pure sensory stroke involving face, arm, and leg. *Neurology* 1965;15:76–80. Fisher CM. Thalamic pure sensory stroke: A pathologic study. *Neurology* 1978;28:1141–1144. Fisher CM. Pure sensory stroke and allied conditions. *Stroke* 1982;13:434–447. Fisher CM. A lacunar stroke, the dysarthria-clumsy hand syndrome. *Neurology* 1967;17:614–617. Fisher CM, Cole M. Homolateral ataxia and crural paresis, a vascular syndrome. *Journal of Neurology Neurosurgery and Psychiatry* 1965;28:48–55. Fisher CM. Ataxic hemiparesis. *Archives of Neurology* 1978;35:126–128. Fisher CM. Capsular infarcts. *Archives of Neurology* 1979;36:65–73. Fisher CM. Lacunar strokes and infarcts: A review. *Neurology* 1982;32:871–876.

18. Fisher CM. Pathology and pathogenesis of intracerebral hemorrhage in pathogenesis and treatment of cerebrovascular disease. In Fields W (ed.), *Proceedings of the Annual*

Meeting of the Houston Neurological Society. Springfield, IL: Charles C. Thomas, 1961, pp. 295–317. Fisher CM. Clinical syndromes in cerebral hemorrhage in pathogenesis and treatment of cerebrovascular disease. In Fields W (ed.), *Proceedings of the Annual Meeting of the Houston Neurological Society.* Springfield, IL: Charles C. Thomas, 1961, pp. 318–342.

19. Fisher CM, Picard E, Polak A, Dalal P, Ojemann R. Acute hypertensive cerebellar hemorrhage: Diagnosis and surgical treatment. *Journal of Nervous and Mental Diseases* 1965;140:38–57. A clinical-pathological discussion of a case seen at MGH: Fisher CM, Richardson EP. Sudden headache and vertigo in a man with hypertension. Case 35-1967. *New England Journal of Medicine* 1967;277:423–428.

20. Fisher CM. Pathological observations in hypertensive cerebral hemorrhages. *Journal of Neuropathology and Experimental Neurology* 1971;30:536–550.

21. Fisher CM, Roberson GH, Ojemann RG. Cerebral vasospasm with ruptured saccular aneurysm: The clinical manifestations. *Neurosurgery* 1977;1:245–248. Fisher CM, Kistler JP, Davis JM. Relation of cerebral vasospasm to subarachnoid hemorrhage visualized by computerized tomographic scanning. *Neurosurgery* 1980; 6(1):1–9. Kistler JP, Crowell RM, Davis KR, Heros R, Ojemann RG, Zervas NT, Fisher CM. The relation of cerebral vasospasm to the extent and location of subarachnoid blood visualized by CT scan: A prospective study. *Neurology* 1983;33:424–437.

22. Fisher CM. Gore I. Okabe N. White PD. Atherosclerosis of the carotid and vertebral arteries – Extracranial and intracranial. *Journal of Neuropathology and Experimental Neurology* 1965;24:455–476.

23. Fisher CM, Ojemann RG. A clinico-pathological study of carotid endarterectomy plaques. *Revue Neurologique (Paris)* 1986;39:273–299.

24. [Fisher CM] A new vascular syndrome: "The subclavian steal." *New England Journal of Medicine* 1961;265:912.

25. Fisher CM, Ojemann RG, Roberson GH. Spontaneous dissection of cervicocerebral arteries. *Canadian Journal of Neurological Science* 1978;5:9–19.

26. Fisher CM. Clinical syndromes in cerebral arterial occlusion. In Fields W (ed.), *Proceedings of the Annual Meeting of the Houston Neurological Society.* Springfield, IL: Charles C. Thomas, 1961, pp. 151–181. Fisher CM, Karp HR, Adams RD. Cerebrovascular diseases. In Harrison TR, Adams RD, Bennett I Jr, Resnik WH, Thorn GW, Wintrobe MM (eds.), *Principles of Internal Medicine,* 3rd ed. New York: McGraw-Hill, 1958, pp. 1560–1606.

27. An account of Fisher's publications and that of others on the topic of atrial fibrillation has been included in Caplan LR. Atrial fibrillation, past and future: From a stroke non-entity to an over-targeted cause. *Cerebrovascular Diseases* 2018;45:149–153.

28. Fisher CM, The treatment of atrial fibrillation. Letter to the editor. *Lancet* 1972;299:1284.

29. Hinton RC, Kistler JP, Fallon JT, Friedlich AL, Fisher CM. Influence of etiology of atrial fibrillation on incidence of systemic embolism. *American Journal of Cardiology* 1977;40:509–513.

30. Fisher CM. Headache in cerebrovascular disease. In Vinken PJ, Bruyn GW (eds.), *Handbook of Clinical Neurology, vol. 5: Headaches and Cranial Neuralgias.* Amsterdam: North Holland, 1968, pp. 124–156.

31. Fisher CM. Migraine accompaniments versus arteriosclerotic ischemia. *Transactions of the American Neurological Association* 1968;93:211–213.

32. Fisher CM. Late-life migrainous accompaniments as a cause of unexplained cerebral attacks. Charcot lecture, 1979, Hôpital de la Salpêtrière, 293–324. Fisher CM. Late-life

migraine accompaniments as a cause of unexplained transient ischemic attacks. *Canadian Journal of Neurological Sciences* 1980;7:9–17. Fisher CM. Late-life migraine accompaniments: Further experience. *Stroke* 1986;17:1033–1042.

33. Fisher CM. An unusual case of migraine accompaniments with permanent sequellae. *Headache* 1986;26:266–270. Fisher CM. Cerebral ischemia: Less familiar types. *Clinical Neurosurgery* 1971;18:267–336.

34. Fisher CM. Some neuro-ophthalmological observations. *Journal of Neurology Neurosurgery and Psychiatry* 1967;30:383–392.

35. Fisher CM. Oval pupils. *Archives of Neurology* 1980;37:502–503.

36. Fisher CM. Dilated pupil in carotid occlusion. *Transactions of the American Neurological Association* 1966;91:230–231.

37. Fisher CM. Ocular bobbing. *Archives of Neurology* 1964;11:543–546.

38. Fisher CM. Ocular palsy in temporal arteritis. *Minnesota Medicine* 1959;42:1258–1268, 1430–1437, 1617–1630.

39. Fisher M. An unusual variant of acute idiopathic polyneuritis (syndrome of ophthalmoplegia, ataxia, and areflexia). *New England Journal of Medicine* 1956;255:57–65.

CHAPTER THIRTY

LOUIS CAPLAN

Call me Ishmael . . .
. . . and I only am escaped alone to tell thee.
                    —Herman Melville, *Moby-Dick*

Although my contributions to the history of stroke are meager, I (Louis R. Caplan) decided to include my autobiography in this volume. I have functioned mostly like Ishmael: as a scribe, witness, simplifier, disseminator, and describer of the stroke-related ideas and events that have transpired during the last 50 years or so when the most changes occurred. My story includes a glimpse into medicine, neurology, and stroke as it changed during the twentieth century. It is an autobiographical sketch that has not appeared elsewhere. It seemed awkward to write the memoir in anything but the first person, although that is discouraged by publishers.

I was born in Baltimore, Maryland, on the last day of 1936, in the midst of a depression. My father was forced to leave school during World War I and drove a jitney bus taxi to help provide for his parents and seven older siblings. After the war, Carl took a two-month course at the Max Morris School of Pharmacy and was granted a license to practice pharmacy, although he had never finished high school. He was self-educated. My mother's family had emigrated from the Ukraine. My grandfather had created a jewelry business in downtown Baltimore. He was tragically murdered during his mid-forties during a robbery at the store. His two sons took over the business, one having to leave medical school after his first year of matriculation. After graduating from high school, my mother worked at the jewelry store during her whole life. I helped out at the store after school and on Saturdays.

Two of my uncles were active in World War II. Dr. Ephraim Lisansky, who was married to my mother's youngest sister, had the wartime duty of tracking *Anopheles* mosquitos, the carriers of *Plasmodium* parasites, the cause of malaria. More individuals died of malaria and other infections than from warfare. Uncle Eph was an internist by training. When he returned from the war he became the single most important role model for me. Eph insisted that I take the A course at the Baltimore City College (high school) as he had years before. The course curriculum was very exacting; five years of teaching was condensed into four years, making it possible to enter some colleges in the second year or to waive some of the college requirements. The curriculum consisted of five years of Latin and two years each of French and German, advanced calculus, physics, chemistry, biology, and literature and history courses. I took readily to the challenge; my grade average was greater than 95, near the top of the class.

When it came to applying to college, I was on my own. My parents knew nothing about the process. Older boys whom I respected had attended Brown University and told me that was the place to go. In the early spring I took a train trip with a high school friend to visit Brown, Amherst, and Williams. I applied to Brown for early admission and to other schools, including Duke and Princeton, for regular admission. I was stunned and very disappointed to receive a rejection in the mail. I was convinced that if Brown rejected me, so would all the other schools, so I wrote Brown that the university had made a serious mistake and my application should be reconsidered. My relatives and friends said that I had shown incredible chutzpah in doing so. To everyone's surprise, I received a letter from Brown that they would reconsider. Ultimately, they did accept me, but by then I had decided to attend Williams College in rural Massachusetts.

When I began college, I planned to be a chemical engineer and so elected advanced physics, chemistry, and math as well as English literature and economics. I was good when working with chemical formulas and electrical diagrams on paper but was all thumbs in the science labs. An early essay (freshmen had to write one each week) was graded as an F, with a note that my writing was a disaster and needed high-level corrective remediation. I told my mother to hold my room at home for me because I might not make it at school. All my classmates were very smart and almost two thirds had been to prep school and had been well schooled in writing. I had not realized that English teachers on purpose characteristically scared freshmen by seriously downgrading essays. I played freshman basketball, tennis, and baseball and spent most of my time with sports and studying. During my sophomore year I continued chemistry and became fascinated by my history and English courses, taught by outstanding teachers. When I had to declare a major, I chose history, emphasizing American history and literature, but also included chemistry. By the end of the junior year I seriously considered a career in academic chemistry or history. Uncle Eph convinced me that medicine was my best choice. As a physician I could practice, research, teach, or write and could readily switch from one to another depending on my druthers and results. I added biology courses and German (a medical school requirement), continued chemistry, and stuck with my history major courses. During the last three years in college I stopped competing on college teams but was active in intramural athletics, played golf and tennis, and studied very hard. I was elected junior Phi Beta Kappa and won the history prize at graduation. At Williams I had learned to write simply and directly and to communicate well verbally. Those skills stood me in good stead in the years to come.

I entered the freshman medical school class at the University of Maryland in Baltimore. Tuition was $1,000 per year, which I covered from college prize money and summer and weekend earnings. I lived at home and spent nearly all my time in class or studying. We had full year courses in the basics: anatomy, physiology, and pathology. In my sophomore year I moonlit doing autopsies at a nearby community hospital. The most influential medical class was in neuroanatomy, taught by two well-known Dutch neuroscientists, Walle Nauta and Hans Kuypers, who were performing research at Walter Reed Army Hospital. Nauta was a master of metaphor and simile. He composed stories about the interrelationships of various neural groups and tracts, making nervous systems fascinating and understandable. During medical school my special interests were internal medicine and cardiology. I took my neurology rotation and some internal medicine in London at Guy's Hospital and Queen Square. I applied for internal medicine internships and residencies during my senior year. I graduated from the University of Maryland summa cum laude as the class valedictorian and chair of the Alpha Omega Alpha medical honorary society.

I matched with the Boston City Hospital for medical internship and junior residency. The pay was $120 per month plus a room in the house officer building and three meals daily in the cafeteria. The events surrounding my first rotation are reflective of medicine at BCH in 1962. There was no orientation. When I picked up my room key, the clerk said I was to be in charge of the male side of the emergency room beginning July 1. I spoke to the intern who was then working in the ER for guidance. He only had a minute to talk. He said, "It's simple: if they are sick, admit them; if they are well send 'em home; if minor issues, treat 'em. That's all you need to know." I learned the ER triage system. If they walked in, they were sent to room 1; if carried in on a stretcher, room 3; if they were on their feet but needed assistance, room 2. There were no labs or X-rays in the ER. Only your eyes and ears and brain and very experienced nurses who knew the ropes. Similarly, ward duty was trial by fire. I once was entrusted with 45 sick women on the ward when my co-intern went home for a family matter. Supervision was only by a senior resident and staff internist during a 90-minute quick ward round each morning. Weekend duty was Friday morning until Monday night. During my internship and junior medical residency, a neurology conference was held each Friday. These sessions and a rotation on the Harvard Neurology Unit at BCH, chaired by Derek Denny-Brown, cemented my decision to become a neurologist. But first I had to serve my obligatory military duty. During my junior residency year I had met and wooed an ER nurse, Brenda Fields, and we were married in November 1963.

I was assigned duty as a captain in the US Army at Tripler Army Hospital in Honolulu, Hawaii. My wife and I purchased a small home in Ewa Beach on the leeward side of Oahu. I worked in the internal medicine clinic at the hospital. I traveled to and from the hospital on a navy shuttle across Pearl Harbor. The neurologist who consulted on neurological inpatients and held regular outpatient clinics learned of my interest and asked me to attend the neurology clinics and consult on complex inpatients After I began to attend the clinics, he absented himself and I seemed to be in charge, although I had had very little formal neurological training. Brenda did visiting nurse duties. Our first two children were born in Hawaii.

While in the army, I applied for neurology residence on the Harvard Neurological Unit at BCH and was accepted as one of the five residents chosen each year. My neurology training began July 1966. I have written in much detail about the neurology unit in the biography of C. Miller Fisher, so will not repeat it here [1]. Training included a full year of neuropathology. Denny-Brown expected that when you completed the three-year program and were a fully trained neurologist, you should be able to, without preparation, discuss any neurological condition in depth, including its background history, nature of the condition, evaluation, treatment, and research. Denny-Brown retired after my second year of residency and Norman Geschwind assumed directorship of the neurological unit. He stimulated my interest in higher cortical brain function.

During my neurology residency I had decided to focus on stroke. The reasons were several: (1) I had had four years of internal medicine training and experience, and my training especially in cardiology and hematology were important in relation to stroke; (2) stroke at that time was a neglected topic; much was to be learned and there were opportunities for research and improvement in patient care; and (3) strokes were by nature localized lesions within the brain; analysis of the clinical features especially in reference to cognition, memory, speech, and behavior allowed important insights into how the brain worked, a topic that fascinated me. During my senior year

I applied for a stroke fellowship with Miller Fisher at the Massachusetts General Hospital (MGH). I received a very brief note from Miller Fisher saying I was welcome to come: Be at work on July 1, 1969.

My year as Fisher's cerebrovascular disease fellow changed my life [1]. I was the only fellow. I had a direct tutorial. I spent three to five hours each day, six days per week, mostly at the bedside with Miller Fisher. His teaching style was Socratic. His forte was teaching how to learn, how to extract the maximum from each patient encounter. During the first six months of the fellowship, he never directly conveyed his thoughts and opinions. He did not want me to parrot back what he had told me. We saw one or two patients together each evening and some others during the day. I saw nearly every stroke patient who was hospitalized at MGH during that year, attended brain cuttings, and participated in all of the conferences. In addition to Miller Fisher, Raymond Adams and E. P. Richardson were master teachers. They emphasized the importance of in-depth knowledge of anatomy and pathology – the basics. During the preceding three years I had been nurtured by Denny-Brown, who was a Sherringtonian physiologist. No neurology trainee could have been better prepared for a future career in academic neurology and stroke than I.

Before my stroke fellowship I was offered a position as a staff neurologist at the Beth Israel Hospital (BIH) in Boston. Pressure was exerted to forgo my MGH fellowship and join BIH directly. The hospital waited for me to complete the stroke fellowship and in July 1970 I became an attending neurologist at BIH. I was the second trained neurologist on the full-time staff. The first neurologist had been appointed several years earlier. Some internists commented that "we already have one, why do we need another?" Many internists during those days felt confident in handling most neurological issues. Neurology at BIH was a subdivision of internal medicine. A dozen full-time internists comprised the staff, most subspecialists. Private practitioners admitted patients to the hospital and cared for them while hospitalized. For two months per year I attended on the internal medical wards. (I had passed my internal medical board exams during my neurology training and was a board-certified internist.). During six months of the year I was the attending physician for the neurology inpatients. I also saw neurology consultations of private physicians. I was appointed chief of the neurology outpatient clinic. As one of my Harvard University duties, I was assigned to be the only neurologist for the newly formed Harvard Community Health Plan (HCHP). This meant I took care of all their neurology inpatients, outpatients, and patients referred to the ER at BIH. The princely salary for my HCHP duties was $2,000 per year. I was also appointed as an attending physician at the Boston Children's Hospital, across the street from the BIH. Another Harvard responsibility was teaching the Longwood area (BIH, Brigham and Women's Hospital, Boston Children's Hospital) Harvard neurology trainees during rotations through the BIH. I was also expected to produce and publish research. In July 1970, at age 33, I had finally become a staff physician with an impossible load of responsibilities. There were by then five young children at home for whom I needed to provide. I worked from 7 am to 11 pm most days and was on duty many nights and weekends, so my time with my children and wife was limited. I was allowed to enrich my extremely meager BIH/Harvard pay by having my secretary bill for private patient visits and consultations.

I gained considerable experience during the BIH years caring for almost all of the stroke patients. An interchange with Howard Bleich, a nephrologist colleague, during my first years at BIH changed my career. The internal medicine department at BIH instituted a clinical decision analysis program that offered consultations regarding difficult cases. Led by Bleich and Warner Slack, an internist who had some training as a neurologist, the unit began to use computers to aid decisions. Bleich published an influential report in 1971 in the prestigious *New England Journal of Medicine* about the use of computers in aiding clinical diagnosis [2]. The report described a computer diagnostic program designed to help physicians manage patients with electrolyte and acid-base disorders. The program directed a dialogue during which physicians supplied clinical and laboratory information. When the interchange was completed, the program produced an evaluation note and references. The program taught physicians what data was needed, how to make accurate acid-base diagnoses, and how to calculate the nature and quantity of fluids needed for treatment. Flushed with this success, Bleich urged me to create a computerized program that would diagnose all neurological conditions. I replied that the heterogeneity of neurological conditions and the anatomy was too complex and that I could not comply with the request. After much back and forth, I agreed to try to write a diagnostic program for stroke limited only to the probability of the patient having one of the stroke subtypes but not about the anatomy.

I was introduced to a premed MIT student who knew about computers but knew nothing about stroke, while I had absolutely no knowledge about computers and diagnostic programs. We worked together in formulating a potential diagnostic program. The only viable choice for determining probabilities was to use a Bayesian analysis. This required two pieces of information: (1) the frequency of each stroke subtype in the population being studied and (2) the frequency of each data item in each stroke subtype. How many patients with intracerebral hemorrhage have headache before their stroke? How many have headache at onset? How many have seizures? How many have sudden maximal at onset symptoms? In how many does the deficit accrue gradually? How many have preceding hypertension? How many smoked? And other questions. Some subtypes – for example, lacunar strokes – were newly described and lacked information on these and other items. I surveyed four experienced neurologists who had special interests in stroke about the various frequencies, and also speculated about the frequencies myself. The probabilities were all over the ballpark. I concluded that we had no reliable data and needed to acquire it to aid clinical diagnosis. The idea for the Harvard Stroke Registry was born.

I contacted J. P. Mohr. He had preceded me as Fisher's stroke fellow. We had had identical stroke training and thought alike. He had returned from his military requirement in Washington and had taken over direction of the stroke fellowship at MGH from Fisher. Mohr and I and Bleich and Slack met regularly to choose items to be collected and diagnostic criteria for each stroke subtype. I examined every stroke patient at BIH and entered the data myself on paper. Mohr took responsibility for entering the same data at MGH. The data entry sheet consisted of 86 items, including risk factors, activity at onset, course, major findings, on examination spinal fluid data, and neurologists' initial impression. The completed data sheets were sent to the computer medicine lab at BIH. Information was entered into a large PDP-15 computer using a miniature information and retrieval system. The computer was housed in a special area with tight temperature control. When the five-year data was collected and analyzed, Mohr and his fellows and I and our computer colleagues sent a report of the results among the 694 patients to the *New England Journal*. It was summarily rejected with the comment that "computers would never have an important role in medicine." The diagnostic criteria and the frequencies from the Harvard Stroke Registry were published in the journal *Neurology* [3]. This was the first published registry in any medical field. Table 30.1 is a representative table from the registry. I became convinced that prospectively collected data was needed in many medical fields as an important aid to diagnosis and management. Computerized registries became an emphasis during my future career. The other emphasis during my eight years at BIH was

TABLE 30.1. *Nature of onset for each type of stroke*

Onset.	Large Artery Thrombosis. Thrombosis %	Lacune %.	Embolism %.	Hematoma %.	Aneurysm or AVM %
Sudden.	40	28	79	34	80
Stepwise or Stuttering	34	32	11	3	3
Smooth or Gradual	13	20	5	63	14
Fluctuating.	12	10	5	0	3

From Mohr J, Caplan L, Melski J, Duncan G, Goldstein R, Kistler J, Pessin M, Bleich H. The Harvard Cooperative Stroke Registry: A prospective registry. *Neurology* 1978;28:754–762, p. 758, table 4.

on disease of the vertebrobasilar circulation [4]. I published a widely read report on the top of the basilar syndrome in the journal *Neurology*. In 1975 I was made the chief of the neurology section at BIH. When the Harvard Neurological Unit from the Boston City Hospital moved to BIH, neurology became a department at BIH and my teaching and clinical responsibilities diminished. I became unhappy with the methods of the new regime and received no support for my research or clinical activities.

Beginning in 1977, I received several offers from academic centers outside Boston. In 1978, I moved to Chicago to accept an attractive offer to head the neurology department at the Michael Reese Hospital, a 2,000-bed urban medical center. The position included a professorship at the University of Chicago. I became the cochair of the University of Chicago neurology residency program with Dr. Barry Arneson, an MGH alumnus. My first major activity was to recruit Dan Hier, who had just finished his neurology residency at MGH. Dan, like me, was interested in stroke and higher cortical function. Our family lived in Evanston, on the North Shore. I commuted by train and shuttle to the hospital. I had to leave the hospital by 5:30 pm to catch the last reasonable train home. I seldom worked weekends. We had our sixth child (fifth boy) in 1980. Our three oldest children were in high school. I had more time to spend with my family than in Boston earlier. I continued to believe heavily in computer registries. One of the University of Chicago neurology residents, Gordon Banks, was also a computer guru. He was able to create a computer program on an Apple personal computer for registration of the Michael Reese Stroke Registry, and we collected data on all ischemic stroke cases at Michael Reese [5].

The National Institute of Neurological Diseases and Stroke (NINDS) by then had also become convinced of the utility of acquiring prospective data about stroke and funded the Stroke Data Bank (SDB). (The Harvard Stroke Registry was voluntary and not funded.) The patients in the Harvard Registry were predominantly Caucasian. The Stroke Data Bank centers were chosen partly to accrue a racially mixed population. CT scanning had become available and it was hoped that subtype diagnosis would be more accurate. Anatomical CT scan data was also collected. I was one of the principal investigators (PIs) in the SDB, which was generously funded. The PIs spent a full year traveling back and forth to Bethesda and the National Institutes of Health to agree on data items, entry sheets, and plans of analysis before beginning data collection [6]. I began a stroke training program and recruited one fellow each year. Among the fellows was Rob Stein, who was the coauthor of the first edition of *Stroke: A Clinical Approach* [7], and Phil Gorelick, who went on to have an accomplished career as a neuro-epidemiologist focusing on cerebrovascular disease. Brain hemorrhages were common at Michael Reese and became a focus of interest, as did drug-related stroke [8]. I and coauthors drew attention to the frequency of paradoxical brain emboli related to a patent foramen ovale [9]. I became very interested in racial and sex differences in the distribution of cerebrovascular lesions.

In the early 1980s Michael Reese began to have economic difficulties as a large portion of their base moved to the suburbs. The close relationship between the hospital and the University of Chicago began to come apart. In 1984 I received an offer to return to Boston that I could not refuse. My wife's parents were in Boston and she and I were anxious to return. I was offered the position of neurologist-in-chief at the then New England Medical Center (NEMC) and chair of the department of neurology at Tufts University. I spent the next 15 years at Tufts. Michael Pessin had already begun a stroke service at NEMC. He had been a stroke fellow at MGH with supervision by Miller Fisher, Mohr, and Phillip Kistler. Dana DeWitt, an early stroke fellow who had been with me at Michael Reese Hospital, was added to our stroke attending staff. We began to attract stroke research fellows from Europe, Asia, and South America. There were often four to seven fellows working at one time. All were funded by their own countries. They were highly motivated to learn as much as possible about cerebrovascular disease and to collaborate on many research projects. In the mid-1980s NEMC had the largest stroke service in the United States and elsewhere. One project was to prospectively collect posterior circulation ischemic stroke patients into the NEMC posterior circulation stroke registry. Ultimately, more than 400 patients were entered; the data was reviewed in conferences each week to ensure accuracy and completeness [10]. Other projects were to clarify, analyze, and write reviews of various stroke infarct and hemorrhage syndromes [11]. I continued my interest in racial and sex differences in the distribution of vascular and brain lesions.

The other major project during my Tufts years was involvement in early thrombolysis research. I joined a consortium of investigators: Mike Pessin and I in Boston; Werner Hacke, Herman Zeumer, Klaus Poeck, Berndt Ringelstein, Andreas Ferbert, and Helmet Bruckmann in Aachen, Germany; Greg del Zoppo and Shirley Otis from Scripps Clinic in La Jolla, California; Tony Furlan from Cleveland Clinic in Ohio; and Etsuo Mori from Japan. We met to plan investigations with thrombolytic drugs in stroke patients. Later these investigators were joined by others, including Lawrence Wechsler, Carlos Kase, J. P. Mohr, and Edward Feldmann, in performing early trials. Streptokinase, urokinase, and rt-PA were the most common agents used. In these early studies, acute stroke patients were screened clinically and by CT scans, and then catheter angiography was performed [12]. If an intracranial arterial occlusion was shown, thrombolytic drugs were given either intraarterially into the clots or intravenously. Follow-up angiography was performed after treatment to assess recanalization. These studies showed that thrombolytic agents could often open blocked arteries. Opening of the arteries correlated with better outcomes than when the arteries remained occluded. These studies were observational and not randomized trials. They showed the potential effectiveness of thrombolysis and its safety.

During my time at NEMC, I did much traveling in the United States, Europe, and Asia, at conferences and giving talks and bedside rounds at many institutions. During the mid-1990s, NEMC and Tufts began to have severe economic difficulties. Expensive modern new buildings were constructed despite declining revenues. Admissions diminished. Tufts Medical School and our neurology department split training of residents with the Lahey Clinic and St. Elizabeth's Hospital. I was tired of the administrative burden of being a chair. A philanthropist supported a move to the Beth Israel Deaconess Medical Center (BIDMC) and Harvard Medical School. The Beth Israel Hospital had recently merged with the Deaconess Hospital. In 1998, I was back where I began my career. After Steve Warach departed for Washington, I assumed the directorship of the stroke unit, a position I held for a decade. I accepted no other administrative burdens, except membership on some Harvard professorial committees. I wanted to teach, do research, train residents and stroke fellows, and write.

Early work at BIDMC consisted of collecting research data using MRI in patients with hyperacute brain ischemia. Warach and Gottfried Schlaug, stroke unit clinicians, had engineering and MRI research training, and Robert Edelman, of the radiology department, was a pioneer in magnetic resonance angiography (MRA). The stroke service was able to garner access to an MRI machine, and stroke fellows and staff utilized a full MRI/MRA diagnostic program and recorded extensive information on all incoming patients with acute brain ischemia. The data was stored on hard discs and was analyzed and reported. At BIDMC, I became interested in neurological and cardiac complications of cardiac surgery, and collaborated with Denis Barbut of New York and the Northern New England Cardiovascular Disease Study Group in analyzing frequencies and causes [13]. I became active in some early stem cell research. At BIDMC we were the first to inject fetal stem cells into stroke cavities. With Sean Savitz, a former BIDMC neurology resident and stroke fellow, I helped write early reports on stem cell research and its promise, drawbacks, and controversies [14].

Much of the time during the years at BIDMC were spent training stroke fellows and international trainees. European countries now had their own

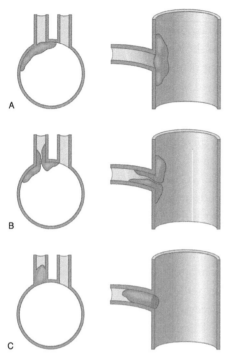

30.1. Drawing showing the arterial pathology in atheromatous branch disease. A, plaque in parent artery obstructing a branch; B, a junctional plaque extending into the branch; C, a microatheroma formed at the orifice of a branch. From Caplan LR, *Caplan's Stroke: A Clinical Approach*, 5th ed. Cambridge: Cambridge University Press, 2016, p. 39, figure 2.33, with permission.

stroke training programs and stopped funding full-year American fellowships. Instead, we hosted mostly neurology trainees from Hong Kong, China, Korea, Japan, India, and Thailand. I traveled often to these countries and continued to collaborate with European, Asian, and South American stroke clinicians and researchers. In later years I concentrated on clinical care and writing.

My Main Contributions

1. Posterior circulation stroke: The two monographs on this topic [15] are my magnum opus. Each took years to write. Other important reviews [16] and reports are listed [11].

2. Registries and data banks: J. P. Mohr and I published the first stroke registry [3]. I created stroke registries at each work location [5,6,10] and was instrumental in stimulating other national and international colleagues to make registries and data collections.

3. Racial and sex differences in the distribution of brain and vascular lesions [17]

4. Binswanger disease: early description and clinical, imaging, and pathological features [18]

5. Intracranial atheromatous branch disease: introduced and popularized the concept [19] (Figure 30.1)

6. Coexistence and complementary effects of hypoperfusion and embolism: ineffective washout of emboli is an important factor in occlusive large artery disease [20]

7. Cardiac encephalopathy [21]: first description

8. Dissection of neck and intracranial arteries [22]

9. Posterior reversible encephalopathy syndrome: first description and characterization of clinical features, etiology, and outcomes [23]

10. Clinical diagnosis: three editions of *The Effective Clinical Neurologist* and five editions of *Caplan's Stroke: A Clinical Approach* emphasize the methods of clinical diagnosis. Definition of stroke entities [24] and characterization of many stroke syndromes [11]

11. Treating the individual patient: Pitfalls of "evidence-based medicine" [25]

12. Cerebrovascular complications of pregnancy and the puerperium [26]

13. Non-stroke entities ("Caplan's syndrome"), HSV2 sacral radiculoneuritis [27]

14. Creating a full cerebrovascular disease library that emphasized the origin, evolution, and nature of conditions; five editions of *Caplan's Stroke: A Clinical Approach*, three editions each of *Uncommon Causes of Stroke* and *Stroke Syndromes*, two editions of *Primer of Cerebrovascular Diseases, Brain Embolism, and Intracerebral Hemorrhage*

NOTES AND REFERENCES

1. A longer account of the fellowship and Fisher's career and contributions is found in Caplan LR. *C. Miller Fisher: Stroke in the 20th Century*. New York: Oxford University Press, 2020.

2. Bleich HL. The computer as a consultant. *New England Journal of Medicine* 1971;284:141–147.

3. Mohr J, Caplan L, Melski J, Duncan G, Goldstein R, Kistler J, Pessin M, Bleich H. The Harvard Cooperative Stroke Registry: A prospective registry. *Neurology* 1978;28:754–762.

4. Caplan LR. Occlusion of the vertebral or basilar artery: Follow-up analysis of some patients with benign outcome. *Stroke* 1979;10:277–282. Caplan L. Top of the basilar syndrome: Selected clinical aspects. *Neurology* 1980;30:72–79.

5. Caplan L, Hier D, D'Cruz I. Cerebral embolism in the Michael Reese Stroke Registry. *Stroke* 1983;14:530–540. Among the discoveries was the first recognition of the importance of the size of the left atrium in cardiogenic brain embolism: Caplan LR, D'Cruz I, Hier DB, et al. Atrial size, atrial fibrillation and stroke. *Annals of Neurology* 1986;19:158–161.

6. The Stroke Data Bank published many reports, among which were Foulkes MA, Wolf PA, Priced TR, Mohr JP, Hier DB. The Stroke Data Bank: Design, methods, and baseline characteristics. *Stroke* 1988;19:547–554. Shinar D, Gross C, Mohr J, Price T, Caplan L, et al. Inter-observer variability in the assessment of neurologic history of examination in the stroke data bank. *Archives of Neurology* 1985;42:557–565.

7. Caplan LR, Stein RW. *Stroke: A Clinical Approach*. Boston: Butterworth, 1986.

8. Caplan L, Banks G, Thomas C. Central nervous system complications of addiction of "T's and Blues." *Neurology* 1982;32:623–628. Harrington H, Heller A, Dawson D, Caplan L, Rumbaugh, C. Intracerebral hemorrhage and oral amphetamine. *Archives of Neurology* 1983;40:503–507.

9. Jones HR, Caplan L, Come P, et al. Cerebral emboli of paradoxical origin. *Annals of Neurology* 1983;13:314–319.

10. Representative reports from the NEMC-P Circulation Registry include Caplan LR, Chung C-S, Wityk RJ, et al. New England Medical Center posterior circulation stroke registry: I. Methods, data base, distribution of brain lesions, stroke mechanisms, and outcomes. *Journal of Clinical Neurology* 2005;1:14–30. Caplan LR, Wityk RJ, Pazdera L, et al. New England Medical Center posterior circulation stroke registry: II. Vascular lesions. *Journal of Clinical Neurology* 2005;1:31–49. Glass TA, Hennessey PM, Pazdera L, Chang H-M, Wityk RJ, DeWitt LD, Pessin MD, Caplan LR. Outcome at 30 days in the New England Medical Center Posterior Circulation Registry. *Archives of Neurology* 2002;59(3):369–376. Caplan LR, Wityk RJ, Glass TA, et al. New England Medical Center Posterior Circulation Registry. *Annals of Neurology* 2004;56:389–398.

11. Representative descriptions and reviews of brain infarcts: Caplan LR, DeWitt LD, Pessin MS, Gorelick PB, Adelman LS. Lateral thalamic infarcts. *Archives of Neurology* 1988;45:959–964. Caplan LR, Schmahmann JD, Kase CS, et al. Caudate infarcts. *Archives of Neurology* 1990;47:133–143. Caplan LR, Kelly M, Kase CS, et al. Infarcts of the inferior division of the right middle cerebral artery: Mirror image of Wernicke's aphasia. *Neurology* 1986;36:1015–1020. Helgason C, Caplan LR, Goodwin J, Hedges T. Anterior choroidal artery territory infarction: Case reports and review. *Archives of Neurology* 1986;43:681–686. Amarenco P, Rosengart A, DeWitt LD, Pessin MS, Caplan LR. Anterior inferior cerebellar artery territory infarcts: Mechanisms and clinical features. *Archives of Neurology* 1993;50:154–161. Chaves CJ, Caplan LR, Chung C-S, et al. Cerebellar infarcts in the New England Medical Center Posterior Circulation Registry. *Neurology* 1994;44:1385–1390. Representative examples of brain hemorrhage syndromes: Stein R, Kase C, Hier D, Caplan L, Mohr J, et al. Caudate hemorrhage. *Neurology* 1984;34:1549–1554. Caplan L, Neely S, Gorelick P, Caplan L, Goodwin J. Lateral brainstem tegmental hemorrhage. *Neurology* 1982;32:252–260. Chung C-S, Caplan LR, Han W, Pessin MS, et al. Thalamic haemorrhage. *Brain* 1996;119:1873–1886. Chung C-S, Caplan LR, Yamamoto Y, et al. Striatocapsular haemorrhage. *Brain* 2000;123:1850–1862.

12. The early investigations of thrombolytic therapy are reviewed in del Zoppo GJ, Poeck K, Pessin MS, et al. Recombinant tissue plasminogen activator in acute thrombotic and embolic stroke. *Annals of Neurology* 1992;32:78–86. Wolpert SM, Bruckmann H, Greenlee R, et al. Neuroradiologic evaluation of patients with acute stroke treated with recombinant tissue plasminogen activator. The rt-PA Acute Stroke Study Group. *American Journal of Neuroradiology* 1993;14:3–13. Pessin MS, del Zoppo GJ, Furlan AJ. Thrombolytic treatment in acute stroke: Review and update of selected topics. In *Cerebrovascular Diseases, 19th Princeton Conference, 1994.* Boston: Butterworth-Heinemann, 1995, pp. 409–418.

13. Barbut D, Caplan LR. Brain complications of cardiac surgery. *Current Problems in Cardiology* 1997;22(9):449–480. Caplan L. Protecting the brains of patients after heart surgery (editorial). *Archives of Neurology* 2001;58:549–550. Likosky DS, Leavitt BJ, Marrin CAS, Malenka DJ, Reeves AG, Weintraub RM, Caplan LR, et al. for the Northern New England Cardiovascular Disease Study Group. Intra- and postoperative predictors of stroke after coronary artery bypass grafting. *Annals of Thoracic Surgery* 2003;76:428–435.

14. Savitz SI, Dinsmore J, Wu J, Henderson GV, Stieg P, Caplan L. Neurotransplantation of fetal porcine cells in patients with basal ganglia infarcts: A preliminary safety and feasibility study. *Cerebrovascular Diseases* 2005;20:101–107. Savitz S, Rosenbaum DM, Dinsmore JH, Wechsler LR, Caplan LR. Cell transplantation for stroke. *Annals of Neurology* 2002;52:266–275.

15. Caplan LR. *Posterior Circulation Disease: Clinical Findings, Diagnosis, and Management.* Boston: Blackwell Scientific, 1996. Caplan LR. *Vertebrobasilar Ischemia and Hemorrhage: Clinical Findings, Diagnosis, and Management of Posterior Circulation Disease.* Cambridge: Cambridge University Press, 2014.

16. Caplan L. Posterior circulation ischemia: Then, now, and tomorrow. The Thomas Willis Lecture – 2000. *Stroke* 2000;31:2011–2013. Savitz SI, Caplan LR. Current concepts: Vertebrobasilar disease. *New England Journal of Medicine* 2005;352:2618–2626.

17. Gorelick P, Caplan L, Hier D, Patel D, Parker S. Racial differences in the distribution of anterior circulation occlusive cerebrovascular disease. *Neurology* 1984;34:54–59.

Gorelick PB, Caplan LR, Hier DB, et al. Racial differences in the distribution of posterior circulation occlusive disease. *Stroke* 1985;16:785–790. Feldmann E, Daneault N, Kwan E, Ho K, Pessin MS, Langenberg P, Caplan LR. Chinese-white differences in the distribution of occlusive cerebrovascular disease. *Neurology* 1990;40:1541–1545. Caplan LR, Gorelick PB, Hier DB. Race, sex and occlusive vascular disease: A review. *Stroke* 1986;17:648–655.

18. Caplan L, Schoene W. Clinical features of subcortical atherosclerotic encephalopathy (Binswanger disease). *Neurology* 1978;28:1206–1215. Caplan, L. Binswanger's disease. In Fredericks JAM (ed.), *Handbook of Clinical Neurology, vol. 46: Neurobehavioral Disorders.* Amsterdam: Elsevier, 1985, pp. 317–321. Caplan LR. Binswanger's disease. *Current Opinion in Neurology and Neurosurgery* 1988;1:57–62. Caplan LR. Binswanger's disease – Revisited. *Neurology* 1995;45:626–633.

19. Fisher, C.M. Basilar artery branch occlusion: A cause of pontine infarction. *Neurology* 1971;21:900–905. Caplan LR. Intracranial branch atheromatous disease. *Neurology* 1989;39:1246–1250.

20. Caplan LR, Hennerici M. (Hypothesis) Impaired clearance of emboli (washout) is an important link between hypoperfusion, embolism, and ischemic stroke. *Archives of Neurology* 1998;55:1475–1482.

21. Caplan LR. Cardiac encephalopathy. *(Current Treatment Options in) Cardiovascular Medicine* 2004;6:171–178. Caplan LR. (Hypothesis) Cardiac encephalopathy and congestive heart failure – A hypothesis about the relationship. *Neurology* 2006;66:99–101.

22. Caplan LR, Baquis GD, Pessin MS, et al. Dissection of the intracranial vertebral artery. *Neurology* 1988;38:867–877. Caplan LR. (Review) Dissections of brain-supplying arteries. *Nature Clinical Practice (Neurology)* 2008;4(1):34–42. Chaves C, Estol C, Esnaola MM, Gorson K, O'Donoghue M, De Witt LD, Caplan LR. Spontaneous intracranial internal carotid artery dissection: Report of 10 patients. *Archives of Neurology* 2002;59(6):977–981. Caplan LR, Biousse V. (State of the Art) Cervicocranial arterial dissections. *Journal of Neuro-Ophthalmology* 2004;24(4):299–305. Caplan LR, Estol CJ, Massaro AR. Dissection of the posterior cerebral arteries. *Archives of Neurology* 2005;62:1138–1143.

23. Hinchey JA, Chaves CJ, Appignani B, Breen JC, Pao L, Wang A, Pessin MS, Lamy C, Mas J-L, Caplan LR. A reversible posterior leukoencephalopathy syndrome. *New England Journal of Medicine* 1996;334:494–500.

24. Albers G, Caplan LR, Easton JD, et al. Transient ischemic attack. Proposal for a new definition. *New England Journal of Medicine* 2002;347:1713–1716. Amarenco P, Bogousslavsky J, Caplan LR, Donnan GA, Hennerici M. Classification of stroke subtypes. *Cerebrovascular Diseases* 2009;27(5):493–501. Amarenco P, Bogousslavsky J, Caplan LR, Donnan GA, Wolf ME, Hennerici MG. The ASCOD phenotyping of ischemic stroke (updated ASCO phenotyping). *Cerebrovascular Diseases* 2013;36:1–5. Sacco LR, Kasner SE, Broderick JP, Caplan LR, et al. (AHA/ASA Expert Consensus Document) An updated definition of stroke for the 21st century: A statement for healthcare professionals from the American Heart Association/American Stroke Association. *Stroke* 2013;44:2064–2089.

25. Editorial. TIAs: We need to return to the question, What is wrong with Mr. Jones? *Neurology* 1988;38:791–793; Caplan L. (Editorial) Evidence based medicine: Concerns of a clinical neurologist. *Journal of Neurology, Neurosurgery, and Psychiatry* 2001;71:569–576. Caplan L. (Invited commentary) Is the promise of randomized control trials ("evidence-based medicine") overstated? *Current Neurology &*

Neuroscience Reports 2002;2:108. Caplan LR. Evidence and the effective clinical neurologist. The 2009 H. Houston Merritt Lecture. *Archives of Neurology* 2011;68:1252–1256.

26. Siderov E, Feng W, Caplan LR. Stroke in pregnant and postpartum women. *Expert Reviews in Cardiovascular Therapy* 2011;9:1235–1247. Edlow JA, Caplan LR, O'Brien K, Tibbles C. Diagnosis of acute neurological emergencies in pregnant and postpartum women. *Lancet Neurology* 2013;12:175–185. Digre KB, Varner M, Caplan LR. Eclampsia and stroke during pregnancy and the puerperium. In Caplan LR (ed.), *Uncommon Causes of Stroke*, 2nd ed. Cambridge: Cambridge University Press, 2008, pp. 515–528.

27. Caplan L, Kleeman F, Berg S. Urinary retention probably secondary to herpes genitalis. *New England Journal of Medicine* 1977;297:920–921. Caplan LR. "Caplan's syndrome" – Revisited and lessons learned. *Practical Neurology* 2005;5(5):304–307.

IMAGING

CHAPTER THIRTY ONE

CEREBRAL ANGIOGRAPHY

Egas Moniz performed the first successful cerebral angiogram on June 28, 1927. Since then, remarkable achievements in studies of the cerebral circulation have been obtained. Most astonishing is that after more than 90 years, cerebral angiograms are performed daily at the largest hospitals of the world, adding an application that Moniz barely could imagine: interventional angiography for acute treatment of stroke.

António Caetano de Abreu Freire Egas Moniz was born in the small rural village of Avanca in a picturesque region of coastal lagoons in the north of Portugal. He graduated in medicine from the University of Coimbra in 1899 and soon decided to pursue a university career. In 1902, he obtained his PhD with the thesis "The Sexual Life: Pathology."

Moniz was elected to the monarchic parliament in Lisbon in 1900. He fulfilled his teaching duties at the University of Coimbra simultaneously with political activities in Lisbon. From 1902 on, he also found time to visit the Hôpital de la Salpêtrière in Paris during his summer vacations as regularly as possible, until the 1930s.

During the first 20 years of the twentieth century Moniz was better known in Portugal as a politician than as a physician. At parliament, he demonstrated all his oratory skills and his ability to argue. He carefully prepared his interventions, making him respected by his comrades and feared by his opponents.

In 1911, the Faculty of Medicine of Lisbon was founded and he was appointed the new chair in neurology. This position forced him to resign his position in the republican parliament to fully dedicate himself to medicine. This period did not last long. Lisbon was a small town and the political turmoil of the early period of the new republican regimen could not allow him to remain uninvolved.

Moniz temporarily left his duties at the School Hospital in Lisbon to become leader of parliament and, soon after, in March 1918, he became the Ambassador of Portugal in Madrid, Spain. In October of that year, he was appointed Minister of Foreign Affairs. When World War I ended, he was appointed leader of the Portuguese delegation to the Peace Conference in Versailles. In early 1919 the political situation in Portugal was very unstable, so he considered his position unsustainable and decided to end his political activities. He embraced medicine and resumed his position as professor of neurology.

At that time, a major problem in neurology was the diagnosis and location of space-occupying lesions, mainly tumors. Moniz was aware of the work of Jean-Athanase Sicard, a French radiologist and neurologist who introduced lipiodol, a radio-opaque oxidized poppy seed oil, into the cisterna magna to radiologically identify blockage of the spinal canal [1].

Moniz discussed with Sicard the possibility of opacification of cerebral vessels. The French neurologist had already tried to inject lipiodol in animals, but the results were discouraging since the greasy product occluded smaller vessels. Returning to Lisbon, Moniz aimed to find an innocuous substance to visualize the cerebral circulation on X-rays.

Aside from technical limitations of brain surgery, identification and location of space-occupying lesions was based only on clinical grounds. That was clearly insufficient to preclude surprises during surgery.

During the years of 1918 and 1919, Walter Dandy introduced ventriculography and pneumoencephalography into the radiographic identification of brain tumors [2]. These procedures included the injection of air or other gases such as helium or oxygen by lumbar puncture or through a burr hole in the skull to allow visualization of the cerebral ventricles and their distortions. Patients were restrained in a rotating chair to allow movement in several positions including upside down, which was very uncomfortable and difficult to manage. Patients developed long-lasting headaches and often vomited.

Egas Moniz entertained the idea of diagnosing space-occupying intracranial lesions by visualizing the cerebral circulation. The distortions of the normal "map" would allow identification of lesions. To inject a chemical fluid directly into the carotid arteries seemed a reckless idea, so Moniz performed a cautious sequence of experiments in order to identify the lowest concentration able to be adequately visualized. He began by visualizing contrast media in different concentrations that were dropped in a few rubber tubes attached to a card and exposed to X-ray films through a hemi-skull. The next step was to obtain human heads from the morgue, inject the carotid arteries, and expose them to X-rays.

For the first time, the cerebral circulation was depicted accurately. Segments never before identified were seen, some of them named by Moniz: carotid siphon and sylvian group. He then moved to living animals and the choice fell on dogs, mainly because their heads had adequate dimensions for this purpose and were easy to obtain from the city authority that caught stray dogs.

Although the first attempt in living beings allowed him to see the cerebral circulation, the chemical product was too toxic and all the animals died. So, Moniz progressively reduced the concentrations of strontium bromide, and, finally, after many attempts, animals survived and angiograms were obtained safely. The final step foreseen by him was to apply the procedure to human beings.

Moniz was aware of the risks, so he waited for a patient with a desperate situation to justify the uncertainty of the results. Finally, the opportunity arrived: a man with intracranial hypertension, suspected of having a brain tumor but without neurological signs to allow localization. The procedure showed the cerebral circulation, but the patient convulsed and died in a few hours. This caused Moniz great distress and he paused his research.

A few months later, he decided to resume his experiments. He posited that the reason for the failure was the excessive concentration of contrast. He made another attempt using a lower concentration. This time, on June 27, 1927, he was successful. The patient had a pituitary tumor and was already blind because of intracranial hypertension. The angiogram clearly showed distortions caused by the tumor. The patient had no procedural complications.

The next week, Moniz took the train to Paris to present his success at a meeting of the Societé Neurologique. This was intended as a tribute to the school where he learned neurology. His lecture was well accepted and Moniz recalled it in his memories, including the laudatory comments by Joseph Babinski, Sicard, Souques, and Roussy, the president of the society [3].

Angiography required exposing the carotid artery to puncture and then injecting contrast with a syringe. Moniz did not have these skills. Almeida Lima (1903–1985) was the neurosurgeon who performed all the procedures invented by Moniz throughout his life, from angiography to leucotomy.

Progressively, cerebral angiography achieved worldwide acceptance, but Moniz and his team continued investigating. By chance in one of the patients suspected of having a brain tumor, carotid injection showed that no dye flowed above the carotid bifurcation. The carotid artery was occluded [4]. Moniz and Lima soon understood that cerebral angiography was not just a way of identifying brain tumors. The vessels themselves deserved attention, and this method showed a large field of application. For the following years a new window of progress was open: the diagnosis of carotid occlusions hitherto unknown, as well as several other abnormalities: intracranial vessel occlusions, aneurysms, and arteriovenous malformations.

Soon after, Moniz published two works: the first one in 1931 devoted to the diagnosis of tumors with a foreword by Joseph Babinski [5] and the second in 1934, dealing with the study of cerebral vessels [6], both published by the prestigious Parisian house Masson.

In Portugal, angiography was expanded by several investigators who used this technique in opacifying the aorta and limb vessels. Moniz's later research involved leukotomy in patients with psychosis [7], and for this research, rather than angiography, he was awarded the Nobel Prize in Physiology or Medicine in 1949.

Surgical exposure of the carotid arteries was a drawback to the performance of angiography, and so several attempts were made to puncture the carotid artery through the intact skin. This method had some failures and complications. An easier and safer procedure was needed.

In 1947, a catheter method was used by Stig Radner, a Swedish radiologist from Lund [8]. After exposure of the radial artery a catheter was introduced in retrograde direction via the brachial, axillary, and subclavian arteries into the vertebral artery and contrast was injected through the catheter. Radner initially applied his technique in 142 instances in patients of all ages without untoward effects of the catheterization [7]. He then reported the results of vertebral artery angiography among over 200 patients [9]. In one patient a subclavian injection defined a tumor [10].

Despite research on catheter use by Radner and later Seldinger, cerebral angiography during the 1950s to early 1970s was performed mostly by neurosurgeons and some neurologists. Radiologists were accustomed to sitting in front of lit boxes to review X-ray films. They were not accustomed or trained to perform cut-downs or inject needles into the body. Arteriography was performed either by cut-down or by percutaneous injection using a syringe or insertion of a through-the-needle catheter [11]. Both methods had disadvantages: The cut-down method was time-consuming and the percutaneous technique required a large bore needle that produced a vascular hole. Perivascular bleeding was a risk.

During the late 1960s when one of the editors of this volume (LRC) was a stroke fellow, cerebral angiography was a risky endeavor. The unanesthetized patient lay on their back on a hard X-ray table. The patient's occiput was extended to allow maximal neck exposure. LRC would direct a large bore needle with a central cannula [12] through the neck until it hit bone, attempting to impale the carotid artery against the vertebral column. Then the needle was drawn back until red blood shot out, spurting toward the ceiling. A syringe with a needle and attached catheter was inserted into the cannula and contrast was hand-injected. LRC would then rush around the table to hand pull the X-ray films. If rapid circulation was predicted, films were pulled and exposed quickly, and if circulation was posited to be slow, then films were pulled more leisurely. Only an anteroposterior or lateral projection could be filmed at any one time, so that multiple injections were needed. Sometimes both carotid arteries or a vertebral artery was studied using the same injection technique. At times the technique resulted in dissection of the arterial wall, and brain infarction occasionally resulted.

Sven Ivar Seldinger was a young radiologist at the Karolinska Institute in Stockholm when he found a solution [13]. The main principle of his procedure consisted "in the catheter being introduced on a flexible leader through the puncture hole after withdrawal of the puncture needle" [14]. The major advantage of the Seldinger technique is that it allowed for the insertion of a catheter that was larger in diameter than the needle. At the time, Seldinger's chief at the department of radiology at the Karolinska Hospital did not think that the new technique that allowed accessing all the arteries in the human body was sufficient to form the basis for a thesis. Seldinger had to work on a different project, the development of percutaneous cholangiography.

Seldinger's technique is now used for nearly all endovascular work. Interventional radiology would not have been developed without this technique. Seldinger was chosen in 1992 to be the first recipient of the "Pioneer in Interventional Radiology Award" by the American Society of Cardiovascular and Interventional Radiology [13].

During the 1960s and 1970s, use of the Seldinger technique for cerebral angiography was instrumental in the development of a new radiology specialty, neuroradiology. Neuroradiologists gradually replaced neurologists and neurosurgeons in performing catheter angiography. Further expansion of the field came in the late 1970s and 1980s when brain imaging with CT and MRI became available.

One of the most important leaders in the development of neuroradiology and cerebral angiography was Juan Manuel Taveras. Taveras was born in Moca, in the Dominican Republic, in September 1919 [15]. His father was a schoolteacher. Taveras was an excellent student and often served as a tutor for other students. He was given music lessons, and as a teenager played clarinet in a dance band. As a medical student, he worked his way through school playing clarinet, saxophone, and flute in orchestras and jazz bands. He received MD degrees from the University of Santo Domingo in 1943 and from the University of Pennsylvania in 1949. After completing a radiology residency at the Graduate Hospital of the University of Pennsylvania, he joined the staff at the Columbia-Presbyterian Medical Center in New York and was appointed director of radiology at the Neurologic Institute of New York.

During his 13-year New York tenure he was able to change practice. All neuroradiologic procedures at the Neurologic Institute were performed and interpreted by neuroradiologists. He coauthored, with Ernest Wood, the first English-language textbook of neuroradiology, which included detailed sections on performance and interpretation of cerebral angiograms [16]. Angiography was the main diagnostic tool in detecting and localizing brain tumors and showing various mass effects. Arterial anatomy was also clarified as were common locations of vascular occlusions in the neck and head. The Taveras-Wood text became the standard textbook for a generation of American radiologists, neurologists, and neurosurgeons.

In 1965, Taveras was appointed professor and chairman of radiology and director of the Edward Mallinckrodt Institute of Radiology at Washington University School of Medicine in St. Louis. In 1971, Juan was appointed professor of radiology at Harvard Medical School and radiologist-in-chief at the Massachusetts General Hospital. During his 17-year tenure in Boston, he built a department with cutting-edge equipment and operational systems that attracted and trained future radiology and neuroradiology leaders. After formal retirement, Juan continued active practice in Boston and in Mexico City and Santo Domingo, traveling there almost monthly [15].

After its development in 1927, cerebral dye catheter angiography remained for 50 years the main diagnostic tool for detecting intracranial pathology until the introduction of brain CT scanning in 1975. During the 1960s until the early 1980s many vascular surgeons insisted on full opacification of the neck and intracranial vasculature, "an arch and 4." The high load of dye and the time taken for injections and catheterizations led to procedural complications, estimated at between 2 and 5 percent of procedures. Clinicians argued for a more eclectic approach, avoiding large arch injections and mainly studying the clinically involved artery and its branches, opacifying other vessels only when indicated [17].

Computers allowed modification of catheter-based cerebral angiography. Digital subtraction angiography (DSA), in which a pre-contrast image was acquired, then subtracted from subsequent post-contrast images, was made possible during the 1970s. During DSA examinations images were created in several planes using much less dye than in the past. Later, introducing the dye intravenously avoided the risk of arterial catheterization. During intravenous DSA examinations, a noncontrast (mask) image of the region was taken. Then images were taken in succession while contrast material was being injected. The mask image was then subtracted from the contrast images pixel by pixel. The resulting subtraction images showed only the filled vessels. The subtraction images could be viewed in real time.

When CT and later MRI became available, preliminary study of the brain-supplying circulation using either MRA or CTA greatly limited the need for catheter-based angiography. When indicated because of unclear results from these noninvasive studies, intravenous DSA could be performed.

By the turn of the century, arterial catheter angiography became mostly limited to dye injection into an artery by an interventionalist when a therapeutic intervention (e.g., stent placement, mechanical thrombus removal, or ablation of an aneurysm or vascular malformation) involving that artery was planned. Catheter angiography became more therapeutic than diagnostic [18].

NOTES AND REFERENCES

1. Sicard JA, Forestier J. Méthode radiographique d'exploration de la cavité épidurale par la lipiodol. *Rev. Neurol.* 1921;28:1264–1266.

2. Dandy WE. Ventriculography following injection of air into the cerebral ventricles. *Ann. Surg.* 1918;68:5–11. Walter Dandy and his career are discussed in Chapter 57 on brain aneurysm treatment.

3. Moniz E. *Confidências de um investigador científico*. Lisbon: Ática, 1948 (reprint 1999). Oliveira V. *Egas Moniz: The Legacy of His Life and Work*. Lisbon: By the Book, 2019.

4. Moniz E. *Trombosis y otras obstrucciones de las carotidas*. Barcelona: Salvat, 1941. Oliveira V. The history of carotid occlusions: The contribution of Egas Moniz. *J. Stroke Cerebrovasc. Dis.* 2018;27(12):3626–3629.

5. Moniz E. *Diagnostique des tumeurs cérébrales ses applications et épreuve de l'encephalographie artérielle*. Paris: Masson Éditeurs, 1931.

6. Moniz E. *l'angiographie cérébrale, ses applications et résultats en anatomie, physiologie et clinique*. Paris: Masson Éditeurs, 1934.

7. Moniz E. *Tentatives opératoires dans le traitement de certaines sychoses*. Paris: Masson Éditeurs, 1936.

8. Radner, S. Intracranial angiography via the vertebral artery: Preliminary report of a new technique. *Acta Radiol.* 1947;28(5–6):838–842.

9. Radner S. Vertebral angiography by catheterization: A new method employed in 221 cases. *Acta Radiol. Suppl.* 1951;87:1–134.

10. Radner, S. Subclavian angiography by arterial catheterization: Visualization of metastatic tumor in the upper thoracic aperture. *Acta Radiol.* 1949;32(5–6):359–364.

11. Bull JW. A review of cerebral angiography. *Proc. R. Soc. Med.* 1949;42(11):880–890.

12. The needle and the technique for its use was introduced by Paul New at Massachusetts General Hospital. New PF, Baker E. Technique of arterial puncture: A new needle-cannula for arteriography. *J. Neurosurg.* 1963;20:390–396.

13. Doby T. A tribute to Sven-Ivar Seldinger. *AJR* 1984;142:1–4.

14. Seldinger SI. Catheter replacement of the needle in percutaneous arteriography: A new technique. *Acta Radiol.* 1953;39:368–376. Sternbach G. Sven Ivar Seldinger: Catheter introduction on a flexible leader. *J. Emerg. Med.* 1990;8(5):635–637.

15. Huckman MS. In memoriam Juan Manuel Taveras (1919–2002). *Am. J. Neuroradiol.* 2002;23:1065–1068.

16. Taveras JM, Wood EH. *Diagnostic Neuroradiology*. Baltimore, MD: Williams & Wilkins, 1964.

17. Caplan LR, Wolpert S. Conventional cerebral angiography in occlusive cerebrovascular disease. In Wood JH (ed.), *Cerebral Blood Flow: Physiologic and Clinical Aspects*. New York: McGraw-Hill, 1987, pp. 356–384.

18. Therapeutic aspects of angiography are discussed in Chapters 55 (angioplasty and stenting), 56 (clot removal), 57 (aneurysms), and 59 (AVMs).

CHAPTER THIRTY TWO

COMPUTED TOMOGRAPHY

QUEST FOR A WAY TO SAFELY IMAGE THE BRAIN USING X-RAYS

In December 1895, German physicist Wilhelm Conrad Roentgen announced that a form of radiation that he dubbed X-rays could penetrate solid substances and produce an outline of their interior contents. The use of X-rays became widespread and greatly improved physician's diagnostic capabilities; doctors could look at broken bones, lungs, the heart, or the intestines. However, X-rays were very limited in showing the brain. The skull was radio dense and the fluid surrounding the brain made it appear as a homogenous density without any structural details [1]. The first X-ray image of the brain reported at the end of the nineteenth century was fraudulent. It was an image of a cat's intestine filled with a mercuric compound, radiographed in a brain-shaped pan. The famous American inventor Thomas Edison attempted to image the brain. His fame was such that reporters and the general public waited outside his laboratory for two weeks in anticipation of the good news. His efforts were unrewarding [2].

Walter Dandy, a trainee of Harvey Cushing, began experimenting during the early years of the twentieth century with ways to see the brain and its cerebrospinal fluid contents. Cerebrospinal fluid in the ventricles and subarachnoid space was replaced with air injected either directly into the ventricles (ventriculography) or into the lumbar subarachnoid space (pneumoencephalography). Ventriculography and pneumoencephalography allowed neurologists and neurosurgeons for the first time to visualize brain lesions, especially tumors, using X-rays [3,4]. The air injection into the lumbar spinal fluid produced severe headache, nausea, and often vomiting. Patients were turned and twisted, often using a special chair in order to induce the air to go into the various ventricles and into the fluid around the brain [5]. This technique showed the cerebral ventricles and displacement of the brain but did not show the internal aspects of the brain.

During the second quarter of the twentieth century, clinicians and researchers tried to see the brain better by opacifying the arteries and veins that supplied and drained the brain of blood. Egaz Moniz, a neurosurgeon in Lisbon, introduced contrast directly into arteries of the neck, mostly with the intent of diagnosing brain tumors [6]. He was surprised that some injections showed that a carotid artery was occluded in the neck. Moniz used a cutdown over the artery in the neck to introduce dye contrast. This technique was replaced during the middle years of the twentieth century by direct puncture of the carotid and vertebral arteries using specialized needles. Anteroposterior and lateral view images were produced by hand-pulling of the films after injecting dye. During the 1960s and 1970s, direct injections were superseded by introducing contrast through catheters placed in the femoral and brachial arteries, the so-called Seldinger technique [7]. Ultimately, newer filming techniques allowed digital contrast angiography using smaller amounts of dye. Angiography was capable of showing vascular abnormalities (aneurysms, vascular malformations, and obstructions, irregularities, and stenoses) but could not show the internal contents of the brain.

THE ORIGINS OF CT SCANNING OF THE BRAIN AND SKULL

In 1979, the Nobel Prize in Physiology or Medicine was jointly awarded to Allan M. Cormack and Godfrey N. Hounsfield; neither was a physician. Both conducted independent research and were unaware of each other's work. The Nobel committee noted: "Ordinary X-ray examinations of the head had shown the skull bones, but the brain had remained a gray, undifferentiated fog. Now, suddenly, the fog had cleared" [1].

Allan M. Cormack was a nuclear physicist at the University of Cape Town. When the hospital physicist resigned, he was asked to supervise radioactive isotope doses used for cancer therapy at the Groote Schuur Hospital. He realized that the method used to calculate dosing was imprecise and was developed assuming that the body was a homogenous medium. His primary aim was to calculate the radiation attenuation coefficients of different parts of the body. He recognized that determining the tissue-density distribution in the body was highly mathematical. He formulated equations, conducted various experiments, and managed to reconstruct an accurate cross-section of an irregularly shaped object. He reported his findings in two articles published in 1963 and 1964. Using a simple desktop calculator as the "computer," he produced the first computerized tomograms ever made. He was aware of the potential of his method to produce X-ray or positron camera images of cross-sectional slices of the body. Computers of his time were not capable of executing the enormous calculations the procedure required, so that he did not use or construct any apparatus of practical diagnostic importance [8,9].

In 1962, the Beatles singing group signed with Electric & Music Industries (EMI). The band was a worldwide success and the company earned many millions of dollars, so much that they didn't know what to do with the money earned. One of the scientists working with the company was Godfrey Hounsfield, who led the team that built the first all-transistor computer in 1958. The company gave Hounsfield freedom to conduct his independent research and funded it with the profits made by the Beatles. The Beatles, the most successful band in history, indirectly contributed to the development of CT scanning [9].

Hounsfield's idea was to take multiple radiographic images around an object and to reconstruct it using a computerized technique. The first prototype of the machine made by Hounsfield used a gamma-ray radiation source because he could not afford an X-ray source. The radiation source was placed in a lead box with a pinhole through which a single beam of radiation was projected onto the object and recorded on a detector on the opposite side placed on a lathe bed. The radiation beam was moved across the entire object. The disk under the object was then rotated by one degree and the beam was passed again. This process was repeated until a rotation of 180 degrees was achieved. Hounsfield took approximately 28,000 measurements, digitized them, and recorded them on paper tape. The gamma source used was very slow and the machine had to operate continuously for nine days to obtain the image. The computer itself took two and a half hours to process the data and produce the image. Hounsfield later shifted to an X-ray tube, which yielded more detailed images in shorter time. The process now took about nine hours and the picture was that of an animal brain, showing gray and white matter. He realized that formalin used to preserve the specimen enhanced the image and produced exaggerated results. He then imaged fresh bullocks' brains, but the ventricles of those brains were filled with blood due to the method used for killing them and did not produce satisfactory images. He then traveled to Jewish kosher slaughtering houses where the animals were killed by bleeding and so the brains had little blood. He carried the brains across London [2,8,10,11]. After obtaining satisfactory results using animal brains, Hounsfield built an improved prototype for clinical use.

Concurrently, William Oldendorf, a clinical and research neurologist practicing at the University of California at Los Angeles also strove to invent an apparatus that could scan a head using transmitted X-ray beams and then reconstruct a radiographic cross-section that would delineate the distribution of tissue structures based on regional radio density. Oldendorf developed a model using domestic materials that ranged from a frying pan to his son's discarded train set. In 1961, he published his first paper on the project and after two years obtained a patent on his projected device [12]. In the prototypic scanner that he sketched, a gamma-ray source and detector were placed opposite to each other with a simulated head in the middle. The source and detector arrangement could revolve 360 degrees around the head. A capacitance circuit was used to imitate these internal points. Having isolated one such internal point or a discrete region of the simulated head, other regions could be successively observed by providing a relative linear movement between the simulated head and the axis of rotation. This process would yield a line through the simulated head. When many such lines parallel to each other were produced, the entire interior of the head could be effectively studied. Although Oldendorf's concept was revolutionary, he was told that such a machine had a probable cost of $250,000. X-ray manufacturers were unwilling to risk the capital and denied his request for backing. He never was able to bring his scanner into practice. Due to his work on the scanner concept he was awarded the Lasker Prize in 1975. Sadly, his efforts were overlooked by the Nobel Prize committee and he was not recognized as the third contributor to the invention of CT scanning along with Cormack and Hounsfield.

The first CT scanner (the EMI Mark I) was installed at the Atkinson Morley Hospital in Wimbledon under the direction of James Ambrose, a neuroradiologist [13]. The first CT scans were known as EMI scans based on the company that made the scanner. CT stood for computed (computerized) tomography (*tomos*, slices; *graphy*, write). The apparatus was designed to image the brain and had a small opening just for the head. The first tomographic examination took place on October 1, 1971, in a 41-year-old woman with a suspected brain tumor. A cystic lesion in the frontal lobe was easily distinguished, for it was much darker than the surrounding healthy tissue. The scan took about four and a half minutes and the image was reconstructed in about 20 seconds [13]. Hounsfield presented his results at a seminar at the British Institute of Radiology on April 1972 and published his findings in various journals, including the *British Journal of Radiology* [14]. The company EMI could not keep up with mass production of CT scanners. Other technology giants began making CT scanners [11].

Hounsfield continued to work on modifying scanners. Faster scanning systems led to the development of complete body scanners that could image constantly moving organs like the heart and the brain. The first full body scan was of Hounsfield himself. Hounsfield was appointed Commander of the Order of the British Empire in 1976 and was knighted in 1981. The Hounsfield scale is used as a measurement tool for radiodensity. Hounsfield also made contributions in the development of magnetic resonance imaging (MRI) [11].

The first EMI scanner in North America was installed at the Mayo Clinic in 1973, and the second scanner was in operation at Massachusetts General Hospital (MGH) in Boston in July 1973. During less than a full year, 750 patients were scanned at MGH. The findings on the CT scanner corelated well with the pathology findings in 10 patients who were scanned [15]. The first scans were difficult to read and the results sometimes misleading. The publications from MGH used the designation computerized axial tomography, accounting for the term "CAT" scanning; later, CT was the term adopted.

THE EVOLUTION OF CT BRAIN SCANNING

The first-generation scanners consisted of a single radiation beam and a single detector that had a translation motion across the object followed by rotation by a degree and another translation motion until 180 degrees was scanned. The pictures were often grainy, and small lesions were easy to miss. The second-generation scanners used multiple detectors and a fan beam instead of a single beam. The third generation had a row of fixed multiple detectors forming a complete circle that remained stationary while the beam moved. This was followed by the helical scanner that could rotate 360 degrees (the earlier models could rotate only 180 degrees as the wires in the circuit would entangle otherwise). As the scanner completed one rotation, the patient was moved through it, giving a resultant helical motion. Modern scanners function at a tremendous speed; the entire body was scanned in less than a minute. The more advanced scanners produce images with better lesion definition.

By the mid-1980s, most hospitals in the United States and Europe had CT scanners. These were in general use in evaluating patients with head trauma and individuals suspected of having a stroke or harboring a brain tumor or subdural hematoma. Their use in patients with acute strokes was mostly to exclude hemorrhages, tumors and, non-stroke lesions [16]. An intracerebral hemorrhage could easily be distinguished from a brain infarct, and the location and size of the bleed was shown as well as displacement of normal brain structures.

During the 1990s, a non-contrast CT scan was part of the required protocol for evaluating patients in the National Institute of Neurological Diseases and Stroke (NINDS) trial in the United States and the European Cooperative Acute Stroke (ECASS) Trials, which assessed the effectiveness and safety of intravenous thrombolysis. After publication of these trials, guidelines incorporated the need for performing and interpreting an acute non-contrast CT scan as quickly as possible after the patient presented to the hospital. Well-delineated brain infarcts were seldom found within the first three to five hours after symptom onset. Early scans could show thrombi or slowed flow within intracranial arteries as hyperdense artery signs. Subtle early signs of brain ischemia were sometimes evident. Scans could exclude intracerebral hemorrhage and important non-stroke lesions. Aneurysmal subarachnoid hemorrhages were identified.

When MRI scanning became more widely available during the late 1980s and 1990s, it became evident that acute ischemic lesions could be identified earlier and more precisely using MRI rather than CT (Chapter 27). During these same years, vascular imaging using MR angiography or CT angiography became widely used to identify the presence, location, and extent of occluded neck and intracranial arteries. Since the effectiveness of intravenous and intraarterial treatments to open arteries depended heavily on the details of the causative vascular process and its anatomy, stroke clinicians urged that vascular and brain imaging should be performed acutely and together to guide treatment. Acute multimodal MRI and CT protocols were designed to evaluate patients presenting with acute brain ischemia. Since CT scanners were often located near emergency rooms and were much more accessible for acute scanning and were less costly, most hospitals opted for CT protocols rather than MRI. MRI testing took longer and was not as readily accessible in many medical centers.

Doctors evaluating patients in the NINDS trial had devised and published a score for quantifying neurological deficits, the NINDS score. This score quickly became integrated into common use as a way of quantifying and comparing the severity of neurological deficits between medical centers and before and after treatments. It became important to similarly quantify abnormalities on brain scanning. The Calgary stroke group in Alberta, Canada, devised a system for quantifying and rating ischemia on acute CT scans. Led by Alastair Buchan, Michael Hill, Andrew Demchuk, and Phillip Barber, they dubbed the system the Alberta Stroke Program Early CT Score (ASPECTS) [17]. Soon most CT stroke protocols suggested including measurement of the ASPECTS and NINDS scores in each patient studied.

CT ANGIOGRAPHY AND VENOGRAPHY AND MULTIMODAL CT

During the past quarter of a century, helical multiple row detectors replaced early generation CT scanners. These helical (spiral) scanners could scan larger volumes of tissue than early scanners in shorter times. The introduction of 64 detector row helical CT scanners further shortened examination times and reduced the volume of intravenous non-ionic contrast material needed to study contrast traveling through vascular beds. Volumetric data acquisition and better computerized image manipulation improved CT angiographic image displays into three-dimensional reformations. Images of the arteries in the neck and intracranial arteries were produced that closely approximated the images obtained from digital subtraction cerebral angiography. The veins that drained blood from the brain could also be imaged well. The shortened time of the exam reduced potential radiation exposure.

Max Wintermark, a neuroradiologist originally educated in Switzerland, and his Stanford University colleagues were among investigators who developed and evaluated the use of CT angiography in patients suspected of having cerebrovascular disease and strokes. He and his colleagues were active in studying the technical aspects of producing high-quality CT angiograms. They also created images of cerebral perfusion (perfusion computed tomography (PCT)) by generating maps of cerebral blood flow (CBF), cerebral blood volume (CBV), and mean transit time (MTT). The technical aspects of these measurements had been developed first using MRI. Wintermark and colleagues developed automated, color-coded images that aided clinicians in visualizing brain regions of reduced blood flow [18]. Michael Lev and his colleagues at MGH in Boston were also among the first to describe the utility of computed tomography angiography (CTA) and multimodal imaging in the evaluation of patients with brain ischemia [19].

As experience was gained in attaining reperfusion in patients with intracranial vascular occlusions, it became clear that timing was crucial. The earlier treatment was delivered, the better the chance of reperfusion and saving threatened and ischemic brain from infarction. Complete and thorough evaluation of the brain, heart, blood, and supplying vessels took precious time. The race was on to develop very rapid evaluation using CT scanners that would prove adequate for practical decisions on treatment. Neurologists and neuroradiologists at Samsung Medical Center in Seoul, Korea, developed a procedure they called "triphasic perfusion computed tomography" [20]. A plain CT of the head that was optimal to show the middle cerebral arteries was chosen. Contrast was infused and images were created sequentially at three designated times: a very early phase showing the main intracranial anterior circulation arteries, a middle phase, and a late phase. The earliest phase showed whether there was an intracranial occlusion and where it was located. The latter two phases showed images of branching and collateral flow. This information was enough to guide decisions on reperfusion.

The Neurology and Neuroradiology Group in Calgary, Alberta, more than a decade later, used advanced technology to build on the concept introduced in Korea. A non-contrast CT scan was adequate to calculate an ASPECT score. Then a calculated infusion of contrast followed by saline was injected and images from the skull base to the vertex were created in three phases after contrast material injection: during the peak arterial phase, the equilibrium/peak venous phase, and the late venous phase. Later, a subsequent injection was performed and blood flow, blood volume, and blood transit data was used to produce cerebral perfusion maps. This data was very helpful in guiding acute reperfusion decisions [21].

By the end of the first quarter of the twenty-first century, acute CT-based protocols (CT and CTA) or, in advanced centers, CT, CTA, and CT perfusion had replaced MRI-based protocols for evaluation of patients suspected of having acute strokes. CTA evaluation of the aorta [22] and of the coronary arteries and heart [23] was also important in evaluating patients with cardio-vascular disease.

NOTES AND REFERENCES

1. The Nobel Prize in Physiology or Medicine 1979. NobelPrize.org. Available at www .nobelprize.org/prizes/medicine/1979/ceremony-speech.

2. Doctor Klioze. History of computerized tomography (CT scanner). Available at www .youtube.com/watch?v=9SUHgtREWQc.

3. Dandy WE. Ventriculography following injection of air into the cerebral ventricles. *Annals of Surgery* 1918;68:5–11.

4. Dandy WE. Roentgenography of the brain after the injection of air into the spinal canal. *Annals of Surgery* 1919;70:397–403.

5. Robertson EG. Some physical aspects of encephalography. *Brain* 1947;70:59–74. Robertson EG. *Pneumoencephalography*. Oxford: Blackwell, 1957.

6. Moniz E. L'encephalographie arterielle, son importance dans la localisation des tumeurs cerebrales. *Revue Neurologique (Paris)* 1927;2:72–89. Moniz E. *L'angiographie cérébrale, ses applications et résultats en anatomic, physiologie et clinique* (Cerebral angiography, its applications and results in anatomy, physiology, and clinic). Paris, 1934.

7. Seldinger SI. Catheter replacement of the needle in percutaneous arteriography: A new technique. *Acta Radiologica* 1953;39(5):368–376.

8. The Scanner Story (part 1 of 2 of documentary covering early CT development). YouTube. Available at www.youtube.com/watch?v=u_R47LDdlZM.

9. Allan M. Cormack, Nobel Lecture: Early Two-Dimensional Reconstruction and Recent Topics Stemming from It. NobelPrize.org. Available at www.nobelprize .org/prizes/medicine/1979/cormack/lecture/.

10. Goodman LR. The Beatles, the Nobel Prize, and CT scanning of the chest. *Radiology Clinics of North America* 2010;48:1–7.

11. Godfrey N. Hounsfield, Nobel lecture: Computed medical imaging. NobelPrize.org. Available at www.nobelprize.org/prizes/medicine/1979/hounsfield/lecture.

12. Mishra SK, Singh P. History of neuroimaging: The legacy of William Oldendorf. *Journal of Child Neurology* 2010;25:508–517. Oldendorf WH. Isolated flying spot detection of radiodensity discontinuities: Displaying the internal structural patterns of a complex object. *IRE Transactions Biomedical and Electronic* 1961;8:68–72. Oldendorf WH, inventor. Radiation energy apparatus for investigating selected areas of the interior of objects obscured by dense material. US patent 3106640. October 8, 1963.

13. Ambrose J. Computerized transverse axial scanning (tomography). 2. Clinical application. *British Journal of Radiology* 1973;46:1023–1047.

14. Hounsfield GN. Computerized transverse axial scanning (tomography): Part I. Description of system. *British Journal of Radiology* 1973;46:1016–1022.

15. New PFJ, Scott WR, Schnur JA, Davis KR, Taveras JM. Computerized axial tomography with the EMI scanner. *Radiology* 1974;110:109–123. Kistler JP, Hochberg FH, Brooks BR, Richardson EP, New PJ, Schnur J. Computerized axial tomography: Clinicopathologic correlation. *Neurology* 1975;25:201–209.

16. Caplan LR. Computed tomography and stroke. In McDowell FH, Caplan LR (eds.), *Cerebrovascular Survey Report to the National Institute of Neurological and Communicative Disorders and Stroke (NINCDS)*. Revised 1985, pp. 61–74.

17. Barber PA, Demchuk AM, Zhang J, Buchan AM. Validity and reliability of a quantitative computed tomography score in predicting outcome of hyperacute stroke before thrombolytic therapy. ASPECTS Study Group. Alberta Stroke Programme Early CT Score. *Lancet* 2000;355:1670–1674. Pexman JHW, Barber PA, Hill MD, Sevick RJ, Demchuk AM, Hudon ME, et al. Use of the Alberta Stroke Program Early CT Score (ASPECTS) for assessing CT scans in patients with acute stroke. *American Journal of Neuroradiology* 2001;22:1534–1542. Hill MD, Demchuck AM, Tomsick T, Palesch YY, Broderick JP. Using the baseline CT scan to select acute stroke patients for IV-IA therapy. *AJNR American Journal of Neuroradiology* 2006;27:1612–1616.

18. Tong E, Wintermark M. CTA-enhanced perfusion CT: An original method to perform ultra-low-dose CTA-enhanced perfusion CT. *Neuroradiology* 2014;56 (11):955–964. Wintermark M, Sincic R, Sridhar D, Chien JD. Cerebral perfusion CT: Technique and clinical applications. *Journal of Neuroradiology* 2008;35(5):253–260. Leiva-Salinas C, Jiang B, Wintermark M. Computed tomography, computed tomography angiography, and perfusion computed tomography evaluation of acute ischemic stroke. *Neuroimaging Clinics of North America* 2018;28(4):565–572.

19. Lev MH, Nichols SJ. Computed tomographic angiography and computed tomographic perfusion imaging of hyperacute stroke. *Topics in Magnetic Resonance Imaging* 2000;11(5):273–287. Delgado Almandoz JE, Romero JM, Pomerantz SR, Lev MH. Computed tomography angiography of the carotid and cerebral circulation. *Radiologic Clinics of North America* 2010;48(2):265–281.

20. Lee KH, Cho S-J, Byun HS, et al. Triphasic perfusion computed tomography in acute middle cerebral artery stroke: A correlation with angiographic findings. *Archives of Neurology* 2000;57:990–999. Lee KH, Lee SJ, Cho SJ, et al. Usefulness of triphasic perfusion computed tomography for intravenous thrombolysis with tissue-type plasminogen activator in acute ischemic stroke. *Archives of Neurology* 2000;57:1000–1008.

21. Menon BK, Campbell BC, Levi C, et al. Role of imaging in current acute ischemic stroke workflow for endovascular therapy. *Stroke* 2015;46:1453–1461. Menon BK, d'Esterre CD, Qazi EM, et al. Multiphase CT angiography: A new tool for the imaging triage of patients with acute ischemic stroke. *Radiology* 2015;275:510–520.

22. . Chatzikonstantinou A, Krissak R, Flüchter S, Artemis D, Schaefer A, Schoenberg SO, Hennerici MG, Fink C. CT angiography of the aorta is superior to transesophageal echocardiography for determining stroke subtypes in patients with cryptogenic ischemic stroke. *Cerebrovascular Diseases* 2012;33:322–328.

23. Rubin GD, Leipsic J, Joseph Schoepf U, Fleischmann D, Napel S. CT angiography after 20 years: A transformation in cardiovascular disease characterization continues to advance. *Radiology* 2014;271(3):633–652.

CHAPTER THIRTY THREE

MAGNETIC RESONANCE IMAGING

The story of the development of magnetic resonance as an imaging device applicable for human diagnosis is colorful and exemplifies the triumphs, errors, and luck often involved in great discoveries. The story of the awarding of the Nobel Prize for the development of MR is fascinating.

EARLY DISCOVERIES AND EXPLORATIONS

In 1937, Columbia University professor Isidor I. Rabi discovered a phenomenon that he dubbed nuclear magnetic resonance (NMR). Rabi recognized that atomic nuclei show their presence by absorbing or emitting radio waves when exposed to a strong magnetic field. Felix Bloch and Edward Purcell received the 1952 Nobel Prize for Physics for showing that atomic nuclei in a magnetic field absorb and reemit electromagnetic radiation.

Nuclear magnetic resonance was first used to determine the structure of chemical compounds. Raymond Damadian, a physician, believed that while a medical practitioner can impact thousands of lives, a researcher impacts millions. He did his undergraduate studies in chemistry and graduated from Albert Einstein Medical School. His internship and residency in internal medicine were at Downstate Medical Center in Brooklyn. He was fascinated by how the kidney maintained the proper electrical state of the body by balancing the electrically active ions sodium and potassium. After his residency he worked as a postdoctoral fellow in nephrology [1].

He was approached by Freeman Winder Cope of Pennsylvania to collaborate with him in order to study how potassium ions accumulated in the cells of the body using NMR technology for chemical analysis. Damadian obtained a bacterium from the Dead Sea, called *Halobacter halobium*, which contained about 20 times more potassium than found in normal cells. Cope put the bacteria in a test tube, wrapped an antenna around the test tube, and put it in the NMR machine. He measured the exact amount of K^+ ions in that cell of the bacterium within seconds using NMR. This fascinated Damadian, for the conventional chemistry methods of analysis would have taken him days to achieve the same result. Damadian considered using NMR to detect differences between normal and cancerous tissues [1].

During the late 1970s, nuclear magnetic resonance was renamed magnetic resonance (MR) because of the negative connotations that "nuclear" invited, and has been referred to as simply MR during the last 25 years. The "I" (for "imaging") was added by the medical community to identify MR as an imaging technology [1]. Magnetic resonance is a technology widely used by chemists to study the properties of different atoms and molecules. It is basically like chatting with the nuclei of the atoms: You send them a "hey" and they reply back with a "hi." In proton MR we chat with the hydrogen atoms, which combine with other atoms such as oxygen and carbon to form water (60% of our body is water) or fat. A hydrogen atom is like a tiny magnet itself as its nucleus consists of a proton (positively charged) surrounded by an electron (negatively charged). As the proton spins around its axis it produces a magnetic field. Since different atoms produce this field in different directions, the net effect is zero. If you place these atoms in an external magnetic field, they align themselves parallel to the direction of the field, analogous to asking a group of students to line up. After this alignment is achieved, the "hey" signal or a radiofrequency pulse is applied, which causes some nuclei to turn by 90 degrees and some by 180 degrees, just like asking some students to face left or right. After the radiofrequency pulse is stopped, just like a group of unattended students, the atoms begin to realign themselves in their original lower energy state, parallel to the magnetic field. As they return to their original positions, they emit energy that is received as the "hi" signal. Since the hydrogen atoms in different molecules have different degrees of freedom (freer in a water molecule as compared to a complex molecule like fat), they emit different measured signals. Different body organs have different amounts of water and fat; similarly, there is a difference in the water content between the normal and cancerous tissues.

After working with bacteria, Damadian acquired rats bearing Walker sarcoma tumors. He excised the tumor, put the sample in an MR machine, and compared the MR signals with that of normal tissues. The differences were dramatic. He confirmed his finding by experimenting on rats containing other tumors and published a paper entitled "Tumour Detection by Nuclear Magnetic Resonance" in the March 19, 1971, journal *Science*. The challenge for him was to convert the test tube–sized MR scanner into a full-sized human scanner [1].

Paul Lauterbur held a PhD in magnetic resonance and was the cofounder of the company NMR Specialties, in New Kensington, Pennsylvania. NMR Specialties devised equipment for potential customers. On September 2, 1971, Leon Saryan, a postdoctoral fellow at Johns Hopkins, went to NMR Specialties to confirm the findings of Raymond Damadian's *Science* paper. Lauterbur observed Saryan's experiment and saw the differences between the signals of normal and malignant tissue. Saryan brought samples from rats and Lauterbur saw the significance in the measurements and thought of devising a method to noninvasively measure the signals from tissues of the human body [2].

The same evening an idea occurred to him and he sketched it on a paper napkin. He wanted to create images from MR signals. He thought of using a gradient magnetic field instead of a constant magnetic field. Because the frequencies of MR signals depended on the local magnetic field, there might be a way to locate them in a nonuniform magnetic field. He thought of creating two-dimensional pictures through this method and then stacking them to create a three-dimensional image. Paul named his technique "zeugmatography," from the Greek word *zeugma*, "that which is used for joining" [2].

Although both Lauterbur and Damadian were in contact with each other, they did not collaborate to build the first MRI scanner. Sadly, a bitter rivalry ensued between them.

Lauterbur conducted experiments on test tubes containing water and, using his gradient field approach, obtained pictures. He submitted a manuscript containing these pictures to the journal *Nature* but was rejected. He then appealed to the journal by highlighting the medical applications of the technique and its importance in detection of cancers. His paper was subsequently accepted and published in 1973 [3]. He did not cite Damadian's experiments [1]. Lauterbur obtained an image of a clam that his daughter had collected at the beach. The clam was big enough to be imaged and small enough to fit in the 4 millimeters of available space. This was the first MRI image of a live organism [4]. He later obtained an image of the thorax of a mouse [2].

To proceed further with his experiments, he needed a human-sized magnet. He finally acquired funds from the National Cancer Institute, a part of the National Institutes of Health, and asked for a 60-centimeter magnet (28-inch bore), but instead got a 45-centimeter (18-inch) magnet. The coils used to transmit and receive MR signals had to be improved. So, the coils were enlarged, leaving only 42 centimeters (16 inches) of available space, which would not accommodate any human being [2]. Nevertheless, he developed important methods and techniques to improve MRI imaging. Today, the MRI machines use gradient fields along the x, y, and z axes in order to obtain images in different planes [2].

FIRST HUMAN MR SCANS

Peter Mansfield was a physicist who worked at the University of Nottingham, England. Mansfield used MR gradients to study the structures of solids. After he presented a paper at a conference in Krakow in 1973, he was questioned by John Waugh, who asked if he was aware of similar work that had been published by Lauterbur a month earlier in *Nature*. Mansfield was unaware of Lauterbur's work. Intrigued, he searched the library for Lauterbur's paper upon his return to Nottingham. He noted a large contrast between their approaches. It might be easier to use his multiple pulse technique on liquids than on solids [5]. Point-by-point imaging would be very slow. Imaging speed would be a major concern for medical imaging. He thought of "line scanning," in which a whole line of data is obtained in a one-shot experiment. Line scanning could be modified further to obtain an entire plane at a time [5].

There were also size limitations. The only human object that could fit within the diameter of 1.5 centimeters was a finger. His and his students' fingers were too large; he found a person with thin fingers and several images of his fingers were obtained. This first human MR scan was performed in 1976 [5].

Meanwhile, Raymond Damadian set out to build a MR machine that could scan the human body. His team tried to build a magnet large enough to accommodate a human. To build the magnet, he needed superconducting coils measuring around 30 miles, which would cost around $150,000. He had about $15,000 available. He called his friend Steve Lane, who told him that Westinghouse was stopping production of superconducting magnets. He had some 30 miles of superconducting wires that he could give him for $15,000. Precisely the length he needed, for the amount he had! Damadian and colleagues built their MR scanner and named it "Indomitable" [1].

Damadian entered the Indomitable on June 24, 1977. His goal was to stay in the machine for about 30 minutes. He entered the machine with a blood pressure cuff on his arm, an EKG machine attached to his chest, and a cardiologist standing by his side in case of an emergency. They tried for hours but could not receive any signal [1]. Perhaps they did not receive a signal because Damadian was "too fat" for the coil and was loading it down. A thinner colleague, after observing Damadian for any ill-effects from being in the machine, entered the machine on July 2, 1977 [1]. He was in the machine for hours, finishing at 4:45 am. The scan of his torso produced

106 picture elements (pixels) in about five hours (today an MRI generates 65,000 pixels in minutes). A thinner individual who was scanned was moved inch by inch, while another colleague simultaneously drew an image on the graph paper from the signal they were receiving. They named the scan "Mink 5" after test subject Larry Minkoff; it was an image of the heart, lungs, aorta, heart, and chest wall at the thoracic level of T8 [1].

Around this time, Paul Lauterbur reported his setback with his inadequately sized magnet [1]. Raymond Damadian eventually worked on reducing the scan time and built a company named FONAR for the commercial production of MR machines [1].

Peter Mansfield's magnet arrived on the last working day before Christmas in 1977. It came in the late afternoon, during a Christmas party. Mansfield unloaded it with two students whom he managed to drag out of the party and assembled it the next day [5]. After the entire machine was set up and adjustments made, Mansfield volunteered to be scanned. He climbed into the machine and asked his teammates Peter Morris and Ian Pykett to operate it when he called out. The door of the machine was closed; it was very dark for they didn't have time to install a light inside. The wiring of the electric bulb would have interfered with the signals of the machine. Mansfield was shut in the magnet in complete darkness with his face between two large coils. He couldn't touch the coils as they would get really hot after about 10 minutes. His wife and Morris's fiancée were waiting outside, ready to pull him out in case of an emergency [5]. A week before his scan, Mansfield had received a note from Tom Budinger, a medical scientist working at the University of California, San Francisco, who had made a calculation that suggested that the gradient strength that Mansfield was planning to use for his abdominal image was dangerous as it could trigger cardiac fibrillation. But Mansfield did not accept Tom's result: He had done his own calculations, which he trusted, and proceeded with the scan [5].

After he had positioned himself in the magnet, he signaled Peter to send the first pulse. There was a loud click from within the magnet, but he felt nothing, so he signaled to carry on the scan. After about 50 minutes in the sweltering heat, he got out, sweating profusely, but the scan went well. This was the first scan of the human abdomen (Damadian's scan was of the chest region) [5]. The scan was performed the night before they were due to fly to Blacksburg, Virginia, to attend the Experimental MR Conference meeting held in April 1978. They took pictures of their results and carried the roll of film to the United States. Mansfield had the film developed at a photographic shop close to the conference center, just in time to present his findings at the conference [5]. Mansfield, like the other two, committed his life to further develop MRI scanning. He founded a company named General Magnetic and worked on reducing the acoustic noise during the MRI procedure.

THE NOBEL PRIZE

A physicist, a chemist, and a medical doctor pioneered the field of magnetic resonance imaging. There were many more individuals who deserve credit for this magnificent discovery. The 2003 Noble Prize for Physiology or Medicine was jointly awarded to Paul Lauterbur and Peter Mansfield [6]. Alfred Nobel's will states that the prize can be jointly awarded to three persons and that the physiology prize should be awarded for the most important "discovery," while that in physics and chemistry should be given for important "methods." Raymond Damadian discovered differences between abnormal and normal tissues, while the other two developed methods for obtaining images. Why was Damadian excluded from the prize [1,7]? Some believe that the exclusion was related to his differences with Lauterbur and his firm belief in creation science as opposed to evolution [1,8]. The deliberations of the Nobel Prize committee are kept secret for 50 years. We won't know until 2053 the reasons that led to this decision [7].

Damadian became furious at his exclusion and bought full-page advertisements in the *Washington Post*, the *New York Times*, and the *Los Angeles Times* to protest the decision. He mounted a letter-writing campaign directed at Stockholm aimed at correcting what he called "this shameful wrong." Lauterbur and Mansfield remained silent on the issue [8].

Disputes arose in the past over the Nobel Prize committee's decisions. The decision to award Egas Moniz the Nobel Prize for "prefrontal leukotomy" was highly condemned. Similarly, Paul Herman Müller was awarded the prize for his discovery of DDT, the pesticide that killed insects that spread typhus and malaria and seemed instrumental in saving millions of lives. Later it was realized that DDT took a terrible toll on birds, fish, and other wildlife [8].

In 1923, Fredrick G. Banting and John J. R. Macleod received the Nobel Prize for the discovery of insulin. Macleod, who was the department head at the University of Toronto where the work was done, was not even on the campus when the experiments were conducted. It was Banting and a medical student, Best, in collaboration with biochemist James B. Collip, who actually discovered insulin. Banting strongly felt about Best's contribution and shared half of his Nobel winnings with him. Inspired by Banting, Macleod split his award money with Collip [8].

Damadian's contributions were acknowledged through various other awards. He was awarded the nation's highest honor in technology, the United States Medal of Technology, by President Ronald Reagan. His name was included in the National Inventors Hall of Fame. The Indomitable was put on display at the Smithsonian Institute in Washington [1].

INTRODUCTION OF MRI INTO CLINICAL MEDICINE

During the 1970s, the preliminary research made it crystal clear that MRI had the potential to provide images and information that could be very useful in treating patients with neurological conditions. An MRI image is a computerized map or image of radio signals emitted by the human body. This new modality had the ability to create three-dimensional images so that axial, coronal, and sagittal images could be displayed. This was not available with CT scanning. MRI was potentially safer than CT because CT scan used ionizing radiation while MRI used harmless radio waves. But the powerful magnetic fields used during MRI imaging could change the position of metallic implants, which could be problematic in individuals with metallic brain, heart, and other implants.

During the 1970s a team led by John Mallord, a professor of physics at the University of Aberdeen in the United Kingdom, built the first full-body MRI scanner. On August 28, 1980, this machine was used to obtain the first clinically useful MRI image of a patient's internal tissues. Shown were a primary chest tumor, an abnormal liver, and secondary cancer in the patient's bones [9]. This machine was later used at St. Bartholomew's Hospital in London.

Once it became clear that MRI had clinical and commercial potential, device makers went into rapid action mode to produce clinically useful, safe MRI scanners. The early period of MRI was dominated by the "field-strength war." What was the best field strength for MRI [9]? The strength of the MRI magnetic field was denoted in tesla units after Nicola Tesla, a Serbian physicist, engineer, and inventor. The first MRI machines operated at low fields, and many of the prototypes had strengths of about 0.15 teslas. Researchers doubted that imaging at higher field strengths would be possible because higher radio frequencies would not penetrate the human body. This prediction proved wrong. MR images taken at low field strengths were crude, blurry, and mostly worse than CT images. Scientists working for the research and development divisions of companies producing MR equipment were asked: "How do you get better image quality?" They had a simple answer: "Increase field strength." From analytical applications that used magnetic resonance to study chemicals, researchers found that the signal-to-noise ratio increased when the field strength was increased. The better the signal-to-noise ratio, the better the image. Higher field strengths required higher gradient strengths to reduce chemical-shift artifacts created by these fields, which led to better spatial resolution [9]. Paul Bottomley, a physicist, joined the General Electric Company Research Center in 1980. His research team built the first high-field device using a 1.5-tesla magnet. They were able to overcome problems of coil design, penetration, and signal-to-noise ratio to build the first effective, clinically useful whole-body MRI scanner [9].

TAILORING MRI TO DIAGNOSE AND TREAT PATIENTS WITH STROKE AND CEREBROVASCULAR DISEASE

What imaging sequences would provide clinically important information? After much trial and error during the 1980s and 1990s, clinicians and researchers arrived at a strategy to use different relaxation times (T1 and T2) and other sequences to ideally show the information needed to optimally diagnose and treat stroke patients. The first aim was to identify brain infarcts. During the 1960s and 1970s, the results of work on relaxation, diffusion, and chemical exchange of water in cells and tissues of various types appeared in the scientific literature [9]. Scientists at device-making companies applied this information to select the optimal T1 and T2 times to create useful and accurate brain images. T1, also referred to as the spin-lattice relaxation time, was the time that it took for the net nuclear magnetization vector to reach thermal equilibrium with the surrounding environment (the lattice) [10]. Physicists recognized that the components of the magnetization vector become out of phase, resulting in decay of net magnetization. T2, also referred to as the transverse relaxation time, was the time it took for the components of the magnetization vector to decay [10]. MRI images were denoted T1-weighted and T2-weighted images.

MRI machines were studied at Massachusetts General Hospital in Boston during the early 1980s. MRI displays were especially important in showing images of the brainstem and cerebellum, regions often not shown well by early generation CT scanners. MRI also made it easier to visualize lesions in different planes by providing sagittal, coronal, and horizontal sections. Reports confirmed the utility of MRI, especially in vascular lesions of the cerebellum and brainstem [11]. MRI was used to study animals with various experimental stroke protocols.

Later diffusion-weighted images (DWI) and fluid-attenuated inversion Recovery (FLAIR) images were added to the armamentarium. Brain infarction caused changes in the diffusion of water molecules. DWI was able to show even very early brain infarcts. FLAIR images are inversion recovery T2-weighted spin echo sequences. This sequence suppressed cerebrospinal fluid effects on the images so as to bring out hyperintense lesions, such as those found in more established brain infarcts [12].

The second important aim was to show recent and old brain hemorrhages. Calcium and blood collections produce hyperdense areas on CT scans. These tissues are "susceptible" to produce artifacts that alter magnetization on MRI images. Researchers devised susceptibility weighted imaging (SWI) that was very sensitive to venous blood, hemorrhage, and iron storage. SWI used a fully flow-compensated, long echo, gradient recalled echo (GRE) pulse sequence to acquire images. This exploited the "susceptibility" differences between tissues and used the phase image to detect these differences. The magnitude and phase data were combined to produce an enhanced contrast magnitude image. A different technique was the use of so-called T2*-weighted images, which were created as a post-excitation refocused gradient echo (GRE) sequence. SWI and T2*-weighted images could show deoxygenated hemoglobin, methemoglobin, hemosiderin, and even old brain hemorrhages. Hyperacute and older hemorrhages could be readily detected by MRI [13].

Selection of optimal treatment of stroke patients required information about disease within the arteries that supplied the brain and the veins that drained the brain in addition to knowledge about infarcts and hemorrhages within the brain parenchyma. During the 1970s and 1980s the most common way to show the arteries in the neck was dye contrast catheter angiography, an invasive technique. High-quality CT angiography was not readily available until the mid-1990s. Blood flow in arteries and veins could potentially be shown using MRI. Researchers eliminated all signals that arose from structures except vessels that carried pulsatile flow using velocity-dependent phase contrast, electrocardiographic gating, and image subtraction. Using these techniques, background structures became transparent, enabling the three-dimensional vascular tree to be imaged by projection to a two-dimensional image plane. Image acquisition and processing were accomplished using conventional two-dimensional Fourier transform magnetic resonance imaging techniques [14]. The first blurry magnetic resonance angiography (MRA) images were published in 1985 [15]. At first, images of the carotid and vertebral arteries in the neck were acquired separately from intracranial imaging. Robert Edelman, a general radiologist, and Steven Warach were among early researchers who collaborated with stroke clinicians to deliver clearer, more accurate vascular images [16]. By the early 1990s, clinically useful MRI and MRA images of the head and neck could be acquired during the same scanning period [17]. Contrast using a gadolinium compound (Gd-DTPA) could also be administered to improve the quality of the MRA images.

The next advances concerned producing images of the ischemic penumbra, that is, brain regions that had diminished blood flow but were not yet infarcted. The penumbra represented the at-risk brain tissue threatened to become infarcted if blood flow was not restored. Brain perfusion was imaged using dynamic contrast-enhanced MR scanning. Ultrafast imaging after Gd-DTPA injection was used to calculate regional cerebral blood volume (rCBV) and regional cerebral blood flow (rCBF) to produce so-called perfusion-weighted images [18]. These images showed regions of reduced blood flow when compared to comparable portions of the brain. Perfusion was found to be complex. There were multiple possible measurements used to capture the severity of hypoperfusion, including the relative mean transit time (rMTT), which analyzed the rate of passage of the bolus of gadolinium through the ischemic region; the time to peak, that is, the time it took for maximum perfusion (TMax); and the relative cerebral blood flow and cerebral blood volumes in the ischemic area. Within an ischemic zone, perfusion was often found to be heterogeneous, showing severe hypoperfusion in one area and less hypoperfusion in another region.

MRI protocols that included diffusion and perfusion-weighted imaging along with T2 and T2*-weighted images and MRA became routinely used in many stroke centers to rapidly evaluate stroke patients. Doctors could by the mid- to late 1990s safely and quickly diagnose old and recent brain hemor-rhages, determine the presence and location of new and old brain infarcts, recognize narrowing and occlusion of arteries that supplied brain infarcts, and show the adequacy of brain perfusion in areas around the brain infarct that were threatened by further brain ischemia. Vascular malformations and aneur-ysms could also be identified.

Researchers and clinicians explored a way of imaging perfusion without the need for contrast infusion. Gadolinium had risks for potentially serious skin complications in patients with renal disease, and gadolinium could accumulate in body tissues. A radiofrequency pulse could be delivered to the arterial blood column in the neck, giving the blood a magnetic label. Continuous arterial spin labeling (ASL) perfusion magnetic resonance imaging was developed during the early years of the twenty-first century. This technique used mag-netically labeled arterial blood water as a tracer to display maps of blood flow and to obtain quantifiable measurements of cerebral blood flow [19].

After perfusion imaging was performed, it took additional time to calculate and display perfusion scans, delaying comparison of the diffusion-weighted scan abnormalities with the perfusion information from scanning. Clinicians and researchers working at Stanford University under the leadership of Greg Albers, Michael Moseley, and Maarten Landsberg created an automated method of displaying data derived from perfusion imaging. Rapid Processing of Perfusion and Diffusion (RAPID) software automatically produced decon-voluted mean transit time and time when the residue function reached its maximum (TMax) sequences [20]. This software was used in clinical trials of reperfusion treatment [21].

REFERENCES

1. Kinley J, Damadian R. *Gifted Mind: The Dr. Raymond Damadian Story, Inventor of the MRI.* Green Forest, AZ: Master Books, a Division of New Leaf Publishing Group, 2015.
2. Dawson MJ. *Paul Lauterbur and the Invention of MRI.* Cambridge, MA: MIT Press, 2013.

3. Lauterbur PC. Image formation by induced local interactions: Examples employing nuclear magnetic resonance. *Nature* 1973;242:190–191.

4. Lauterbur PC. Magnetic resonance zeugmatography. *Pure Appl. Chem.* 1974;40 (1–2):149–157.

5. Mansfield, P. *The Long Road to Stockholm: The Story of Magnetic Resonance Imaging – An Autobiography.* Oxford: Oxford University Press, 2013.

6. The Nobel Prize in Physiology or Medicine 2003. NobelPrize.org. Available at www .nobelprize.org/prizes/medicine/2003/mansfield/facts/.

7. Dreizen P. The Nobel Prize for MRI: A wonderful discovery and a sad controversy. *Lancet* 2004 Jan 3;363(9402):78.

8. Prize Fight. *Smithsonian.* Available at www.smithsonianmag.com/science-nature/ prize-fight-95652491/.

9. Rinck PA. *The History of MRI.* Berlin: ABW, 2003. Rinck PA. *Magnetic Resonance in Medicine: The Basic Textbook of the European Magnetic Resonance Forum,* 12th ed. BoD Germany.

10. Sood R, Moseley M. Technical introduction to MRI. In Davis S, Fisher M, Warach S (eds.), *Magnetic Resonance Imaging in Stroke.* Cambridge: Cambridge University Press, 2003, pp. 55–67.

11. Kistler JP, Buonanno FS, DeWitt LD, Davis LD, Brady KR, Brady TJ, Fisher CM. Vertebral-basilar posterior cerebral territory stroke delineation by proton nuclear magnetic resonance Imaging. *Stroke* 1984;15:417–426.

12. Warach S, Chien D, Li W, Ronthal M, Edelman RR. Fast magnetic resonance diffusion-weighted imaging of acute human stroke. *Neurology* 1992;42:1717–1723. Warach S, Gaa J, Siewert B, Wielopolski P, Edelman RR. Acute human stroke studied by whole brain echo planar diffusion-weighted magnetic resonance imaging. *Ann. Neurol.* 1995;37:231–241.

13. Linfante I, Llinas RH, Caplan LR, Warach S. MRI features of intracerebral hemorrhage within 2 hours from symptom onset. *Stroke* 1999;30:2263–2267. Fiebach, JB, Schellinger PD, Gass A, et al. Stroke magnetic resonance imaging is accurate in hyperacute intracerebral hemorrhage. *Stroke* 2004;35:502–506.

14. The principles of magnetic resonance angiography (MRA) are discussed in Edelman RR, Meyer J. MR angiography of the head and neck: Basic principles and clinical applications. In Davis S, Fisher M, Warach S (eds.), *Magnetic Resonance Imaging in Stroke.* Cambridge: Cambridge University Press, 2003, pp. 85–101.

15. The first publication of MRA was Wedeen VI, Meuli RA, Edelman RR, Frank LR, Brady TJ, Rosen BR. Projective imaging of pulsatile flow with magnetic resonance. *Science* 1985;230:946–948.

16. Edelman RR, Mattle HP, Wallner B, Bajakian R, Kleefield J, Kent C, Skillman JJ, Mendel JB, Atkinson DJ. Extracranial carotid arteries: Evaluation with "black blood" MR angiography. *Radiology* 1990;177:45–50. Edelman RR, Chien D, Kim D. Fast selective black blood MR imaging. *Radiology* 1991;181:655–660. Edelman RR, Mattle HP, Atkinson DJ, et al. MR angiography. *AJR* 1990;154:937–946.

17. Warach S, Li W, Ronthal M, Edelman R. Acute cerebral ischemia: Evaluation with dynamic contrast-enhanced MR imaging and MR angiography. *Radiology* 1992;182:41–47.

18. Rother J, Guckel F, Neff W, Schwartz A, Hennerici M. Assessment of regional cerebral blood flow volume in acute human stroke by use of a single-slice dynamic susceptibility contrast-enhanced magnetic resonance imaging. *Stroke* 1996;27:1088–1093. Sorensen

AG, Buonanno F, Gonzalez RG, et al. Hyperacute stroke: Evaluation with combined multisection diffusion-weighted and hemodynamically weighted echo-planar MR imaging. *Radiology* 1996;199:391–401. Schlaug G, Benfield A, Baird AE, et al. The ischemic penumbra operationally defined by diffusion and perfusion MRI. *Neurology* 1999 53:1528–1537. Fisher M, Prichard JW, Warach S. New magnetic resonance techniques for acute ischemic stroke. *JAMA* 1995;274:908–911.

19. Wang Z, Wang J, Connick TJ, et al. Continuous ASL (CASL) perfusion MRI with an array coil and parallel imaging at 3T. *Magn. Reson. Med.* 2005;54:732–737. Fernandez-Seara MA, Wang Z, Wang J, et al. Continuous arterial spin labeling perfusion measurements using single shot 3D GRASE at 3 T. *Magnetic Resonance Med.* 2005;54:1241–1247. Ances BM, McGarvey ML, Abrahams JM, et al. Continuous arterial spin labeled perfusion magnetic resonance imaging in patients before and after carotid endarterectomy. *J. Neuroimaging* 2004;14:133–138.

20. Kleinman JT, Zaharchuk G, Mlynash M, et al. Automated perfusion imaging for the evaluation of transient ischemic attack. *Stroke* 2012;43:1556–1560.

21. Lansberg MG, Lee J, Christensen S, et al. RAPID Automated Patient Selection for Reperfusion Therapy: A pooled analysis of the Echoplanar Imaging Thrombolytic Evaluation Trial (EPITHET) and the Diffusion and Perfusion Imaging Evaluation for Understanding Stroke Evolution (DEFUSE) study. *Stroke* 2011;42:1608–1614.

CHAPTER THIRTY FOUR

CEREBROVASCULAR ULTRASOUND

Ultrasound is a field that exemplifies the important marriage of physics and mathematics to medicine. Ultrasonography is among the top four major discoveries in medicine during the twentieth century, along with electron microscopy, nuclear magnetic resonance, and computed tomography. The discovery of the principle behind medical ultrasonography and its evolution into everyday medical practice is told through the story of remarkable individuals, intertwined careers, and life sagas.

EARLY PRINCIPLES AND RESEARCH

Christian Andreas Doppler (1803–1853) discovered the principal concept that underlies ultrasound in 1842. The son of a stonemason, Doppler was born in Salzburg, Austria, a decade after the death of another famous individual from the same city, Wolfgang Amadeus Mozart. Doppler studied astronomy and mathematics in Salzburg and Vienna, and at age 38 went to work at the Prague Polytechnic in Czechoslovakia [1–3]. His major discovery came from star gazing. The report was entitled "Über das farbige Licht der Doppelsterne und einiger anderer Gestirne des Himmels" (On the colored light of the binary stars and some other stars of the heavens) [4]. Doppler studied brightness emanating from binary stars (two stars orbiting a common central mass). He discovered that the observed frequency of a sound or light wave was affected by the relative motion of the source and the observer (in other words their positions in relation to one another); this became known as the *Doppler effect*.

Another nineteenth-century physicist, Armand Hippolyte Louis Fizeau, became involved in studying aspects of the Doppler effect, known by the French as the *Doppler-Fizeau effect*. Fizeau developed the formal mathematical theorem underlying the principles of this effect. In 1848, he discovered the frequency shift of a wave when the source and receiver were moving relative to each other [5]. An easily understood example of the Doppler effect is the experience one has when an ambulance passes by. The frequency and loudness of the ambulance siren increases as it comes near, and then diminishes as it passes away. To a person inside the ambulance, the frequency of sound remains exactly the same.

The initial use of ultrasound in medicine was therapeutic, to treat peripheral nerve injuries among wounded soldiers of World War I. Ultrasound was studied only later as a potential diagnostic tool. The title of the "Father of diagnostic ultrasonography" could arguably be given to Karl Theodore Dussik, an Austrian-born physician who was trained in neurology and psychiatry. He moved to the United States during the late 1930s and collaborated with his physicist brother, Friedrich Dussik [6]. The brothers built the first system that attempted visualization of brain structures with ultrasound, which they reported in 1942. The aim was to diagnose brain tumors. In 1947, Dussik introduced the term "hyperphonography," a through-transmission ultrasonic technique believed to produce echo-images from the cerebral ventricles. Dussik's belief that low-frequency ultrasound could be used to visualize the interior of the body inspired further development of echocardiography and echoencephalography during the 1960s. The latter was used to diagnose midline shifts in patients with large strokes and tumors until the 1970s when computed tomography replaced echoencephalography for this indication and more.

Dean Franklin and colleagues used Doppler shifts of ultrasound to study blood flow in canine blood vessels and published their results in 1961 [7,8]. Ultrasound energy was used to detect interfaces among structures of different densities and to detect moving targets such as circulating red blood cells. The authors wrote: "The Doppler shift of ultrasound, scattered from moving elements within a stream of blood, is related to the velocity of blood flow. A flowmeter based on this principal has been constructed and was used to record blood flow through intact vessels of dogs" [7,8]. The early flowmeters were unidirectional, depicting blood flow and movements in one direction. Japanese pioneers of ultrasonography, including the prestigious Osaka group, also developed early elements of cardiac assessment techniques and ultrasonic measurements of blood flow in peripheral blood vessels during the 1950s and 1960s that later led to the development of echo-based imaging techniques used today in cardiac and cerebrovascular ultrasound laboratories [9–12].

DEVELOPMENT OF ULTRASOUND TO STUDY THE BLOOD VESSELS IN THE NECK

An outstanding scientist, Merrill P. Spencer, then director of the Virginia Mason Research Center in Seattle, Washington, started to apply ultrasound to detect decompression air bubbles during the 1960s. Spenser was born in Pawnee, Oklahoma, in 1922. His father was a government agent who worked with native Americans. After medical school, Merrill served as a flight surgeon in the US Army Air Corp in postwar Germany from 1951 through 1962. A major interest engendered in relation to wartime was a condition dubbed the "bends," which developed in divers. After his army service, he devoted the remainder of his professional life to the physiology of human blood flow. He sought to construct a device that could measure and display that physiology. He became an associate professor of physiology and pharmacology at Bowman Gray School of Medicine, where he taught and performed research in the dynamics of blood flow. He moved to Seattle in 1963 to become director of the Virginia Mason Research Center for seven years, where he established a hyperbaric laboratory. He founded the Institute of Applied Physiology and Medicine (IAPM) where he pioneered development of a Doppler ultrasound device that could detect nitrogen bubbles to predict and study the bends in divers. He collaborated with an avid diver, John Lindbergh [13], a son of the famous aviator Charles Lindbergh, and their work redefined US Navy diving decompression tables still in use for sport diving [14]. This work also set the stage for later use of ultrasound that blossomed during the 1990s to detect microembolic signals in stroke patients. Spencer partnered with engineers and industry to form Spencer Technologies, which became a leader in developing ultrasound devices used in many US and international medical centers.

The 1960s also marked the emergence of the father of clinical neurosonology in the United States, William Markley McKinney (1930–2003). A Southern gentleman and a visionary, McKinney was born in Roanoke, Virginia. After college he joined the US Navy in 1951 to become operations officer on a destroyer in Korea where he was in charge of submarine detection using ultrasound [15]. He then attended medical school at the University of Virginia, graduating in 1959. In 1963, he joined the Bowman Gray School of Medicine in Winston-Salem, North Carolina (now Wake Forest University Baptist Medical Center), the institution where he remained for the rest of his medical career. McKinney was recruited by James F. Toole to establish the Center for Medical Ultrasound in 1963 at Bowman Gray. McKinney organized an educational program for echoencephalography in 1964, and set up the first neurosonology course in 1975, two years before he helped launch the American Society of Neuroimaging. McKinney and his followers and colleagues educated generations of physicians and technicians in ultrasonography.

The next major breakthrough occurred during the 1970s when an array of diagnostic devices developed in Seattle, Washington, reached clinical application in stroke patients. Eugene Strandness, professor and chief of vascular surgery at the University of Washington, was a visionary for the clinical use of diagnostic ultrasound in medicine. He collaborated with engineers and physicists who created continuous and pulsed wave ultrasound systems for measuring blood flow waveforms and velocities and created images of arteries [16].

A probe or transducer was held over the artery being studied and recorded the ultrasonic information. This information was then converted into electrical energy, either for developing an image (B-mode scan) or for generating Doppler curves of blood-flow velocity. After numerous modifications, Strandness, together with scientists John Reid and Donald Baker, utilized gray-scale structural imaging and Doppler-swift based assessment of blood flow together.

These images of the artery were combined in a so-called duplex ultrasound system that showed graphs of flow velocities at various sites along the arteries of the neck [16,17]. By the early 1980s, Doppler technology could reliably detect moderate and severe vascular occlusive disease in the carotid and vertebral arteries in the neck. Sequential ultrasound studies allowed physicians to study the natural history of the development and progression of these occlusive lesions and to correlate the occurrence and severity of disease with stroke risk factors, symptoms, and treatment. This revolutionized the noninvasive detection of carotid atherosclerosis and stenosis measurements in patients at risk of stroke.

John M. Reid and Donald Baker were scientists who played major roles in influencing stroke applications of ultrasound. Reid was born in Minneapolis, Minnesota, in 1926. He worked as a navy electronics technician (1944–1946). After the war, he received a master's degree in electrical engineering from the University of Minnesota, and a PhD in electrical engineering from the University of Pennsylvania in 1965. He devoted his entire career to medical uses of ultrasound. Reid collaborated on the continuous wave and pulse Doppler and duplex imaging devices with Donald Baker, an electrical engineer. Baker was born in Skagway, Alaska, in 1932. From 1951, he served for four years in the US Air Force in the Korean War. He spent two years working at the Air Force Cambridge Research Center investigating the detection of low-flying aircrafts and airborne bombers based on returned radar signals. During military service he acquired knowledge of various electronic applications and different radar devices. Discharged from the air force in 1955, Baker entered the University of Washington in Seattle and received a doctorate in electrical engineering in 1960.

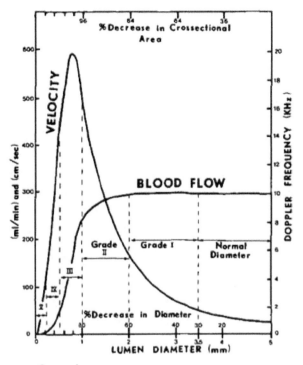

34.1. Spencer's curve.

Reid participated in forming the Institute of Applied Physiology and Medicine in Seattle with Merrill Spencer and was also affiliated with the Providence Hospital from 1971 to 1981. He helped build the first clinical ultrasound scanner during the 1950s at the University of Minnesota, and the first echocardiograph device in the United States with cardiologist Claude Joyner at the University of Pennsylvania during 1957–1965. He helped create a duplex scanner device with Strandness. Reid collaborated with Merrill Spencer and Baker during the 1970s on Doppler-based systems to assess carotid artery blood flow and hemodynamic experiments modeling carotid artery stenosis [18,19]. The latter experiment, published in 1979, made popular what is now known as Spencer's curve (Figure 34.1), a classic hemodynamic model that helps clinicians interpret cerebrovascular ultrasound studies and influenced development of diagnostic criteria for extra- and intracranial disease as well as reperfusion and reocclusion in acute stroke [20]. The major early contributors to the development of extracranial ultrasound – Spencer, Reid, Baker, and McKinney – all were in the military during or after World War II, stimulating their interest in ultrasound.

One of the earliest and long-sustained efforts involving ultrasound of neck arteries was to understand early, preclinical signs of atherosclerosis using B-mode imaging (intima media thickness), a measurement offered in most duplex scanner software packages.

TRANSCRANIAL ULTRASOUND OF INTRACRANIAL ARTERIES AND THE BRAIN

Noninvasive assessment of intracranial vessels remained a challenge since the ultrasound frequencies used for imaging vessels in the neck could not effectively penetrate through the skull; transducers in use were not suitable for this purpose. A major breakthrough was reported in 1982, when a brilliant scientist, Rune Aaslid, a Norwegian-born engineering cyberneticist and physiologist, developed a two-megahertz frequency pulsed wave Doppler system that could successfully insonate proximal intracranial arteries [21]. Aaslid was part of an illustrious Trondheim group in Norway that greatly influenced the development of ultrasound in general. One of his collaborators, Alf Brubakk, recalls that "there is a mad student who claims he can make a mathematical model of the cardiovascular system. This is how I met Rune Aaslid.... In 1970, when our project was initiated, there was no digital computer that could solve the non-linear equations involved in our model. Rune built our own analogue computer that we named Jenny" [22]. Aaslid had the ability and tenacity to take on very complex tasks. Later, Rune also became a pilot and flew his plane between continents as well as for sightseeing around Mount Rainier in the Seattle area.

Aaslid termed his technique transcranial Doppler (TCD) [21,23]. The TCD technique involved placing transducer probes in three regions: the orbit, the foramen magnum, and a region of the thinnest section of the squamous portion of the temporal bone. An early clinical application studied by Aaslid in collaboration with a group of Norwegians, Swiss neurosurgeons, and German pioneers was in subarachnoid hemorrhage patients. Blood in the subarachnoid space stimulated arteries at the base of the brain to constrict (vasospasm), increasing blood flow velocities within these vessels. TCD could detect and quantitate the severity of vasoconstriction [24]. When Aaslid edited his first textbook on TCD in 1986, he was already working with Merrill Spencer in Seattle, sparking interest in the new technology in the United States and worldwide. Their work led to the ability to timely intervene in cerebral vasospasm and much more. Multiple research groups confirmed the value of TCD monitoring of subarachnoid hemorrhage patients. Further clinical research established the utility of TCD in assessing cerebral circulatory arrest and detection and grading of the severity of intracranial arterial stenoses and occlusions.

Later clinical applications of TCD included detection, localization, and quantification of cerebral embolization in real time and detection of right to left cardiac and pulmonary shunts. Further progress, led by clinicians and researchers in Europe, led to the introduction of three-dimensional-display vascular maps that allowed better orientation of the insonation to the location of the artery being studied. Specially designed helmets and headbands were made to hold probes in place, facilitating monitoring of arteries over time. These improvements allowed the introduction of duplex scanning of intracranial arteries. Power Doppler technology, used in imaging neck vessels, was also applied to transcranial duplex scanning [25]. B-mode images of the intracranial arteries were produced and color-coded scans were obtained from intracranial arteries during transcranial sonography [26]. Solutions containing microbubbles were injected intravenously to obtain contrast-enhancement of the transcranial ultrasound signals and so improve the diagnostic capability of transcranial ultrasound scans [26]. Brain parenchyma and ventricles could also be imaged [27-29].

The ability of TCD to detect brain hypoperfusion and cerebral embolization in real time captured the attention of research groups from United Kingdom, the Netherlands, Germany, the United States, and other countries [30–33]. By the turn of the twenty-first century, TCD technology had evolved toward multi-gate sampling and digital platforms that increased processing speeds. Under the mentorship of Kirk Beach, Mark Moehring, then at Spencer Technologies in Seattle, developed power motion Doppler (PMD) for emboli tracking, window finding, vessel identification, and more complete TCD investigations [34]. When Moehring showed the newly developed TCD system to Aaslid, Rune was surprised that the middle cerebral artery could be found as shallow as at 3 centimeters in depth! This was truly a testament that power motion Doppler was a useful aid even for the most experienced sonographer. During the next decade PMD displays were adopted by all major TCD companies and became the standard for multi-depth display of flow direction and signal intensity.

Studies of real-time emboli detection with TCD exploded during the 1990s, increasing knowledge about risk factors, mechanisms, and ways to protect the brain from embolism in a variety of settings, including carotid revascularization, repairs of ascending aorta aneurysms, detecting right-to-left shunts and paradoxical embolism, and tailoring therapies [31,32]. The utility of TCD for detection of intracranial atherosclerosis was studied in Chinese communities by Lawrence Wong. He and his collaborators used TCD to detect, grade, and monitor the severity of intracranial atherosclerosis in China, Southeast Asia, and beyond [35].

TCD also shone light on the hemodynamics and physiology of cerebral blood flow and its response to various pathological conditions. David Newell and Rune Aaslid pioneered TCD studies of autoregulation and cerebral blood flow [36,37]. TCD assessed blood flow velocity changes at a constant angle of insonation and measured vasomotor reactivity. Reserve capacity for augmenting blood flow in patients with arterial occlusions was studied using TCD and vasodilator stimuli [38]. The most common technique involved injection of acetazolamide or inhalation of a gas mixture containing carbon dioxide. These promoted vasodilatation in normal arteries. Blood flow velocities were monitored using TCD. In normal patients and those with good "vasomotor reactivity," cerebral blood flow increased. When collateral vessels were already maximally dilated, they failed to further augment flow. Reduced cerebrovascular reserve capability was correlated with increased stroke risk in patients with severe occlusive carotid artery disease [39]. The reduced blood flow reserve capacity reflected a tenuous circulation at risk.

TCD hemodynamics were also studied during acute brain ischemia. During the acute stroke phase, carbon dioxide builds up in patients with apnea, sleep disordered breathing, and hypoventilation. The increased carbon dioxide level augmented blood flow in vessels that retained their reactivity. Ischemic vessels lost their reactivity. The result was direction of blood flow away from ischemic regions, an entity that Alexandrov dubbed the "reversed Robin Hood syndrome" [40]. This stealing of blood away from where it was most needed was one cause of clinical deterioration. Knowledge of this phenomenon represented a target for noninvasive ventilatory correction.

TCD technology was also used to study cerebral veins and dural sinuses [41]. Vein locations varied and were difficult to visualize. Some venous structures such as the superior sagittal sinus were far away from usual insonating windows. Power-based and color-coded duplex sonography could show the major veins and dural sinuses, especially after bubble ultrasound contrast injections. Dural sinus occlusions could be diagnosed and followed by sequential TCD studies [42].

The therapeutic potential of ultrasound in stroke was also explored. Could ultrasound enhance thrombolysis? Ultrasound was shown to have the potential to physically loosen fibrin bridges within red blood clots, allowing erythrocytes to escape and the clot to dissolve [43]. TCD was used effectively to diagnose and localize intracranial arterial occlusions and to monitor spontaneous or treatment-related recanalization. Preliminary small studies suggested that continuous monitoring of the middle cerebral artery using TCD ultrasound during thrombolysis might augment the lytic effect of the thrombolytic agent [44].

ULTRASOUND DIAGNOSIS IN CLINICAL TRIALS

Cerebrovascular ultrasound emerged as an important tool in clinical trials. The most exemplary design, standardization, training, and implementation of TCD was achieved in sequential clinical trials known as the Stroke Prevention in Sickle Cell (STOP) program under the leadership of Robert J. Adams, then at the Medical College of Georgia [45]. Sickle cell disease patients were monitored periodically by TCD measurement of time-averaged maximum mean flow velocities (TAMM). Those with high values were selected to receive blood transfusions. The STOP trials showed a primary stroke risk reduction of 90 percent when children were transfused according to TCD results. This benefit was sustained if children with abnormal TAMMs continued to receive blood transfusions.

Standardized carotid ultrasonography was successfully adopted by James F. Toole and the Asymptomatic Carotid Stenosis (ACAS) trialists to determine patient eligibility for a study of carotid artery surgery [46]. A nonstandardized approach to obtaining ultrasound data in the North American Symptomatic Carotid Endarterectomy Trial (NASCET) led to underestimation of its role and prognostic implications [47] and highlighted the importance of prior training and standardization of the ultrasound examinations and interpretations [48].

In London, Hugh Markus and his collaborators showed through prospective studies and the CARESS trial the mechanism of how dual antiplatelet therapy reduced artery-to-artery embolism [49] and how emboli detection could identify the highest-risk patients with asymptomatic carotid stenosis [50].

Preliminary small studies suggested that continuous monitoring of the middle cerebral artery using TCD ultrasound during thrombolysis might augment the lytic effect of the thrombolytic agent. A randomized trial was designed to test this capability. CLOTBUST patients were randomly assigned to receive continuous two-megahertz TCD or dummy monitoring. The primary combined end point was complete recanalization assessed by TCD or dramatic clinical recovery. Complete recanalization or dramatic clinical recovery within two hours after the administration of a tPA bolus occurred in 31 patients in the target group (49%), compared with 19 patients in the control group (30%; P = 0.03). At three months, 22 out of 53 (42%) patients in the target group and 14 out of 49 in the control group (29%) had favorable outcomes. The results of this trial suggested that continuous transcranial Doppler could augment tPA-induced arterial recanalization [51,52].

NEUROSONOLOGY SOCIETIES AND ULTRASOUND TRAINING AND STANDARDIZATION

Professional societies were formed to provide leadership, advocacy, training, and credentialing in the rapidly growing field of cerebrovascular ultrasound. The American Society of Neuroimaging was formed in 1977 and continually offered neurosonology proficiency examinations for physicians since the 1980s [53]. In Europe, David Russel at Oslo University Hospital, Norway, initiated creation of the European Society of Neurosonology and Cerebral Hemodynamics (ESNCH) in 1993 [54]. American, European, Australasian, and South American ultrasound experts continue to provide tutorials at national meetings of neurosonological societies and in conjunction with stroke meetings.

Other important clinicians and researchers not mentioned earlier deserve credit for furthering the field of diagnostic and therapeutic ultrasound in cerebrovascular disease [55].

REFERENCES

1 Biography of Christian Doppler, Mathematician and Physicist. ThoughtCo.com. www .thoughtco.com/christian-doppler-biography-4174714.

2 Eden, A. *The Search for Christian Doppler*. Wien: Springer-Verlag, 1992.

3 Eden A. *Christian Doppler: Leben und Werk*. Salzburg: Landespressebureau, 1988

4 Doppler C. Über das farbige Licht der Doppelsterne und einiger anderer Gestirne des Himmels. *Abh. Kgl. Böhm Ges. Wissensch. (Prag.)* 1842:465–482.

5 Houdas Y. Doppler, Buys-Ballot, Fizeau. Historical note on the discovery of the Doppler's effect. *Ann. Cardiol. Angéiol.* 1991;40(4):209–213. PMID 2053764.

6. Shampo MA, Kyle RA. Karl Theodore Dussik: Pioneer in ultrasound. *Mayo Clin. Proc.* 1995;70:1136.

7. Fields WS, Lemak NA. *The History of Stroke*. New York: Oxford University Press, 1989, pp. 129–149.

8. Franklin DL, Schlegel WA, Rushner RF. Blood flow measured by Doppler frequency shift of back-scattered ultrasound. *Science* 1961;134:564–565.

9. Veyrat C. Cardiovascular applications of the Doppler technique: A long way from birth to scientific acceptance. *J. Am. Soc. Echocardiogr.* 1999;12:278–284.

10. Satomura S, Tamura A, Kido Y. Study of blood flow in vessels by ultrasonics. *Abst. Meeting Acoust. Soc. Jpn.* 1958 Oct:81–82.

11. Satomura S. Study of the flow patterns in peripheral arteries by ultrasonics. *J. Acoust. Soc. Jpn.* 1959;15:151–158.

12. Kato K, Kido Y, Motomiya M, Kaneko Z, Kotani H. On the mechanism of generation detected sound in ultrasonic flowmeter. *Memoirs Inst. Sci. Res. Osaka Univ.* 1962;19:51–57.

13. Spencer MP, Cambell SD, Sealey JL, Henry FC, Lindbergh J. Experiments on decompression bubbles in the circulation using ultrasonic and electromagnetic flow meters. *J. Occupational Med.* 1969;11:38–44.

14. Seidel S. Merrill P. Spencer, M.D. 1922–2006 eulogy. *J. Neuroimaging* 2007;17:1–3.

15. Toole JF. In memorium. William Markley McKinney (1930–2003). *Neurology* 2004;62:536–537.

16. Barber FE, Baker DW, Nation AW, Strandness DE Jr, Reid JM. Ultrasonic duplex echo-Doppler scanner. *IEEE Trans. Biomed. Eng.* 1974;21:109–113.

17. Strandness DE. *Duplex Scanning in Vascular Disorders*. New York: Raven Press, 1990.

18. Reid JM, Spencer MP. Ultrasonic Doppler technique for imaging blood vessels. *Science* 1972;176:1235–1236.

19. Spencer MP, Reid JM. Quantitation of carotid stenosis with continuous wave Doppler ultrasound. *Stroke* 1979;10:326–330.

20. Alexandrov AV. The Spencer's curve: Clinical implications of a classic hemodynamic model. *J. Neuroimaging* 2007;17:6–10.

21. Aaslid R, Markwalder TM, Nornes H. Noninvasive transcranial Doppler ultrasound recording of flow velocity in basal cerebral arteries. *J. Neurosurgery* 1982;57:769–774.

22. Bribakk AO. Career perspective: Alf O. Brubakk – Looking back to see ahead. *Extrem. Physiol. Med.* 2025;4:4. https://doi.org/10.1186/s13728-015-0023-z.

23. Aaslid R (ed.). *Transcranial Doppler Sonography*. Wien: Springer-Verlag, 1986.

24. Sloan MA, Alexandrov AV, Tegeler CH, Spencer MP, Caplan LR, Feldmann E, et al. Assessment: Transcranial Doppler ultrasonography: Report of the Therapeutics and Technology Assessment Subcommittee of the American Academy of Neurology. *Neurology* 2004;62:1468–1481.

25. Griewing B, Doherty C, Kessler CH. Power Doppler ultrasound examination of the intracerebral and extracerebral vasculature. *J. Neuroimaging* 1996;6:32–35.

26. Bartels E. *Color-Coded Duplex Ultrasonography of the Cerebral Vessels*. Stuttgart: Schattauer, 1998. Baumgartner RW. Transcranial color duplex sonography in cerebrovascular disease: A systematic review. *Cerebrovas. Dis.* 2003;16:4–13. Krejza J, Baumagartner RW. Clinical applications of transcranial color-coded duplex sonography. *J. Neuroimaging* 2004;14:215–225.

27. Bogdahn U, Becker G, Schlief R, et al. Contrast-enhanced transcranial color-coded real-time sonography. *Stroke* 1993;24:676–684.

28. Schoning M, Buchholz R, Walter J. Comparative study of transcranial color duplex sonography and transcranial Doppler sonography in adults. *J. Neurosurgery* 1993;78:776–784.

29. Becker G, Seufert J, Bogdahn U, Reichmann H, Reiners K. Degeneration of substantia nigra in chronic Parkinson's disease visualized by transcranial color-coded real-time sonography. *Neurology* 1995 Jan;45(1):182–184.

30. Padayachee TS, Bishop CCR, Gosling RG, et al. Monitoring middle cerebral artery blood flow velocity during carotid endarterectomy. *Br. J. Surg.* 1986;73:98–100.

31. Steiger HJ, Schaffler L, Boll J, Liechti S. Results of microsurgical carotid endarterectomy: A prospective study with transcranial Doppler and EEG monitoring, and selective shunting. *Acta Neurochir. (Wien)* 1989;100:31–38.

32. Spencer MP, Thomas GI, Nicholls SC, Sauvage LR. Detection of middle cerebral artery emboli during carotid endarterectomy using transcranial Doppler ultrasonography. *Stroke* 1990;21:415–423.

33. Ackerstaff RGA, Janes C, Moll FL, et al. The significance of emboli detection by means of transcranial Doppler ultrasonography monitoring in carotid endarterectomy. *J. Vas. Surg.* 1995;21:415–423.

34. Moehring MA, Spencer MP. Power M-mode transcranial Doppler ultrasound and simultaneous single gate spectrogram. *Ultrasound Med. Biology* 2002;28:49–57.

35. Wong KS, Li H, Chan YL, Ahuja A, et al. Use of transcranial Doppler ultrasound to predict outcome in patients with intracranial large-artery occlusive disease. *Stroke* 2000;31(11):2641–2647. Wong KS, Li H, Lam WW, Chan YL, Kay R. Progression of middle cerebral artery occlusive disease and its relationship with further vascular events after stroke. *Stroke* 2002;33(2):532–536. Wong KS, Gao S, Chan YL, et al. Mechanisms of acute cerebral infarctions in patients with middle cerebral artery stenosis: A diffusion-weighted imaging and microemboli monitoring study. *Ann. Neurol.* 2002;52(1):74–81. Wong KS, Li H. Long-term mortality and recurrent stroke risk among Chinese stroke patients with predominant intracranial atherosclerosis. *Stroke* 2003;34(10):2361–2366.

36. Aaslid R, Newell DW, Stooss R, Sorteberg W, Lindegaard KF. Assessment of cerebral autoregulation dynamics from simultaneous arterial and venous transcranial Doppler recordings in humans. *Stroke* 1991;22(9):1148–1154.

37. Newell DW, Aaslid R, Lam A, Mayberg TS, Winn HR. Comparison of flow and velocity during dynamic autoregulation testing in humans. *Stroke* 1994;25(4):793–797.

38. Piepgras A, Schmiedek P, Leinsinger G, et al. A simple test to assess cerebrovascular reserve capacity using transcranial Doppler sonography and acetazolamide. *Stroke* 1990;21:1306–1311. Dahl A, Russell D, Rootwelt K, Nyberg-Hansen R, Kerty E. Cerebral vasoreactivity assessed with transcranial Doppler and regional cerebral blood flow measurements. Dose, concentration, and time of the response to acetzolamide. *Stroke* 1995;26:2302–2306. Valdueza JM, Draganski B, Hoffman O, Dirnagl U, Einhaupl KM. Analysis of CO_2 vasomotor reactivity and vessel diameter changes by simultaneous venous and arterial Doppler recordings. *Stroke* 1999;30:81–86.

39. Yonas H, Smith HA, Durham SR, Pentheny SL, Johnson DW. Increased stroke risk predicted by compromised cerebral blood flow reactivity. *J. Neurosurgery* 1993;79:483–489.

40. Alexandrov AV, Sharma VK, Lao AY, Tsivgoulis G, Malkoff MD, Alexandrov AW. Reversed Robin Hood syndrome in acute ischemic stroke patients. *Stroke* 2007;38:3045–3048.

41. Becker G, Bogdahn U, Gehlberg C, et al. Transcranial color-coded real-time sonography of intracranial veins: Normal values of blood flow velocities and findings in superior sagittal sinus thrombosis. *J. Neuroimaging* 1995;5:87–94. Valdueza JM, Schmierer K, Mehraein S, Einhäupl KM. Assessment of normal flow velocity in basal cerebral veins: A transcranial Doppler ultrasound study. *Stroke* 1996;27:1221–1225.

42. Valdueza JM, Schultz M, Harms L, Einhäupl KM. Venous transcranial Doppler ultrasound monitoring in acute dural sinus thrombosis: Report of two cases. *Stroke* 1995;26:1196–1199. Canhão P, Batista P, Ferro JM. Venous transcranial Doppler in acute dural sinus thrombosis. *J. Neurol.* 1998;245:276–279.

43. Polak JF. Ultrasound energy and the dissolution of thrombus. *N. Engl. J. Med.* 2004;18 (351):2154–2155.

44. Alexandrov AV, Demchuk AM, Felberg RA, et al. High rate of complete recanalization and dramatic clinical recovery during tPA infusion when continuously monitored with 2-Mhz transcranial Doppler monitoring. *Stroke* 2000;31:610–614. Eggers J, Koch B, Meyer K, Konig I, Seidel G. Effect of ultrasound on thrombosis of middle cerebral artery occlusion. *Ann. Neurol.* 2003;53:797–800.

45. Adams R, McKie V, Nichols F, et al. The use of transcranial ultrasonography to predict stroke in sickle cell disease. *N. Engl. J. Med.* 1992;326:605–610. Adams RJ, McKie VC, Hsu L, et al. Prevention of first stroke by transfusions in children with sickle cell anemia and abnormal results on transcranial Doppler ultrasonography. *N. Engl. J. Med.* 1998;339:5–11. Adams RJ, Brambilla D, Optimizing Primary Stroke Prevention in Sickle Cell Anemia (STOP 2) Trial Investigators. Discontinuing prophylactic transfusions used to prevent stroke in sickle cell disease. *N. Engl. J. Med.* 2005;353:2769–2778.

46. Howard G, Baker WH, Chambless LE, Howard VJ, Jones AM, Toole JF. An approach for the use of Doppler ultrasound as a screening tool for hemodynamically significant stenosis (despite heterogeneity of Doppler performance). A multicenter experience. Asymptomatic Carotid Atherosclerosis Study Investigators. *Stroke* 1996;27:1951–1957.

47. Eliasziw M, Rankin RN, Fox AJ, Haynes RB, Barnett HJ. Accuracy and prognostic consequences of ultrasonography in identifying severe carotid artery stenosis. North American Symptomatic Carotid Endarterectomy Trial (NASCET) Group. *Stroke* 1995;26:1747–1752.

48. Ringelstein EB. Skepticism toward carotid ultrasonography: A virtue, an attitude, or fanaticism? *Stroke* 1995 Oct;26(10):1743–1746.

49. Markus HS, Droste DW, Kaps M, et al. Dual antiplatelet therapy with clopidogrel and aspirin in symptomatic carotid stenosis evaluated using doppler embolic signal detection: The Clopidogrel and Aspirin for Reduction of Emboli in Symptomatic Carotid Stenosis (CARESS) trial. *Circulation* 2005;111(17):2233–2240.

50. Markus HS, King A, Shipley M, et al. Asymptomatic embolisation for prediction of stroke in the Asymptomatic Carotid Emboli Study (ACES): A prospective observational study. *Lancet Neurol.* 2010;9(7):663–671.

51. Alexandrov AV, Molina CA, Grotta JC, et al. Ultrasound-enhanced systemic thrombolysis for acute ischemic stroke. *N. Engl. J. Med.* 2004;351:2170–2178.

52. Alexandrov AV, Köhrmann M, Soinne L, et al., CLOTBUST-ER Trial Investigators. Safety and efficacy of sonothrombolysis for acute ischaemic stroke: A multicentre, double-blind, phase 3, randomised controlled trial. *Lancet Neurol.* 2019;18:338–347.

53. Information is found on the website of the organization (www.asnweb.org). Charles Tegeler of Wake Forest University and Andrei Alexandrov served as directors for 30 years. The ASN also developed and successfully launched neurovascular specialist examinations for sonographers under the leadership of Alexander Razumovsky.

54. The organizers of the first and subsequent meetings included an illustrious group of ultrasound experts who focused their research on stroke: E. Bernd Ringelstein, Jurgen Klingelhofer, Eva Bartels (Germany), and Rob G. A. Ackerstaff (Netherlands).

55. Neurosurgeons: Karl Frederick Lindegaard (Oslo), Albrecht G. Harders (Freiburg), David Newell (Seattle), and Neil Martin (Los Angeles); neurologists: Gerhard-Michael von Reutern (Bad Nauheim), Michael Hennerici (Mannheim), Manfred Kaps (Giessen, Germany), Michael Sloan (Baltimore), Elietta Zanette (Rome), Viken Babikian (Boston), J. Phillip Kistler (Boston), Brian Chambers (Melbourne), Nathan Bornstein (Israel), Jean-Pierre Touboul (Paris), Mattthias Sturznegger (Switzerland), and Laszlo Csiba (Debrecen); vascular surgeons: Andrew Nicolaides (London), Ali F. AbuRhama (Charlottesville), and Tanja Rundek (Miami); radiologists: Ed Bluth (New Orleans), Daniel O'Leary (Boston), and Ed Grant (Los Angeles). And Katsuro Tachibana (Fukuoka), Hiroshi Furuhata (Tokyo), Fabienne Perren (Geneva), Georgios Tsivgoulis (Greece), Jurgen Klingelhoffer (Germany), Leandra Pourcelot (France), and R. G. A. Ackerstaff (Utrecht, Netherlands).

CHAPTER THIRTY FIVE

CEREBRAL BLOOD FLOW, RADIONUCLIDES, AND POSITRON EMISSION TOMOGRAPHY

The development of radionuclides and positron emission tomography (PET) resulted from important discoveries and advancements in physics, chemistry, physiology, mathematics, and computer science, notably, the discovery of computerized tomography by Hounsfield (see Chapter 32) [1]. PET was the first-ever technique to allow mapping of brain perfusion and metabolism in three dimensions. Understanding of cerebral blood flow (CBF) and metabolism coupled with technological advancements made it possible to functionally image the brain in healthy and diseased individuals. PET studies critically contributed to deciphering the mechanisms underlying cerebrovascular disease and stroke, which led to a revolution in clinical practice [2].

PHYSIOLOGY OF CEREBRAL BLOOD FLOW

Cerebral blood flow, also termed "perfusion," represents the quantity of blood that passes through brain capillaries to deliver oxygen and glucose to brain cells. Neurons depend on a continuous supply given their lack of energy reserves. Blood flow also removes wastes. CBF is commonly expressed in units of milliliters per 100 grams of brain tissue per minute. The normal average CBF is 50 ml/100 g/min; blood flow is four times higher in gray than in white matter. Studying perfusion is paramount in ischemic strokes because they are caused by insufficient perfusion, temporary (transient ischemic attack) or long-lasting (stroke), potentially causing tissue infarction or selective neuronal loss.

CBF is essentially stable across a wide range of systemic blood pressures and local cerebral perfusion pressures (CPP) attributable to arterial vasodilation and vasoconstriction. Beyond maximal diameter changes, autoregulation is overridden and CBF becomes linearly dependent on CPP. CBF changes widely in response to direct vasoactive compounds such as $PaCO_2$, PaO_2, and vasoactive drugs.

CBF changes locally in the brain in relation to changes in neuronal activity. The concept that blood flow within the brain is intimately related to brain function dates to one century before PET was invented. In 1878, Angelo Mosso, a prominent Italian physiologist, measured an increase in brain pulsations from the right prefrontal cortex during an arithmetic task performed by a subject with a bony skull defect. The physiological relationship between brain function and blood flow was first explored in 1890 by Charles Roy and Charles Sherrington [3,4]. They concluded the following:

> There are, then, two more or less distinct mechanisms for controlling the cerebral circulation, viz. – firstly, an intrinsic one by which the blood supply of various parts of the brain can be varied locally in accordance with local requirements, and secondly, an extrinsic, viz. – the vasomotor nervous system, whose action affects the amount of blood passing through the brain in virtue of the dependence of the latter circulation on the general arterial blood-pressure [as noted above, the latter statement proved to be largely inaccurate]. Presumably, when the activity of the brain is not great, its blood-supply is regulated mainly by the intrinsic mechanism and without notable interference with the blood supply of other organs and tissues. When, on the other hand, the cerebral activity is great, or when the circulation of the brain is interfered with, the vasomotor nerves are called into action, the supply of blood to other organs of the body being thereby trenched upon. [5]

Despite this promising beginning, interest in the relationship between brain function and blood flow almost ceased during the first quarter of the twentieth century. This was due to the lack of sophisticated tools and the influence of Sir Leonard Hill, an eminent British physiologist who opposed the relationship between blood flow and function. In his 1896 book, *The Physiology and Pathology of Cerebral Circulation: An Experimental Research*, Hill rejected Roy and Sherrington's claims as false. He considered his own experiments to be more accurate [3,4].

There was no serious challenge to Hill's views until a remarkable clinical study of a patient, Walter K., was reported by John Fulton in the 1928 issue of the journal *Brain*. Walter K. had a vascular malformation lying over his visual cortex. He remarked to his physicians that a noise (i.e., a bruit) that he perceived in the back of his head increased in intensity when he was using his eyes. He said that he had often noticed this during the preceding several years but had "never thought much of it." Fulton noticed that when the patient began to use his eyes after a period of prolonged rest in a dark room, there was a prompt and noticeable increase in the intensity of his bruit. Activity of his other sense organs had no effect on the bruit. Fulton became well known for localizing cerebral function in primates. With Fulton's work and reputation, the blood flow function theory reemerged [3,4,6].

DISCOVERY OF THE POSITRON AND ARTIFICIAL RADIOACTIVITY

Paul Dirac predicted in 1931 that the universe consisted not only of matter but of antimatter as well. On August 2, 1932, Caltech physicist Carl Anderson discovered the positron, the first particle of antimatter to be identified. He had built a cloud chamber to study cosmic rays, high-energy particles that rained down from space. His instrument included a magnet, which allowed Anderson to determine whether the particles passing through were positively or negatively charged, and a lead plate to slow the particles down. He took hundreds of photographs of tracks taken by cosmic ray particles. The curve of the trajectory of one of the particles suggested that it was positively charged yet far less massive than a proton. An editor at the journal *Physical Review* suggested the name "positron," since the particle was identical to the electron except for the opposite charge [7]. The discovery earned Anderson the 1936 Nobel Prize in Physics [8]. After Anderson's discovery physicists searched through their files of cloud-chamber photographs and identified positron tracks they had previously misidentified. The Joliot-Curies, who had earlier missed the neutron, saw that they had also missed the positron. They started up their cloud chamber again and looked for the new particle in other experimental arrangements [9].

The radiochemist Iréne Joliot-Curie was a battlefield radiologist, activist, politician, and daughter of two of the most famous scientists in the world, Marie and Pierre Curie [10]. Jean Frédéric Joliot, born in Paris on March 19, 1900, was a graduate of the École de Physique et Chimie of the city of Paris. In 1925, he became an assistant to Marie Curie at the Radium Institute and married Iréne in 1926. He performed research on the structure of the atom, in collaboration with his wife. They worked on the projection of nuclei, an essential step in the discovery of the neutron and the positron [11]. Their most important discovery was that of artificial radioactivity in 1934. They found that certain light elements emitted positrons when bombarded by alpha particles emitted from Polonium. When an aluminum foil was irradiated on a polonium preparation, the emission of positrons did not cease immediately after the source was removed. The aluminum foil remained radioactive and decayed like a naturally occurring radioactive element. They observed the same phenomenon with boron and magnesium. New radio elements were formed by transmutation of boron, magnesium, and aluminum, named *radionitrogen, radiosilicon,* and *radiophosphorus* [12]. These two physicists received the 1935 Nobel Prize for Chemistry for their very important discovery of artificial radioactive elements [11].

Marie Curie made the following statement regarding these newly discovered radio elements: "One could only hope that in the future one could obtain by means of tubes generating accelerated particles radio-elements of which the intensity of the radiation would be comparable to that of natural radio-elements. These new substances could then have medical applications and probably other practical applications" [1].

In 1930, Ernest Lawrence and colleagues in Berkeley, California, conceived the idea of a machine in which particles were accelerated between two D-shaped magnets, called a cyclotron, in order to produce progressively higher-energy protons and deuterons that could then bombard elements to explore the nature of the atomic nucleus. The magnets in their first cyclotron were 4 inches in diameter, and their subsequent machines had 10-, 37-, and 60-inch magnets. Between 1930 and 1934, their group produced radioactive cobalt and other radionuclides by bombarding the metal components of their cyclotrons. They did not recognize the artificial radioactivity because the power supply to their cyclotron and their radiation detection instruments was shut off every evening. The report of the discovery of artificial radioactivity by the Joliot-Curies caused great disappointment within the cyclotron team because they had failed to be the first to show that one could make practically any element radioactive [13].

The Berkeley investigators then used their cyclotron to produce artificial radionuclides in quantities meaningful for performing biological experiments [1]. They produced large quantities of artificial radioisotopes, including carbon-11, nitrogen-13, oxygen-15, and fluorine-18, each of which would later prove of great significance to biomedical research [13]. During the 1930s, biologists, physiologists, and physicians flocked to Berkeley to use the newly produced radioelements as tracers. The first use of positron-emitting radionuclides in humans was done in 1945, using $C^{[11]}$ labeled to carbon monoxide to study its fate in man [1].

POSITRON EMISSION AND DETECTION

The nuclei of naturally occurring radioelements and artificially produced radionuclides are unstable. To achieve stability they emit subatomic particles, a phenomenon called radioactive decay. The half-life is the time it takes for half of the unstable nuclei present in a sample to decay (e.g., $F^{[18]}$, $t^{1/2}$ = 109.5 minutes). An atom can undergo an alpha, beta, or positron decay. Positron emission from the nucleus is secondary to the conversion of a proton into a neutron. As a positron travels through matter, it loses energy and undergoes deflection due to its interaction with other atoms and takes a very tortuous path before coming to rest. This limits the spatial resolution of PET scan in human beings to 1–2 millimeters at best, depending on the radionuclide. A positron eventually combines with an electron when both are at rest. They annihilate and give off electromagnetic radiation in the form of two photons (gamma rays). The amount of energy released is calculated by Einstein's equation $E = mc^2$. Two photons each of 0.511 MeV (the rest mass equivalent of each particle) are emitted at 180° to each other. The photons are emitted in opposite directions to conserve momentum, which is close to zero before annihilation [14].

The Gieger-Muller tube was the only external counting device available to detect high-energy radionuclides such as radioactive iodine until 1949. The tube responded to only approximately 2 percent of the total gamma-ray emission from a radioactive source and could not detect 0.511-MeV photons. The groundwork for a better detector was accomplished at the turn of the century by Ernest Rutherford, who visually counted the scintillations produced by interactions of alpha particles with zinc sulfide crystals. Heinz Kallman reported in 1948 that photomultiplier tubes could detect these scintillations individually and amplify them for electronic counting. By 1949 Cassen, Curtis, and Reed reported the use of calcium tungstate as detectors of higher-energy gamma photons. The resulting development of the scintillation detector during this period was crucial for the later advancement of dual and single photon cameras [1,15].

CEREBRAL BLOOD FLOW AND ENERGY METABOLISM

The first quantitative measurements of cerebral blood flow and metabolism, 35 years before PET emerged, were made in the macaque monkey by Paul Dumke and Carl Schmidt with their bubble flowmeter, published in 1943. This meter was a coiled tube of constant cross-sectional area that was intercalated into a single cerebral artery that had been surgically isolated. An air bubble was introduced into the tube and its velocity measured. Cerebral blood flow was calculated from this velocity and the tube's cross-sectional area. This procedure required extensive surgery and was limited to anesthetized animals [16,17].

The average blood flow in the human brain was first determined in 1944 by Seymour S. Kety, who was then working with Schmidt. Kety's method was to observe the rate at which the brain was saturated or desaturated with an inert gas. The subject inhaled 15 percent nitrous oxide for 10 minutes, during which the concentration of nitrous oxide was monitored by drawing samples of peripheral arterial blood and jugular venous blood. The area between the arterial and the venous saturation curves yielded a measure of the average blood flow. Kety also measured the difference in oxygen content of the arterial and venous blood, which is normally about 0.7 milliliter of oxygen per milliliter of blood. Multiplying flow by oxygen difference yielded the average cerebral metabolic rate of oxygen ($CMRO_2$), which is normally about 3.5 milliliters of oxygen/100 g/min [18].

In 1961, Niels A. Lassen, David H. Ingvar, and Erik Skinhøj at Bispebjerg Hospital in Copenhagen and at the University of Lund in Sweden developed a new radioactive-isotope technique to directly measure blood flow in areas within the human cerebral cortex. The method involved the use of $Xe^{[133]}$, a radioactive isotope of the inert gas xenon. The radioactive gas was dissolved in sterile saline solution and a small volume was injected into the internal carotid artery as part of conventional angiography. The arrival and subsequent wash-out of the radioactivity from many brain regions was followed for one minute with a gamma-ray camera consisting initially of a few, and subsequently of a battery of 254, externally placed scintillation detectors, arrayed like a helmet over the head. Each detector was collimated to scan approximately one square centimeter of brain surface. Information from the detectors was processed by a small digital computer and following exponential curve stripping was displayed in graphical form on a color television monitor, with each CBF level being assigned a different color or hue. Owing to the attenuation of radiation from structures deeper in the brain, the gamma radiation almost exclusively originated from the superficial convexity of cortex. The radioactive-xenon technique provided a picture of perfusion of the cerebral cortex directly below the detector array, information that for the first time allowed functional neuronal activity during sensory-motor, perceptual, or cognitive tasks to be generated according to Sherrington's law [18].

The resting pattern of blood flow in the brain of a normal subject was found to be highly characteristic and reproducible. It served as a point of departure for the interpretation of the functional patterns recorded during different tasks. Lassen and colleagues found an increase in CBF of about 20 percent in the visual association cortex when the subject was presented with a visual stimulus. Similarly, auditory stimuli resulted in an increase in blood flow to the primary auditory cortex. The effects of tactile stimulation were studied by Per Roland in Copenhagen in collaboration with Lassen. Voluntary movements of the hand were studied by Jes Olesen in Copenhagen in collaboration with Lassen [18].

Bo Siesjo and his coworkers at the University Hospital in Lund studied the effects of anxiety and pain on cerebral blood flow. They studied rats awakening from anesthesia after they had been paralyzed by a muscle-relaxant drug of the curare type. The stress of the animals' waking in a state of paralysis gave rise to an enormous increase in CBF. The increase could be diminished by removing the adrenals and could be completely abolished with drugs that blocked epinephrine receptors. This research showed the role of stress hormones like epinephrine on cerebral blood flow [18].

Another method for measuring regional cerebral blood flow with great spatial resolution and precision in animals was autoradiography [19]. This method involved the systemic administration of a radiolabeled compound of interest. When the compound reached the organ of interest the animal was sacrificed and the organ removed, sliced, and placed on X-ray film, enabling researchers to assess the distribution of radiolabeled compound [4]. Kety and colleagues developed an autoradiography method using trifluoroiodomethane ($CF_3I^{[131]}$). They showed a local increase in cerebral blood flow in the visual pathways of cats upon retinal stimulation by strobe lights. The $CF_3I^{[131]}$ was later modified for use with $C^{[14]}$ autoradiography and a nonvolatile tracer, first [$C^{[14]}$] antipyrine and then [$C^{[14]}$] iodoantipyrine. Kety's method was later adapted for use in humans with $H_2O^{[15]}$ and PET was the equivalent of autoradiograms in vivo [16,17].

Cerebral blood flow serves regions of the brain and is sensitive to systemic factors, but energy metabolism is a function of individual cells. Measurement of energy metabolism could be used to provide better resolution and specificity in response to altered neuronal functional activity [16,20]. Kety's student, Louis Sokoloff, studied the compound 2-deoxyglucose (DG), a reversible competitive inhibitor of glucose-6-phosphate, an important part of the glycolytic pathway. In 1969, he began research with [$C^{[14]}$] DG, a safer and longer-lasting radiotracer, and developed quantitative autoradiography of cerebral glucose utilization (CMRglc) in the rat. CMRglc increased in light-stimulated primary visual cortex with exquisite details, including the functional columns. In 1976, Sokoloff collaborated with radiochemists Alfred Wolf and Joanna Fowler and synthesized 2-[$F^{[18]}$] fluoro-2-deoxy-D-glucose (FDG), one of the most widely used radiotracers today [3,20].

THE EVOLUTION OF PET SCANNERS

In 1953, well before computerized tomography was invented, physicist Gordon Brownell and neurosurgeon William Sweet at Massachusetts General Hospital designed a positron scanner for localization of brain tumors. This device consisted of two sodium iodide detectors mounted in columns on an adjustable platform that moved in a rectilinear fashion. A printing mechanism recorded the coincidence counting rate on carbonized paper. They used radionuclides copper-64 and arsenic-75 [1,3,13].

In 1956, David Kuhl, a resident at the University of Pennsylvania, modified Cassen's scintillation detector and developed the photoscanner. In his design, a radioisotope emission-activated glow lamp provided grayscale images with greater sensitivity and resolution than ever before. Kuhl developed several single photon emission computed tomography (SPECT) devices known as Mark II, Mark III, and Mark IV in 1964, 1970, and 1976, respectively. These early devices predated X-ray CT, developed in 1971 by Godfrey Hounsfield. Kuhl improved the machines to measure physiologic function in three dimensions and to develop cross-sectional reconstructions. These machines are considered the forerunners of SPECT, PET, and CT technology [3].

In the mid-1950s, Ter-Pogossian and colleagues at Washington University in St. Louis worked with oxygen-15 (half-life 2.5 minutes), produced by a cyclotron built in the early 1940s in the physics department. They studied mice with mammary adenocarcinomas, using autoradiography to map the distribution of the injected oxygen-15. These early experiments stimulated interest in the use of short-lived radioactive gases and led in 1955 to building of the first medical cyclotron located on the grounds of Hammersmith Hospital in London. This was followed by installations at Massachusetts General Hospital and Washington University's Mallinckrodt Institute of Radiology in 1965. Subsequently, the US Department of Energy later funded hospital cyclotrons at UCLA, the University of Chicago, and Memorial Sloan Kettering Institute in New York. Existing cyclotrons at UC Berkeley and Ohio State continued to be used to produce radionuclides of biological importance [13]. Worldwide, medical cyclotrons were also soon installed at McGill University, in Montreal, Canada, and at the Frederic Joliot Clinical Research Hospital at Orsay, France.

Even before the introduction of positron imaging devices, the group led by Mark Raichle at St. Louis started to use oxygen-15 labeled water, carbon monoxide, and oxy-hemoglobin to measure in humans regional CBF, cerebral blood volume (CBV), mean transit time (MTT), oxygen extraction fraction (OEF), and $CMRO_2$ by curve stripping of data acquired using single probe detectors. This technique required intracarotid injection as part of carotid angiograms and was invasive. Raichle was later instrumental in investigating the brain regions active at rest and in response to various situations and stimuli.

Inspired by the introduction of the X-ray CT scan by Hounsfield in 1972, Ter-Pogossian and colleagues realized that if an image of the density of a transverse section of the body could be reconstructed from the measured attenuation of highly focused X-ray beams projected through the section, then the distribution of a radionuclide within the section could also be accurately and quantitively reconstructed from its emissions. This resulted in the design and construction of a machine for positron emission tomography, christened positron emission transaxial tomography (PETT). The term "transaxial" was later dropped [4].

Ter-Pogossian and coworkers built an apparatus that incorporated the features of Kuhl's device and a positron detection system similar to that developed by Brownell. The prototype PETT basically consisted of 24 NaI scintillation detectors placed in a hexagonal array. Each opposing pair of detectors was connected in coincidence such that events were accepted only when two photons were recorded by the two detectors simultaneously. The subject under study was placed on a computer-controlled rotating platform in the center of the hexagon. The data collected from the 12 pairs of detectors was used to reconstruct an image of the cross-section distribution of activity by a computer-applied algorithm. They chose a Fourier-based algorithm developed by the Biomedical Computer Laboratory at the Washington University School of Medicine. The overall resolution of PETT was first evaluated using three capillary tubes containing a solution of $Cu^{[64]}$, placed in an 18-centimeter-diameter cylindrical phantom filled with water. Animal studies were then conducted in dogs through two sets of experiments using $H_2O^{[15]}$, $N^{[13]}H_3$ and $C^{[11]}O$-hemoglobin [21].

The prototypical tabletop models, PETT I and PETT II, were then expanded to the clinically applicable PETT III whole-body camera that consisted of 48 NaI detectors placed in a hexagonal array with eight detectors on a side. The detector assembly scanned simultaneously in linear and rotational directions for the necessary linear and angular sampling of the data. The detection field of view was large enough to accommodate any position of the human body. The unit had sufficient detection efficiencies to complete scans in two to four minutes with 500,000–2,000,000 counts collected from 10 to 15 mCi of injected material. This capability was important for the imaging of short-lived isotopes $C^{[11]}$, $N^{[13]}$, and $O^{[15]}$. PETT III was used extensively for both patient and animal studies [1,22].

PETT III was sold to Brookhaven National Laboratory to acquire funds to build a better scanner at Washington University. Ter-Pogossian and his group along with Raichle conducted animal and human studies with carotid injections of $O^{[15]}$ labeled water, carbon monoxide, and oxy-hemoglobin to measure quantitatively in humans the regional CBF, cerebral blood volume (CBV), mean transit time (MTT), oxygen extraction fraction (OEF), and the cerebral metabolic rate of oxygen ($CMRO_2$) by curve stripping of data acquired with other external detectors. They became pioneers in the use of $O^{[15]}$ radioisotopes. They showed the physiological coupling of regional CBF and $CMRO_2$ in healthy subjects [23]. Eventually, PETT V and PETT VI were developed. PETT VI was commissioned in 1980 and was developed strictly for the brain. It could handle very high count rates and gave quick measurements. The majority of techniques for brain mapping were developed on PETT VI. It was decommissioned as a human instrument in 1993 but is still used for animal studies [24]. In parallel, Michael Phelps at UCLA developed the ECAT PET scanner with an industrial partner, and the first-ever commercial ECAT scanner, which could acquire a single brain 20-millimeter-thick axial slice at a time. It was delivered to a research center in Orsay, France, in late 1977 and was routinely used in human studies in early 1978.

CEREBROVASCULAR DISEASE AND BRAIN FUNCTION USING PET

The first major discoveries from PET in cerebrovascular diseases and stroke were derived from oxygen-15 based studies and were published in 1981. The most widely used technique was developed by Terry Jones at Hammersmith Cyclotron Unit in London, and involved continuous inhalation of carbon dioxide, which labeled circulating water, followed by continuous inhalation of molecular oxygen, which labeled both circulating hemoglobin and water, until equilibrium between inflow and radioactive decay was reached (about eight minutes later) [25]. This technique allowed mapping of CBF and also the OEF and the $CMRO_2$. This technique together with alternative oxygen-15 based techniques, notable using an intravenous bolus of labeled water to map perfusion, were extensively used in the 1980s and 1990s to study brain disorders and to map focal activations in healthy and damaged brain. These studies opened the way to major physiological discoveries as well as to functional MRI [2].

Robert Harold Ackerman, director of the Massachusetts General Hospital's neurovascular laboratory, was a pioneer in stroke imaging and prevention. In his seminal 1981 article, "Positron Imaging in Ischemic Stroke Disease Using Compounds Labeled with Oxygen 15: Initial Results of Clinicophysiologic Correlations," he reported alterations in brain tissue metabolism following stroke that are still highly relevant to current, novel "late window" (6–24 hours post onset) treatment trials. He reported that in acute stroke, PET data on oxygen metabolism correlated better with tissue viability than data reflecting cerebral blood flow [26,27].

Jean-Claude Baron, a young neurologist from Paris, initially trained by Robert Ackerman at MGH, started PET investigations on healthy subjects, acute/subacute stroke patients, and patients with continuing symptoms distal to carotid occlusion at the Orsay PET center in Paris in early 1978. He documented focal uncoupling of blood flow and oxygen metabolism after ischemic stroke. His work showed that some stroke patients had increased perfusion, post-recanalization hyperperfusion with low OEF, so-called luxury perfusion [28], which had been predicted by Niels Lassen in 1966 [29]. He also noted inverse uncoupling, focal hypoperfusion with high OEF, both in non-recanalized acute stroke patients [30] and in unstable patients with chronic carotid artery occlusion, which he termed "misery perfusion" [28]. He showed its reversibility following extra-intra-cranial artery bypass as a means to recanalize brain distal to chronic carotid occlusion [28]. He considered misery perfusion the hallmark of reversible cerebral ischemia, accounting for "hemodynamic" transient ischemic attacks in patients with chronic severe stenosis or occlusion of large cerebral arteries [28]. This condition in acute human stroke patients was the PET equivalent of the viable "ischemic penumbra" described by Lindsay Symon and his colleagues in baboons [31]. These studies were instrumental in fostering clinical trials testing therapies to reperfuse the penumbra. In 1981, Baron reported a new observation: reduced CBF and $CMRO_2$ in the cerebellar hemisphere contralateral to acute supratentorial strokes. He considered that the cerebellar findings reflected loss of excitatory input to granule cells via the cortico-ponto-cerebellar pathway, as a remote effect of the stroke-induced damage [32]. This was the first demonstration of the existence of von Monakow's "diaschisis" concept from the early twentieth century. Baron named this intriguing phenomenon "crossed cerebellar diaschisis." Other examples of diaschisis were subsequently uncovered using PET.

During the early 1990s, as director of the INSERM at Caen, France, Baron noted marked between-patient heterogeneity in the physiology of patients with acute carotid territory ischemia. Some patients showed persistent penumbra; in others, the penumbra had very early progressed to irreversible damage, invariably predicting poor outcome. Patients who had spontaneously recanalized before PET scanning invariably had excellent outcomes [33]. These findings led clinicians to advocate the use of physiological imaging instead of time-since-stroke-onset to triage patients for reperfusion therapies and randomized trials [34].

Wolf-Dieter Heiss, an Austrian-born neuroscientist and the director of the Max-Planck-Institute for Neurological Research in Germany, initially investigated neuronal function in relation to local perfusion in cat models of ischemic stroke. He showed the brain's ability to survive blood flow reductions according to the length of time the brain was ischemic and the severity of the ischemia [35]. These findings together with Lindsay Symon's research on the ischemic penumbra and Robert Crowell's research in monkeys at MGH [36] became the basis for the development of effective therapy for stroke. Using PET, Heiss and Baron documented survival of the penumbra up to 24 hours and beyond in a fraction of acute stroke patients [33,37]. Their work, among others', many years later led to thrombectomy being licensed up to 24 hours in selected patients. Heiss's work also helped in recognition of patterns of functional activation in healthy controls and patients and contributed to the understanding of deficits and compensatory brain mechanisms [38].

PET VERSUS OTHER IMAGING MODALITIES IN RECENT DECADES

PET scanning had characterized the physiology of brain ischemia and brain metabolism. The results were quantitative and provided benchmarks for future research. During the late 1980s and afterward, the advent of diffusion/perfusion MRI and advanced CT techniques replaced PET as a clinical tool for evaluating stroke patients, following their validation against PET in stroke patients. Brain PET has largely remained a research tool for analyzing brain function and metabolism, currently by means of PET/MR "hybrid" scanners. Practical issues limited the use of PET in the clinic. Most PET isotopes have rapid decay and so need to be synthesized on demand. PET machines were complex and expensive to maintain and often needed oversight by trained physicists, so costs were high. The images derived were grainy and lacked anatomical detail as seen with MRI or CT. During the late years of the twentieth century, technical advances in MRI and CT made it possible to generate data that approximated PET. As applied to cerebrovascular diseases, nuclear medicine and PET had shown the way, but MRI and CT technology proved more practical in the clinic. However, hybrid PET/CT using FDG labeled with the two-hour half-life $F^{[18]}$, allowing transport to any hospital, has become a routine clinical tool to investigate suspected cancer patients as well as in the etiological investigation of suspected neurodegenerative conditions.

NOTES AND REFERENCES

1. Rich DA. A brief history of positron emission tomography. *J. Nucl. Med. Technol.* 1997 Mar 1;25(1):4–11.

2. Baron J-C, Jones T. Oxygen metabolism, oxygen extraction and positron emission tomography: Historical perspective and impact on basic and clinical neuroscience. *NeuroImage* 2012 Jun 1;61(2):492–504.

3. Portnow LH, Vaillancourt DE, Okun MS. The history of cerebral PET scanning. *Neurology* 2013 Mar 5;80(10):952–956.

4. Raichle ME. A brief history of human brain mapping. *Trends Neurosci.* 2009 Feb 1;32 (2):118–126.

5. Roy CS, Sherrington CS. On the regulation of the blood-supply of the brain. *J. Physiol.* 1890 Jan;11(1–2):85–158.

6. Fulton JF. Observations upon the vascularity of the human occipital lobe during visual activity. *Brain* 1928 Oct 1;51(3):310–320.

7. Positron discovered. August 2, 2016. *Physics Today*. Available at https://physicstoday .scitation.org/do/10.1063/PT.5.031277/abs/.

8. The Nobel Prize in Physics 1936. NobelPrize.org. Available at www.nobelprize.org/ prizes/physics/1936/anderson/biographical/.

9. Rhodes R. *The Making of the Atomic Bomb*. Simon and Schuster, 2012.

10. The Nobel Prize. Women who changed science: Irene Joliot-Curie. NobelPrize.org. Available at www.nobelprize.org/womenwhochangedscience/stories/irene-joliot-curie.

11. The Nobel Prize in Chemistry 1935. NobelPrize.org. Available at www.nobelprize.org/prizes/chemistry/1935/joliot-fred/biographical/.

12. Joliot F, Curie I. Artificial production of a new kind of radio-element. *Nature* 1934 Feb 1;133(3354):201–202.

13. Wagner HN. A brief history of positron emission tomography (PET). *Semin. Nucl. Med.* 1998 Jul 1;28(3):213–220.

14. Bailey DL, Townsend DW, Valk PE, Maisey MN (eds.). *Positron Emission Tomography: Basic Sciences*. London: Springer-Verlag, 2005.

15. Blahd WH. History of external counting procedures. *Semin. Nucl. Med.* 1979 Jul;9(3):159–163.

16. Sokoloff L. Historical review of developments in the field of cerebral blood flow and metabolism. In Fukuuchi Y, Tomita M, Koto A (eds.), *Ischemic Blood Flow in the Brain*. Keio University Symposia for Life Science and Medicine, vol. 6. Tokyo: Springer, 2001. https://doi.org/10.1007/978-4-431-67899-1_1.

17. Seymour Kety, MD, interviewed by Ayub Ommaya, MD. 2015. YouTube. Available at www.youtube.com/watch?v=VZL9jVWL-bY.

18. Lassen NA, Ingvar DH, Skinhøj E. Brain function and blood flow. *Sci. Am.* 1978 Oct;239(4):62–71.

19. Heistad DD, Kontos HA. Cerebral circulation. In Terjung R (ed.), *Comprehensive Physiology*. Available at https://onlinelibrary.wiley.com/doi/10.1002/cphy.cp020305.

20. Louis Sokoloff, MD, interviewed by Ayub Ommaya, MD. 2016. YouTube. Available at www.youtube.com/watch?v=oURD-neou8A&index=91&list=PLWscsgSk-BepdDVWmKLowNlDTR4ZxWYSm.

21. Ter-Pogossian MM et al. A positron-emission transaxial tomograph for nuclear imaging (PETT). *Radiology* 1975;114(1):89–98. doi:10.1148/114.1.89.

22. Hoffmann EJ, Phelps ME, Mullani NA, Higgins CS, Ter-Pogossian MM. Design and performance characteristics of a whole-body positron transaxial tomograph. *J. Nucl. Med.* 1976 Jun;17(6):493–502.

23. Raichle ME, Grubb RL, Gado MH, Eichling JO, Ter-Pogossian MM. Correlation between regional cerebral blood flow and oxidative metabolism: In vivo studies in man. *Arch. Neurol.* 1976 Aug;33(8):523–526.

24. Marcus E. Raichle, MD, interviewed by Sidney Goldring, MD. 2016. YouTube. Available at www.youtube.com/watch?v=XsDIpyaumIo.

25. Jones T, Chesler DA, Ter-Pogossian MM. The continuous inhalation of oxygen-15 for assessing regional oxygen extraction in the brain of man. *Br. J. Radiol.* 1976 Apr;49(580):339–343.

26. Lev MH, Romero JM, Schwamm LH, Cudkowicz ME, Brink JA. Robert H. Ackerman, MD, MPH (1935–2018). *AJNR Am. J. Neuroradiol.* 2019;40(3):E12–E13.

27. Ackerman RH, Correia JA, Alpert NM, Baron J-C, Gouliamos A, Grotta JC, et al. Positron imaging in ischemic stroke disease using compounds labeled with oxygen 15: Initial results of clinicophysiologic correlations. *Arch. Neurol.* 1981;38(9):537–543.

28. Baron JC, Bousser MG, Rey A, Guillard A, Comar D, Castaigne P. Reversal of focal "misery-perfusion syndrome" by extra-intracranial arterial bypass in hemodynamic cerebral ischemia. A case study with [15]O positron emission tomography. *Stroke* 1981;12:454–459.

29. Lassen NA. The luxury-perfusion syndrome and its possible relation to acute metabolic acidosis localised within the brain. *Lancet* 1966;2(7473):1113–1115.

30. Baron JC, Bousser MG, Comar D, Soussaline F, Castaigne P. Noninvasive tomographic study of cerebral blood flow and oxygen metabolism in vivo: Potentials,

limitations, and clinical applications in cerebral ischemic disorders. *Eur. Neurol.* 1981;20 (3):273–284.

31. Astrup J, Symon L, Branston NM, Lassen NA. *Thresholds of Cerebral Ischemica.* New York: Springer, 1977.

32. Baron JC, Bousser MG, Comar D, Castaigne P. "Crossed cerebellar diaschisis" in human supratentorial brain infarction. *Trans. Am. Neurol. Assoc.* 1981;105:459–461.

33. Marchal G, Serrati C, Rioux P, Petit-Taboué MC, Viader F, de la Sayette V, et al. PET imaging of cerebral perfusion and oxygen consumption in acute ischaemic stroke: Relation to outcome. *Lancet* 1993 Apr 10;341(8850):925–927.

34. Baron JC, von Kummer R, del Zoppo GJ. Treatment of acute ischemic stroke: Challenging the concept of a rigid and universal time window. *Stroke* 1995;26 (12):2219–2221.

35. Heiss WD, Rosner G. Functional recovery of cortical neurons as related to degree and duration of ischemia. *Ann. Neurol.* 1983;14(3):294–301.

36. Jones TH, Morawetz RB, Crowell RM, Marcoux FW, FitzGibbon SJ, DeGirolami U, et al. Thresholds of focal cerebral ischemia in awake monkeys. *J. Neurosurg.* 1981;54 (6):773–782.

37. Heiss WD, Huber M, Fink GR, Herholz K, Pietrzyk U, Wagner R, et al. Progressive derangement of periinfarct viable tissue in ischemic stroke. *J. Cereb. Blood Flow Metab.* 1992;12(2):193–203.

38. Wolf-Dieter Heiss. Wikipedia. 2020. Available at https://en.wikipedia.org/w/index .php?title=Wolf-Dieter_Heiss&oldid=934049598.

CHAPTER THIRTY SIX

CARDIAC IMAGING AND FUNCTION

The heart is a major source of brain embolism. Many stroke patients have coexistent coronary and valvular heart disease. Strokes can also cause secondary cardiac pathologies. Evaluation of the heart is an integral part of the care of stroke patients.

During the nineteenth century, implements began to be used to supplement the clinical history and physical examination of the heart. The stethoscope was introduced in 1819 by the French physician René Laennec. Before his time doctors placed their ears directly on the chest to be able to hear cardiac sounds. This proved embarrassing for women. Laennec commented that he recalled the "augmented impression of sound when conveyed through certain solid bodies" [1]. This fact led him to try rolling paper into a cylinder and applying one end to the region of the heart and the other to his ear. He then could "perceive the action of the heart much more clear and distinct than I had ever been able to do by the immediate application of the ear" [1].

Since then, many technological advances were made in cardiac imaging that enhanced knowledge of cardiac structure, function, and disease. The two most commonly performed cardiac tests – electrocardiography and echocardiography – are now considered essential components for the evaluation of stroke patients.

ELECTROCARDIOGRAPHY

The basic concepts that led to the invention of electrocardiography were discovered at the end of the eighteenth century. In 1786, Luigi Galvani, an Italian physician at the University of Bologna, was the first to notice that electrical current could be recorded in skeletal muscles. He recorded electrical activity in dissected muscles of a frog [2]. Galvani´s name was later given to the galvanometer, an instrument used to measure and record electricity. In 1842, Carlo Matteucci, a professor of physics at the University of Pisa, using a frog noted that electrical activity accompanied every heartbeat [3].

In 1887, Augustus Waller, a British physiologist working at St. Mary's Medical School in London, performed an electrocardiogram for the first time in a human. Augustus's father discovered Wallerian degeneration. Augustus Waller was born in Paris, educated in Geneva, and went to Aberdeen to qualify in medicine but later dedicated himself to physiology. To record the heart examination, he used a capillary electrometer and electrodes placed on the chest and back of the subject. The trace from the heartbeat was projected onto a photographic plate that was fixed to a toy train. The electrocardiograms recorded by Waller used five electrodes, one on each of the four extremities and the mouth, with 10 leads derived from the different combinations [4]. Waller often performed electrograms using his dog Jimmie, who would stand with his paws in glass jars of saline. At the time, Waller did not consider the idea of using his invention for clinical practice.

Willem Einthoven, a Dutch physiologist at the University of Leiden, attended Waller's lectures and gained an interest in the subject. He improved the capillary electrometer and named the deflection obtained as ABCD. The term "electrocardiogram" was introduced by Einthoven in 1893 at a Dutch medical meeting [5]. Later in 1895, he implemented a mathematical correction to improve the precision of the instrument that resulted in the curves that are now shown in electrocardiograms. He used the terminal part of the alphabet series (PQRST) to name these corrected deflections, according to the mathematical tradition established by René Descartes. ("N" is used with other meanings in mathematics and "O" is the origin of the Cartesian coordinates [6].) Einthoven also reduced the number of electrodes to three: I, II, and III. The resulting three leads were used to construct Einthoven's triangle [5]. In 1903, Einthoven discussed with manufacturers the possibility of commercializing his invention. Two firms later produced the machine. In 1924, Einthoven was awarded the Nobel Prize in physiology and medicine "for the discovery of the mechanism of the electrocardiogram." Waller had died in 1922 and therefore was not eligible for a joint award.

Sir Edward Schafer of the University of Edinburgh was the first to buy a string galvanometer electrograph for clinical use in 1908. The first electrocardiogram machine was introduced to the United States in 1909 by Alfred Cohn at Mt. Sinai Hospital in New York [7].

Sir Thomas Lewis, of University College Hospital London, was the first person in England to apply electrocardiography to clinical investigation. In 1909 he discovered that delirium cordis, a clinical diagnosis of irregular heartbeat, was a result of atrial fibrillation [8]. He had been a visitor at Einthoven's laboratory. Lewis published an article in the *British Medical Journal* in 1912 concerning clinical and electrocardiographic observations of atrial fibrillation [9]. He claimed at the time that atrial fibrillation was a common clinical condition. Carl Rothberger and Heinrich Winterberg, two German physicians, showed that atrial fibrillation was characterized by three features: an irregular ventricular rate, the absence of P waves, and the presence of peculiar oscillations in the tracing [10].

In 1937, Taro Takemi invented a portable electrocardiograph machine [11]. He was a Japanese physician who was later a member of the research team that investigated the effects of the atomic bomb in Hiroshima in 1945.

The American Heart Association and the Cardiac Society of Great Britain in 1938 defined the standard positions, and wiring, of the chest leads V1–V6. The "V" represents voltage [12]. Emanuel Goldberger in 1942 created the augmented limb leads and aVR, aVL, and aVF.

In 1949, Norman Jeff Holter, a biophysicist working at the University of California, created a backpack that could record the electrocardiogram and transmit the signal of a person carrying it continuously for 24 hours or more. He had created a portable cardiac telemetry device. At that time, the backpack weighed 75 pounds [13]. In 1979, the Association for the Advancement of Medical Instrumentation (AAMI) bestowed on Holter the Laufman-Greatbatch Award. His system was progressively refined with time resulting in smaller and lighter devices that were later combined with digital recording, and now widely used to record ambulatory electrocardiograms.

In 1954, the American Heart Association published their recommendation for standardization of the 12-lead electrocardiogram [14]. In 1968, Henry Marriott introduced the Modified Chest Lead 1 (MCL1) to monitor patients in coronary care. Continuous monitoring of the heart rhythm is currently performed in most stroke units. During the 1990s, implantable loop recorders were introduced by Krahn. They were used to record heart rhythm for up to three years and could be interrogated transcutaneously [15].

Several clinical trials performed at the beginning of the twenty-first century showed that long-term cardiac monitoring performed in patients with cryptogenic stroke improved the probability of detecting atrial fibrillation.

ECHOCARDIOGRAPHY

The concept of echo reflection was first introduced by Lazzaro Spallanzani at the end of the eighteenth century. He showed that bats used reflected echoes of inaudible sound to navigate [16]. In 1880, Pierre and Marie Curie in France discovered piezoelectricity and consequently the possibility of creating ultrasonic waves [17].

In 1946, André Denier, a French physiotherapist, suggested the use of ultrasound to visualize structures located inside the human body [16]. In May 1953, Inge Edler and Hellmuth Hertz met to discuss the possibilities of using ultrasound for investigating the heart [18]. Edler was a cardiologist at Lund University in Sweden and was responsible for the cardiology department. Hertz was a physicist, son of a Nobel Prize winner in physics (Gustav Hertz), and nephew of the man whose name was used to describe wave frequencies (Heinrich Hertz) [16]. The main goal at the time was to use the invention to diagnose mitral regurgitation. Inge Edler as the director of the cardiology department was responsible for the preoperative evaluation of valvular heart disease. He intended to find a way to study the presence of mitral valve disease using noninvasive means. They were the first to use M-mode echocardiography. At the time Edler called this technique "ultrasound cardiography" (UCG). Hertz was the first person to be examined. In order to know exactly what cardiac structures he was studying with the ultrasound examination, Edler started by studying patients who were dying. He initially marked the location and direction of the ultrasonic beam, and after the patient died, he performed an autopsy to correlate his examination findings. Edler reported several of his findings with the echocardiogram in a review article that was published in the *Acta Medica Scandinavica* in 1961 [18]. Elder and Hertz are cited as the fathers of echocardiography.

Japanese investigators during the same time were interested in developing Doppler technology to use in the heart. Doppler technology made it possible to measure and quantify the speed and direction of blood flow within the heart [16,18].

The first American report on the use of diagnostic ultrasound to study the heart was published in the journal *Circulation* in 1963 by Joiner, Reid, and Bond [19]. Joiner was a cardiologist at the University of Pennsylvania and Reid was a graduate student there. Because at that time the ultrasound examination of the brain was called "echoencephalography," the examination of the heart was called "echocardiography." In 1960, contrast echocardiography was introduced at the University of Rochester by Gramiak and Shah [18].

The initial echocardiograms were produced by placing a probe or transducer on the chest wall over the heart (transthoracic echocardiography (TTE)).

Transesophageal echocardiography (TEE), which involved the placement of a probe in the esophagus, was mainly developed by European investigators and introduced in the late 1960s [18]. Since the left atrium of the heart lies just in front of the esophagus, TEE allowed better imaging of the left atrium and left atrial appendage, areas where clots often formed.

The first academic course dedicated solely to cardiac ultrasound was taught in Indianapolis in January 1968. The first book on echocardiography was published in 1972 [20]. Introduction of echocardiography and ambulatory cardiac rhythm monitoring in the 1970s and 1980s contributed greatly to the detection of cardioembolic sources of embolism. The rheumatic and infective valvular diseases that were previously described as sources of cardiac embolism, as well as left ventricular segmental disease sometimes with the presence of thrombi, could now be well documented. Atrial septal characteristics like a patent foramen ovale and atrial septum aneurysms were shown to be frequent in patients with strokes of undetermined etiology. Pierre Amarenco in France showed that protruding aortic atheromas found during transesophageal echocardiography and necropsy were prevalent in ischemic stroke patients [21]. Several other minor cardioembolic sources were documented, such as mitral annulus calcification and mitral valve prolapse with myxomatous degeneration.

CARDIAC CT AND CARDIAC MRI

Since the end of the twentieth century and the beginning of the twenty-first century, both cardiac CT and cardiac MRI have also been used to image the heart in the context of evaluation of stroke patients [22]. These exams complement the images obtained by echocardiography. Cardiac MRI, in particular, has helped to uncover possible new stroke etiologies that were not traditionally considered, such as atrial cardiopathy and ventricular cardiomyopathies. Currently, studies are evaluating the possibility of using cardiac CT at the time of patient's admission to the emergency department to document the early presence of cardiac thrombi. Although not now used in routine clinical practice, both of these exams are considered in patients with a cryptogenic stroke when suspicion of a cardioembolic etiology is high.

REFERENCES

1. Nuland S. René Laennec. In *Doctors: The Biography of Medicine*. New York: Vintage Books, 1988, pp. 200–237. Laennec R. *De l'auscultation mediate*. Paris: Brosson et Chaudé libraires, 1819.
2. AlGhatrif M, Lindsay J. A brief review: History to understand fundamentals of electrocardiography. *J. Community Hosp. Intern. Med. Perspect.* 2012 Apr 30;2(1).

3. Matteucci C. Sur un phenomene physiologique produit par les muscles en contraction. *Ann. Chim. Phys.* 1842;6:339–341.

4. Waller AD. On the electromotive changes connected with the beat of the mammalian heart, and of the human heart in particular. *Phil. Trans. R. Soc. Lond. B* 1889;180:169–194.

5. Einthoven W. The different forms of the human electrocardiogram and their signification. *Lancet* 1912;1:853–861.

6. Henson JR. Descartes and the ECG lettering series. *J. Hist. Med. Allied Sci.* 1971;26 (2):181–186.

7. Burnett J. The origins of the electrocardiograph as a clinical instrument. *Med. Hist. Suppl.* 1985;5:53–76. PubMed PMID: 3915524; PubMed Central PMCID: PMCPMC2557409.

8. Lewis T. Report CXIX. Auricular fibrillation: A common clinical condition. *Br. Med. J.* 1909;2(2552):1528.

9. Lewis T. A Lecture on the evidences of auricular fibrillation treated historically: Delivered at University College Hospital. *Br. Med. J.* 1912;1:57–60.

10. Rothberger CJ, Wiiterberg H. Vorhofflimmem und Arhythmia perpetua. *Wien Klin. Wochenschr.* 1909;22:839–844.

11. Taro Takemi. Wikipedia. Available at https://en.wikipedia.org/wiki/Taro_Takemi.

12. Barnes AR, Pardee HEB, White PD, et al. Standardization of precordial leads. *Am. Heart J.* 1938;15:235–239.

13. Holter NJ, Generelli JA. Remote recording of physiologic data by radio. *Rocky Mountain Med. J.* 1949:747–751.

14. Wilson FN, Kossmann CE, Burch GE, Goldberger E, Graybiel A, Hecht HH, et al. Recommendations for standardization of electrocardiographic and vectorcardiographic leads. *Circulation* 1954;10(4):564–573.

15. Krahn AD, Klein GI. Yee R, Norros C. Maturation of the sensed electrogram amplitude over time in a new subcutaneous implantable loop recorder. *PACE* 1997;20:1686–1690.

16. Feigenbaum H. *Echocardiography*. Philadelphia: Lea & Febiger, 1972. Chapter 34 discusses the use of ultrasound in cerebrovascular disease.

17. Curie P, Curie J. Developpement, par pression de l'electricite polaire dans les cristaux hemiedres a faces inclinees. *Comptes Rendus* 1880;91:291–295.

18. Feigenbaum H. Evolution of echocardiography. *Circulation* 1996;93:1321–1327. Edler I, Lindström K. The history of echocardiography. *Ultrasound Med. Biol.* 2004;30 (12):1565–1644. Edler I, Gustafson A, Karlefors T, Christensson B. Ultrasound cardiography. *Acta Med. Scand. Suppl.* 1961;370:5–123.

19. Joyner CR Jr, Reid JM, Bond JP. Reflected ultrasound in the assessment of mitral valve disease. *Circulation* 1963;27:503–511.

20. Feigenbaum H. *Echocardiography*. Philadelphia: Lea & Febiger, 1972.

21. Amarenco P, Duyckaerts C, Tzourio C, Henin D, Bousser M-G, Hauw J-J. The prevalence of ulcerated plaques in the aortic arch in patients with stroke. *N. Engl. J. Med.* 1992;326:221–225. Amarenco P, Cohen A, Baudrimont M, Bousser M-G. Transesophageal echocardiographic detection of aortic arch disease in patients with cerebral infarction. *Stroke* 1992;23:1005–1010.

22. Fonseca AC, Ferro JM, Almeida AG. Cardiovascular magnetic resonance imaging and its role in the investigation of stroke: An update. *J. Neurol.* 2021 Jan 13. doi: 10.1007/s00415-020-10393-6.

CHAPTER THIRTY SEVEN

STROKE-RELATED TERMS

Apoplexy was the first term used [1]. The term *apoplexia* ("struck down with violence," "to strike suddenly") was probably first used by Hippocrates [2]. The term was used when individuals developed rapid loss of consciousness and/or various manifestations of brain dysfunction. The "apoplexy" concept was used to describe varied disorders, later identified as acute cerebral events, vascular and nonvascular, as well as noncerebral acute occurrences such as myocardial infarction, pulmonary embolism, and intoxications, among others [1].

Stroke. The first recorded use of the word "stroke" in the English literature was in 1599 when "an excellent Cinnamome water for the stroke of Gods hande" was recommended [3,4]. The word conveyed the sudden and seemingly random nature of the acute event. William Cole is usually cited as the first person to use the word in a medical communication. Cole was a British physician and contemporary of Thomas Sydenham and John Locke. Cole wrote an essay on apoplexy that was published in 1689. He avowed that apoplexy was a disorder of the brain: "When the persons affected have not time allowed them to declare their perceptions 'tis evident that the stroke is impressed on the animal faculty ... which must argue the cause to reside about the original of it, the Brain, since from thence only that faileure can so generally be affected" [5].

The term *stroke* was variously applied to indicate an injury to the nervous system or eye caused by an abnormality of the blood vessels supply. In 1970 the World Health Organization published a definition still used today: "rapidly developing clinical signs of focal (or global) disturbance of cerebral function, lasting more than 24 hours or leading to death, with no apparent cause other than that of vascular origin" [6]. The WHO used a simple definition of stroke in 1971: "A sudden onset of disturbance of focal brain function due to the blockage or rupture of blood vessels" [7]. In 2013, a committee of the American Heart/American Stroke Association updated the definition. They urged classification by stroke subtype if known. The following definitions were suggested. Ischemic stroke: An episode of neurological dysfunction caused by focal cerebral, spinal, or retinal infarction. Central nervous system infarction: Brain, spinal cord, or retinal cell death attributable to ischemia, based on (1) pathological, imaging, or other objective evidence of cerebral, spinal cord, or retinal focal ischemic injury in a defined vascular distribution or (2) clinical evidence of cerebral, spinal cord, or retinal focal ischemic injury based on symptoms persisting $\geq$24 hours or until death, and other etiologies excluded. Intracerebral hemorrhage: A focal collection of blood within the brain parenchyma or ventricular system that is not caused by trauma. Stroke caused by subarachnoid hemorrhage: Rapidly developing signs of neurological dysfunction and/or headache because of bleeding into the subarachnoid space which is not caused by trauma. Stroke caused by cerebral venous thrombosis: Infarction or hemorrhage in the brain, spinal cord, or retina because of thrombosis of a cerebral venous structure. Symptoms or signs caused by reversible edema without infarction or hemorrhage do not qualify as stroke. Definition of stroke, not otherwise specified: An episode of acute neurological dysfunction presumed to be caused by ischemia or hemorrhage, persisting $\geq$24 hours or until death, but without sufficient evidence to be classified as one of the above [6].

The terms *cerebrovascular accident* (CVA), *accident cérébrovasculaire* (French) and *accidente cerebrovascular* (Spanish) were also widely used but are discouraged. The disorder is not an accident but is related to knowable pathology, and these terms are vague and nonspecific. During the 1970s and 1980s, various terms based on timing were used to modify *stroke*: completed stroke, stroke-in-evolutions, progressive stroke, stroke in progress. These terms were variously defined and variously applied. Classification in one or the other of these time courses did not reflect whether or not a brain infarct had occurred or the cause and mechanism of the brain ischemia, or the prognosis for further brain ischemia [8]. When modern brain and vascular imaging became widespread, these terms were abandoned.

Transient ischemic attack (TIA). Stroke has always implied some persistent neurological injury and deficit. But what should temporary episodes of ischemia be called? The textbooks of Sir William Osler, Sir William Gowers, and Kinnier Wilson all mention temporary warnings before a stroke but are very sparse on details [9]. C. Miller Fisher, at the First Princeton Conference on

Cerebrovascular Diseases, held in 1954, brought the issue of transient attacks to the attention of the attendees:

> If a satisfactory history can be obtained . . . one finds in a great many cases that there had been a warning prior to the stroke. The warnings may go back weeks or months. There may have been only one or as many as 500. Some of these very interesting cases lying in the wards are described simply as "had a stroke this morning" but in going into the details, many premonitory symptoms may be elicited. I have seen a man with eight attacks a day for two months, each attack characterized by numbness around the lip, numbness of the thumb and index finger and drooping of the lip. Attacks occurred in physicians' offices. Finally the patient awakened one morning with a massive hemiplegia from which there has been practically no recovery. [10]

During the first two Princeton conferences, held in 1954 and 1957, warning spells before strokes were discussed and various terms for these temporary episodes were suggested: intermittent vascular insufficiency, ischemic recurrent attacks, recurrent focal cerebral ischemic attacks, transient cerebral ischemia, and transient ischemic attacks [10,11]. At the Fourth Princeton Conference, held in 1965, the conference attendees agreed on the term *transient ischemic attack* (TIA) [12]. An Ad Hoc Committee on Cerebrovascular Disease in 1975 stated that transient ischemic attack is defined as a "cerebral dysfunction of ischemic nature lasting no longer than 24 hours with a tendency to recur" [13]. The 24-hour definition was arbitrarily chosen. Later analyses showed that most TIAs lasted less than one hour [14–16]. Loeb and colleagues proposed a general term, "reversible ischemic attacks" (RIA), defined as "A focal neurologic deficit that lasts for less than 24 hours, is presumed to be of vascular origin, and is confined to an area of the brain or eye perfused by a specific artery" [17].

With the advent of CT and later MRI, it became evident that a surprising number of patients with clinical TIAs had brain infarcts in regions appropriate to the transient neurological symptoms [18,19]. The term suggested for this occurrence was "cerebral infarction with transient signs" (CITS) [18]. Other acronyms were introduced if the transient episodes lasted longer than 24 hours or if some deficit remained: SFR: stroke with full recovery; RIND: reversible ischemic neurological deficit; and PRIND: partially reversible neurological deficit [20].

A group of nationwide US stroke experts met regularly from 2000 to 2002 to discuss redefining TIA terminology and to reach a consensus on a new definition, treatment guidelines, and risk factors [14,15]. They chose a new definition of TIA consonant with available information from series of cases and from brain imaging: "Transient ischemic attack is a brief period of neurological dysfunction caused by focal brain or retinal ischemia with clinical symptoms typically lasting less than an hour, and without evidence of acute infarction" [15].

After publication of a 2009 position paper from the American Heart/ American Stroke organizations, TIA has been defined as a neurological deficit typically lasting less than one hour with no evidence of stroke on imaging [21].

Clinicians sought information about how often patients with TIAs had strokes. How soon after the last TIA? Was the frequency of stroke after TIA different if there was imaging evidence of a relevant brain infarct? Because clinicians with experience and training in cerebrovascular disease were in short supply and technology for acute imaging assessment was limited, doctors sought a useful score that could predict the occurrence of stroke in the days after TIA. Triage of TIA patients using this score could determine who should be urgently evaluated in the hospital or dedicated clinic and who could be seen on a nonurgent basis. The ABCD2 score was most commonly used and studied. ABCD2 was tallied as follows: age > 60; BP > 140/90; diabetes: one point; speech disturbance, one point; unilateral weakness, two points; duration of symptoms: 10–59 minutes, 1 point; > 60 min, two points. The maximum score was seven points. Low scores were predicted to be associated with a low frequency of acute stroke. Hospital admission and urgent evaluation and treatment were usually recommended for scores greater than four.

Pierre Amarenco, a professor of neurology in Paris, recruited stroke experts to organize a study of TIA patients. Amarenco had previously made important stroke contributions regarding the aorta as a source of brain embolism and about cerebellar infarction. The TIA registry recruited patients who had had a TIA or minor stroke within the previous seven days and evaluated them at sites that had systems dedicated to urgent evaluation of patients. Between 2009 and 2011, the registry enrolled 4,789 patients at 61 sites in 21 countries. More than three quarters of patients were evaluated by stroke specialists within 24 hours after symptom onset [22,23]. Patients with imaging evidence of relevant brain infarction (technically, minor strokes) had a higher frequency of strokes than those with negative studies [24]. Higher scores on ABCD2 did corelate with more frequent strokes, but an important number of patients with low scores also developed strokes [22,23,25].

Because the etiology and evaluation of patients with TIAs and minor strokes were identical and those with either had an important risk of developing new brain infarction, Kidwell and Warach suggested using the term "acute ischemic cerebrovascular syndrome" to include both TIA and minor stroke patients [26].

REFERENCES

1. Pound P, Bury M, Ebrahim S. From apoplexy to stroke. *Age and Ageing* 1997;26:331–337. Writings about apoplexy are reviewed at length in Chapter 8.
2. Adams F. *The Genuine Works of Hippocrates: Translated from the Greek.* Baltimore, MD: Williams and Wilkins, 1939. Hippocrates's contributions to stroke are discussed in Chapter 1.

3. *Oxford English Dictionary*, 2nd ed. Oxford: Clarendon Press, 1989.

4. Barnhart RK. *The Barnhart Dictionary of Etymology*. New York: HW Wilson, 1988.

5. Cole W. *A Physico-Medical Essay Concerning the Late Frequency of Apoplexies Together with a General Method of Their Prevention and Cure: In a Letter to a Physician*. Oxford: The Theater, 1869. Reprint: New York: Classics of Neurology & Neurosurgery Library, 1995.

6. Sacco LR, Kasner SE, Broderick JP, Caplan LR, et al. (AHA/ASA Expert Consensus Document) An updated definition of stroke for the 21st century: A statement for healthcare professionals from the American Heart Association/American Stroke Association. *Stroke* 2013;44:2064–2089.

7. Cerebrovascular diseases: Prevention, treatment, and rehabilitation. WHO Technical Report Series No. 469, 1971.

8. Caplan LR. Are terms such as completed stroke or RIND of continued usefulness? *Stroke* 1983;14:431–433. Caplan LR. Terms describing brain ischemia by tempo are no longer useful. A polemic (with apologies to Shakespeare). *Surg. Neurol.* 1993;40:91–95.

9. These texts are mentioned and discussed in Chapter 14.

10. Luckey H, ed. *Cerebral Vascular Diseases: Transactions of a Conference Held under the Auspices of the American Heart Association, Princeton, New Jersey, January 24–26, 1954*. New York: Grune & Stratton, 1955, pp. 95–96.

11. Wright IS, Millikan C, eds. *Cerebral Vascular Diseases: Transactions of the Second Conference Held under the Auspices of the American Heart Association, Princeton, NJ, January 16–18, 1957*. New York: Grune & Stratton, 1958.

12. Siekert RG, Whisnant JP, eds. *Cerebrovascular Disease: Fourth Conference*. New York: Grune & Stratton, 1965.

13. A classification and outline of cerebrovascular disease. *Stroke* 1975;6:564–616.

14. Easton JD, Albers GW, Caplan LR, Saver JL, Sherman MD (for the TIA Working Group). (Discussion) Reconsideration of TIA terminology and definitions. *Neurology* 2004;62(6):S29–S34.

15. Albers G, Caplan LR, Easton JD, et al. Transient ischemic attack: Proposal for a new definition. *N. Engl. J. Med.* 2002;347:1713–1716.

16. Mohr JP. Historical perspective. *Neurology* 2004 62(suppl 6):S3–S6.

17. Loeb C, Priano A, Albano C. Clinical features and long-term follow-up of patients with reversible ischemic attacks (RIA). *Acta Neurologica Scandinavica* 1978;57:471–480.

18. Bogousslavsky J, Regli F. Cerebral infarction with transient signs (CITS): Do TIAs correspond to small deep infarcts in internal carotid artery occlusion? *Stroke* 1984;15:536–539.

19. Waxman S, Toole JF. Temporal profile resembling TIA in the setting of cerebral infarction. *Stroke* 1983;14:433–437.

20. Bernstein EF, Browse NL. The CHAT classification of stroke. *Ann. Surg.* 1989;209 (2):242–248.

21. Easton JD, Saver JL, Albers GW, et al. Definition and evaluation of transient ischemic attack: A scientific statement for healthcare professionals from the American Heart Association/American Stroke Association Stroke Council; Council on Cardiovascular Surgery and Anesthesia; Council on Cardiovascular Radiology and Intervention; Council on Cardiovascular Nursing; and the Interdisciplinary Council on Peripheral Vascular Disease. *Stroke* 2009;40:2276–2293.

22. Amarenco P, Lavallée PC, Labreuche J, et al. for the TIAregistry.org Investigators. One-year risk of stroke after transient ischemic attack or minor stroke. *N. Engl. J. Med.* 2016;374:1533–1542.

23. Amarenco P, Lavallée PC, Monteiro Tavares L, et al. for the TIAregistry.org Investigators. Five-year risk of stroke after TIA or minor ischemic stroke. *N. Engl. J. Med.* 2018;378:2182–2190.

24. Giles MF, Albers GW, Amarenco P, et al. Early stroke risk and ABCD2 score performance in tissue- vs time-defined TIA: A multicenter study. *Neurology* 2011;77:1222–1228.

25. Lou M, Safgdar A, Edlow J, et al. Can ABCD2 score predict the need for in-hospital intervention in patients with transient ischemic attacks? *Int. J. Emerg. Med.* 2010;3:75–80. Amarenco P, Labreuche J, Lavallée PC. Patients with transient ischemic attack with $ABCD^2$ <4 can have similar 90-day stroke risk as patients with transient ischemic attack with $ABCD^2$ ≥4. *Stroke* 2012;43:863–865. Al-Khaled M, Eggers J. Early hospitalization of patients with TIA: A prospective, population-based study. *J. Stroke Cardiovasc. Dis.* 2014;23:99–105.

26. Kidwell CS, Warach S. Acute ischemic cerebrovascular syndrome: Diagnostic criteria. *Stroke* 2003;34:2995–2998.

CHAPTER THIRTY EIGHT

EPIDEMIOLOGY AND RISK FACTORS

Epidemiological studies sought to understand what behaviors and health conditions led to heart disease and strokes [1]. If one knew the factors that led to these conditions, heart attacks and strokes could be prevented by controlling these adverse conditions. During the first half of the twentieth century, coronary artery atherosclerosis with occlusions of the coronary arteries became a widely accepted cause of heart attacks and cardiac deaths. Cardiologists and internists wanted to try to understand what presaged coronary artery disease. They urged the US Congress to support community studies that could yield important information about heart disease precursors. Since many strokes were caused by emboli from the heart and impaired heart function, the information gleaned would also be important for stroke. Atherosclerosis, the cause of coronary artery disease, was also the major cause of disease of the arteries that supply the brain.

Framingham, Massachusetts, a relatively small western suburb of Boston, was chosen as the initial research site. Thomas Dawber was the first doctor chosen to lead this research. The original cohort, founded in 1948, consisted of 5,209 men and women who lived in Framingham. Requirements for entry were a minimum age of 30 to a maximum age of 62 at the time of first examination, and no history of heart attack or stroke [2]. Due to lukewarm interest at first, doctors, nurses, and healthcare workers volunteered for the study to set an example for others. The individuals in the original cohort were examined at routine intervals; lifestyle practices and habits such as smoking, alcohol intake, and exercise were recorded as well as conditions such as hypertension, diabetes, and high cholesterol levels. Family histories were noted. Cholesterol levels and other blood constituents were tested, and electrocardiograms and chest X-rays were performed. During the ensuing years, various other tests were added in the Framingham Study, including brain imaging, vascular imaging, and genetics. A second cohort that consisted of the children of the initial cohort was founded in 1971. The Generation Three Cohort, founded in 2002, was a third-generation study composed of children of the offspring cohort and/or grandchildren of the original cohort participants. The minimum age for entry was 20 [2].

Although originally conceived as a "heart study," it soon became clear that many of the findings also applied to cerebrovascular disease and stroke. Phillip Wolf and, later, Carlos Kase and Sudha Seshadri analyzed the large body of information to determine precursors of stroke. The Framingham Study coined the term "risk factors" and generated enough data to allow calculations as to the probability of developing a heart attack or stroke depending on a number of key variables [2].

Most Framingham residents were Caucasian. Other studies sought a broader population base. The Atherosclerosis Risk in Communities (ARIC) study was initiated in 1987. The ARIC study first entered 4,000 adults aged 45–64 years who lived in four communities in the United States: Forsyth County, North Carolina; Jackson, Mississippi; and the suburbs of Minneapolis, Minnesota, and Washington County, Maryland [3]. These were racially diverse communities, in contrast to Framingham. The intent was to follow the cohort to study the causes of cardiovascular disease according to race, sex, place, and time. Examinations included ultrasound scanning of neck and lower limb arteries; analysis of blood lipids, including cholesterol and its high- and low-density components; and clotting factors and functions. The initial study examinations and data collections took place in 1987–1989, the second in 1990–1992, the third in 1993–1995, the fourth in 1996–1998, and the fifth in 2011–2013. During these extensive examinations, information was obtained on demographics, medical history, medication use, and health behaviors. The ARIC study published over 1,000 journal articles in diverse areas of clinical and population research. Information from the ARIC study has become an important resource for the study of heart disease, stroke, kidney disease, diabetes, and cognitive decline [3]. Rebecca Gottesman and colleagues mined the massive epidemiological and imaging results in ARIC to study the effects of vascular risk factors on cognitive function in the aging population [4].

The World Health Organization (WHO) established the MONICA (Multinational Monitoring of Trends and Determinants in Cardiovascular Disease) project during the early 1980s in many regions around the world to monitor trends in cardiovascular diseases and to relate these to risk factor changes in the population over a 10-year period [5]. Kjell Asplund of the University of Umea in Sweden led the investigations. There were 32 MONICA collaborating centers in 21 different countries. Ten million men and women aged 25–64 years were monitored. The data collection was completed during the late 1990s, and the main results were published in the following years. The data is still being used for analysis [5]. Epidemiological data about heart disease and stroke has also been collected in very diverse geographical locations, for example, Oslo, Norway; Western Australia; China; and Olmstead County, Minnesota.

Ruth Bonita, a New Zealand epidemiologist [6], and, later, Valery Feigin, a Russian-born neurologist and epidemiologist, were leaders in an epidemiological study based in New Zealand entitled ARCOS: Auckland Regional Community Stroke Study [7]. Stroke was very common in New Zealand and there was little information about the access and quality of stroke services, especially for Maori and Pacific people who were at high risk of stroke and who had deficient healthcare. New Zealand was a small country and data was readily collected and analyzed. The aim of this study was to quantify the impact of stroke in Auckland, to refine methods for assessing this impact, and to identify whether factors such as socioeconomic circumstances, ethnicity, case mix, and quality of healthcare delivery influence variations in impact.

Some epidemiological studies entered selective groups of patients, for example, the Nurses Health Study [8] and the British Doctors study [9]. Some studies focused on specific health and risk factors. The Nurses Study yielded unique information about sex hormones; smoking was the focus of the British Doctors study. The National Health and Nutrition Examination Survey (NHANES) program concentrated on nutrition [10]. NHANES was conducted by the National Center for Health Statistics; it used sequential surveys to study nutrition and health in adults and children in the United States and to track changes over time. The survey combined interviews, physical examinations, and laboratory testing. The first NHANES survey was in 1971; in 1999 the surveys became an annual event. The first report was published in 2001 [10]. Some studies were designed to study specific issues. For example, the Reasons for Geographic and Racial Difference in Stroke (REGARDS) aimed at trying to explain why the Southeastern part of the United States had an unusually high frequency of strokes (the "stroke belt") [11]. Another study (the Hawaiian Heart Study) was designed to determine the reason for differences in the frequency of heart disease and stroke in Japanese men in Japan, Hawaii, and the United States [12].

Much epidemiological information was gleaned from stroke patients hospitalized in academic hospitals in large cities. It also became important to collect community-wide information. Stroke-specific epidemiological information was collected from projects that included data from community-based hospital registries in the Lehigh Valley of Pennsylvania, North Carolina, Oregon, New York, and Oxfordshire in the United Kingdom [13]. The data collection from this study that covered North Carolina, Oregon, and New York included over 4,000 patients.

Jack Whisnant [14] took advantage of the data information systems at the Mayo Clinic to study the epidemiology of stroke at the clinic and in surrounding Olmstead County over a number of epochs [15]. He reviewed extensive epidemiological data to understand why the frequency of stroke declined during the third quarter of the twentieth century [16]. A subsequent detailed review tracked changes in stroke and risk factor incidence during the latter years of the twentieth century and the first decade of the twenty-first century [17].

Information from these studies alerted doctors and the public to the importance of risk factors that promoted atherosclerosis and led to heart disease, heart attacks, and strokes. High blood pressure was found to be the most important risk for stroke. The risk of stroke depended heavily on the severity and duration of the elevated blood pressure. Diabetes, high cholesterol, cigarette smoking, obesity, lack of exercise, and a strong family history of stroke and coronary heart disease have also been established as conditions and behaviors that increase the risk for stroke. The epidemiological information gained from these studies and surveys has contributed to clinical practice guidelines and policy statements for doctors and the public [18]. Attention by the public and family practice physicians, internists, and neurologists to translating the epidemiological information into practice was one of the most important explanations for this decline in stroke mortality and incidence. Some recent trends – for example, the increase in the frequency of obesity and diabetes – cause considerable concern. Stroke prevalence is still high, especially among older age groups and some racial groups: African Americans and Hispanics. People are living longer, and closer surveillance and the availability of brain imaging account for more strokes being recognized.

Important contributors to our knowledge of stroke epidemiology include John Kurtzke [19], Milton Alter [20], and Phillip Gorelick [21].

NOTES AND REFERENCES

1. Some material in this chapter has been previously published in Caplan LR. *Caplan's Stroke*, 5th ed. Cambridge: Cambridge University Press, 2016. Caplan LR. (Historical perspectives) The last 50 years of cerebrovascular disease: Part I. *International Journal of Stroke* 2006;1(2):104–110. Caplan LR. (Historical perspectives) Caplan's short rendition of stroke during the 20th century: Part II. *International Journal of Stroke* 2006;1(4):228–234.
2. Dawber TR. *The Framingham Study: The Epidemiology of Atherosclerotic Disease*. Cambridge, MA: Harvard University Press, 1980. Kannel WB, Dawber TR, Sorlie

P, Wolf PA. Components of blood pressure and risk of atherothrombotic brain infarction: The Framingham Study. *Stroke* 1976;7:327–331. Wolf PA, D'Agostino RB, Belanger AJ, Kannel WB. Probability of stroke: A risk profile from the Framingham Study. *Stroke* 1991;22:312–318.

3. The ARIC study has produced more than 1,000 reports. ARIC Investigators. The Atherosclerosis Risk in Communities (ARIC) study: Design and objectives. *American Journal of Epidemiology* 1989;129:687–702. Chambless LE, Heiss G, Shahar E, Earp M J, Toole J. Prediction of ischemic stroke risk in the Atherosclerosis Risk in Communities Study. *American Journal of Epidemiology* 2014;160(3):259–269. Bekwelem W, Jensen PN, Norby FL, Soliman EZ, Agarwal SK, Lip GYH, Pan W, Folsom AR, Longstreth WT, Alonso A, et al. Carotid atherosclerosis and stroke in atrial fibrillation: The Atherosclerosis Risk in Communities Study. *Stroke* 2016;47(6):1643–1646.

4. Gottesman RF, Albert MS, Alonso A, et al. Associations between midlife vascular risk factors and 25-year incident dementia in the Atherosclerosis Risk in Communities (ARIC) Cohort. *JAMA Neurology* 2017;74(10):1246–1254.

5. WHO MONICA Project principal investigators. The World Health Organization MONICA project (Monitoring Trends and Determinants in Cardiovascular Disease: A major international collaboration. *Journal of Clinical Epidemiology* 1988;41:105–114. WHO MONICA Project principal investigators. WHO MONICA Project: Geographic variation in mortality from cardiovascular diseases: Baseline data on selected population characteristics and cardiovascular mortality. *World Health Statistics Quarterly* 1987;40:171–184.

6. Ruth Bonita. Passionate about prevention. *Lancet Neurology* 2009;8:312.

7. Krishnamurthi RV, Basrker-Collo S, Parag V, et al. Stroke incidence by major pathological type and ischemic subtypes in the Auckland Regional Community Stroke Studies. *Stroke* 2018;49:3–10.

8. The Nurses Health Study was launched in 1976. The cohort consisted of 121,700 married registered nurses. The second Nurses Health Study began in 1989 and enrolled 116,430 nurses; and the third cohort began in 2010 and has ongoing enrollment. During 40 years, these studies generated long-term results about lifestyle, hormonal factors, and health-related information across the life course and an extensive collection of various biological specimens. Bao Y, Bertoia ML, Lenart EB, Stampfer MJ, Willett WC, Speizer FE, Chavarro JE. Origin, methods, and evolution of the Three Nurses' Health studies. *American Journal of Public Health* 2016;106:1573–1581. Colditz GA, Philpott SE, Hankinson SE. The impact of the Nurses Health Study on population health, prevention, translation, and control. *American Journal of Public Health* 2016;106:1540–1545.

9. The British Doctors Study enrolled 40,701 British male doctors in 1951. Doll R, Hill AB. The mortality of doctors in relation to their smoking habits. *British Medical Journal* 1954;328:1529–1533. 2004;2281519. Doll R, Peto R, Boreham J, Sutherland I. Mortality from cancer in relation to smoking: 50 years observations on British doctors. *British Journal of Cancer* 2005;92:426–429.

10. The National Health and Nutrition Examination Survey (NHANES) information and survey results are available at www.entnet.org/content/national-health-and-nutrition-examination-survey-nhanes.

11. The Stroke Belt in the Southeastern United States has been extensively researched: Gillum RF, Ingram DD. Relation between residence in the Southeast region of the United States and stroke incidence: The NHANES 1 epidemiologic follow-up study.

American Journal of Epidemiology 1996;144:665–673. Howard VJ, Cushman M, Pulley L, et al. The Reasons for Geographic and Racial Differences in Stroke (REGARDS) study: Objectives and design. *Neuroepidemiology* 2005;25:135–143. Howard VJ, McClure LA, Glymour MM, Cunningham SA, Kleindorfer DO, Crowe M, Wadley VG, Peace F, Howard G, Lackland DT. Effect of duration and age at exposure to the stroke belt on incident stroke. *Neurology* 2013;80:1655–1661.

12. Kagan A, Harris BR, Winkelstein W Jr, et al. Epidemiologic studies of coronary heart disease and stroke in Japanese men living in Japan, Hawaii and California: Demographic, physical, dietary and biochemical characteristics. *Journal of Chronic Diseases* 1974;27:345–364. Kagan A, Popper JS, Rhoads GG, Yano K. Dietary and other risk factors for stroke in Hawaiian Japanese men. *Stroke* 1985;16:390–396.

13. The community-wide studies cited were: Oxfordshire Community Stroke Project: Incidence of stroke in Oxfordshire: First year's experience of a community stroke registry. *British Medical Journal* 1983;287:713–717. Alter M, Sobel E, McCoy RC, Francis ME, Davanipour Z, Schofer F, Levitt LP, Meehan EF. Stroke in the Lehigh Valley: Incidence based on a communitywide hospital registry. *Neuroepidemiology* 1985;4:1–15. Yatsu FM, Becker C, McLeroy K, et al. Community hospital-based stroke programs: North Carolina, Oregon, and New York. I. Goals, objectives, and data collection procedures. *Stroke* 1986;17:276–284. Becker C, Howard G, McElroy KR, Yatsu FM, Toole JF, Coull B, Feibel J, Walker MD. Community hospital-based stroke programs: North Carolina, Oregon, and New York II: Description of Study Population. *Stroke* 1986;17:285–293.

14. Brown RD, Rocca WA. Jack P. Whisnant, MD, FAAN (1924–2015). *Neurology* 2015;85:1832–1833.

15. Whisnant JP, Fitzgibbons JP, Kurland LT, et al. Natural history of stroke in Rochester, Minnesota, 1945 through 1954. *Stroke* 1971;2:11–22. Matsumoto N, Whisnant JP, Kurland LT, et al. Natural history of stroke in Rochester, Minnesota, 1955 through 1969: An extension of a previous study 1945 through 1954. *Stroke* 1973;4:20–29. Stroke epidemiology and prevention are highlighted in Whisnant JP (ed.), *Stroke: Populations, Cohorts, and Clinical Trials*. Boston: Butterworth-Heinemann, 1993.

16. Whisnant JP. The decline of stroke. *Stroke* 1984;15:160–168.

17. Koton S, Schneider AL, Rosamond WD, Shahar E, Sang Y, Gottesman RF, Coresh J. Stroke incidence and mortality trends in US communities, 1987 to 2011. *Journal of the American Medical Association (JAMA)* 2014;312:259–268.

18. Gorelick PB. Alter M (eds.). *Handbook of Neuroepidemiology*. New York: Marcel Dekker, 1994. Kasner SE, Gorelick PB. *Prevention and Treatment of Stroke*. Philadelphia: Butterworth-Heinemann, 2014.

19. Frohman EM, Stuve O, Frohman TC, Lisak R. In memoriam: John F. Kurtzke, MD (1926–2015): A founding father of neuroepidemiology and pioneer of modern clinical trial design. *JAMA Neurology*. 2016;73(4):482–483.

20. Kelley RE, Azizi A. In memoriam: Milton Alter, MD, PhD (1929–2016). *Neurology* 2016;87:2012.

21. Kirby T. Phillip B. Gorelick: Cshanging neurological practice in the USA. *Lancet Neurology* 2016:15:361. Gorelick PB. Adaptation of neurological practice and policy to a changing US health-care landscape. *Lancet Neurology* 2016:15:444–450.

CHAPTER THIRTY NINE

DATA BANKS AND REGISTRIES

During the middle years of the twentieth century, clinicians advanced their knowledge of clinical phenomenology by personally studying and describing small groups of patients. In 1935, Charles Aring and Houston Meritt studied a group of patients coming to necropsy at the Boston City Hospital to clarify the differential diagnosis between brain hemorrhages and infarcts [1]. Dalsgaard-Nielsen analyzed the relationship between clinical and postmortem diagnosis in all autopsied cases of "cerebral apoplexy" seen in the neurology department of the Frederiksberg hospital in Denmark from 1940 through 1953. He discussed the clinical characteristics that might allow differentiation between hemorrhage and thromboembolism [2]. The excellent filing and record systems at the Mayo Clinic in Rochester, Minnesota, facilitated analyses by Jack Whisnant and Leonard Kurland and their colleagues of the characteristics of stroke patients in Olmstead County, Minnesota, during several epochs (1945–1954 and 1954–1969) [3]. These studies were all retrospective and selected specified data items to analyze. The data collection depended on information already collected in the hospital records.

During the 1970s and 1980s, technological advances in imaging and laboratory analyses made it possible to define the clinical and laboratory features of nonfatal, even minor, strokes and cerebrovascular lesions. With better knowledge of clinical and morphologic features, clinicians naturally sought more quantitative data. How often did intracerebral hemorrhages, carotid artery occlusion, or lacunar infarcts occur? How often did each of the clinical symptoms and signs occur in each subtype of stroke? Clinicians recognized that valid, statistically meaningful data could not be collected unless large numbers of patients with a wide spectrum of representative cases were collected, studied, and analyzed. The advent of computers in medicine in the 1970s greatly facilitated the storage and analysis of large quantities of complex data. To be certain that the desired information was recorded, the data was collected prospectively and entered on data forms or directly into a computer program.

The Harvard Cooperative Stroke Registry in the early 1970s was the first computer-based registry of prospectively studied stroke patients [4]. Each of the 694 stroke patients was examined by one of the originators of the registry, J. P. Mohr or Louis Caplan. They and their colleagues collected data about the frequency of various findings in patients with various stroke subtypes. For example, what risk factors preceded development of lacunar strokes, intracerebral hemorrhage, and brain embolism? How many patients with ischemic stroke had preceding headaches, headaches at onset, or headaches after development of stroke? How was the headache frequency and pattern different between patients with lacunar infarcts, large-artery atherothrombotic strokes, and brain hemorrhages? The initial patients were entered in the Harvard Stroke Registry before high-sensitivity CT scanning was available, but many of these patients had catheter angiography that identified causative vascular lesions.

The National Institute of Neurological and Communicative Disorders and Stroke (NINCDS) decided to sponsor a computer-based registry similar to the Harvard Stroke Registry. CT scanning had improved and become more widely available, and data was sought that would include racial and geographic diversity. The Harvard Stroke registry had included only Boston-based patients who were almost exclusively Caucasian. The pilot Stroke Data Bank was a preliminary feasibility study carried out at four US sites: University of Maryland in Baltimore, Maryland; University of South Alabama in Mobile, Alabama; Boston University; and Duke University in Durham, North Carolina [5]. The Southern centers contributed many Black patients among the 1,158 patients entered and analyzed. The leaders of this study included J. P. Mohr, Carlos Kase, Tom Price, and Philip Wolf. After the success of the pilot study, the Stroke Data Bank study was organized by the NINCDS and was to be centered in four US centers: Boston University, Michael Reese Hospital in Chicago, the University of Maryland, and Columbia University [6]. The principal investigators (Wolf, Dan Hier/Caplan, Price, and Mohr) met for a full year to decide on entry items, criteria, and aims of the data bank collection. A total of 1,805 thoroughly evaluated patients were enrolled in the Stroke Data Bank between July 1983 and June 1986 [6]. Two thirds of these patients were admitted within 24 hours after stroke onset. These registries published extensive detailed information about risk factors, clinical onset and course, neurological signs, and imaging and laboratory results.

Stroke registries and databases were later developed around the world and provided more quantitative information about clinical and laboratory phenomena and diagnoses [7]. Some registries collected and analyzed subtypes of stroke such as brain embolism [8], subarachnnoid and intracerebral hemorrhage [9], or strokes in the posterior circulation of the brain [10]. Neurological researchers at the University of Cincinnati led by Tom Brott and Joe Broderick contributed valuable epidemiological information by analyzing and reporting the frequencies and risk factors for brain hemorrhages that occurred in Blacks and whites in their region [9]. Studies performed in a designated area of northern Manhattan, among multiracial Latinx, Black, and white residents provided very important epidemiological data about stroke occurrence and risk factors among the different groups [11].

Data banks and registries created very large data sets that yielded very valuable information about the frequency of various stroke subtypes, risk factors, natural history, and response to various treatments.

NOTES AND REFERENCES

1. Aring CD, Merritt HH. Differential diagnosis between cerebral hemorrhage and cerebral thrombosis. *Archives of Internal Medicine* 1935;56:435–456. This study is the topic of Chapter 25.

2. Dalsgaard-Nielsen T. Survey of 1000 cases of apoplexia cerebri. *Acta Psychiatrica Neurologica Scandinavica* 1955;30:169–185.

3. Whisnant JP, Fitzgibbons JP, Kurland LT, Sayre GP. Natural history of stroke in Rochester, Minnesota, 1945 through 1954. *Stroke* 1971;2:11–22. Matsumoto N, Whisnant JP, Kurland LT, Okazaki H. Natural history of stroke in Rochester, Minnesota, 1955 through 1969: An extension of a previous study 1945 through 1954. *Stroke* 1973;4:20–29.

4. Mohr J, Caplan L, Melski J, Duncan G, Goldstein R, Kistler J, Pessin, M, Bleich H. The Harvard Cooperative Stroke Registry: A prospective registry. *Neurology* 1978;28:754–762. This registry and the role of Caplan is discussed in Chapter 30.

5. Kunitz S, Gross CR, Heyman A, Kase CS, Mohr JP, Price TR, Wolf PA. The pilot Stroke Data Bank: Definition, design, and data. *Stroke* 1984;15:740–746.

6. Foulkes MA, Wolf PA, Price TR, Mohr JP, Hier DB. The Stroke Data Bank: Design, methods, and baseline characteristics. *Stroke* 1988;19:547–554.

7. Examples of International Stroke Registries include Australia: Chambers BR, Donnan GA, Bladin PF. Patterns of stroke: An analysis of the first 700 consecutive admissions to the Austin Hospital Stroke Unit. *Australia and New Zealand Journal of Medicine* 1983;13:57–64. Switzerland: Bogousslavsky J, Mille GV, Regli F. The Lausanne Stroke Registry: An analysis of 1,000 consecutive patients with first stroke. *Stroke* 1988;19:1083–1092. France: Moulin T, Tatu L, Crepin-Leblond T, Chavot D, Bergès S, Rumbach T. The Besancon Stroke Registry: An acute stroke registry of 2,500 consecutive patients. *European Neurology* 1997;38:10–20. Germany: Heuschmann PU, Kolominsky-Rabas PL, Misselwitz B, Hermanek P, Leffman C, Janzen RW, Rother J, Buecker-Nott HJ, Berger K. Predictors of in-hospital mortality and attributable risks of death after ischemic stroke: The German Stroke Registers Study Group.

Archives of Internal Medicine 2004;164:1761–1768. Greece: Vemmos KN, Takis CE, Georgilis K, Zakopoulos NA, Lekakis JP, Papamichael CM, Zis VP, Stamatelopoulos S. The Athens stroke registry: Results of a five-year hospital-based study. *Cerebrovascular Diseases* 2000;10:133–141.

8. Caplan LR, Hier DB, D'Cruz I. Cerebral embolism in the Michael Reese Stroke Registry. *Stroke* 1983;14:530–536.

9. Researchers in Cincinnati were leaders in epidemiological studies of stroke patients. Their research focused on brain and subarachnoid hemorrhage and on differences between frequencies in Black and white patients. Broderick J, Brott T, Tomsick T, Huster G, Miller R. The risk of subarachnoid and intracerebral hemorrhages in blacks as compared with whites. *The New England Journal of Medicine* 1992;326:733–736. Broderick JP, Brott T, Tomsick T, Miller R, Huster G. Intracerebral hemorrhage is more than twice as common as subarachnoid hemorrhage. *Journal of Neurosurgery* 1993;78(2):188–191. Broderick J, Brott T, Tomsick T, Huster G. Lobar hemorrhage in the elderly: The undiminishing importance of hypertension. *Stroke* 1993;24 (1):49–51. Broderick J, Brott T, Kothari R, Miller R, Khoury J, Pancioli A, Tomsick T, Mills D, Minneci L, Shukla R. The Greater Cincinnati/Northern Kentucky Stroke Study: Preliminary first-ever total incidence rates of stroke among blacks. *Stroke* 1998;29:415–421.

10. Caplan LR, Wityk RJ, Glass TA, Tapia J, Pazdera L, Chang HM, Teal P, Dashe JF, Chaves CJ, Breen JC, Vemmos K, Amarenco P, Tettenborn B, Leary M, Estol C, Dewitt LD, Pessin MS. New England Medical Center Posterior Circulation Registry. *Annals of Neurology* 2004;56:389–398.

11. The Northern Manhattan Study (NOMASS) provided important epidemiological information among various racial groups in New York City. Sacco RL, Boden-Albala B, Abel G, Lin IF, Elkind M, Hauser WA, Paik MC, Shea S. Race-ethnic disparities in the impact of stroke risk factors: The northern Manhattan stroke study. *Stroke* 2001;32:1725–1731. Dhamoon MS, Sciacca RR, Rundek T, Sacco RL, Elkind MSV. Recurrent stroke and cardiac risks after first ischemic stroke: The Northern Manhattan Study. *Neurology* 2006;66:641–646. Elkind MSV, Sciacca RR, Boden-Albala B, Rundek T, Paik MC, Sacco RL. Moderate alcohol consumption reduces risk of ischemic stroke: The Northern Manhattan Study. *Stroke* 2006;37:13–19. Suk SH, Sacco RL, Boden-Albala B, Cheun JF, Pittman JG, Elkind MS, Paik MC. Abdominal obesity and risk of ischemic stroke: The northern Manhattan stroke study. *Stroke* 2003;34:1586–1592. Jacobs BS, Boden-Albala B, Lin IF, Sacco RL. Stroke in the young in the northern Manhattan stroke study. *Stroke* 2002;33:2789–2793. Sacco RL, Gan R, Boden-Albala B, Lin IF, Kargman DE, Hauser WA, Shea S, Paik M. Leisure-time physical activity and ischemic stroke risk: The northern Manhattan stroke study. *Stroke* 1998;29:380–387.

CHAPTER FORTY

PEDIATRIC STROKE

INTRODUCTION

Pediatric stroke had its origins from three fields: adult stroke, pediatric neurology, and thrombotic disorders [1]. Each discipline evolved from different directions and provided unique but complementary perspectives. From the sixteenth to nineteenth century, autopsies showed brain hemorrhages and brain softenings or porencephaly underlying "infantile paralysis." The vascular basis of apoplexy established in adults was eventually realized in children. From 1900 to 1950, classification of neurological impairment associated with pediatric stroke subtypes emerged, including congenital hemiplegia and acquired apoplexy, arterial versus venous thrombosis, and, in the pre-immunization era, a strong association with childhood infections. From 1950 to 2000, development of computed tomography and magnetic resonance imaging in the 1970s and 1980s provided in vivo imaging signatures of pediatric stroke from acute onset to chronic recovery. Neuroimaging improved the ability to detect stroke across the pediatric age spectrum. The images provided by analysis of tomographic and magnetic resonance imaging (MRI) sequences accelerated the ability to detect, characterize, and understand pediatric stroke. An increasingly detailed landscape of pediatric stroke and its recognizable subtypes emerged: primary brain hemorrhage, brain arterial occlusion with focal infarction, and intracranial venous occlusion. Noninfectious etiologies causing stroke were increasingly recognized, including cardiogenic, arteriopathic, prothrombotic, and hematological disorders. Networks of collaborators accelerated discovery. Two major developments launched the field of pediatric stroke as an important pediatric neurology subspecialty: neuroimaging and the formation of collaborative networks of clinician-researchers.

The relative rarity of pediatric stroke in any single institution had limited the ability to enroll large numbers of children into clinical research studies. Beginning in the 1990s, pediatric stroke collaborative networks were formed, grew rapidly, and connected patients and their families with investigators. Investigations ranging from coagulation laboratory studies on thrombosis to translational research in neonatal stroke began to elucidate how the molecular and cellular events underlying pediatric stroke differed from those in adults. Advocacy groups focusing on pediatric stroke facilitated the agenda. These interactions shaped current knowledge about the mechanisms and impact of stroke on the developing brain.

The current approach to pediatric stroke treatment developed gradually during the past four decades. This began using observational studies in children with unacceptably high recurrence rates when no antithrombotic treatment was provided. Use of antithrombotic treatments was forged by partnerships between pediatric neurologists, pediatric hematologists, neuroradiologists, and adult neurovascular specialists. Experience derived from other pediatric thrombotic disorders provided the rationale and dosing guidelines for antithrombotic treatment based on studies involving systemic arteries and veins in neonates, infants, and children. Evidence from adult stroke trials provided supportive safety and effectiveness data. Selective extrapolation of these findings to the pediatric stroke population followed.

EARLY HISTORY OF PEDIATRIC STROKE

Stroke in infants, both zones of "softening" and hemorrhage into the brain, were observed as early as the seventeenth century at necropsy. From the seventeenth to nineteenth centuries, isolated cases of infants and children with hemiplegia were reported. The carefully documented clinical presentations of such cases set the stage for identifying the major subtypes of pediatric stroke, from congenital hemiplegia to apoplexy in infancy and later childhood. Postmortem examination of pediatric brains revealed structural and pathological findings that explained the clinical findings. While recognition of brain softening and cavitation related to apoplexy was evolving in adults, similar postmortem findings in infants and children were described. These pediatric cases appeared in the pediatric and pathology literature under a number of terms, including "cerebral apoplexy," "acute infantile hemiplegia," "acute hemiplegia of childhood," "congenital hemiplegia," and "hemiplegic cerebral palsy."

MILESTONES ACROSS THE CENTURIES

Seventeenth Century

Thomas Willis (1621–1675), at Oxford University, documented the first cases of pediatric stroke. Between 1660 and 1672, Willis wrote all of his neurological works, including extensive descriptions of apoplexy and other brain disorders in adults. Willis saw many children in his clinical practice and performed pediatric autopsies. Among his cases was a child with postmortem findings of intracranial hemorrhage, likely the earliest published childhood instance of venous sinus thrombosis, with "septic thrombosis" of the vein of Galen and straight sinus [2].

Nineteenth Century

Jean Cruveilhier (1794–1874) published his *Anatomie pathologique du corps humain* (two volumes, 1829–1835, 1835–1842), which contained hand-colored lithographic plates, several of which depicted immature brains with focal atrophy, hemiatrophy, and porencephaly [3]. Sir Richard Quain (1800–1887) collected and published a large clinical series of apoplexy. He reported two illustrative case histories of apoplexy in childhood along with demographic and some general observations on the causes of the disease and the age-related frequency of its occurrence [4]. Quain summarized the reasons for the rarity of apoplexy in infants and children compared to adults as follows:

> In early life we find the skull less resisting, and the blood-vessels more elastic and yielding, than in the adult, where the one becomes dense and rigid, and the others frequently the seat of deposit or degeneration. In the young subject, the energies of the system are directed to nutrition and growth; in the adult, the chief call is on the brain and nervous system, which then has to bear the wear and tear of life. The heart, in the progress of life, becomes larger and more powerful, it is subjected to greater excitement, and becomes oftener the seat of disease – all interfering with the circulation through the brain. These, and other causes, make a wide difference in the comparative frequency of apoplectic disease. [4]

Probably, the first well-described case of arterial ischemic stroke in a child was documented in 1882 by a German physician, Otto Huebner [5]. He evaluated a 2.5-year-old child who had had the sudden onset of fever, convulsions, and ensuing aphasia and paralysis. The child died one year later, and postmortem examination showed three zones of focal brain atrophy involving both cerebral hemispheres, an embolism filling the middle cerebral artery (MCA) from its origin to its bifurcation, and destruction of both descending pyramidal tracts in the pons [6]. In a single childhood case,

Huebner illustrated the combination of findings that we recognize as the fingerprint of arterial ischemic stroke, namely, thrombotic occlusion of an intracranial artery, corresponding cerebral infarction, and Wallerian degeneration of the descending corticospinal tracts.

The first significant case series of infantile spastic hemiplegia due to cerebral (vs. spinal) causes was published in 1885 by Sarah J. McNutt, the first woman member of the American Neurological Association. She reported seven children with infantile spastic hemiplegia and reviewed 34 prior cases that described the distribution of postmortem findings, including porencephalic cysts, brain softenings, and brain hemorrhages. Huebner's case is among those in her summary table. McNutt concluded that "it is not now sufficient to divide infantile paralyses simply into those of a cerebral and those of a spinal origin. Of the cerebral variety we must discriminate whether from tumor or from tubercle, or from embolus, or from a clot" [6].

In 1889, Sir William Osler described a series of 120 children with hemiplegia and another 20 with diplegia in his treatise on "cerebral palsy" [7]. Osler summarized the then current state of understanding of infantile hemiplegia: "Infantile hemiplegia is probably the result of a variety of different processes, of which the most important are: Haemorrhage during a paroxysm of whooping cough; post-febrile processes (embolic, endoarterial changes); encephalitis; and thrombosis of the cerebral veins" [7].

One year later, Bernard Sachs and Frederick Peterson published a large series that contained a thorough analysis of 140 infants and children with "infantile cerebral paralysis." The analysis was initially read at the New York Academy of Medicine on April 3, 1890 [8]. The series included a predominance of males (87 males; 53 females). The hemiplegic pattern of paralysis predominated (105, hemiplegia; 24, diplegia; 11, paraplegia). They observed that the hemiplegic pattern occurred more often when acquired at three to four years of age. Sachs correlated the presence of mental deficits to the age of onset and pattern of paralysis. Sachs and Peterson noted that each pattern of paralysis could result from a variety of brain pathologies. They cautioned that, since porencephaly and sclerosis were the end stage of a variety of brain pathologies, they were not useful in assigning etiologies. They noted the relative specificity of brain hemorrhage ($n = 23$), thrombosis ($n = 95$), and embolism ($n = 7$) to the hemiplegic subtype of cerebral palsy [8]. They wrote that "the first fact that is brought about with great distinctness is that haemorrhage, thrombosis and embolism, the conditions which give rise to adult apoplexy, are also found to be a frequent cause for the cerebral palsies of early life." And he closes his paper with a visionary message of hope for stroke rehabilitation: "as for the condition of mental enfeeblement, much can be done by careful manual and mental training. This should be begun at an early day" [8].

In 1895, Sachs published one of the first definitive textbooks devoted to pediatric brain disorders [9]. In this 666-page textbook he emphasized that vascular lesions were nearly always found in cases of acquired childhood paralysis.

In 1895, Sigmund Freud at age 39, while a lecturer in neuropathology at the University of Vienna, published *Die Infantile Cerebrallähmung* (Infantile Cerebral Paralysis) in which he emphasized the thrombotic and vascular components of cerebral paralysis in infants and children [10]: "It has further been determined that a large number of cases of infantile cerebral palsy is caused by the same factors that bring about the majority of cases of cerebral paralysis of adults: by tearing, embolism, and thrombosis of cerebral vessels" [10].

Luther Emmett Holt (1855–1924) included in his 1897 textbook of pediatrics a 13-page section on "infantile cerebral paralysis" [11]. He noted that "spastic diplegia, or paraplegia" was four times more common than "hemiplegia," in contrast to Sachs's observations of approximately equal proportions. He attributed this discrepancy to death in the first two years of infancy for the more severe forms so that such children did not survive to be followed in a general neurology clinic such as the one that Sachs attended. Holt also focused on pediatric cerebral venous thrombosis, dividing it into "cachectic" and "septic" forms. He summarized the challenges inherent in treating children with these conditions: "The course and the result of cerebral paralysis depend upon the extent of injury to the brain, its nature and the age at which it is inflicted – all these being conditions which are beyond the power of the physician to modify or control. The treatment of cerebral palsy is therefore extremely unsatisfactory" [11].

Twentieth Century

New tools began to refine understanding of pediatric stroke. With the advent of cerebral angiography and then brain imaging, it became possible to distinguish cerebral hemorrhage from infarction and arterial from venous occlusions and to study the clinical and imaging course in children with milder, nonfatal disease.

First half of the twentieth century, 1900–1950. Highlights included a focus on venous thrombosis and infection in an era before the availability of antibiotics or immunizations, and better clinical and neuropathological characterization of stroke in previously healthy children. In 1927, Frank Ford and A. J. Schaffer published a comprehensive review of the role of infection in childhood hemiplegia. They divided infantile hemiplegias into those following acute infectious diseases and those in apparently healthy children [12]. They summarized the operative or autopsy findings among 70 patients from the

Harriet Lame Home into focal cortical softening, scarring atrophy, and cystic changes with or without thrombosis. The findings were summarized as follows: "It seems possible to state definitely that the infantile hemiplegias that are associated with the acute infectious diseases are due to vascular lesions." They "depend almost invariably on arterial thrombosis, hemorrhage and embolism of the cerebral vessels."

> Those which occur early in the course of the illness are, in the majority of cases, due to invasion of the blood stream by the primary organism or by some secondary invader. The palsies that develop during convalescence are the result of the vascular lesions in the cerebral arteries which Wiesel and others have described. These complications are common to all severe infections and are not in any sense specific, although apparently specific changes in the nervous system may be produced by variola, vaccinia, varicella, and perhaps by measles and mumps.

Regarding coagulation disorders, they stated: "Another possible factor in the production of vascular lesions is change in the coagulability of the blood ... with arterial thromboses and mural thrombi on the endocardium, which give rise to emboli" [12].

In 1932, Roy Simpson reviewed 42 cases of cerebral thrombosis in infants and children seen during the previous 10 years on the wards of the Hospital for Sick Children in Toronto [13]. He recognized iatrogenic reasons for cerebral venous thrombosis. In many children, the diagnosis had not been made clinically but discovered only at autopsy following death from sepsis. Simpson made a cautionary observation about the then common practice of intravenous access utilizing the superior sagittal sinus:

> Particularly I wish to draw attention to the finding of several instances of thrombosis of the superior longitudinal sinus, in association with intravenous therapy by this route. In only three cases, though, was there evidence of infection of the thrombus, the others being aseptic and probably due to disturbance of the endothelial lining of the wall of the sinus. One's impression after having done many sinus punctures is that thrombosis frequently occurs and cures itself spontaneously by recanalization. This impression is gained by being unable to obtain blood after one or more previous punctures, but after several days have elapsed to obtain again a free flow in apparently the identical area. [13]

Pediatrician Hertha Ehlers and neuropathologist Cyril Courville described internal cerebral vein thrombosis in 26 infants. They included drawings showing the locations of the associated deep white and gray matter infarction and hemorrhage including intraventricular hemorrhage. They introduced the concept of multiple coexisting risk factors for venous thrombosis. In many children, venous thrombosis was not due solely to systemic illness (e.g., dehydration) or infection (septic thrombosis related to otitis media and mastoiditis), but to an interplay between these two conditions [14].

Second half of the twentieth century, 1950–2000. Great advances in clinical and research capabilities in the field of pediatric stroke were reached during the second half of the twentieth century. Differentiating vascular pathologies became feasible. With the availability and application of contrast cerebral arteriography in pediatrics, hemiplegia due to vaso-occlusive causes became diagnosable. Noninfectious etiologies were more accurately categorized, including cardiogenic, arteriopathic, prothrombotic, and sickle cell anemia (and other hematological disorders). The field was transformed by the launching of collaborations and networks of investigators working together.

During the 1950s and 1960s, study of pediatric cerebral venous thrombosis continued. Treatment of children with anticoagulants and antibiotics was advised for the first time [15]. The prenatal onset of MCA occlusion was reported and attributed to placental embolism [16]. In a hallmark study, the importance of cerebrovascular disease as a cause of death in children was emphasized by neurologist and neuropathologist Betty Banker (1921–2010) [17]. Banker reported that, among 555 consecutive pediatric autopsies at Boston Children's Hospital, 48 (8.7%) died with cerebral occlusive disease, over half of whom had cerebral venous thrombosis, many with "phlebothrombosis." Banker provided support for the pathogenesis of neonatal stroke as arising from placental emboli, stating: "Occlusion of major arteries with infarction is not an uncommon occurrence in the neonatal period. The pathogenesis of these lesions appears to be in some way related to an abnormality of the placenta" and that "it is possible that the occlusions resulted from multiple emboli, the source of which was an infarcted placenta. It is also possible that the thrombotic lesions were the result of placental tissue degradation and the release of thromboplastin into the fetal circulation" [17].

In 1969, Jean Aicardi and colleagues published a seminal descriptive paper on "acute hemiplegia in infancy and childhood," based on 122 children with acute onset hemiplegia treated at the Hôpital Saint Vincent de Paul in Paris [18]. Jean François Marie Aicardi (1926 –2015) was a French pediatric neurologist and epileptologist [19]. He was born in November 1926 in Rambouillet, 50 kilometers from Paris, the seventh of nine children. At the Lycée Hoche in Versailles, he characterized himself as "an average student with no burning interest in any particular subject, notably not maths." A vague attraction to biology led him to consider a career in medicine. He earned his MD from the University of Paris for a thesis on convulsive disorders in the first year of life. He was inspired to study neurology by Raymond Garcin and to study child neurology by Stéphane Thieffry. He spent an inspirational year as a research fellow at Harvard Medical School and the Children's Hospital Medical Center in Boston. There he was mentored by Cesare Lombroso. He was exposed to North American research methods and their rigor. Thereafter he rejoined Thieffry in Paris in what was to become the first child neurology unit in France at both Hôpital des Enfants Malades and Hôpital Saint Vincent DePaul. Aicardi joined the Institut National de la Santé et de la Recerche Médicale (INSERM) where he was Mâitre de Recherche from 1969 to 1991 and research director from 1986 to 1991. He authored several textbooks, all written in English. Most of his work was done in Paris, but in later years he also held posts in Miami, Florida (as visiting scientist), at the Institute of Child Health (as honorary professor of child neurology), and at Great Ormond Street Hospital (as honorary consultant neurologist) in London [19].

Aicardi considered acute hemiplegia in his study as persisting for one month to exclude Todd's paresis and migraine [18]. He excluded cardiac-related conditions and congenital hemiplegia in order to limit the study to children "in which a deficit is fortuitously recognized in an infant previously considered healthy." He sought to differentiate hemiplegia due to seizures from other forms. He compared 89 children with convulsive versus 33 with nonconvulsive hemiplegia by cause, course, and prognosis. Cerebral angiography, done in 55 of the patients, was abnormal in 25 percent of the nonconvulsive group and in none of the convulsive group; 21 children in the latter group had had previous convulsions. This study clearly indicated that in some children, acute and persistent hemiplegia was due to prolonged seizures with brain damage rather than a vascular cause [18]. During the 1990s, Aicardi played a critical role in fostering transatlantic collaborations.

Larger and more in-depth case series of strokes in infants and children emerged during the 1960s and 1970s. Prognosis and outcomes could now be estimated in children with arterial ischemic stroke. In a review published in 1978, Gerry Golden observed: "The child with an acute cerebrovascular accident has an advantage over the adult in one respect, that of increased potential for recovery resulting from functional and perhaps anatomical plasticity" [20].

In 1970, a Columbia University neurology group reported outcomes in 41 children with acute hemiplegia. They defined predictors of poor prognosis as age below two years and seizures at the onset of symptoms [21]. They described five distinct arteriopathic patterns in childhood hemiplegia in 15 affected children: (1) basal vascular occlusive disease with telangiectasia, (2) basal vascular occlusive disease without telangiectasia, (3) stenosis of the origin of the internal carotid artery, (4) distal branch occlusion over the convexity, and (5) very small artery disease [21].

In 1971, the first book on acute childhood hemiplegia was written by Werner Isler, a Swiss pediatric neurologist with neurosurgical training [22]. This monograph contained chapters on vascular malformations, arterial occlusions, venous occlusions, and other brain conditions underlying hemiplegia. Isler's liberal use of case histories and extensive reporting of cerebral angiography enriched the book. Isler published additional papers on vaso-occlusive infarction and cerebrovascular disease in young children and made the insightful statement in 1980: "I firmly believe that our understanding of cerebrovascular disease in children would greatly profit by efficient coordination of observations made worldwide. We on our part are happy and willing to contribute to it as much as we possibly can" [23].

Angiography provided pathophysiological insights into venous thrombosis, including dynamic flow characteristics. Doppler ultrasound and angiographic evidence of sagittal sinus compression in neonates led to the concept that head molding during labor and delivery could result in newborn sinovenous occlusion and thrombosis [24].

In 1986, the first of many publications appeared from Fenella Kirkham, a pioneer in the field of pediatric stroke [25]. Kirkham was an undergraduate at Girton College, Cambridge, and followed up her second MB with a BA in history and philosophy of science in 1975. Her clinical training was at King's College Hospital, where she was awarded a bachelor in medicine (MB) in 1978 and a bachelor in surgery (BChir) in 1979 [26]. She particularly enjoyed child health and neurology and went directly into pediatrics. In 1982, she undertook a research project on coma in childhood at Guy's Hospital, funded by the British Heart Foundation. She trained as a pediatric neurologist. She held an honorary clinical post at Great Ormond Street Hospital until 1999, when she moved to Southampton University Hospitals Trust as a consultant pediatric neurologist. She was appointed professor at University College London Institute of Child Health in 2006.

Early in her career Kirkham became interested in brain ischemia and in methods of detecting the adequacy of cerebral blood flow. She obtained grants from the British Heart Foundation to study monitoring of cerebral perfusion and function in the unconscious child and, later, to study methods of ensuring adequate cerebral perfusion during cardiopulmonary bypass. She studied the role of seizures and status epilepticus in causing secondary deterioration after acute insults. Her research interests include sickle cell disease and focal brain ischemia [26].

Kirkham reported the first use and value of transcranial pulsed Doppler ultrasound in the diagnosis of proximal MCA stenosis in an 11-year-old with transient ischemic episodes. In 1983, the first reports of CT scanning investigating stroke emerged in neonates and children [27]. In a Swedish study, 26 children with stroke were studied over 10 years; 15 had hemorrhagic and 11 had ischemic stroke [28]. This study reported mortality rates of 36 percent for hemorrhagic stroke and 18 percent for ischemic stroke. Persistent disabilities were found in 75 percent of patients. The authors emphasized: "A child with stroke must without delay be transported to a hospital with access to neurosurgical expertise and neuroradiological facilities such as CAT scan and angiography" [28].

In 1985, Charles Raybaud and colleagues provided a thorough review of CT features of pediatric ischemic stroke [29]. They contrasted pediatric and adult strokes. They wrote that in children "the site of the infarct may result from pathologies more particular to children (e.g. basal ganglia infarction due to arteritis of the carotid siphon and its branches)" [29]. This description likely represents the first reference to a condition still frequently recognized in children with stroke and later dubbed "transient cerebral arteriopathy" and still later "focal cerebral arteriopathy."

In the mid-1980s acute neonatal stroke emerged as an important subtype of pediatric stroke. Pediatric neurologists at the University of Massachusetts wrote: "Neonatal stroke should be considered as a cause of seizures in a full-term newborn in spite of a normal obstetrical history and a non-focal neurological examination ... 7/50 full term neonates with seizures had them due to cerebral infarction" [30].

In 1988, the first edition of a textbook on pediatric stroke was published by Steven Roach and his colleague, Anthony Riella [31]. This and subsequent editions have served generations of physicians as a comprehensive resource for those who care for children. Roach continued to teach, energize, and facilitate growth of the field.

During the 1990s, pediatric stroke emerged as a subspecialty within pediatric neurology, with the development of national and international collaborations and registries, particularly in Canada, Germany, and Switzerland. A critical feature was the development of training programs in pediatric stroke that served as a catalyst for clinical research and increased the number of physicians who provided specialized expertise, primarily within children's hospitals. Jean Aicardi introduced Gabrielle deVeber in Canada to Fenella Kirkham in London, as he recognized their common interest in pediatric stroke.

Gabrielle deVeber was born in Sudbury, Ontario, Canada. She is a direct descendant of Sir Richard Quain, who wrote about apoplexy in the early nineteenth century [4]. Her father was a pediatric hematologist-oncologist. She initially chose a career in physical and occupational therapy, earning her degree in 1981 at the University of British Columbia. She moved on to three years of medical school. Her pediatric residency was completed at the Hospital for Sick Children in Toronto in 1986. DeVeber completed training in adult neurology at the University of Western Ontario in 1987 and in child neurology, with a clinical fellowship in pediatric neurorehabilitation and electromyography (EMG) at Massachusetts General Hospital. There she was mentored by Ray Adams, C. Miller Fisher, and Verne Caviness. She then spent four years as a child neurologist at McMaster University where she acquired an understanding of clinical epidemiology and biostatistics. She then began her long-term relationship with the Hospital for Sick Kids in Toronto. During 1995–1998, deVeber had a stroke-thrombosis fellowship in Maureen Andrew's hematology lab with support from the Ontario Heart and Stroke Foundation.

DeVeber began to receive external requests for advice about care for child with stroke. Cases and consultations poured in from Canada, the United States, and many international sites. This led her to develop an international consortium for pediatric stroke that would have research, clinical, and therapeutic trial capabilities. In 2003, deVeber and a small, international group of child neurologists started the International Pediatric Stroke Study (IPSS), a prospective, multicenter registry for neonates and children with ischemic stroke. She initiated and directed several large multicenter collaborative studies, including the Canadian Pediatric Ischemic Stroke Registry. The IPSS is a large international study of childhood stroke with over 6,000 enrolled children at over 75 enrolling centers spanning 18 countries in Asia, Europe, and North and South America. The central organization and database is at Sick Kids Hospital in Toronto. Since 2009, deVeber has been senior scientist and professor at the Child Health Evaluative Sciences program of the University of Toronto. Important in deVeber's career has been her collaboration with Donna Ferriero and Heather Fullerton at the University of California at San Francisco and Fenella Kirkham in the United Kingdom.

From 1992 on, deVeber and Kirkham forged a strong collaborative friendship. They started outpatient pediatric stroke clinics, and then fledgling inpatient clinical stroke services at their pediatric hospitals in Toronto and London. Around the same time, young investigators in the United States began to establish strong clinical and research interests in pediatric stroke. They began to publish case reports and case series of pediatric strokes. As neonatology emerged in the United States, Europe, and England, more focus was directed on perinatal and neonatal stroke by Joseph Volpe, Donna Ferriero, Rebecca Ichord, Linda de Vries, and others. De Vries began her research career publishing seminal papers on intraventricular hemorrhage and cystic encephalomalacia. In 1997 she and her colleagues published the first of many pivotal papers on neonatal stroke [32]. De Vries remained a world leader in neonatal stroke and helped begin clinical trials for this condition.

A fundamental component of pediatric stroke advancement was attention directed to the hematological aspects of pediatric stroke. Collaboration with those who worked in the field of pediatric thrombosis led to applications to pediatric stroke. In 1992, the first pediatric thrombosis–pediatric stroke partnership began in Canada, under the leadership of Gabrielle deVeber and Maureen Andrew (with whom deVeber later spent a three-year fellowship). During that year the world's first national multicenter registry was launched.

DeVeber and Andrew initiated the Canadian registry at all 15 academic pediatric hospitals in Canada. The Canadian national health care system enabled the consistent referral of children with serious conditions for care at these hospitals, so a population-based perspective was achieved. The Canadian Pediatric Ischemic Stroke Registry collected data on over 1,200 Canadian newborns, infants, and children with arterial ischemic stroke or sinovenous thrombosis and defined the epidemiology and clinical and radiographic features of these conditions [33]. Between 1980 and 2000, over 1,000 manuscripts were published on pediatric stroke compared to fewer than 25 in the preceding 100 years.

The IPSS was established in 2003 by 11 original coinvestigators (pediatric neurologists, hematologists, and epidemiologists) as an international registry with the long-term goal of developing multinational clinical trials in pediatric ischemic stroke. The number of enrolling centers increased to 106 sites located in 34 countries, including Australia, Canada, Chile, China, Georgia, Germany, Malaysia, Thailand, the United Kingdom, the United States, and many others. A central IPSS office was established at the Hospital for Sick Children in Toronto to manage the website and database. IPSS investigators established consensus-based diagnostic definitions for stroke subtypes, etiologic investigations, study outcomes, and treatment approaches. International collaborations led to reports, therapeutic trials, and guidelines on diverse topics in pediatric stroke, including sickle-cell disease and transfusion management, sinovenous thrombosis, thrombophilia, anticoagulant treatment, thrombolysis, mechanical thrombectomy, and others.

REFERENCES

1. Much of this chapter is adapted and published in Ashwal S (ed.), *Founders of Child Neurology*, 2nd ed. Elsevier, 2021.

2. Willis T. Of the pia mater. In *The Anatomy of the Brain*. Reprint. Tuckahoe, NY: USV Pharmaceutical Corp., 1971. Williams AN, Sunderland R. Thomas Willis: The first paediatric neurologist? *Arch. Dis. Child.* 2001;85(6):506–509.

3. Cruveilhier J. *Anatomie pathologique de corp humaine; descriptions figures lithographies et colores des diverses alterations morbides dont le corp humain est susceptible.* Paris: JB Bailliere, 1842.

4. Quain R. *Observations on Cerebral Apoplexy at Different Periods of Life.* London, 1849.

5. Otto Huebner's career and his recurrent artery are discussed in Chapter 12.

6. McNutt SJ. Seven cases of spastic infantile hemiplegia. *Am. J. Med. Sci.* 1885;177 (1):58–78.

7. Osler W. *The Cerebral Palsies of Childhood: A Clinical Study from the Infirmary for Nervous Diseases.* London: P. Blakiston, 1889. Osler and his textbook of mediicne are discussed at length in Chapter 14.

8. Sachs B, Peterson F. A study of the cerebral palsies of early life, based upon an analysis of one hundred and forty cases. *J. Nerv. Ment. Dis.* 1890;17:295–332.

9. Sachs B. *A Treatise on the Nervous Diseases of Children*. London: Balliere, Tindall and Cox, 1895.

10. Freud S. *Infantile Cerebral Paralysis* (1895). Trans. L. A. Russin. Coral Gables, FL: University of Miami Press, 1968.

11. Holt LE. *The Diseases of Infancy and Childhood: For the Use of Students and Practitioners of Medicine*. D. Appleton and Company, 1897.

12. Ford FR, Schaffer AJ. Hemiplegia. *Arch. Neurol. Psychiatry* 1927;18(3):323–347.

13. Simpson R. Thrombosis of the cerebral vessels in infants. *Can. Med. Assoc. J.* 1932;26 (3):317–319.

14. Ehlers H, Courville C. Thrombosis of internal cerebral veins in infancy and childhood. *J. Pediatr.* 1936;8:600–623.

15. Mitchell RG. Venous thrombosis in acute infantile hemiplegia. *Arch. Dis. Child.* 1951;27(131):95–104.

16. Clark RM, Linelle EA. Case report: Prenatal occlusion of the internal carotid artery. *J. Neurol. Neurosurg. Psychiatry* 1954;17(4):295–297.

17. Banker BQ. Cerebrovascular disease in infancy and childhood. 1. Occlusive vascular disease. *J. Neuropathol. Exp. Neurol.* 1961;21:127–140.

18. Aicardi J, Amsili J, Chevrie JJ. Acute hemiplegia in infancy and childhood. *Developmental Med. Child Neurol.* 1969;11(2):162–173.

19. Stephenson JBP. In memoriam: Professor Jean Aicardi (1926–2015). *Pediatr. Neurol.* 2016;54:3–4. Also published in the Child Neurology Society Archives. Available at www.childneurologysociety.org/docs/default-source/default-document-library/con nectionsfinal-oct-2014.pdf?sfvrsn=4309d28_0.

20. Golden GS. Vascular diseases of the brain and tics, twitches and habit spasms. *Curr. Probl. Pediatr.* 1978;8(6):1–41.

21. Solomon GE, Hilal SK, Gold AP, Carter S. Natural history of acute hemiplegia of childhood. *Brain* 1970;93(1):107–120.

22. Isler W. *Acute Hemiplegias and Hemisyndromes in Childhood*. London: William Heinemann Medical Books, 1971.

23. Isler W. Cerebrovascular diseases in the first three years of life. *Brain Dev.* 1980;2 (2):95–105.

24. Newton TH, Gooding CA. Compression of superior sagittal sinus by neonatal calvarial molding. *Radiology* 1975;115(3):635–640.

25. Kirkham FB Neville B, Levin S. Bedside diagnosis of stenosis of middle cerebral artery. *Lancet* 1986;5(1):197–198.

26. Fenella Kirkham. University College London. Available at www.ucl.ac.uk/child-health/people/fenella-kirkham.

27. Hill A, Martin DJ, Daneman A, Fitz CR. Focal ischemic cerebral injury in the newborn: Diagnosis by ultrasound and correlation with computed tomographic scan. *Pediatrics* 1983;71(5):790–793.

28. Eeg-Olofsson O, Ringheim Y. Stroke in children: Clinical characteristics and prognosis. *Acta Paediatr. Scand.* 1983;72(3):391–395.

29. Raybaud CA, Livet MO, Jiddane M, Pinsard N. Radiology of ischemic strokes in children. *Neuroradiology* 1985;27(6):567–578.

30. Levy SR, Abroms IF, Marshall PC, Rosquete EE. Seizures and cerebral infarction in the full-term newborn. *Ann. Neurol.* 1985;17(4):366–370.

31. Roach ES, Riella AR. *Pediatric Cerebrovascular Disorders*. Mt. Kisco, NY: Futura Publishing, 1988.

32. de Vries LS, Regev R, Dubowitz LM. Late onset cystic leucomalacia. *Arch. Dis. Child.* 1986;61(3):298–299. de Vries LS, Groenendaal F, Eken P, van Haastert IC, Rademaker KJ, Meiners LC. Infarcts in the vascular distribution of the middle cerebral artery in preterm and fullterm infants. *Neuropediatrics* 1997;28(2):88–96. Roelants-van Rijn AM et al. Neonatal diffusion-weighted MR imaging: Relation with histopathology or follow-up MR examination. *Neuropediatrics* 2001;32(6):286–294.

33. deVeber GA et al. Epidemiology and outcomes of arterial ischemic stroke in children: The Canadian Pediatric Ischemic Stroke Registry. *Pediatr. Neurol.* 2017;69:58–70. deVeber GA et al. Cerebral sinovenous thrombosis in children. *N. Engl. J. Med.* 2001 345(6):417–423.

CARE

CHAPTER FORTY ONE

CARE OF STROKE PATIENTS

One of the most important therapeutic advances during the last decades of the twentieth century in the treatment of patients with acute stroke was the development of stroke services, stroke centers, stroke nurses, stroke specialists, and stroke units.

STROKE UNITS

During the nineteenth and first two thirds of the twentieth century, nearly all acute stroke patients were cared for in the general wards and rooms of hospitals. There were very few stroke specialists and no stroke nurse specialists. Some rehabilitation units, almost entirely outside the acute hospitals, specialized in stroke rehabilitation. During the 1960s and 1970s, neurology departments began to split off from departments of internal medicine within academic medical centers in the United States and Europe. When this occurred, hospitals with neurology departments began to place stroke patients and other patients with neurological diseases on neurology wards and private rooms, while other stroke patients continued to be treated on medical services scattered throughout the hospitals. During the 1970s and 1980s, hospitals placed very sick patients requiring frequent monitoring and care into specialized intensive care units (ICUs). Cardiac, surgical, and medical ICUs were first formed. Neurosurgeons and neurologists in large medical centers were successful in creating neuroscience ICUs manned with nurses specially trained to care for very ill patients with acute neurological disorders, including stroke. A new neurological specialty, neurology intensivists, began to grow.

A number of factors during the 1980s and 1990s conspired to promote the development and proliferation of specialized stroke units. CT, MRI, ultrasound, and vascular imaging capabilities made it clear that strokes were complex and composed of very diverse etiologies and pathophysiologies. Specific diagnoses could be made quickly and safely but required special training, expertise, and experience. Funding for trials made it possible in academic medical centers to hire nursing coordinators who could ensure that all eligible patients were entered and met study criteria. The development of managed care strategies in hospitals in the United States forced more rapid and efficient care and throughput of stroke patients. Newer therapies, surgeries, percutaneous interventions, and especially thrombolysis made it advantageous to segregate stroke patients in ICUs and specialized stroke units.

These specialized stroke units were composed of nurses with experience and training in stroke, internists, and stroke neurologists. These stroke units were able to deliver specialized nursing care; attention to management of blood pressure, fluid volumes, and other physiological and biochemical factors; protocols and practices to facilitate rapid and thorough evaluation and treatment, monitor treatment, carry out randomized therapeutic trials, and prevent complications; and education about stroke and its prevention to patients and their families and caregivers [1–3]. They also promoted an upbeat, optimistic view of stroke recovery, in contrast to the situation previously present on medical wards where stroke patients were often considered undesirable patients with hopeless outcomes.

Once these units began to proliferate, first in Europe and then in the United States, it became clear that they were an important major advance. Dedicated stroke units were convincingly shown to decrease mortality, limit stroke morbidity, and allow more patients to retain their independence and to return home after stroke [4–6]. During the three years between the two large European thrombolytic trials (ECAS I [7] and ECAS II [8]), neurologists in the hospitals engaging in these trials developed dedicated stroke units. These units attended to the general medical care of the stroke patients and prevention of complications. As a result, the morbidity in both the thrombolytic treatment group and placebo groups improved dramatically in the ECAS II trial, and the good results in the placebo-treated group exceeded that of any prior thrombolytic trial [8]. The milieu and the care in dedicated stroke units leads to better outcomes. Mortality is reduced. More patients return home and fewer are transferred to chronic hospitals and nursing homes. Short-term and long-term functional outcomes are also improved. There is now a general agreement that stroke units work.

ROLE OF STROKE NURSES

Nurses who work in acute stroke care units have a wide-ranging role that includes assessment, identification, and monitoring, as well as rehabilitation, psychological support, and end-of-life care. They are responsible for monitoring patients on presentation, immediately following treatment, and throughout the inpatient stay. The physiological parameters that require regular monitoring are blood glucose, blood pressure, cardiac rate and rhythm, hydration and nutrition, level of consciousness, respiratory rate, and oxygen saturation of hemoglobin and temperature. If a patient's condition deteriorates, nurses may provide initial interventions, and in hyperacute or critical settings they may be responsible for ongoing interventions such as the titration of antihypertensives and active cooling [9].

Nurses are responsible for assessing and regularly reviewing a patient's ability to care for themself and to address any needs. Assessing the risks of deep vein thrombosis, pressure ulcers, and malnutrition should also be undertaken by nurses on admission and regularly thereafter so that appropriate care can be provided. Early rehabilitation is a core element of acute stroke care and should begin as soon as the patient becomes clinically stable. It includes mobilization, optimal positioning, continence care, oral care, and pain management [9].

Many stroke patients have low mood, anxiety, and depression. Nurses working in acute stroke services are well placed to provide early psychological support, such as brief interventions and motivational interviewing. Nurses can administer stroke-specific screening for depression to identify patients who require further psychological support [9].

STROKE CENTERS AND ACUTE STROKE-READY HOSPITALS

The Brain Attack Coalition (BAC), formed in 1996, is a multidisciplinary organization in the United States that includes most major medical organizations involved with stroke care. BAC members determined that two levels of stroke centers should be established: a primary stroke center (PSC) and a comprehensive stroke center (CSC). A primary stroke center would stabilize and provide emergency care for patients with acute stroke. These centers then either would transfer the patient to a comprehensive stroke center or would admit the patient and provide further care, depending on the patient's need and that center's capabilities. A comprehensive stroke center typically would include tertiary care medical centers and hospitals with the infrastructure and personnel necessary to perform highly technical procedures and provide all needed levels of care [10].

The major elements of a primary stroke center are acute stroke teams, written care protocols, emergency medical services, emergency department, stroke units, neurological services, and various support services such as a stroke center director, neuroimaging capabilities, laboratory services, outcome and quality improvement activities, and continuing medical education. A stroke unit is required only in those primary stroke centers that provide ongoing inpatient care for patients with stroke [10].

Studies have the affirmed the benefits of primary and comprehensive stroke centers in improving the outcomes for admitted patients. The Joint Commission and other national, regional, and state agencies have developed and implemented certification programs for PSCs and CSCs [10].

To address the concerns of providing acute stroke care in all settings, the BAC in 2013 proposed a new designation for hospitals that are not PSCs yet can provide timely, evidence-based care to most patients with an acute stroke: the Acute Stroke Ready Hospital (ASRH). The ASRH would provide initial diagnostic services, stabilization, and emergent care and then transfer the patients to a PSC or CSC. An ASRH would not require a stroke unit [11].

MOBILE STROKE UNIT

The concept of a mobile stroke unit (MSU) was first published by Fassbender et al. in 2003 as a way of "bringing treatment to the patient rather than patient to the treatment." All MSUs have the basic components to provide assessment and treatment of acute ischemic infarcts, including standard ambulance equipment and medications, a computed tomography (CT) scanner, point-of-care laboratory equipment, telemedicine capabilities and tPA. In addition to the staff of a standard ambulance, the unit also has a physician, either in person or through telemedicine, and a member trained as a CT technologist. In the first generation of MSUs, standard ambulances could not house all the necessary components, but miniaturization of technology has now allowed all necessary components to fit into a standard ambulance. The team members work to quickly and effectively diagnose or exclude stroke and determine IV tPA eligibility. Care at the location of the patient eliminates the delays associated with in-hospital care such as triage of multiple patients, competing obligations of the hospitalist, availability of a CT scanner, and attention of emergency department nurses and technicians [12].

REFERENCES

1. Indredavik B, Bakke F, Solberg R, Rokseth R, Haaheim LL, Holme I. Benefit of a stroke unit: A randomized controlled trial. *Stroke* 1991 Aug;22(8):1026–1031.
2. Indredavik B, Slørdahl SA, Bakke F, Rokseth R, Håheim LL. Stroke unit treatment: Long-term effects. *Stroke* 1997 Oct;28(10):1861–1866.

3. Díez-Tejedor E, Fuentes B. Acute care in stroke: Do stroke units make the difference? *Cerebrovasc. Dis.* 2001;11(suppl 1):31–39.

4. Birbeck GL, Zingmond DS, Cui X, Vickrey BG. Multispecialty stroke services in California hospitals are associated with reduced mortality. *Neurology* 2006 May 23;66 (10):1527–1532.

5. How do stroke units improve patient outcomes? A collaborative systematic review of the randomized trials. Stroke Unit Trialists Collaboration. *Stroke* 1997 Nov;28 (11):2139–2144.

6. Collaborative systematic review of the randomised trials of organised inpatient (stroke unit) care after stroke. Stroke Unit Trialists Collaboration. *BMJ* 1997 Apr 19;314 (7088):1151–1159.

7. Hacke W, Kaste M, Fieschi C, et al. Intravenous thrombolysis with recombinant tissue plasminogen activator for acute hemispheric stroke. The European Cooperative Acute Stroke Study (ECASS). *JAMA* 1995;274:1017–1025.

8. Hacke W, Kaste M, Fieschi C, et al. Randomised double-blind placebo-controlled trial of thrombolytic therapy with intravenous alteplase in acute ischaemic stroke (ECASS II). *Lancet* 1998;352:1245–1251.

9. Clare CS. Role of the nurse in acute stroke care. *Nurs. Stand.* 2020 Apr 1;35(4):68–75.

10. Alberts MJ, Hademenos G, Latchaw RE, Jagoda A, Marler JR, Mayberg MR, et al. Recommendations for the establishment of primary stroke centers. Brain Attack Coalition. *JAMA* 2000 Jun 21;283(23):3102–3109.

11. Alberts MJ, Wechsler LR, Jensen MEL, Latchaw RE, Crocco TJ, George MG, et al. Formation and function of acute stroke-ready hospitals within a stroke system of care recommendations from the Brain Attack Coalition. *Stroke* 2013 Dec 1;44 (12):3382–3393.

12. Towner J, Pieters T, Schmidt T, Pilcher W, Bhalla T. A history of mobile stroke units and review of literature. *Am. J. Interv. Radiol.* 2018;2(9):1–5.

CHAPTER FORTY TWO

NEUROCRITICAL CARE

You say you want a revolution
Well, you know
We all want to change the world
  "Revolution 1," The Beatles

INTRODUCTION

When Werner Hacke, the 39-year-old newly appointed chair of neurology at the University of Heidelberg in Germany, strode into the 12-bed Neuro-Intensive Care Unit in 1987, it was the start of something new. Neurocritical care began in the 1980s with convergence of the evolution of critical care and advances in the diagnosis and management of severe brain injury. Although many people contributed to that convergence, three stand out: Allan Ropper at Massachusetts General Hospital (MGH), Dan Hanley at Johns Hopkins Hospital, and Werner Hacke. Bold, confident, and with a take-no-prisoners focus on aggressive treatment, Hacke was the embodiment of neurocritical care, especially for acute stroke. The roots of neurocritical care can be traced to the surgical wards of Johns Hopkins Hospital in Baltimore early in the twentieth century.

EVOLUTION OF CRITICAL CARE

Postoperative and Respiratory Units

Walter Dandy, a young protégé of neurosurgeon Harvey Cushing, believed that patients after surgery would benefit if managed in a specific postoperative environment, one efficiently staffed day and night by specialized nurses and doctors. He created the first three-bed intensive care unit (ICU) at Hopkins in 1923 [1]. Other hospitals created similar postoperative units. More than anything, the deadly respiratory failure during the poliomyelitis epidemics was the impetus for the development of critical care. The first tank respirator, invented by Scottish physician John Dalziel in 1832, used negative pressure to expand the lungs but was hand-operated and inefficient [2]. In 1929, engineer Philip Drinker and physiologist Louis Shaw at Harvard developed a better tank respirator, which used electrically operated pumps to create the negative pressure [3]. Their new "iron lung," tested first at Children's Hospital in Boston, was used extensively throughout the United States to provide ventilatory support during the poliomyelitis epidemics of the 1940s [4]. This led to the establishment of dedicated respiratory units – the first real intensive care units – to treat patients with respiratory failure. Many neurologists were at the forefront of managing these patients, including W. Ritchie Russell at the University of Oxford, A. B. Baker at the University of Minnesota, and Fred Plum at the University of Washington [5].

Positive Pressure Mechanical Ventilation

Many patients with poliomyelitis had impaired airway control from bulbar muscle weakness. The large number of these bulbar patients in Copenhagen in 1952 prompted anesthesiologist Bjørn Ibsen to try a different approach. Fresh from his anesthesia training at MGH, where Henry Beecher encouraged him to question dogma [6], Ibsen performed tracheotomies and supported patients with intermittent positive pressure using bag ventilation. With dedicated but exhausted medical students bagging patients around the clock, positive pressure ventilation cut mortality from 80 to 40 percent [7]. Advances in endotracheal intubation (e.g., the curved Macintosh laryngoscope blade and cuffed endotracheal tube), coupled with the first positive pressure mechanical ventilator [8], made respiratory support central to intensive care, supporting polio patients and those with myasthenia gravis and Guillain-Barré syndrome. The Batten Respiratory Unit at the Institute of Neurology and National Hospital for Nervous Diseases in Queen Square, London, opened in 1954 to treat such patients and those with stroke, spinal cord disorders, and encephalitis [9]. Mechanical ventilation also supported a new group of patients – those with cardiac arrest.

Defibrillation and Cardiopulmonary Resuscitation

Claude Beck, another Cushing protégé, was bewildered when, after a patient suddenly became pulseless at the end of a case, he observed the attending surgeon calmly remove his gloves to call the Baltimore Fire Department. Fifteen minutes later, burly firefighters burst in and tried, unsuccessfully, to revive the patient. Beck believed that surgeons should be able to deal with such emergencies themselves [10]. In 1947, after two decades of collaborating with cardiovascular physiologist Carl Wiggers from Western Reserve University in Cleveland, Beck performed the first successful defibrillation of a patient with intraoperative ventricular fibrillation [11]. He reported the first out-of-hospital resuscitation in 1956 [12]. Both were accomplished with direct cardiac massage (requiring an open thoracotomy) and defibrillation with placement of the paddles directly onto the heart. The first successful human closed-chest defibrillation, also in 1956, was reported by Paul Zoll of Boston's Beth Israel Hospital [13]. Closed-chest massage (chest compressions) followed in 1960 [14]. When combined with mouth-to-mouth breathing, introduced by Peter Safar in 1957, the new, life-saving approach was called "cardiopulmonary resuscitation" [15].

Safar, an Austrian anesthesiologist who immigrated to the United States in 1950, played a leading role in establishing critical care and, indirectly, neurocritical care. After his 11-year-old daughter tragically died following an asthma-induced respiratory arrest, he understood that saving the heart and lungs was of little value if the brain was not protected. He promoted cardiopulmonary *cerebral* resuscitation that used induced hypothermia to protect the brain against global ischemia.

Growth of Modern ICUs

Safar at Baltimore City Hospital and Max Weil at USC Medical Center in Los Angeles opened the first modern medical ICUs in 1958. The Baltimore unit was called an "intensive care unit" and emphasized airway and respiration [16]. The Los Angeles unit was called a "shock ward," focusing on acute circulatory failure [17]. The first coronary care unit opened in 1964 at the Royal Infirmary of Edinburgh. The premise was that continuous electrocardiographic monitoring could rapidly identify and promote termination of peri-infarction lethal arrhythmias [18]. A landmark article in 1967 described a nearly 20 percent decline in the post-myocardial infarction mortality rate after implementation of a coronary care unit [19]. The expansion of automated monitoring of vital signs with alarms in the 1960s and introduction of the pulmonary artery catheter in the 1970s allowed doctors to intervene promptly to prevent physiological deterioration. As ICUs opened in hospitals across the United

States and Europe, consistently better outcomes justified their significantly higher costs [20].

Neurologists were by the 1970s increasingly uncomfortable managing multi-organ system failure. A new breed of internists, surgeons, and anesthesiologists emerged to provide this specialized care: the *intensivist*. The Society of Critical Care Medicine was founded in the United States in 1971. The European equivalent, the European Society of Intensive Care Medicine, was founded in 1981.

Not all neurologists were uncomfortable with multi-organ system failure, however. At Johns Hopkins in 1975, David Jackson had trained in both internal medicine and neurology when he was recruited to Case Western Reserve University to become the first director of the newly opened medical intensive care unit, still under construction when he arrived. His research would focus on neurological complications of medical illness, post-cardiac arrest encephalopathy, and the challenging ethical dilemmas that were arising in critical care, particularly in patients with severe brain injury [21].

ADVANCES IN THE DIAGNOSIS AND MANAGEMENT OF SEVERE BRAIN INJURY

Examination of the Comatose Patient

Comatose ventilated patients presented new challenges since, in the past, patients with massive strokes, cardiac arrest, and traumatic brain injury (TBI) typically died. The new resuscitative technology created unique diagnostic, prognostic, and ethical dilemmas for neurologists. Accurate prognostication was difficult with few guidelines. In 1966, Fred Plum and Jerome Posner published *Diagnosis of Stupor and Coma* [22]. Distinguishing patients with severe but potentially recoverable neurological injuries from those "hopelessly unconscious" led neurologists Raymond Adams, Robert Schwab, and Derek Denny-Brown and anesthesiologist Henry Beecher to publish "A Definition of Irreversible Coma" in 1968, establishing standard criteria for "brain death" [23]. The following year, C. Miller Fisher published his classic paper, "The Neurological Examination of the Comatose Patient" [24].

The first CT scans for clinical use were installed at the Mayo Clinic and MGH in 1973. Armed with brain imaging, Allan Ropper, a bright young neurology protégé of Adams and Fisher, began managing patients with large ischemic strokes at MGH and consulting on neurosurgical patients, offering detailed neurological examinations and thoughtful prognostication. Together with anesthesiologist Sean Kennedy, Ropper also managed many of the critical care aspects of neurosurgical patients.

Board-certified in internal medicine, Ropper had gained extensive experience in critical care during his medicine residency at the University of California, San Francisco. Around the same time, Nicholas Zervas, chief of neurosurgery at MGH, urged expansion of the neurosurgery ICU, which abutted the neurology ward. This led to one of the first combined neurology-neurosurgery ICUs in the country, and Ropper was put in charge.

Introduction of plasma exchange therapy in 1978 led to renewed interest in Guillain-Barré syndrome [25]. Ropper began managing these patients, many of whom had respiratory failure and autonomic instability. He also questioned the mechanism of early neurological deterioration in patients with large hemispheric lesions. Ropper opined, based on head CT scans, that horizontal brain displacement was the likely mechanism [26], challenging the vertical shift theory by Donald McNealy and Fred Plum based on autopsy findings [27]. Implicit in this hypothesis was the concept of intracranial pressure gradients, which also provided the rationale for decompressive hemicraniectomy in patients with large hemispheric strokes.

Management of Traumatic Brain Injury

Decompressive hemicraniectomy for large hemispheric strokes was extrapolated from TBI. Raymond Kjellberg and Alberto Prieto reported their experience at MGH with bifrontal decompressive craniectomy to treat elevated intracranial pressure (ICP) in TBI in 1971 [28]. Continuous ICP monitoring in TBI was introduced in 1965 by Swedish neurosurgeon Nils Lundberg [29]. Lundberg had developed the technique in the 1950s at Lund University Hospital as part of his doctoral thesis [30]. While the main treatment for elevated ICP relied on mannitol and hyperventilation, ventricular catheters allowed monitoring and therapeutic draining of cerebrospinal fluid. In 1977, J. Douglas Miller and Donald Becker showed improved outcomes by incorporating ICP into clearly defined treatment algorithms [31]. ICP monitoring would become the cornerstone of neurocritical care.

The CT scan also revolutionized the management of head trauma. For the first time, hematomas could be identified and quickly evacuated. In a landmark paper in 1981, a study showed that early evacuation of subdural hematomas cut mortality from 90 to 30 percent [32]. That study, which emphasized the importance of rapid CT scanning, early operative decompression, and ICP monitoring, made head trauma something worth rallying around.

Bryan Jennett, a British neurosurgeon in Glasgow, Scotland, observed that many patients with head injury seemingly "talked and died," suggesting that additional factors other than their primary injury were important [33]. Recognition of this "secondary brain injury," from ischemia, tissue hypoxia, and a cascade of metabolic events, translated into the need for aggressive critical care to avoid or rapidly correct adverse factors [34]. In the 1990s and early 2000s, prevention of secondary brain injury spurred development of new neuromonitoring tools, including those for cerebral perfusion, brain tissue oxygenation, and brain metabolism. Taken together, this approach became known as "multimodal monitoring."

Even with early surgery and aggressive intensive care, many patients did not survive. Accurate prognostication in the 1970s remained challenging. In 1975, Jennet co-created the Glasgow Coma Scale [35] and, two years later, the Glasgow Outcome Scale [36], standardized scoring systems that facilitated more accurate prognostication and made modern coma research possible. Emphasizing meticulous management in an ICU, the first TBI guidelines were published in 1996 [37].

Decompressive craniectomy for TBI ultimately did not improve outcomes in two randomized controlled trials (DECRA [38] and RESCUicp [39]). This would also be the fate for another intuitive TBI therapy: induced hypothermia.

Induced Hypothermia

Temple Fay, chief of neurosurgery at Philadelphia's Temple University, reported the first series of patients with TBI treated with induced hypothermia in 1945 [40]. However, large randomized trials failed to show an improved outcome with hypothermia [41], with some showing even a worse outcome [42]. Hypothermia would prove more successful in ameliorating anoxic brain injury following cardiac arrest. First applied to post–cardiac arrest patients at Hopkins in 1959 [43] and recommended by Peter Safar as early as 1961 [44], interest in hypothermia for cardiac arrest lay dormant until the 1990s.

The 1990s, designated the "Decade of the Brain" by the US Congress and the National Institutes of Health, stimulated a renaissance in neuroscience research. Animal models of cardiac arrest (particularly, clinically relevant dog models developed in Safar's lab at the University of Pittsburgh) showed improved functional recovery and reduced cerebral histologic deficits with therapeutic hypothermia [45]. In 2002, the Hypothermia after Cardiac Arrest trial demonstrated that therapeutic hypothermia could significantly reduce mortality and improve neurologic outcomes [46]. Today, "targeted temperature management," ranging from 32 to 36°C for 24 hours post–cardiac arrest, is standard of care [47].

Treatment of Ischemic Stroke

The "Decade of the Brain" also saw a revolution in the treatment of ischemic stroke with Werner Hacke as one of its leaders. Hacke joined the University Hospital of Aachen in Germany in 1978. In 1982, he published the first cases of intraarterial thrombolysis for basilar artery occlusion [48]. In 1986, Hacke was a visiting professor at the Scripps Clinic in La Jolla, California, where he collaborated with hematologist Greg del Zoppo on thrombolytic therapy. A year later, parking his Harley Davidson at the front entrance, he walked into the University of Heidelberg's newly opened "Kopfklinik" as chair of the department of neurology.

In Germany, critical care in the 1960s and 1970s evolved mainly as part of anesthesiology, leading the German Society for Anesthesiology in 1977 to change its name to the German Society for Anesthesiology and Intensive Medicine. Neurosurgery ICUs were staffed following this model [49]. However, other specialties were free to adopt their own intensive care units [50]. Many German institutions in the 1970s opened separate neurology ICUs staffed solely by neurologists, beginning in Hamburg, Giessen, Chemnitz, and Aachen, where Hacke had trained, acquiring particular expertise in managing coma and acute respiratory failure stemming from the heroin epidemic in the Netherlands [51].

Emergency care in Germany also differed in that typically there were separately staffed "emergency admission areas" within hospitals for internal medicine, surgery, gynecology and obstetrics, pediatrics, and, in larger teaching hospitals, neurology [52]. When the Kopfklinik, a specialty hospital combining neurology; neurosurgery; ophthalmology; and ear, nose, and troat, opened in September 1987 on the outskirts of Heidelberg, both the neurology ICU and the emergency room were staffed by neurologists alone. Benefiting from this autonomy, neurocritical care flourished at the Kopfklinik in the 1990s, especially for ischemic stroke.

In 1990, Hacke hosted the first international thrombolysis meeting at the Kopfklinik and published the proceedings a year later [53]. German-American collaboration led to open angiography-based studies of the effect of intravenous and intraarterial recombinant tissue plasminogen activator (rt-PA) on recanalization in patients with acute ischemic stroke [54]. In 1995, Hacke and colleagues published the results of ECASS I, the first large randomized controlled trial of intravenous rt-PA for acute ischemic stroke. The NINDS-sponsored trial, also published in 1995, led to FDA-approval of intravenous rt-PA in 1996. ECASS III in 2008, led again by Hacke, extended the time window for intravenous rt-PA for selected patients [55].

Treatment of Intracerebral Hemorrhage

In 1981, Dan Hanley, a quiet, young neurologist at Johns Hopkins (and medical school classmate of Allan Ropper), started managing critically ill patients with ischemic stroke who, up until that point, had been treated exclusively in the medical intensive care unit. Simultaneously, Don Long, chief of neurosurgery, like Nick Zervas at MGH, needed more ICU beds for his rapidly growing service. The plan was to create a combined neurology-neurosurgery ICU, and Hanley was targeted to run it. Board-certified in internal medicine, Hanley had also trained under leaders in critical care, including Joseph Parillo and Henry Masur. After an 18-month anesthesia fellowship, Hanley became the director in July 1983 and, together with anesthesiologist Cecil Borel, began managing complex, critically ill neurological and neurosurgical patients.

In 1986, Werner Hacke gave an inspiring grand rounds at Hopkins, sharing his experience with intraarterial thrombolysis for basilar artery occlusion. Shortly after that, Hanley started using urokinase for similar patients at Hopkins. In 1992, faced with a patient with intraventricular hemorrhage in whom the ventricular catheter kept clotting, he used urokinase to lyse the drain. That's when the novel idea of using thrombolysis to treat patients with intraventricular hemorrhage and intracerebral hemorrhage was born.

In 1996, with funding from the Humboldt Foundation, Hanley took a sabbatical year at the Max Planck Institute in Heidelberg, where he also worked closely with Hacke. They later reported a case series of patients receiving intraventricular rt-PA, resulting in faster clearance of intraventricular blood [56]. Hanley also launched the North American Consortium of Acute Brain Injury (NACABI), a collaborative research network for multicenter trials, including his proposal for the Intraventricular Hemorrhage Lysis Study, a randomized pilot clinical trial to test the effect of intraventricular injection of urokinase.

This research continued back at Hopkins. In 2000, results of that pilot clinical trial confirmed that intraventricular urokinase reduced the 30-day mortality rate in patients with intraventricular hemorrhage [57]. In 2017, Hanley published the results of the Clot Lysis Evaluation of Accelerated Resolution of Intraventricular Hemorrhage (CLEAR-III) trial, comparing intraventricular rt-PA injection to placebo. With treatment, there was a 10 percent reduction in mortality and, for patients with larger initial intraventricular hemorrhage volumes, a better functional outcome [58]. A bedside procedure, intraventricular thrombolysis for intraventricular hemorrhage further emphasized the essential value of meticulous neurocritical care.

Hanley also pursued stereotactic-guided placement of a catheter inside the hematoma, followed by intrahemorrhage thrombolysis to facilitate hematoma lysis and drainage [59]. In a series of Minimally Invasive Surgery Plus rt-PA for ICH Evacuation (MISTIE) trials, he demonstrated that the approach was safe, feasible, and effective in reducing hematoma volume and peri-hematoma edema [60]. However, a larger efficacy trial failed to show an improved outcome [61].

Hanley also studied the potential for endoscopic evacuation of intracerebral hemorrhages. Ludwig Auer, an Austrian neurosurgeon, reported the first randomized trial of endoscopic hematoma evacuation in 1989, showing a lower mortality rate with evacuation [62]. In 2016, Hanley published the results of the Intraoperative Computed Tomography–Guided Endoscopic Surgery for Brain Hemorrhage trial. Compared with the medical arm from the MISTIE trial, the surgical group showed a trend toward a favorable outcome [63].

Decompressive Craniectomy for Malignant Hemispheric Stroke

Three years after Kjellberg and Prieto's 1971 report of bifrontal decompressive craniectomy for TBI, Henrique Ivamoto and colleagues, emphasizing the importance of intracranial pressure gradients, reported the results of hemicraniectomy in a patient with a malignant right hemispheric stroke [64]. Other reports followed in the 1980s and early 1990s. Hacke showed that standard management with osmotic agents to treat elevated ICP in these patients was rarely effective, with a mortality rate close to 80 percent [65]. In 1995, Hacke's group reported the largest open, nonrandomized, prospective trial: 32 patients treated with hemicraniectomy and 21 with maximal medical therapy. The survival rate was 66 percent in the surgery group versus 24 percent in the medical group [66.]

In 1996, at the second annual NACABI meeting in Heidelberg, Allan Ropper proposed a randomized controlled trial for patients with malignant hemispheric strokes, comparing early versus late hemicraniectomy (with the latter receiving maximal medical therapy). This formed the basis of HeADDFIRST, the first NINDS-sponsored pilot clinical trial that compared hemicraniectomy with maximal medical therapy and showed a trend toward reduced mortality with decompression [67]. Clear evidence of hemicraniectomy's superiority was subsequently shown in three European randomized trials, including DESTINY from Heidelberg [68]. A pooled analysis in 2007 demonstrated a dramatic reduction in mortality with hemicraniectomy (78% vs. 29%) with improvement in functional outcome at one year [69]. Decompressive hemicraniectomy has fundamentally changed the way patients with malignant hemispheric strokes are managed.

THE BIRTH OF NEUROCRITICAL CARE

In 1978, the American Academy of Neurology asked David Jackson to organize the first course on "critical care neurology." In 1983, Allan Ropper took over the course and, together with Kennedy and Zervas, collaborated to publish the first book of the new specialty [70]. A year later, Hacke published a similar monograph [71] and the German Neurological Society of Neurological Intensive Care and Emergency Medicine was founded.

In 1986, with support from the Dana Foundation, Dan Hanley established the first funded, two-year, clinical-research neurocritical care fellowship program in the United States. This led to the training of many young physicians committed to knowledge discovery and generation in neurocritical care. Two years later, the AAN created a section on critical care and emergency neurology with Hanley as its first chair.

In 1994, Werner Hacke published *NeuroCritical Care*, a collaborative textbook bringing together German and American authors (Ropper served as guest editor and Hanley as one of the coeditors) [72]. Neurocritical care continued to mature in the 1990s and 2000s, fueled in part by FDA approval of rt-PA for ischemic stroke, which created an imperative to admit patients with stroke early, initiate treatment, and manage complications – culminating with the establishment of the Neurocritical Care Society (NCS) in 2002.

At the inaugural NCS meeting in 2003, Ropper, Hanley, and Hacke were all bestowed "honorary member" status in recognition of their leading roles in establishing the field of neurocritical care. Today, there is considerable evidence that treatment in neurocritical care units leads to better outcomes in acute ischemic stroke, subarachnoid hemorrhage, intracerebral hemorrhage, and traumatic brain injury [73].

NOTES AND REFERENCES

1. Grenvik A, Pinsky MR. Evolution of the intensive care unit as a clinical center and critical care medicine as a discipline. *Crit. Care Clin.* 2009;25(1):239–250.
2. Woollam CHM. The development of apparatus for intermittent negative pressure respiration. (2) 1919–1976, with special reference to the development and uses of cuirass respirators. *Anaesthesia* 1976;31(5):666–685.
3. Drinker P, Shaw LA. An apparatus for the prolonged administration of artificial respiration: I. A design for adults and children. *J. Clin. Invest.* 1929;7(2):229–247.
4. Rosengart MR. Critical care medicine: Landmarks and legends. *Surg. Clin. North Am.* 2006;86(6):1305–1321.
5. Wijdicks EF, Russell WR, Baker AB, Plum F. Pioneers of ventilatory management in poliomyelitis. *Neurology* 2016;87(11):1167–1170.
6. Ibsen B. From anaesthesia to anaesthesiology: Personal experiences in Copenhagen during the past 25 years. *Acta Anaesthesiol. Scand. Suppl.* 1975;61:1–69.
7. Lassen HC. A preliminary report on the 1952 epidemic of poliomyelitis in Copenhagen with special reference to the treatment of acute respiratory insufficiency. *Lancet* 1953;1(6749):37–41.
8. Engstrom CG. Treatment of severe cases of respiratory paralysis by the Engstrom universal respirator. *Br. Med. J.* 1954;2(4889):666–669.
9. Marshall J. The work of a respiratory unit in a neurological hospital. *Postgrad. Med. J.* 1961;37:26–30.

10. Timmermans S. Hearts too good to die: Claude S. Beck's contributions to life-saving. *J. Hist. Sociol.* 2001;14(1):108–131.

11. Beck CS, Pritchard WH, Feil HS. Ventricular fibrillation of long duration abolished by electric shock. *JAMA* 1947;135(15):985.

12. Beck CS, Weckesser EC, Barry FM. Fatal heart attack and successful defibrillation: New concepts in coronary artery disease. *JAMA* 1956;161(5):434–436.

13. Zoll PM, Linenthal AJ, Gibson W, Paul MH, Norman LR. Termination of ventricular fibrillation in man by externally applied electric countershock. *N. Engl. J. Med.* 1956;254(16):727–732.

14. Kouwenhoven WB, Jude JR, Knickerbocker GG. Closed-chest cardiac massage. *JAMA* 1960;173:1064–1067.

15. Safar P. Mouth-to-mouth airway. *Anesthesiology* 1957;18(6):904–906.

16. Safar P, Dekornfeld TJ, Pearson JW, Redding JS. The intensive care unit: A three year experience at Baltimore city hospitals. *Anaesthesia* 1961;16:275–284.

17. Weil MH, Shubin H, Rosoff L. Fluid repletion in circulatory shock: Central venous pressure and other practical guides. *JAMA* 1965;192:668–674.

18. Julian DG. Treatment of cardiac arrest in acute myocardial ischaemia and infarction. *Lancet* 1961;2(7207):840–844.

19. Killip T, 3rd, Kimball JT. Treatment of myocardial infarction in a coronary care unit: A two year experience with 250 patients. *Am. J. Cardiol.* 1967;20(4):457–464.

20. Rogers RM, Weiler C, Ruppenthal B. Impact of the respiratory intensive care unit on survival of patients with acute respiratory failure. *Chest* 1972;62(1):94–97.

21. Jackson DL, Youngner S. Patient autonomy and "death with dignity": Some clinical caveats. *N. Engl. J. Med.* 1979;301(8):404–408.

22. Plum F, Posner JB. *The Diagnosis of Stupor and Coma*. Philadelphia: EA Davis, 1966.

23. A definition of irreversible coma. Report of the Ad Hoc Committee of the Harvard Medical School to Examine the Definition of Brain Death. *JAMA* 1968;205 (6):337–340.

24. Fisher CM. The neurological examination of the comatose patient. *Acta Neurol. Scand.* 1969;45(S36):5–56.

25. Brettle RP, Gross M, Legg NJ, Lockwood M, Pallis C. Treatment of acute polyneuropathy by plasma exchange. *Lancet* 1978;2(8099):1100.

26. Ropper AH. Lateral displacement of the brain and level of consciousness in patients with an acute hemispheral mass. *N. Engl. J. Med.* 1986;314(15):953–958.

27. McNealy DE, Plum F. Brainstem dysfunction with supratentorial mass lesions. *Arch. Neurol.* 1962;7:10–32.

28. Kjellberg RN, Prieto A Jr. Bifrontal decompressive craniotomy for massive cerebral edema. *J. Neurosurg.* 1971;34(4):488–493.

29. Lundberg N, Troupp H, Lorin H. Continuous recording of the ventricular-fluid pressure in patients with severe acute traumatic brain injury: A preliminary report. *J. Neurosurg.* 1965;22(6):581–590.

30. Lundberg N. Continuous recording and control of ventricular fluid pressure in neurosurgical practice. *Acta Psychiatr. Scand. Suppl.* 1960;36(149):1–193.

31. Miller JD, Becker DP, Ward JD, Sullivan HG, Adams WE, Rosner MJ. Significance of intracranial hypertension in severe head injury. *J. Neurosurg.* 1977;47(4):503–516.

32. Seelig JM, Becker DP, Miller JD, Greenberg RP, Ward JD, Choi SC. Traumatic acute subdural hematoma: Major mortality reduction in comatose patients treated within four hours. *N. Engl. J. Med.* 1981;304(25):1511–1518.

33. Reilly PL, Graham DI, Adams JH, Jennett B. Patients with head injury who talk and die. *Lancet* 1975;2(7931):375–377.

34. Becker DP, Miller JD, Ward JD, Greenberg RP, Young HF, Sakalas R. The outcome from severe head injury with early diagnosis and intensive management. *J. Neurosurg.* 1977;47(4):491–502.

35. Teasdale G, Jennett B. Assessment of coma and impaired consciousness: A practical scale. *Lancet* 1974;2(7872):81–84.

36. Jennett B. Outcome of severe damage to the central nervous system: Scale, scope and philosophy of the clinical problem. *Ciba Found. Symp.* 1975;34:3–21.

37. Bullock R, Chesnut RM, Clifton G, et al. Guidelines for the management of severe head injury. Brain Trauma Foundation, American Association of Neurological Surgeons Joint Section on Neurotrauma and Critical Care. *J. Neurotrauma* 1996;13:641–734.

38. Cooper DJ, Rosenfeld JV, Murray L, Arabi YM, Davies AR, D'Urso P, et al. Decompressive craniectomy in diffuse traumatic brain injury. *N. Engl. J. Med.* 2011;364(16):1493–1502.

39. Hutchinson PJ, Kolias AG, Timofeev IS, Corteen EA, Czosnyka M, Timothy J, et al. Trial of decompressive craniectomy for traumatic intracranial hypertension. *N. Engl. J. Med.* 2016;375(12):1119–1130.

40. Fay T. Observations on generalized refrigeration in cases of severe cerebral trauma. *Res. Publ. Assos. Res. Nerv. Dis.* 1945;4:611–619.

41. Cooper DJ, Nichol AD, Bailey M, Bernard S, Cameron PA, Pili-Floury S, et al. Effect of early sustained prophylactic hypothermia on neurologic outcomes among patients with severe traumatic brain injury: The POLAR randomized clinical trial. *JAMA* 2018;320(21):2211–2220.

42. Andrews PJ, Sinclair HL, Rodriguez A, Harris BA, Battison CG, Rhodes JK, et al. Hypothermia for intracranial hypertension after traumatic brain injury. *N. Engl. J. Med.* 2015;373(25):2403–2412.

43. Benson DW, Williams GR Jr, Spencer FC, Yates AJ. The use of hypothermia after cardiac arrest. *Anesth. Analg.* 1959;38:423–428.

44. Safar P, Brown TC, Holtey WJ, Wilder RJ. Ventilation and circulation with closed-chest cardiac massage in man. *JAMA* 1961;176:574–576.

45. Sterz F, Safar P, Tisherman S, Radovsky A, Kuboyama K, Oku K. Mild hypothermic cardiopulmonary resuscitation improves outcome after prolonged cardiac arrest in dogs. *Crit. Care Med.* 1991;19(3):379–389.

46. Hypothermia after Cardiac Arrest Study G: Mild therapeutic hypothermia to improve the neurologic outcome after cardiac arrest. *N. Engl. J. Med.* 2002;346(8):549–556.

47. Donnino MW, Andersen LW, Berg KM, Reynolds JC, Nolan JP, Morley PT, et al. Temperature management after cardiac arrest: An advisory statement by the Advanced Life Support Task Force of the International Liaison Committee on Resuscitation and the American Heart Association Emergency Cardiovascular Care Committee and the Council on Cardiopulmonary, Critical Care, Perioperative and Resuscitation. *Circulation* 2015;132(25):2448–2456.

48. Zeumer H, Hacke W, Kolmann HL, Poeck K. Lokale Fibrinolyse bei Basilaris thrombose. *Dtsch Med. Wochenschr.* 1982;107:728–731.

49. Prien T, Meyer J, Lawin P. Development of intensive care medicine in Germany. *J. Clin. Anesth.* 1991;3(3):253–258.

50. Opderbecke HW. Opinion of the German Society for Anesthesiology and Resuscitation on the organizations of recovery room, emergency station and intensive care in a hospital. *Anaesthesist* 1967;16(9):282–284.

51. Grund JPC, Breeksema JJ. Drug policy in the Netherlands. In Colson R, Bergeron H (eds.), *European Drug Policies: The Ways of Reform*. Routledge, 2017, pp. 128–148.

52. Sefrin P, Weidringer JW. History of emergency medicine in Germany. *J. Clin. Anesth.* 1991;3(3):245–248.

53. Hacke W, Del Zoppo GJ, Hirschberg M. *Thrombolytic Therapy in Acute Ischemic Stroke*. New York: Springer-Verlag, 1991.

54. Del Zoppo GJ, Poeck K, Pessin M, Wolpert SA, Furlan AJ, Ferbert A, et al. Recombinant tissue plasminogen activator in acute thrombotic and embolic stroke. *Ann. Neurol.* 1992;32:78–86.

55. The initiation and evolution of thrombolysis is discussed in detail in Chapter 50.

56. Schwarz S, Schwab S, Steiner HH, Hanley D, Hacke W. Fibrinolysis of intraventricular hematoma with rt-PA. *Nervenarzt.* 1999;70(2):123–130.

57. Naff NJ, Carhuapoma JR, Williams MA, Bhardwaj A, Ulatowski JA, Bederson J, et al. Treatment of intraventricular hemorrhage with urokinase: Effects on 30-day survival. *Stroke* 2000;31(4):841–847.

58. Hanley DF, Lane K, McBee N, Ziai W, Tuhrim S, Lees KR, et al. Thrombolytic removal of intraventricular haemorrhage in treatment of severe stroke: Results of the randomised, multicentre, multiregion, placebo-controlled CLEAR III trial. *Lancet* 2017;389(10069):603–611.

59. Barrett RJ, Hussain R, Coplin WM, Berry S, Keyl PM, Hanley DF, et al. Frameless stereotactic aspiration and thrombolysis of spontaneous intracerebral hemorrhage. *Neurocrit. Care* 2005;3(3):237–245.

60. Hanley DF, Thompson RE, Muschelli J, Rosenblum M, McBee N, Lane K, et al. Safety and efficacy of minimally invasive surgery plus alteplase in intracerebral haemorrhage evacuation (MISTIE): A randomised, controlled, open-label, phase 2 trial. *Lancet Neurol.* 2016;15(12):1228–1237.

61. Hanley DF, Thompson RE, Rosenblum M, Yenokyan G, Lane K, McBee N, et al. Efficacy and safety of minimally invasive surgery with thrombolysis in intracerebral haemorrhage evacuation (MISTIE III): A randomised, controlled, open-label, blinded endpoint phase 3 trial. *Lancet* 2019;393(10175):1021–1032.

62. Auer LM, Deinsberger W, Niederkorn K, Gell G, Kleinert R, Schneider G, et al. Endoscopic surgery versus medical treatment for spontaneous intracerebral hematoma: A randomized study. *J. Neurosurg.* 1989;70(4):530–535.

63. Vespa P, Hanley D, Betz J, Hoffer A, Engh J, Carter R, et al. ICES (Intraoperative Stereotactic Computed Tomography-Guided Endoscopic Surgery) for brain hemorrhage: A multicenter randomized controlled trial. *Stroke* 2016;47 (11):2749–2755.

64. Ivamoto HS, Numoto M, Donaghy RM. Surgical decompression for cerebral and cerebellar infarcts. *Stroke* 1974;5(3):365–370.

65. Hacke W, Schwab S, Horn M, Spranger M, De Georgia M, von Kummer R. "Malignant" middle cerebral artery territory infarction: Clinical course and prognostic signs. *Arch. Neurol.* 1996;53(4):309–315.

66. Rieke K, Schwab S, Krieger D, von Kummer R, Aschoff A, Schuchardt V, et al. Decompressive surgery in space-occupying hemispheric infarction: Results of an open, prospective trial. *Crit. Care Med.* 1995;23(9):1576–1587.

67. Frank JI, Krieger D, Chyatte D. Hemicraniectomy and durotomy upon deterioration from massive hemispheric infarction: A proposed multicenter, prospective, randomized study. *Stroke* 1999;30:243.

68. Juttler E, Schwab S, Schmiedek P, Unterberg A, Hennerici M, Woitzik J, et al. Decompressive Surgery for the Treatment of Malignant Infarction of the Middle Cerebral Artery (DESTINY): A randomized, controlled trial. *Stroke* 2007;38 (9):2518–2525.

69. Vahedi K, Hofmeijer J, Juettler E, Vicaut E, George B, Algra A, et al. Early decompressive surgery in malignant infarction of the middle cerebral artery: A pooled analysis of three randomised controlled trials. *Lancet Neurol.* 2007;6(3):215–222.

70. Ropper AH, Kennedy SF, Zervas NT. *Neurological and Neurosurgical Intensive Care.* Baltimore, MD: University Park Press, 1983.

71. Hacke W. *Neurologische Intensivmedizin.* Erlangen: Permed, 1984.

72. Hacke W, Hanley D, Einaupl DF, Bleck TP, Diringer MN. *NeuroCritical Care.* Berlin: Springer, 1994.

73. Knopf L, Staff I, Gomes J, McCullough L. Impact of a neurointensivist on outcomes in critically ill stroke patients. *Neurocrit. Care* 2012;16(1):63–71.

TREATMENT

CHAPTER FORTY THREE

CLINICAL STROKE TRIALS

Clinical trials have played a key role in the transformation of stroke from a neglected, untreatable condition to a field where some of the most dramatic outcomes are achieved. The development of concepts in stroke clinical trials has largely occurred during the last six decades and is closely linked to development of clinical trial methodology and evidence-based medicine in general. Stroke trials sometimes played a pioneering role in this development.

This chapter focuses on major landmarks that changed clinical practice. Trials of antithrombotics are highlighted. The historical perspective of clinical trials in specific fields of stroke and cerebrovascular diseases (such as acute reperfusion therapies, other vascular interventions, neurosurgery, and rehabilitation) are discussed in more detail in other chapters.

EARLY DEVELOPMENT OF CLINICAL TRIALS IN STROKE IN THE 1950S: THE PRINCETON CONFERENCES

The Princeton conferences on cerebrovascular diseases played an important role, for the first time, by providing a discussion forum for persons interested in stroke. The initiative came from Irving Wright, professor of medicine at Cornell Medical School and New York Hospital. Wright had an interest in anticoagulation therapy, especially in preventing brain embolism from the heart. The first Princeton conference was held on January 24–26, 1954.

Among the 34 participants at the first conference, only five had clinical experience in the field. Few were neurologists. The list of participants included Raymond Adams, C. Miller Fisher, Houston Merritt, Clark Millikan, and Harold Wolff. The proceedings were published and included verbatim accounts of the discussions [1]. The Princeton conference proceedings provide a unique opportunity to follow the thoughts and perceptions of the pioneers and are important historical documents on the early development of modern stroke medicine.

The first Princeton conference covered the burden of stroke, embryology and anatomy of the cerebral circulation, pathology, physiology, brain chemistry, hypertension, atherosclerosis, and neurological signs and symptoms. Therapeutic issues were the focus in only two presentations. One was on neurosurgery of intracranial aneurysms, in which the mode to induce blood pressure lowering was hotly debated. The other was on anticoagulation, presented by Ellen McDevitt, an internist at Cornell. Anticoagulants had been used clinically among patients with acute myocardial infarction, and the frequency of cerebral embolic episodes appeared to be reduced. McDevitt presented uncontrolled data on 57 patients treated with anticoagulants after "cerebrovascular accidents," many of whom had rheumatic heart disease and atrial fibrillation. The need for a controlled trial was recognized. A recurring theme was the lack of precise definitions and delineations of the temporal course of brain ischemia. For which categories of patients would therapy with anticoagulation or other agents be potentially useful?

An important initiative after the first conference was the formation in 1955 of an ad hoc group under the direction of the National Institute of Neurological Diseases and Blindness with the task to develop uniform criteria for the classification and diagnosis of cerebrovascular disease. The "Classification and Outline of Cerebrovascular Diseases" was included in the printed proceedings of the second Princeton Conference, held on January 16–18, 1957 [2], and was published in 1958 [3]. The writing group was chaired by Clark Millikan and included Raymond Adams, Henry Fang, Miller Fisher, Albert Heyman, Ellen McDevitt, Adolph Sahs, and Peritz Scheinberg. The document provided definitions of transient ischemic attacks, cerebral infarction, and cerebral hemorrhage from clinicopathological concepts known at the time. The conference proceedings included a paper by Miller Fisher on "intermittent cerebral ischemia." The proceedings also included definitions of "stroke-in-evolution" and "completed strokes," terms that would foster discussions and debate during the following decades. Several therapeutic options for stroke were discussed, such as blockade of the stellate ganglion, cortisone, and enzymes to treat thrombosis and embolism. Anticoagulants received the most attention. The stage was set for a randomized controlled trial.

THE FIRST RANDOMIZED TRIAL IN STROKE: THE RISE AND FALL OF ANTICOAGULANTS FOR NONCARDIOEMBOLIC ISCHEMIC STROKE AND TIA

The first randomized controlled trial (RCT) in stroke was the Cooperative Clinical Study of Anticoagulant Therapy in Cerebral Thromboses and Transient Ischemic Attacks, published in the journal *Neurology* in 1961 [4]. This trial may have been the very first randomized controlled trial in neurology. In his memoirs, Miller Fisher described many background details on this study as well as providing the study protocol and case record forms [5]. The study compared anticoagulants versus placebo in patients with transient ischemic attacks (TIAs), TIAs followed by a neurological deficit, and progressive stroke. Patients could be included early after the events, but inclusion was possible for up to eight weeks. Anticoagulants were given for six to nine months. Heparin was given initially to some patients. Informed consent was not required. Some even argued that it was better if the patient was not informed as this could potentially influence patient behavior. Overall, 304 patients were included (44 with TIA, 128 with progressive stroke, and 132 with completed stroke). Results suggested that anticoagulants were effective in TIA and progressive stroke, but not in completed stroke.

In retrospect, several features of this first RCT and the initial era of stroke trials stand out. Atrial fibrillation was not highlighted in patient selection. The number of patients, and even more the number of end points, was very small, and statistical tests were not applied. Confidence intervals were unknown. Kaplan-Meier curves were not used. In 1971, 10 years after the publication of the cooperative study, Millikan published a reassessment of anticoagulant therapy in various types of occlusive cerebrovascular disease [6]. The focus on continuing to divide TIA, progressing stroke, and completed stroke was retained, and only crude outcomes were reported. Anticoagulants were recommended for patients with TIA and progressive stroke, and heparin and oral anticoagulants were much used in clinical practice.

The role of anticoagulants in clinical practice in patients with TIA and ischemic stroke, in both the acute phase (including progressive stroke) and long term, was established only much later, well into the era of modern, large, clinical trials and systematic reviews.

THE ASPIRIN TRIALS, THE DAWN OF MODERN CLINICAL TRIAL METHODOLOGY, AND THE DOSE-OF-ASPIRIN CONTROVERSY

The history of aspirin's trajectory from a pain and fever pill to modern use as a drug on the World Health Organization's list of essential drugs in prevention of vascular disease is among the most fascinating in pharmacology and medicine [7]. After anecdotal observations during the 1950s, interest in aspirin as a preventive drug for vascular disease was stimulated by the findings in the late 1960s that aspirin rapidly and irreversibly inhibited platelet aggregation. Sir John Vane's research group was the first to discover the role of prostaglandins in hemostasis. A classical paper in *Nature* was published 1971 on aspirin's inhibition of prostaglandin synthesis [8]. In 1982 John Vane, Bengt Samuelsson, and Sune Bergström were awarded the Nobel Prize for Medicine in recognition of their work.

Clinical trials on aspirin in stroke began in 1972 with a small trial of 178 patients led by Bill Fields and coworkers [9]. After six months, a statistically significant reduction favoring aspirin was shown, but the main driver for the difference was multiple TIAs, one of the end points. During the mid-1970s it became recognized that in order to show relatively small differences in outcomes, trials needed large sample sizes. This insight guided Henry Barnett in the design of the landmark Canadian Cooperative Study Group trial, which randomized 585 stroke patients to receive aspirin or sulfinpyrazone, alone or in combination, for 26 months [10]. Aspirin reduced the risk of stroke or death by 31 percent (P < 0.05), but benefits were sex dependent, and the conclusion was that aspirin was efficacious only for men with threatened stroke. An aspirin dose of 1,300 milligrams was used. The factorial trial design involving two drugs led to much debate on the solidity of the findings on aspirin. Discussions followed on the biological plausibility that aspirin might be of benefit only in men.

Two of the major drivers of stroke therapeutic trials were Barnett and Fields. Henry Joseph Macaulay Barnett (1922–2016) (Figure 43.1) was born in Newcastle-upon-Tyne, England. His family immigrated to Canada when he was three years old. As a boy rambling around marshes at Ashbridge's Bay in

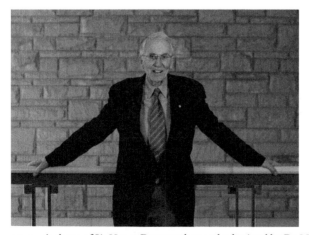

43.1.   A photo of Sir Henry Barnett taken and submitted by Bo Norrving on the occasion of his receiving the Karolinska Prize in 2008.

Toronto, he met two ornithologists who showed him a hoary redpoll through binoculars. From then on, birds, natural science, and eventually medical science captivated him [11]. He graduated from the University of Toronto medical school in 1944. He began clinical work at the University Hospital in London, Ontario, and the University of Western Ontario in 1974. He was an outstanding clinician who was especially interested in stroke. He became the chair of the neurology department and partnered with leading Canadian neurosurgeon Charles Drake in promoting stroke medical treatment and surgery. In midcareer Barnett (known as Barney to colleagues and friends) turned full activities to stroke-related trials, first with aspirin and antiplatelets and then to carotid artery surgery and neurosurgical bypass operations. From its founding in 1986, he was the president and scientific director of the Robarts Research Institute until his retirement in 1995. In 1984 he was made an Officer of the Order of Canada and was dubbed Sir Henry Barnett. He was the third editor of the journal *Stroke* [12].

William Straus Fields (1913–2004) was born in Baltimore, Maryland. He graduated from Harvard College in 1934 and Harvard Medical School in 1938. He was an intern in medicine at Henry Ford Hospital where he was a fellow house officer with C. Miller Fisher. They remained colleagues and close friends for the remainder of their lives. He had a residency in internal medicine at the Royal Victoria Hospital in Montreal and rotated at the Montreal Neurological Institute. He served during World War II as a medical officer on a British destroyer that plied the North Atlantic escorting convoys, favorite targets for German submarines [13]. After the war he settled in Houston, Texas, where he spent his entire career. Fields's career in Houston began in 1949, when he joined Baylor College of Medicine as associate professor of neuropsychiatry. At the time, he was one of three neurologists in Texas. Fields later founded and became the first chairman of Baylor's neurology department. He hosted a number of stroke conferences and became active with Barnett and others in designing and carrying out stroke therapeutic trials. He also authored a book on the history of stroke [14].

In 1985, Carlo Patrono with his research group showed that aspirin had a double action: blocking prostacyclin, which inhibits platelet aggregation, and thromboxane A2, which promotes platelet aggregation. Research in the laboratory showed that 30 milligrams of aspirin daily spared endothelial prostacyclin while still completely blocking thromboxane A2 and prolonging the bleeding time [15]. These findings prompted clinical trials to test the efficacy of low-dose aspirin in cardiovascular disease. In cardiology, the RISC trial randomized 800 men with unstable coronary disease to low-dose (75 mg once daily) aspirin or placebo. RISC measured myocardial infarction (MI) and death during the first three months of treatment and showed a very dramatic 65 percent reduction in event rate over the first month, which was maintained over longer-term follow-up [16]. The Swedish Aspirin Low-Dose Trial (SALT) was the first placebo-controlled study to show that low-dose (75 mg daily) aspirin was effective for secondary prevention after cerebrovascular ischemic events [17]. SALT included 1,360 patients who had had TIAs, minor stroke, or retinal artery occlusion during the preceding three months. The risk of primary outcome events (stroke or death) was reduced by 18 percent.

Almost concurrently, the Dutch TIA trial, carried out across 63 centers, included 3,131 patients with TIA or nondisabling stroke [18]. Participants were randomized to a daily aspirin dose of either 30 milligrams or the standard dose of 283 milligrams. The minimal follow-up period was one year, with five years between the first patient and publication. The results showed an advantage for low-dose aspirin with this disappearing in the last few months of the trial. Side effects were reduced by 17 percent in the 30-milligram dose.

Another large trial was the UK-TIA study that included 2,435 patients with a TIA or minor ischemic stroke [19]. The study found no difference in efficacy between the 300- and 1,200-milligram daily doses of aspirin, but the lower dose was less gastrotoxic. The odds of having a major stroke, myocardial infarction, or vascular death were 15 percent less in the combined aspirin groups compared with the placebo group.

Further data on antiplatelets in stroke was provided by the ESPS-2 trial [20], in which 6,602 patients were randomized to treatment with ASA alone (50 mg daily), modified-release dipyridamole alone (400 mg daily), the two agents in a combined formulation, or placebo. Patients were followed on treatment for two years. In pairwise comparisons, stroke risk compared to placebo was reduced by 18 percent with aspirin alone, 16 percent with dipyridamole alone, and 37 percent with combination therapy.

These trials were hotly debated among the trialists and the scientific community. At almost every major stroke congress in the late 1980s and 1990s a session was devoted to debate trial results and their implications on practice. Views were strongly held and eloquently presented, and views among the different parties did not change over time. The debate was coined "the aspirin wars" [21], and topics included comparison of point estimates of risk reduction and whether brain vessels had a different response to aspirin than vessels elsewhere in the body based on theoretical reasoning.

THE ANTIPLATELET TRIALISTS COLLABORATION AND THE EMERGENCE OF SYSTEMATIC REVIEWS

In 1976, Richard Peto, an epidemiologist at Oxford University, published a landmark paper on "Design and Analysis of Randomised Clinical Trials Requiring Prolonged Observation," in which he introduced new statistical ways to present and visualize results from clinical trials and aggregate the findings into a common estimate [22]. Peto emphasized the routine use of confidence intervals to show the degree of precision of a point estimate and established the "forest plot" using a central cube or diamond, the area of which was related to the size of the trial and the number of end points. In 1980 he published a meta-analysis of six aspirin trials that showed a highly significant 23 percent reduction in vascular disease mortality for those taking aspirin [23].

Soon the Antiplatelet Trialists' Collaboration was formed. The first publication appeared in 1988 [24]. It summarized clinical data on antiplatelet therapies using Peto's methods. Further updates were published in 1994 and 2002 and later extended the findings when new trial evidence appeared [25]. The Antiplatelet Trialists' Collaboration concluded that there was solid evidence that antiplatelet therapy protected a wide range of patients at high risk of occlusive vascular disease and should be considered for almost all with suspected acute myocardial infarction, unstable angina, or a history of myocardial infarction, angina, stroke, TIA, arterial bypass surgery, or angioplasty. Medium-dose aspirin (75–325 mg) was the most widely tested antiplatelet regimen, and no other regimen was significantly more effective in preventing myocardial infarction, stroke, or death. The effect was similar in women and men.

The Antiplatelet Trialists' data showed the need for very large trials (thousands of patients) for therapies in which the effect size was modest, but for which the total benefit was substantial if applied to large patient groups. In cardiology, the landmark trial was ISIS-2, published in the *Lancet* in 1988 [26]. Streptokinase, injected over one hour after the onset of a heart attack, reduced the risk of dying in the next month by more than 20 percent. Taking aspirin had a similarly beneficial outcome. When taken together, the two drugs reduced the relative risk of death by about 40–50 percent. Benefit was shown even for patients treated later than a few hours after onset of myocardial infarction. The trial took three years to complete, and a total of 17,187 patients were randomized in 417 coronary care units in 16 countries [26]. The results changed clinical practice overnight.

The International Stroke Trial (IST) and the Chinese Acute Stroke Trial (CAST) were the first mega stroke trials. In IST, 19,435 patients with suspected acute ischemic stroke entering 467 hospitals in 36 countries were randomized within 48 hours of symptom onset in a factorial design of heparin (two doses), aspirin, both, or neither [27]. In CAST, 21,106 patients with acute ischemic stroke were enrolled in 413 Chinese hospitals at a mean of 25 hours after the onset of symptoms and randomized to aspirin or placebo [28]. CAST and IST together showed that aspirin started early in hospital produced a small but definite net benefit.

THE PATHWAY TO EVIDENCE-BASED MEDICINE

During the 1970s and 1980s, David Sackett, at McMaster University, Canada, and Archie Cochrane in the United Kingdom were pioneers in promoting the need for strengthening the empirical practice of medicine. They urged that the practice of medicine should be based on the best available evidence. They promoted randomized therapeutic trials as the evidence that could be relied on. David Sackett published templates and algorithms for the standardized evaluation of publications of different types (such as observational studies, clinical trials, prognostic studies, diagnostic studies) [29]. Archie Cochrane initiated an openly accessible database where clinicians could rapidly find the most recent and accumulated information of clinical issues, creating the Cochrane database [30].

The principles of Sackett, Cochrane, Peto, and associates were rapidly adopted by stroke scientists, in particular, in the United Kingdom where Charles Warlow played a key role. Charles Picton Warlow was born in 1943. He qualified in medicine at the University of Cambridge. After house officer training at St. George's in London, he became a lecturer at the University of Aberdeen where Stuart Douglas was performing thrombosis research. Douglas kindled Warlow's interest in stroke [31]. Warlow's formative years were spent at Oxford and the Radcliffe Infirmary where he was exposed to Peto and colleagues. In 1987, Warlow was appointed chair of neurology in Edinburgh, where he established and nurtured a fledgling stroke research group into leaders of stroke research in the United Kingdom and Europe. Warlow and colleagues emphasized "pragmatic trials" that did not require pages and pages of entries. Charles Warlow's close circle included Peter Sandercock, Martin Dennis, Rickard Lindley, Joanna Wardlaw, Greame Hankey, Jan van Gijn, Peter Rothwell, and Cathie Sudlow, who in turn inspired stroke scientists to form a global network. The Edinburgh stroke group was instrumental in conducting many medical and surgical stroke trials in Europe. Peter Langhorne was the initial chair of the Cochrane Group, and later Livia Candelise chaired the Cochrane Stroke group.

In 1991 Gordon Guyatt introduced the term "evidence-based medicine" (EBM), which broadened the scope of systematic reviews and statistical evaluation and presentation of evidence. Clinicians were inspired to read and digest primary research studies and systematic reviews [32]. With the rapid accumulation of clinical trials and scientific publications, the focus was directed toward development of trustworthy clinical practice guidelines in which the evidence had been evaluated in a systematic fashion. A new approach to rating evidence quality and the grading strength of recommendations, termed the Grades of Recommendation Assessment, Development, and Evaluation (GRADE) System, was first published in 2004 [33]. GRADE provided a hierarchy of evidence that addressed elements related to the credibility of evidence: study design, risk of bias (study strengths and limitations), precision, consistency (variability in results between studies), directness (applicability), publication bias, magnitude of effect, and dose-response gradients. Further advances related to EBM included standardized reporting of randomized trials (CONSORT statements), observational studies, diagnostic test studies, predictive models, and genetic testing studies. These templates were collected at the EQUATOR website, and adherence to these standards is now mandatory by most scientific journals. A further principle is the requirement of registration of all trial protocols (most commonly used is www.clinicaltrials.gov) before research begins.

STROKE TRIALS OF ANTICOAGULANTS

In the waning years of the twentieth century and thereafter, stroke clinicians began to organize trials of anticoagulants in patients with acute stroke and for preventing stroke in those at risk.

Robert Hart was one of the organizers and leaders of trials of warfarin for stroke prevention in patients with atrial fibrillation [34]. Hart matriculated at the University of Missouri Medical School. After a stroke fellowship in Oregon, he moved to the University of Texas at San Antonio where for 25 years he led their stroke program. He then moved to McMaster University as the DeGroot Chair in Stroke Research. Trials based in San Antonio, Boston, and Europe clearly showed the effectiveness of warfarin in patients with atrial fibrillation [34].

Hart's close neurological and stroke colleagues, David Sherman and J. Donald Easton, worked closely with Hart on anticoagulation trials and were shakers and movers regarding many antiplatelet trials. Sherman grew up on his family's farm in Lexington, Oklahoma. He received his medical degree from the University of Oklahoma in 1967. After an internship at Baylor Affiliated Hospitals in Houston, Texas, and service in the navy, he obtained neurology training at the University of California–San Diego. In 1983, Sherman moved to the University of Texas Health Science Center in San Antonio and in 1986 became the chief of neurology and Ross J. Sibert Research Fund Distinguished Chair.

J. Donald Easton was born in Saskatoon, Saskatchewan, Canada. He graduated from the University of Washington Medical School and was a medical and neurological house officer at the New York Hospital, Cornell University. He became chair of neurology at Brown University in 1986.

Jay P. Mohr led an important trial of warfarin versus aspirin in patients with threatened brain ischemia [35]. Mohr was born in Lynchburg, Virginia. He matriculated at Haverford College and received his medical degree from the

University of Virginia and his neurology training at Columbia University and Massachusetts General Hospital. He had a stroke fellowship with C. Miller Fisher, and after military service at NIH directed the Stroke Service at MGH for a decade. Mohr then moved to Columbia University as the Sciarra Professor of Neurology.

Marc Chimowitz designed and led important studies of trials regarding medical and interventional treatment of intracranial atherosclerosis, including an important study of aspirin versus warfarin [36]. The direct-acting, non-vitamin K–dependent anticoagulants (dabigatran, rivaroxaban, apixaban, edoxaban) were extensively studied in trials mostly in patients with atrial fibrillation and venous thrombosis [37].

THROMBOLYTIC TRIALS

The first thrombolytic trials in Europe were led by Werner Hacke, Markku Kaste, and Cesare Fieschi. Hacke was a pioneer in critical care neurology and chair of neurology at the University of Heidelberg in Germany. Kaste was chief of neurology in Helsinki, Finland, and Fieschi was chief of neurology in Rome. The successive ECASS trials were very important in delineating the safety and effectiveness of intravenous tissue plasminogen activator (tPA) in patients with acute ischemic stroke [38].

In the United States, the National Institute of Neurological Disorders and Stroke (NINDS) trial led to the rapid introduction of tPA into clinical practice [39]. The trial was led by Tom Brott and Joe Broderick of the University of Cincinatti, Clark Haley of the University of Virginia, Pat Lyden of the University of California at San Diego, and Jim Grotta of the University of Texas at Houston, among others.

Geoff Donnan and Steve Davis, Australian neurologists who had trained as stroke fellows at the Massachusetts General Hospital with Robert Ackerman, led stroke trials of thrombolytics in Australia and New Zealand.

Antthony Furlan of the Cleveland Clinic led an important trial of intraarterial thrombolysis [40].

TRIALS OF SURGERY AND OTHER PROCEDURES

The initial stroke trials studied medical treatments. Trial principles were gradually applied to various surgical and endovascular procedures. Barnett showed that a commonly performed surgical procedure, extracranial to intracranial bypass, was not effective in preventing stroke in patients with carotid artery occlusion [41]. During the 1980s trials were designed to study carotid artery surgery. Jim Toole of Bowman Gray Medical School organized a group to study carotid endarterectomy in asymptomatic patients [42], and Barnett organized the North American Symptomatic Carotid Endarterectomy Trial (NASCET), which studied the effectiveness and safety of carotid artery surgery in patients with various degrees of carotid artery stenosis versus medical treatment [43]. When carotid artery stenting was introduced into practice, Tom Brott of the Mayo Clinic and Robert Hobson, a surgeon at the University of Medicine and Dentistry of New Jersey, led studies of carotid artery surgery versus stenting [44]. Other stroke clinicians and surgeons, including Alison Halliday of the Nuffield Department of Surgical Sciences at Oxford, United Kingdom, led studies of carotid interventions in the United Kingdom and Europe [45].

Enrollment of patients into surgical and interventional trials often faced the problem of agreement on equipoise between treatment arms. Many clinicians, surgeons, and interventionalists had strong views on the benefit of certain procedures from clinical experience and observational data, and argued that randomization was unethical. Acceptance of the need for RCTs for nonpharmacological procedures took a longer time than for drug trials. This problem was evident for the use of hemicraniectomy for malignant middle cerebral artery infarction, for which wide acceptance for the procedure was only agreed on after pooling of three concurrent RCTs, each small, which had struggled for patient inclusion [46].

TRIALS OF INTRACRANIAL INTERVENTIONAL PROCEDURES

A major advance in trial methodology was introduced by Mark Chimowitz and his collaborators, Tanya Turan of the University of South Carolina and Colin Derdeyn of the University of Iowa. Chimowitz grew up in South Africa and obtained a medical degree at the University of Capetown. He developed a major interest in mathematics and trained in neurology at Tufts University. After further training in stroke at the Cleveland Clinic, he led stroke groups at the University of Michigan and Emory University before moving to Charleston, South Carolina, to lead stroke research there. Chimowitz organized a trial of stenting versus medical treatment to prevent stroke in patients with severe intracranial occlusive disease. Prior trials that studied surgical treatments pitted surgical procedures against "best medical treatment." Medical treatments were given but no information was gleaned about whether these treatments were effective. In the Stenting versus Aggressive Medical Management for Preventing Recurrent Stroke in Intracranial Stenosis (SAMMPRIS), treatments for hypertension, diabetes, and high cholesterol were adjusted and their effectiveness determined [47]. Lifestyle issues – nutrition, smoking, and sedentary behaviors – were also studied. Physical exercise activities were documented and monitored. Physical activity, which had not received attention in stroke prevention trials, was the strongest predictor of good outcome in the medical arm of the trial [48]. Future trials of elective surgical procedures adopted methodology introduced in SAMMPRIS.

J. P. Mohr led a trial of surgical, interventional, and radiotherapy treatment of patients with intracranial arteriovenous malformations [49].

During the last decade, trials of interventional treatments to remove intracranial large artery occlusions by thrombectomy were pursued and found effective in many patients with acute strokes, opening up a new avenue in acute stroke therapy [50].

REFERENCES

1 Wright I, Millikan CH. *Cerebrovascular Diseases: Transactions of the First Conference Held January 24–26, 1954 at Princeton, New Jersey*. New York: Grune & Stratton, 1954.

2. Wright I, Millikan CH. *Cerebrovascular Diseases: Second Conference*. New York: Grune & Stratton, 1958.

3. NINDS Ad Hoc Committee. A classification and outline of cerebrovascular diseases. *Neurology* 1958;8:188–216.

4. Fisher CM. Anticoagulant therapy in cerebral thrombosis and cerebral embolism: A national cooperative study, interim report. *Neurology* 1961;11:119–131. Baker RN, Broward JA, Fang HC, et al. Anticoagulant therapy in cerebral infarction: Report in cooperative study. *Neurology* 1962;12:823–835.

5. Fisher CM. Anticoagulant study. In *Memoirs of a Neurologist*. Rutland, VT: Sharp, 2006, vol. 3, pp. 173–235.

6. Millikan C. Reassessment of anticoagulant therapy in various types of occlusive cerebrovascular disease. *Stroke* 1971;2:201–208.

7. The story of aspirin is the topic of Chapter 47 and other antiplatelets are considered in Chapter 48.

8. Vane JR. Inhibition of prostaglandin synthesis as a mechanism of action for aspirin-like drugs. *Nat. New Biol.* 1971;231:232–235.

9. Fields WS, Lemak NA, Frankowski RF, Hardy RJ. Controlled trial of aspirin in cerebral ischemia. *Stroke* 1977;8:301–314.

10 Canadian Cooperative Study Group. A randomized trial of aspirin and sulfinpyrazone in threatened stroke. *N. Engl. J. Med.* 1978;299:53–59.

11. Henry J. M. Barnett. Wikipedia. Available at https://en.wikipedia.org/wiki/Henry_J_._M._Barnett.

12. Spence JD, Hachinsky V. Henry J. M. Barnett (1922–2016). *Stroke* 2017;48(1):2–4.

13. Van Horn G, Grotta JC. William S. Fields, MD, Texas medical center pioneer. *Ann. Neurol.* 2004;56(2):314. https://doi.org/10.1002/ana.20167.

14. Fields WS, Lemak NA. *A History of Stroke*. New York: Oxford University Press, 1989.

15. Patrono C, Ciabattoni G, Patrignani P, et al. Clinical pharmacology of platelet cyclooxygenase inhibition. *Circulation* 1985;72:1177–1184.

16. Wallentin LC. Aspirin (75 mg/day) after an episode of unstable coronary artery disease: Long-term effects on the risk for myocardial infarction, occurrence of severe angina and the need for revascularization. Research Group on Instability in Coronary Artery Disease in Southeast Sweden. *JACC* 1991;18:1587–1593.

17. SALT Collaborative Group. The Swedish Aspirin Low-Dose Trial. *Lancet* 1991;338:1345–1349.

18. A comparison of two doses of aspirin (30 mg vs. 283 mg a day) in patients after a transient ischemic attack or minor ischemic stroke: The Dutch TIA Trial Study Group. *N. Engl. J. Med.* 1991;325:1261–1266.

19. Farrell B, Godwin J, Richards S, Warlow C. The United Kingdom Transient Ischaemic Attack (UK-TIA) aspirin trial: Final results. *J. Neurol. Neurosurg. Psychiatry* 1991;54:1044–1054.

20. Diener HC, Cunha L, Forbes C, et al. European Stroke Prevention Study. 2. Dipyridamole and acetylsalicylic acid in the secondary prevention of stroke. *J. Neurol. Sci.* 1996 Nov;143(1–2):1–13.

21. Hart RG, Harrison MJG. Aspirin wars: The optimal dose of aspirin to prevent stroke. *Stroke* 1996;27:585–587.

22. Peto R, Pike MC, Armitage P, et al. Design and analysis of randomised clinical trials requiring prolonged observation of each patient. *Br. J. Cancer* 1977;35:1–39.

23. Peto R. Editorial: Aspirin and myocardial infarction. *Lancet* 1980;1:1172–1173.

24. Antiplatelet Trialists' Collaboration. Secondary prevention of vascular disease by prolonged antiplatelet treatment. *BMJ* 1988;296:320–331.

25. Antiplatelet Trialists' Collaboration. Collaborative overview of randomised trials of antiplatelet therapy – 1. Prevention of death, myocardial infarction and stroke by prolonged antiplatelet therapy in various categories of patients. *BMJ* 1994;308:81–106. Antithrombotic Trialist Collaboration. Collaborative meta-analysis of randomised trials of antiplatelet therapy for prevention of death, myocardial infarction, and stroke in high risk patients. *BMJ* 2002;324:71–86.

26. ISIS-2 (Second international Study of Infarct Survival) Collaborative Group. Randomized trial of intravenous streptokinase, oral aspirin, both, or neither among 17,187 cases of suspected acute myocardial infarction: ISIS-2. *J. Am. Coll. Cardiol.* 1988 Dec;12(6 suppl A):3A–13A.

27. The International Stroke Trial (IST): A randomised trial of aspirin, subcutaneous heparin, both, or neither among 19435 patients with acute ischaemic stroke. International Stroke Trial Collaborative Group. *Lancet* 1997;349:1569–1581.

28. CAST: Randomised placebo-controlled trial of early aspirin use in 20,000 patients with acute ischaemic stroke. CAST (Chinese Acute Stroke Trial) Collaborative Group. *Lancet* 1997 Jun 7;349(9066):1641–1649.

29. Sackett DL, Haynes RB, Tugwell P. *Clinical Epidemiology: A Basic Science for Clinical Medicine.* Boston: Little, Brown, 1985.

30. Cochrane A. *Effectiveness and Efficiency: Random Reflections on Health Services.* The Nuffield Provincial Hospital Trust, 1972.

31. Qiu, J. Charles Warlow: A career of "successive flukes." *Lancet* 2008 Jun;7(6):478.

32 Djulbegovic B, Guyatt GH. Progress in evidence-based medicine: A quarter century on. *Lancet* 2017;390:415–423.

33. GRADE Working Group. The Grades of Recommendation. Assessment, Development and Evaluation Working Group. 2004.

34. The Stroke Prevention in Atrial Fibrillation Investigators. The stroke prevention in atrial fibrillation study: Final results. *Circulation* 1991;84:527–539.

35. Mohr JP, Thompson JLP, Lazar RM, et al. for the Warfarin-Aspirin Recurrent Stroke Study Group. A comparison of warfarin and aspirin for the prevention of recurrent ischemic stroke. *N. Engl. J. Med.* 2001;345:1444–1451.

36. Chimowitz MI, Lynn MJ, Howlett-Smith H, et al. Comparison of warfarin and aspirin for symptomatic intracranial arterial stenosis. *N. Engl. J. Med.* 2005;352:1305–1316.

37. The newer anticoagulants are discussed in Chapter 46.

38. European Investigators published the results of the European Cooperative Acute Stroke Study (ECASS). Hacke W, Kaste M, Fieschi C, et al. Intravenous thrombolysis with recombinant tissue plasminogen activator for acute hemispheric stroke. The European Cooperative Acute Stroke Study (ECASS). *JAMA* 1995;274:1017–1025. Hacke W, Kaste M, Fieschi C, et al. Randomised double-blind placebo-controlled trial of thrombolytic therapy with intravenous alteplase in acute ischaemic stroke (ECASS II). *Lancet* 1998;352:1245–1251.

39. The National Institute of Neurological Disorders and Stroke rt-PA Stroke Study Group. Tissue plasminogen activator for acute ischemic stroke. *N. Engl. J. Med.* 1995;333:1581–1587.

40. Furlan AJ, Higashida RT, Wechsler L, et al. PROACT II. Intra-arterial Pro-urokinase for acute ischemic stroke: A randomized controlled trial. *JAMA* 1999;282;2003–2011.

41. The EC-IC Bypass Study Group. Failure of the extracranial-intracranial arterial bypass to reduce the risk of ischemic stroke. *N. Engl. J. Med.* 1985;313:1191–1200.

42. The Asymptomatic Carotid Atherosclerosis Study Group. Study design for random-ized prospective trial of carotid endarterectomy for asymptomatic atherosclerosis. *Stroke* 1989;20:844–849.

43. NASCET Collaborators. Beneficial effect of carotid endarterectomy in symptomatic patients with high-grade carotid stenosis. *N. Engl. J. Med.* 1991;325:445–453. Barnett HJM, Taylor DW, Eliasziw M, et al. for the North American Symptomatic Carotid Endarterectomy Trial Collaborators. Benefit of carotid endarterectomy in patients with symptomatic moderate or severe stenosis. *N. Engl. J. Med.* 1998;339:1415–1425.

44. Brott TG, Hobson RW II, Howard G, et al. CREST Investigators. Stenting vs endarterectomy for treatment of carotid-artery stenosis. *N. Engl. J. Med.* 2010;363:11–23. Caplan LR, Brott TG. Of horse races, trials, meta-analyses, and carotid artery stenosis (Editorial). *Arch. Neurol.* 2011;68:157–159.

45. Halliday A, Mansfield A, Marro J, et al. Prevention of disabling and fatal strokes by successful carotid endarterectomy in patients without recent neurological symptoms: Randomised controlled trial. *Lancet* 2004;363:1491–1502. Carotid artery surgery is discussed in Chapter 54 and carotid artery stenting in Chapter 55.

46. Vahedi K, Hofmeijer J, Juettler E, et al. Early decompressive surgery in malignant middle cerebral artery infarction: A pooled analysis of three randomised controlled trials. *Lancet Neurol.* 2007;6:215–222.

47. Chimowitz M, Lynn MJ, Derdeyn CP, et al. for the SAMMPRIS Trial Investigators. Stenting versus aggressive medical therapy for intracranial arterial stenosis. *N. Engl. J. Med.* 2011;365:993–1003.

48. Turan TN, Nizam A, Lynn MJ, et al. Relationship between risk factor control and vascular events in the SAMMPRIS trial. *Neurology* 2017;88(4):379–385.

49. Mohr JP, Parides MK, Stapf C, et al. Medical management with or without interven-tional therapy for unruptured brain arteriovenous malformations (ARUBA): A multicentre, non-blinded, randomised trial. *Lancet* 2014;383 (9917):614–621.

50. Trials that evaluated the safety and effectiveness of endovascular management of acute ischemic stroke are discussed in Chapter 56.

CHAPTER FORTY FOUR

HEPARIN

DISCOVERY AND PRODUCTION

The story of heparin began in 1880, with a report by German researcher Adolf Schmidt-Mulheim describing the possibility that mammals harbor indigenous anticoagulants. In 1905, Paul Morawitz reviewed peptone shock research and concluded that the analytical methods available did not enable precise characterization of the anticoagulant. This remained the case until another decade, when further progress was made by William Henry Howell and Jay McLean [1].

Howell was born in Baltimore in 1860 and was educated in local schools where he became interested in chemistry and medicine. During his third year in high school, he accepted a paid appointment as an assistant to a natural science teacher, which gave him the opportunity to perform experiments. In 1879, he entered Johns Hopkins University and fulfilled the requirements of a PhD in biology in 1884. The title of his dissertation was "Experiments upon the Blood and Lymph of the Terrapin, and the Origin of the Fibrin formed in the Coagulation of the Blood" [1]. He examined the molecular components involved in generation of a blood clot and isolated thrombin and fibrinogen. Addition of thrombin to fibrinogen generated a fibrin clot [2].

In 1889, Howell was appointed appointment chairman of the department of physiology at the University of Michigan [1]. He returned to Johns Hopkins University four years later to become the first professor of physiology. He was an outstanding teacher and a devoted experimentalist. He became a charter member of the American Physiological Society. Howell wrote a textbook on human physiology, *A Text-book of Physiology for Medical Students and Physicians*, which was very successful and went through 14 editions [2].

Jay McLean was born in San Francisco in 1890. He lost his father when he was four years old. His mother remarried when he was nine years old. His family was devastated by an earthquake and fire when he was 15 years old. He entered the University of California at Berkeley in 1909, and while there decided to pursue a career in academic surgery at Johns Hopkins Medical School. He wrote in his autobiography, "I deliberately chose the fiercest student competition as Johns Hopkins' matriculants were meticulously chosen" [3].

In 1913, he began his final year at University of California, which was his first year as a medical student, graduating in 1914. He was taught physiology in his first year of medicine, and Howell's textbook of physiology was used. He was fascinated by the subject and its research possibilities. He applied for admission to Johns Hopkins for his second year, but his application was denied. He moved to Baltimore and met with the registrar and the dean, who were surprised to see him and inquired if he had not received the letter denying him admission. He told them that his plan was to work for a year and then try again. Luckily, the next day word was sent to him about an unexpected vacancy and he was admitted to medical school for his second year [3].

He approached Howell and expressed his desire to devote one whole year to physiological research. Howell was determining the value of clot-promoting agents from different tissues. He had obtained a thromboplastic (clot-promoting) substance that was a mixture from macerated brain tissue, called "cephalin." He assigned McLean the task of determining the portion of the crude extract that activated the clotting process and to prepare purified cephalin. McLean took an advance course in German to better read the German chemistry literature. He found some German articles on phosphatides by Alfred Erlandsen and Baskoff in which they described extracts of heart and liver secured by a process similar to that for obtaining cephalin from brain. The heart extract was called "cuorin" and that from the liver was called "hepraphosphatide" [3].

The process of extraction was the same for brain, heart, and liver, yet in the brain, the end product was all cephalin, while in the heart and in the liver, it was something else mixed with cephalin. He saved batches of extracts and on retesting them found that the extract from the liver (more than the heart) possessed a strong anticoagulant action after its contained cephalin had lost its thromboplastic action [3].

Howell was not convinced of McLean's discovery of an anticoagulant. McLean got a beaker full of cat's blood and stirred all of a proven batch of hepraphosphatides into it, placed it on Howell's laboratory table, and asked him to tell him when it clotted. It never did [3]. McLean published his paper,

"The Thromboplastic action of Cephalin," in 1916. He discussed the thromboplastic properties of cephalin and its preparation from liver, heart, and brain. He mentioned that the other phosphatides – cuorin and hepraphosphatide – had no thromboplastic action [4]. He did not conduct further research on the anticoagulants as his research year had ended. He completed medical school [1].

Howell carried on research on anticoagulant hepraphosphatide with T. Emmett Holt. In 1918 Howell and Holt named this substance "heparin" and described a method for its preparation from dried dog liver [5]. Howell published five more papers on heparin from 1923 through 1928 [1].

The original tissue source, dog liver, was unsuitable for large-scale preparation. The purification process was greatly improved in Toronto during the 1930s by Arthur. F. Charles and David. A. Scott, who changed the tissue source from dog or beef liver to beef lung, which was cheaper and gave higher yields. Beef lung became the main source material for heparin production until the 1950s when it was largely replaced by porcine mucosa [6].

Charles H. Best is known for conducting experiments with Frederick Banting that led to the discovery of insulin. This success inspired Best to devote his life to biological research. After receiving his medical degree in 1925 from the University of Toronto, he was granted a traveling fellowship by the Rockefeller Foundation and toured European laboratories. When he returned, he continued research on insulin and glucose and began studies of histamine in lung tissue and choline metabolism. The histamine studies required continuous blood pressure measurement by arterial cannulas, which often clotted. He worked closely with Charles and Scott to improve the manufacturing process for heparin at Connaught Laboratories in Toronto. The method required about 66 separate steps to completion but led to a commercially practical method that used ox lung as a source. By 1937, heparin was available for use on a small scale [1].

The main center for heparin research in Europe during the 1930s was the Karolinska Institute in Stockholm, in the laboratory of Erik Jorpes, who produced his own heparin from beef and horse liver, following a visit to Howell's laboratory in 1929. Production of heparin was later transferred to Vitrum Company in Stockholm [6]. In 1939 in the United States, heparin was first marketed as a pharmaceutical product, "Liquaemin," made by Roche Organon [6]. Even today heparin is largely animal derived. Strategies like microbial production, mammalian cell production, and chemo-enzymatic modification have been proposed to produce a bioengineered heparin [7].

EARLY ANIMAL AND CLINICAL TRIALS

In 1935, D. W. Gordon Murray, a surgeon, collaborated with Best. Together they conducted the first animal and clinical studies on heparin in Toronto.

Similar studies were performed in Stockholm by Clarence Crafoord using material purified by Jorpes and colleagues at the Vitrum company [1,6].

Murray and Best began clinical trials with the crystalline sodium salt of heparin prepared by Charles and Scott's method. Their paper, "Heparin and Thrombosis of Veins Following Injury," was published in 1937. It described very extensive studies on dog veins injured mechanically and chemically in vivo and the efficacy of heparin in preventing thrombosis. They conducted studies in humans by infusing heparin solutions in arm veins and determining the clotting times at six-minute intervals, which rose from 6 to 18 minutes. The purified preparations of heparin did not cause toxic reactions such as weakness, headache, and chills that were observed with earlier, cruder preparations. Crafoord had equally promising results and published (also in 1937) a paper entitled, "Preliminary Report on Postoperative Treatment with Heparin as a Preventive of Thrombosis," a study of the use of heparin in 12 patients for prophylaxis of venous thrombosis [1].

In 1959, Murray and Best reported that heparin prevented postoperative pulmonary embolism. At that time, the rate of pulmonary embolism following major surgery was around 2–7.5 percent, and many patients died of this condition. In their study, 315 patients who were given heparin showed no evidence of pulmonary embolism. They described seven cases of existing pulmonary embolism treated successfully with heparin [6]. Murray built and used the first practical dialysis apparatus originating in North America. Heparin was integral to its success [6].

ANTIDOTE

In 1937, the ability of protamine to reverse the anticoagulant effect of heparin was reported by Chargaff and Olson in New York. Protamine (also known as salmine, as it was obtained from salmon roe) prolonged the effect of insulin. They were expecting protamine to have a similar prolongation effect on heparin, but instead it turned out to be its potent antagonist. Protamine sulfate is used clinically to reverse the effects of heparin [1].

DEVELOPMENT OF LOW-MOLECULAR-WEIGHT HEPARIN

Low-molecular-weight heparin originated in the mid-1970s in the laboratory of Edward Johnson at the National Institute of Biological Standards and Control, United Kingdom. He had been investigating the effect of molecular weight range on the clinical properties of dextran. He carried out similar investigations on heparin and prepared three broadly cut fractions of heparin, of high, medium, and low molecular weight by gel filtration. He organized a volunteer study with his colleague Milica Brozovic in which high- and low-molecular-weight fractions, as well as sodium and calcium salts of unfractionated heparin, were injected subcutaneously into medical students. He published his results in 1976 that showed that low-molecular-weight heparin gave much higher and more prolonged blood levels by anti-Xa assays than either high-molecular-weight or unfractionated heparin. During the late 1970s many pharmaceutical companies prepared and investigated low-molecular-weight heparin as a potential therapeutic agent [6].

USE OF HEPARIN AND LOW-MOLECULAR-WEIGHT HEPARIN AS AN ANTICOAGULANT

The anticoagulant properties of heparin were found to be due to the ability of its components to bind to antithrombin III (AT III). AT III slowly binds to thrombin and serine proteases factors VIIa, IX a, Xa, Xia, and XIIa and neutralizes these compounds. Heparin binds to AT III and accelerates its complex formation with thrombin and coagulation factors Xa and XIa. Heparin also antagonizes thromboplastin and prevents thrombi from reacting with fibrinogen to form fibrin [8].

Unfractionated heparin was most often used during the acute phase of thrombosis and embolism. The necessity of giving the drug parenterally limited its long-term use. Unfractionated heparin was also used during pregnancy in patients who required anticoagulation because of the teratogenic effects of warfarin. Unfractionated heparin was given as an IV bolus, a continuous drip infusion, or, less effectively, subcutaneously. The dose was adjusted to keep the activated partial thromboplastin time (aPTT) at 1.5–2.5 times the mean of normal control values [8].

Unfractionated heparin was given acutely to maintain anticoagulation until vitamin K antagonist anticoagulants reached therapeutic levels. Heparin worked very quickly, while oral anticoagulants like warfarin took days to reach therapeutic levels. Heparin was also used to prevent the initial hypercoagulability that developed with warfarin use [8].

By the onset of the twenty-first century, unfractionated heparin began to be replaced by low-molecular-weight heparins, heparinoids, and synthetic heparin pentasaccharides. Heparinoids are heparin analogs, natural or semi-synthetic sulfated glycosaminoglycans prepared by tissue extraction and blending various components. They are structurally similar and have similar anticoagulant effects as heparin. Synthetic heparin pentasaccharides are molecules synthesized to mimic the active site of naturally occurring heparins. All these compounds bind to AT III and induce in it a conformational change that increases its ability to inactivate coagulation enzymes, including thrombin and activated factor Xa [8].

Low-molecular-weight heparins were shown to have a more favorable bioavailability and pharmacokinetics than standard unfractionated heparin.

They had longer plasma half-lives and fewer hemorrhagic complications than standard heparin because they had less pronounced effect on platelet function and vascular permeability. Low-molecular-weight heparins caused fewer cases of heparin-related thrombocytopenia, heparin-related skin necrosis, and white clot syndromes. While heparin was monitored using partial thromboplastin time (PTT), low-molecular-weight heparins, heparinoids, and synthetic heparin pentasaccharides could be monitored by antifactor Xa activity. High-dose low- molecular-weight heparins and synthetic heparin pentasaccharides were well studied in individuals with lower extremity phlebothrombosis and pulmonary embolism. Low-dose low-molecular-weight heparin showed advantages as an agent to prevent deep vein thrombosis in nonambulatory acute ischemic stroke patients. In the PREVAIL randomized trial, among 1,762 randomized patients, deep venous thrombi were detected in 10 percent of low-molecular-weight heparin patients versus 18 percent of unfractionated heparin patients [8].

The effectiveness of heparins and anticoagulants in ischemic stroke has not been well studied except in regard to atrial fibrillation. Heparin followed by warfarin was often used in patients with cardiogenic embolism who were at high risk for early reembolization, but the benefit of heparin use in preventing recurrent embolism was weighed against the risk of hemorrhagic strokes. The International Stroke Trial was conducted in 3,169 patients with atrial fibrillation, who were randomized to different doses of heparin versus no heparin and to aspirin or no aspirin. The high-dose heparin group, compared with the no-heparin group, had fewer ischemic strokes (2.4% vs. 4.9%) but more hemorrhagic strokes (2.8% vs. 0.4%) and no difference in the rate of being alive and independent at six months after stroke. There were fewer pulmonary emboli in patients treated with heparin [9]. The risk of hemorrhage with early anticoagulation related to the patient's blood pressure, coagulation factors, use of a bolus starting dose, the route and intensity of anticoagulation, and the size of the bland or hemorrhagic infarction on CT or MRI scans. Echocardiography could help decide on the risk of early recurrence [8].

Heparin was also shown to be effective in patients with dural sinus thrombosis. It is also administered to prevent pulmonary embolism in these patients [8]. After 2010, the newer anticoagulants like direct thrombin inhibitors and factor Xa inhibitors began to replace warfarin and heparin because they worked quickly, did not require a heparin bridge, and could be given orally [8].

HEPARIN USE IN INTERVENTIONAL RADIOLOGY AND MECHANICAL THROMBECTOMY

Intravascular procedures using indwelling catheters and sheaths would be impossible without inhibition of the coagulation cascade. The synthetic surfaces of catheters and wires themselves are intrinsically thrombogenic. Tissue damage from vessel punctures, sutures, and other causes releases tissue factor, a powerful trigger for coagulation. Ionic contrast material is also known to be thrombogenic. Heparin, because of its antithrombotic properties, has become indispensable for interventional procedures for clot removal in ischemic stroke [10].

NOTES AND REFERENCES

1. Couch NP. About heparin, or ... whatever happened to Jay McLean? *J. Vasc. Surg.* 1989 Jul;10(1):1–8.
2. Marcum JA. Discovery of heparin: Contributions of William Henry Howell and Jay McLean. *Physiology* 1992 Oct;7(5):237–242.
3. Mclean J. The discovery of heparin. *Circulation* 1959 Jan;19(1):75–78.
4. McLean J. The thromboplastic action of cephalin. *Am. J. Physiol.-Leg. Content* 1916 Aug 1;41(2):250–257.
5. Charles AF, Scott DA. Studies on heparin I. The preparation of heparin. *J. Biol. Chem.* 1933 Oct 1;102(2):425–429.
6. Lever R, Mulloy B, Page C. *Heparin: A Century of Progress.* Berlin: Springer Healthcare, 2012, pp. 4–18.
7. Oduah EI, Linhardt RJ, Sharfstein ST. Heparin: Past, present, and future. *Pharmaceuticals (Basel)* 2016 Jul 4;9(3):38.
8. Caplan L, Saver J. Treatment. In Caplan L (ed.), *Caplan's Stroke: A Clinical Approach,* 5th ed. Cambridge: Cambridge University Press, 2016, pp. 170–177.
9. Saxena R, Lewis S, Berge E, Sandercock PA, Koudstaal PJ. Risk of early death and recurrent stroke and effects of heparin in 3169 patients with acute ischemic stroke and atrial fibrillation in the International Stroke Trial. *Stroke* 2001;32:2333–2337.
10. Resnick SB, Resnick SH, Weintraub JL, Kothary N. Heparin in interventional radiology: A therapy in evolution. *Semin. Interv. Radiol.* 2005 Jun;22(2):95–107.

CHAPTER FORTY FIVE

WARFARIN

EARLY RECOGNITION OF THE MECHANISM OF BLEEDING IN CATTLE

The discovery of warfarin is an example of Pasteur's famous quote: "Chance favors the prepared mind." During the 1920s, in the northern United States and Canada, the livelihood of ranchers declined when cattle started dying. Cows bled to death following minor procedures such as dehorning or castration, and even spontaneously. Herds were decimated. There was no identifiable pathogen or nutritional deficiency. The mystery drew the attention of a Canadian veterinary pathologist, Frank Schofield, who noted that all the affected cattle had eaten moldy silage from sweet clover plants. Sweet clover was a popular source of fodder since it grew in poor soil and was a great source of protein. In damp weather, the silage became infected with molds of *Penicillium nigricans and P. jensi*. Schofield separated good clover hay stalks from spoiled ones and fed them to two different rabbits. The rabbit that consumed the spoiled hay died. Schofield had discovered the anticoagulant properties of spoiled sweet clover hay. The hemorrhagic disease of cattle became known as "sweet clover disease" [1–5].

In 1929, L. M. Roderick found that bleeding in cows was explained by lack of functioning prothrombin, a factor integral to blood clotting. Prothrombin is activated to thrombin, the catalyst for converting fibrinogen to fibrin, and so forming blood clots. Roderick showed that the severity of hemorrhage paralleled the reduction in prothrombin content or activity. By using the precipitation technique developed by the American physiologist and pioneer of blood coagulation, William. H. Howell, Roderick prepared solutions of prothrombin from normal bovine plasma and tested them against blood from animals who had eaten spoiled and unspoiled sweet clover. He showed that sweet clover disease was due to lowering of prothrombin. The disease was reversible upon abstinence from toxic sweet clover hay and by administration of fresh blood. Farmers were advised to stop feeding their cattle moldy sweet clover hay, but the chemical agent responsible for causing the prothrombin deficiency could not be isolated from sweet clover.

The next step was to identify a substance from spoiled sweet clover that could be given to humans to prevent blood clotting. A major contributor was a colorful chemist from the American Midwest, Karl Link. Karl Paul Gerhard Link, the eighth of ten children, was born in LaPorte, Indiana, to Frederika Mohr and George Link, a Missouri Lutheran minister. Link's father had a fine library for the children, and they had a piano brought from Germany, which instilled in them an admiration for literature, music, and poetry. The children spoke German and English. Link had a knack for writing cards and letters; his cards always conveyed time and meteorological data such as the current temperature or the day's weather forecast. He attended the University of Wisconsin where he studied agricultural chemistry, receiving his BS degree in 1922, MS in 1923, and PhD in 1925. He had a postdoctoral fellowship at St. Andrews in Scotland under Sir James Irvine in carbohydrate chemistry, but was evicted from the library over an argument with Irvine. Next, he went to Graz, Austria, and studied under Fritz Pregl, a Nobel laureate and a pioneer in microchemistry. He returned to Madison, Wisconsin, with a microbalance and other instruments and set up his own lab for microchemical analysis. He later went to Zurich, Switzerland, to work in Paul Karrer's organic chemistry lab. He developed tuberculosis and recuperated in Davos. There he began an outlandish dressing style, wearing large bow ties and flannel shirts with knickers and a cape. His hair grew long. He returned to the University of Wisconsin as an assistant professor in 1927 and an associate professor in 1928. He studied carbohydrate chemistry and plant resistance. Link married Elizabeth Feldman in 1930 and came back to the lab in the afternoon after the morning wedding. Elizabeth studied philosophy and German at the university and together they had three children.

Link was first introduced to sweet clover disease in December 1932 by Ross A. Gortner, the head of the biochemistry department at the University of Minnesota. Gortner's department had hit an impasse attempting to isolate the hemorrhagic agent, and since sweet clover disease was a major problem in Minnesota, he offered Link the project. He acquainted Link with the original publications of Roderick. In January 1933, Link began research on sweet clover in collaboration with geneticists R. A. Brink and W. K. Smith. They sought a genetic strain suitable for the Wisconsin climate that had a low coumarin content, for coumarin made the clover plant taste bitter.

Ed Carlson, a farmer, brought a dead cow, a milk can full of unclotted blood, and about 100 pounds of sweet clover to the researchers. The hemorrhagic sweet clover disease of cattle was rampant on his farm. He had been feeding sweet clover hay for years without any difficulties. Several of his cows and bulls had succumbed to incessant bleeding. One cow developed a thigh hematoma that bled profusely following a skin puncture, and the cow died. Two other young cows died, and the bull was bleeding from the nose.

Link was persuaded by his student Eugen Wilhem Schoeffel to delve into the issue. Schoeffel was a German who had come to the United States with a diploma in agricultural chemistry. As Carlson left, Schoeffel hit the ceiling, and as described by Link in his paper, his words were:

> Vat da Hell, a farmer shtruggles nearly 200 miles in dis Sau-wetter, driven by a shpectre and den has to go home vit promises dat might come true in five, ten, fifteen years, maybe never.... Ach!! Gott, how can you do dat ven you haf no money? Dere's no clot in dat blook!... Vat vill he find ven he gets home? Sicker cows. And ven he and his good voman go to church tomorrow and pray and pray and pray, vat vill dey haf on Monday? MORE DEAD COWS!!... if he loses de bull he loses his seed. Mein Gott!! Mein Gott!!

As Link left the laboratory, Schoeffel confronted him and said, "Before you go let me tell you something. Der is a deshtiny dat shapes our ends, it shapes our ends I tell you! I vill clean up and gif you a document on Monday morning." So, Link and his students, Smith, Roberts, and Campbell, began their pursuit of the hemorrhagic agent.

ISOLATING AND SYNTHESIZING THE ACTIVE ANTICOAGULANT COMPOUND

On June 28, 1939, Campbell, after working all night, stumbled onto crystalline dicumarol and isolated about six milligrams of it. Mark A. Stahmann took over the task of mass isolation of the chemical and in about four months accumulated about 1,800 miilgrams of the crystalline compound. C. F. Heubner assumed the task of identifying the structure of the compound. He elucidated the structure of dicumarol to be 3,3′methylenebis (4-hydroxycoumarin). On April Fool's Day, 1940, he synthesized a compound identical to the natural one. This compound was a derivative of coumarin, the agent responsible for the bitter taste of the plant. During the process of spoilage of the sweet clover, coumarin was oxidized to 4-hydroxycoumarin, which on coupling with formaldehyde yielded dicumarol. During the next four years, Link and his students synthesized some hundred related compounds.

In early September 1945, irked by lab work, Link took off and went on a canoe trip with his family. Unfortunately, they were caught in a rainstorm, causing a relapse of Link's tuberculosis. He spent two months at Wisconsin General Hospital and then Lakeview Sanatorium. While recuperating, he became interested in rodent infestations and the urgent need for a rat poison. He contemplated using a coumarin derivative to kill rats. The coumarin derivatives that his lab had synthesized were given numbers based on their chemical structure. A student, L. D. Scheel, was assigned the task of studying the anticoagulant properties of the compounds numbered from 40 to 65. Scheel found that compounds numbered 42 and 63 were more potent than dicumarol as insidious killers of rats and dogs, by causing severe hypothrombinemia without visible bleeding. Dicumarol was not a very effective agent because its action was easily counteracted by vitamin K, which was then abundant in the diet of the rats. Agent numbered 42 was proposed for rodenticidal use in 1948. It was named warfarin ("warf" from the Wisconsin Alumni Research Foundation, which funded their research, and "arin" from "coumarin"). Warfarin became the quintessential rat poison. Its action was not sudden in onset – the sudden death of rats would prevent other rats from eating the bait – and thus bait refusal did not develop in rats.

EARLY USE IN HUMANS

During the 1940s and early 1950s preliminary safety studies were initiated in humans. Clinicians were dubious about using warfarin as an anticoagulant in humans. A tragedy occurred on April 5, 1951, that helped to change minds. An army inductee attempted suicide by consuming warfarin designed for rodent control. He had followed the multiple dosage instructions on the package and consumed 567 milligrams of warfarin in cornstarch over a period of five days. He was admitted to the naval hospital as a case of full-blown sweet clover disease. He walked into the hospital and, following blood transfusion and administration of vitamin K, recovered.

This incident acted as an impetus for the use of warfarin in humans. Collin Schroeder perfected the process of making warfarin sodium, which was found to be about 5–10 times more potent than dicumarol. Mass production was undertaken by Endo Laboratories, in Richmond Hill, New York. The agent was marketed as coumadin sodium (not to be confused with "coumarin"). Coumadin had several advantages over other anticoagulants: it was highly water soluble and could be administered orally, intravenously, intramuscularly, or rectally. The anticoagulant effect could be reversed by administration of vitamin K [6,7].

During the 1940s, anticoagulants were first used in humans to treat leg vein thrombosis and pulmonary embolism [8,9]. In 1960, Barritt and Jordan performed the first randomized trial hoping to show the efficacy of anticoagulant therapy in the treatment of venous thromboembolism [8]. They compared patients treated with heparin and nicoumalone with those not treated with anticoagulants. The trial was stopped when five of the original 19 untreated patients died and none of their 16 treated patients died. Despite the lack of strong evidence, anticoagulation soon became standard therapy for prevention of pulmonary embolism.

The other major condition that clinicians posited could gain from anticoagulation was heart disease. Rheumatic heart disease, especially with atrial fibrillation, was frequently complicated by brain and systemic embolism, and cardiologists began treating these patients with anticoagulants [10–15]. In 1955, President Dwight Eisenhower, while on a holiday in Denver, had a heart attack. He was initially treated with heparin but was eventually started on warfarin at a dose of 35 milligrams per week [16]. The FDA approved warfarin in 1955.

USE IN PATIENTS WITH STROKE

Warfarin was prescribed anecdotally to patients with transient ischemic attacks (TIAs) and progressing strokes during the early 1950s. The first randomized therapeutic trial was organized by the National Institutes of Health during the 1950s. The participating investigators were C. Miller Fisher of the Massachusetts General Hospital in Boston, Harry Fang of Los Angeles, Al Heyman of Duke, Herb Karp of Atlanta, Ellen McDevitt of Cornell University, Clark Millikan of the Mayo Clinic, Adolph Sahs of the University of Iowa, Peritz Scheinberg of Jackson Memorial Hospital at Miami University, and Lawrence Barrows and Jim Toole of the University of Pennsylvania. Fisher was the chairman and director of the coordinating center at MGH where records from the other participating centers were evaluated. Fisher wrote an interim report published in 1961 [17]. To be entered, patients must have had an ischemic episode within eight weeks; they were given a placebo capsule or anticoagulant (dicumerol with or without heparin). At the time of the interim report, 384 patients had been studied. About 70 percent had had episodes within the past seven days. There were 37 deaths among the 182 placebo-treated patients and 38 among the 195 patients who received anticoagulants. Fisher concluded: "Long-term anticoagulation therapy does not appear to reduce the mortality in occlusive cerebrovascular disease and, indeed is associated with an added risk of death due to the hemorrhagic complications. The number of transient cerebral ischemic attacks is reduced by anticoagulation" [17]. A final report on the anticoagulation study was published in 1962, but results had not changed since Fisher's interim report [18]. This was one of the very first therapeutic trials; its makeup and conduction were primitive according to today's trial standards.

One of the most common stroke conditions for which anticoagulants were prescribed during the mid-twentieth century was occlusive disease within the vertebrobasilar circulation. Reports from the Mayo Clinic stroke service in the 1950s and 1960s enthusiastically endorsed anticoagulant treatment of posterior circulation vascular disease [19–21]. Millikan et al. described 21 patients with progressing vertebrobasilar territory strokes who were treated with anticoagulants. Only 3 (14%) died compared with 10 of 23 deaths (43%) in a retrospective search for similar patients not anticoagulated. Attacks stopped in all five patients who had vertebrobasilar TIAs [19,20]. Later, Jack Whisnant described the results among 140 patients with progressive posterior circulation ischemia. Twelve (8.5%) died compared with 23 of 39 deaths (59%) in similar patients not anticoagulated. vertebrobasilar attacks often stopped after anticoagulation [21].

Until the 1990s, the effectiveness of anticoagulation with heparin or warfarin had not been tested in modern randomized therapeutic trials in patients with known pathologies. Prior studies involved only large groups of undifferentiated patients with brain ischemia. Early observational studies had shown the effectiveness of warfarin in patients with rheumatic mitral stenosis who had brain embolism [10–15]. During the latter years of the twentieth century, many trials of stroke prophylaxis in patients with atrial fibrillation who did not have valvular heart disease were performed and showed a dramatic benefit of anticoagulant treatment [22–26]. All trials showed a consistent and considerable risk reduction for stroke in patients treated with warfarin. Warfarin was approximately 50 percent more effective than aspirin in reducing the rate of stroke in patients with nonvalvular atrial fibrillation [27].

Other randomized trials compared warfarin prophylactic treatment with aspirin.

Among patients with ischemic strokes not judged to be cardiembolic, in the Warfarin-Aspirin Recurrent Stroke Study (WARSS) trial, coumadin and aspirin were equally effective in preventing new strokes [28]. The drugs were given within a month of stroke onset, not always acutely, and secondary prevention of new strokes was studied. The number of patients with documented large artery disease was small and vascular studies were not required or reported. The results did not relate well to the use of anticoagulants during the acute stroke.

In the Warfarin-Aspirin for Symptomatic Intracranial Disease (WASID) trial of patients with severe intracranial atherosclerosis, there was no significant difference in the prevention of new strokes between aspirin and warfarin [29]. The study drugs were initiated often weeks after the last ischemic event. Warfarin was difficult to control. In those patients who were maintained within the target therapeutic international normalized ratio (INR) range, warfarin performed better than 1,300 milligrams of aspirin per day. In those who were below the target range, more infarcts developed, and more hemorrhages developed in those above the target INR range [29,30].

Anticoagulants were also investigated to treat patients with dural venous sinus thrombosis. Reports studied the safety and effectiveness of acute treatment with heparins. There was general agreement that they should be given to patients with acute cerebral venous occlusions to prevent new ischemia and pulmonary embolism. Warfarin was customarily prescribed after the acute period, but opinions and customs varied about treatment duration and in which patients [31,32]. Warfarin was also prescribed for patients with hypercoagulability, including those with the antiphospholipid antibody syndrome.

Despite its effectiveness, warfarin use was unpopular with doctors and patients. Frequent blood drawings were needed to adjust the dose. Many food substances and drugs interfered with its activity. Patients had to be careful about what they ate and avoided salads and greens. Even in the very best hands (in coagulation clinics that specialized in monitoring), patients were only on target about three-fourths of the time. When the target level was too low, there was less protection from brain infarction. If the level was too high, serious bleeding could develop. As the twentieth century drew to a close, clinicians and researchers began to search for anticoagulants that would not be vitamin K dependent, that could be given orally, and that would not require as frequent testing and monitoring as warfarin.

NOTES AND REFERENCES

1. Link KP. The discovery of dicumarol and its sequels. *Circulation* 1959 Jan 1;19 (1):97–107.
2. Fields WS, Lemak NA. *A History of Stroke: Its Recognition and Treatment.* New York: Oxford University Press, 1989.
3. Wardrop D, Keeling D. The story of the discovery of heparin and warfarin. *Br. J. Haematol.* 2008 Jun 1;141(6):757–763.
4. Burris RH. Karl Paul Link. In *Biographical Memoirs*, vol. 65. National Academies Press, 1994. Available at www.nap.edu/read/4548/chapter/9.
5. Meek T. This month in 1939: How dead cattle led to the discovery of warfarin. PMLive. June 27, 2013. Available at www.pmlive.com/pharma_news/how_dead_cattle_led_to_the_discovery_of_warfarin_485464.
6. Wessler S, Gitel S. Warfarin: From bedside to bench. *N. Engl. J. Med.* 1984;311:645–652.
7. Deykin D. Warfarin therapy. *N. Engl. J. Med.* 1970;283:691–694.
8. Barritt DW, Jordan MB. Anticoagulant drugs in the treatment of pulmonary embolism: A controlled trial. *Lancet* 1960;275:1309–1312.
9. Ergermayer P. Value of anticoagulants in the treatment of pulmonary embolism: A discussion paper. *J. Roy. Soc. Med.* 1981;74:675–681.
10. Wright IS, Foley WT. Use of anticoagulants in the treatment of heart disease with special reference to coronary thrombosis, rheumatic heart disease with thromboembolic complications and subacute bacterial endocarditis. *Am. J. Med.* 1947;3:718–739.
11. Cosgriff SW. Prophylaxis of recurrent embolism of intracardiac origin: Protracted anticoagulant therapy on an ambulatory basis. *JAMA* 1950;143:870–872.

12. Szekely P. Systemic embolism and anticoagulant prophylaxis in rheumatic heart disease. *Br. Med. J.* 1964:1:1209.

13. McDevitt E. Treatment of cerebral embolism. *Mod. Treat.* 1965;2:52.

14. Fleming HA, Bailey SM. Mitral valve disease, systemic embolism and anticoagulants. *Postgrad. Med. J.* 1971; 47:599–604.

15. Report of the working party on anticoagulant therapy in coronary thrombosis to the Medical Research Council: Assessment of short-term anticoagulant administration after cardiac infarction. *Br. Med. J.* 1969;1:335.

16. Kucharski, A. Medical management of political patients: The case of Dwight D. Eisenhower. *Perspect. Biol. Med.* 1978;22:115–126.

17. Fisher CM. Anticoagulant therapy in cerebral thrombosis and cerebral embolism. A National Cooperative Study, interim report. *Neurology* 1961;11:119–131.

18. Baker RN, Broward JA, Fang HC, Fisher CM, Groch SN, Heyman A. Anticoagulant therapy in cerebral infarction. *Neurology* 1962;12:823–835.

19. Millikan CH, Siekert RG, Shick R. Studies in cerebrovascular disease, III: The use of anticoagulant drugs in the treatment of insufficiency or thrombosis within the basilar arterial system. *Proc. Staff Meet. Mayo Clin.* 1955;30:111–126.

20. Millikan CH, Siekert RG, Whisnant JP. Anticoagulant therapy in cerebrovascular disease: Current status. *JAMA* 1958;166:587–592.

21. Whisnant JP. Discussion. In Millikan C, Siekert R, Whisnant JP (eds.), *Cerebral Vascular Diseases: Third Princeton Conference on Cerebrovascular Diseases.* Orlando, FL: Grune & Stratton, 1961, pp. 156–157.

22. The Boston Area Anticoagulation Trial for Atrial Fibrillation Investigators. The effect of low-dose warfarin on the risk of stroke in patients with nonrheumatic atrial fibrillation. *N. Engl. J. Med.* 1990;323:1505–1511.

23. EAFT (European Atrial Fibrillation Trial) Study Group. Secondary prevention in non-rheumatic atrial fibrillation after transient ischaemic attack or minor stroke. *Lancet* 1993;342:1255–1262.

24. The Stroke Prevention in Atrial Fibrillation Investigators. The stroke prevention in atrial fibrillation study: Final results. *Circulation* 1991;84:527–539.

25. Stroke Prevention in Atrial Fibrillation Investigators. Warfarin versus aspirin for prevention of thromboembolism in atrial fibrillation: Stroke Prevention in Atrial Fibrillation II Study. *Lancet* 1994;343:687–691.

26. Albers GW. Atrial fibrillation and stroke: Three new studies, three remaining questions. *Arch. Intern. Med.* 1994;154:1443–1448.

27. Hart RG, Benavente O, McBride R, et al. Antithrombotic therapy to prevent stroke in patients with atrial fibrillation: A meta-analysis. *Ann. Intern. Med.* 1999;131:492–501.

28. Mohr JP, Thompson JLP, Lazar RM, et al. for the Warfarin–Aspirin Recurrent Stroke Study Group. A comparison of warfarin and aspirin for the prevention of recurrent ischemic stroke. *N. Engl. J. Med.* 2001;345:1444–1451.

29. Chimowitz MI, Lynn MJ, Howlett-Smith H, et al. Comparison of warfarin and aspirin for symptomatic intracranial arterial stenosis. *N. Engl. J. Med.* 2005;352:1305–1316.

30. Koroshetz W. Warfarin, aspirin, and intracranial vascular disease. *N. Engl. J. Med.* 2005;352:1368–1370.

31. Bousser MG, Ross Russell R. *Cerebral Venous Thrombosis.* Philadelphia: WB Saunders, 1997.

32. Ameri A, Bousser MG. Cerebral venous thrombosis. *Neurol. Clin.* 1992;10:87–111.

CHAPTER FORTY SIX

DIRECT ORAL ANTICOAGULANTS

For more than 50 years, vitamin K antagonists (VKAs) were the only available oral anticoagulants. Although several drugs in this class were developed and used clinically (e.g., acenocoumarol, phenprocoumon), warfarin is the best known and most widely used. Warfarin is popularly known by its brand name Coumadin (branded by Endo in the 1950s, acquired by DuPont in 1969 and Bristol Myers Squibb in 2001) [1]. Since it came into use, much has been learned about its mechanism of action, pharmacology, and pharmacodynamics. VKAs are multitargeted and lower the activity of four vitamin K–dependent coagulation factors that promote blood clotting, factors II, VI, IX, and X, and two anticoagulant proteins, protein C and protein S. Remarkably, it took until 2004 for the liver enzyme that is inhibited by VKAs, vitamin K epoxide reductase (VKORC1), to be molecularly identified [2]. As the VKAs have a narrow therapeutic window and individuals vary widely in responsiveness, its effect must be monitored using the prothrombin time (PT) test. It took years of clinical and laboratory investigation to standardize and optimize the monitoring of VKAs to achieve the best possible outcomes with respect to thrombosis prevention and a low bleeding rate. This was achieved by development of the international normalized ratio (INR), which is derived from the PT. Anticoagulation or Coumadin clinics that employ nurses and pharmacists skilled in managing warfarin have greatly improved the care of patients on warfarin. VKAs, however, can still be difficult to use safely, particularly in elderly patients with comorbidities and diminished cognition.

After clinical trials in the early 1990s showed that VKAs prevent stroke in greater than 60 percent of patients with nonvalvular atrial fibrillation, many more patients were now candidates for long-term anticoagulation. Many physicians were wary of prescribing warfarin, particularly in the elderly, fearing a major or life-threatening bleed. In addition, some patients declined warfarin therapy.

At the end of the twentieth century, new oral anticoagulants (NOACs), selective for a specific coagulation factor, either thrombin or factor Xa, were developed. These small-molecule inhibitors were synthesized based on knowledge of the three-dimensional structures of thrombin and factor Xa, reversibly binding to their active sites. Thrombin plays a central role in blood clotting by converting fibrinogen to fibrin as well as by activating coagulation factors V, VIII, XI, and XIII. Factor Xa was also an attractive target for the design of NOACs as it is positioned just above thrombin in the common pathway of coagulation.

Ximelagatran, a prodrug of the thrombin inhibitor melagatran, was the first NOAC or direct oral anticoagulant (DOAC) to be taken through clinical development. A prodrug was required to allow it to be absorbed by the upper gastrointestinal tract. Preclinical studies showed that ximelagatran had a wider therapeutic window as compared to warfarin. Pharmacologic studies in humans showed that it produced a predictable anticoagulant response with few food or drug interactions. In randomized phase III clinical trials, ximelagatran administered twice daily at fixed doses was as effective and safe as warfarin in the prevention of stroke in nonvalvular atrial fibrillation [3], the treatment of venous thromboembolism, and the prevention of venous thromboembolism following total hip or knee replacement. AstraZeneca, the developer of the drug, had confidence in its drug development program and its potential to transform oral anticoagulation. But due to hepatotoxicity, ximelagatran was not approved by the US FDA when it applied for multiple indications in 2004. While it briefly gained approval in Europe for the prophylaxis of venous thromboembolism (VTE) following hip or knee replacement surgery, ximelagatran was withdrawn from the market in 2006 due to instances of serious liver injury. The ximelagatran development program, nevertheless, provided "proof of principle," that fixed doses of a DOAC without coagulation monitoring could be as effective and safe as warfarin in preventing and treating thrombosis in adults with adequate renal function (i.e., creatinine clearance > 30 mL/min). The experience also provided a road map for the development of other DOACs and the need for close surveillance of liver function in early phase clinical trials.

The demise of ximelagatran in 2004 due to hepatotoxicity opened the field for several DOACs that were at early stages of clinical development. Hepatotoxicity turned out to be specific to ximelagatran and was not a class effect of the oral thrombin or factor Xa inhibitors in development. Dabigatran etexilate (Pradaxa, developed by Boehringer Ingelheim) is also an oral prodrug that is rapidly converted to dabigatran, a reversible direct thrombin inhibitor, after ingestion. Peak blood concentrations are achieved one to two hours after oral administration, and the half-life of dabigatran in the circulation is 12–14 hours; about 80 percent is cleared by the kidneys. A large clinical trial (RE-LY) compared dabigatran and warfarin in over 18,000 patients with nonvalvular atrial fibrillation at risk of stroke [4]. Two doses of dabigatran etexilate were compared with warfarin; the stroke rate in patients on dabigatran at a dose of 150 milligrams twice daily was around 30 percent lower than warfarin with similar bleeding rates; the 110-milligram twice-a-day dose had similar efficacy to warfarin, but had a significantly lower bleed rate. The rates of bleeding in the brain (hemorrhagic stroke) with the 110- and 150-milligram dabigatran etexilate doses were around 70 percent lower than warfarin. Based on the results of the RE-LY trial, dabigatran etexilate was approved in 2010 in the United States and other countries for stroke prevention in atrial fibrillation.

Rivaroxaban (Xarelto, developed by Bayer), apixaban (Eliquis, developed by Bristol Myers Squibb), and edoxaban (Savaysa, developed by Daiichi Sankyo) are small molecules that selectively inhibit coagulation factor Xa. A high percentage of these drugs is absorbed after oral administration, and peak blood concentrations are achieved in a few hours. The drugs have similar half-lives, in the range of 7–13 hours and approximately 30 percent is eliminated by the kidney.

In the ROCKET-AF trial, which included over 14,000 patients, rivaroxaban administered at a fixed dose once daily was as effective as warfarin in reducing stroke and systemic embolism with a similar rate of major bleeding [5]. The ARISTOTLE study compared apixaban at a fixed dose twice daily to warfarin for stroke prevention in over 18,000 patients; apixaban had a similar risk of ischemic stroke, but major bleeds were reduced by 30 percent compared to warfarin [6]. The ENGAGE trial of over 14,000 patients using edoxaban also showed favorable outcomes compared to warfarin [7]. As in the RE-LY trial with dabigatran, the rates of intracranial hemorrhage were about 50 percent less with all of the oral factor Xa inhibitors compared to warfarin.

Rivaroxaban, apixaban, and edoxaban were approved by the FDA for patients with atrial fibrillation in 2011, 2012, and 2015, respectively. As all of the DOACs were compared to warfarin, it has been tempting to do cross-trial comparisons of the agents versus one another, although the trials had different designs, different severity of patient risk factors, and different end points.

Given the large numbers of patients with atrial fibrillation requiring indefinite (or lifelong) anticoagulation, being first to be marketed was a commercial advantage for dabigatran. While uptake was substantial among cardiologists, there was hesitancy among internists or general practitioners, who remained more comfortable prescribing warfarin, especially if their patients had access to anticoagulation clinics that oversaw monitoring and medication adherence. Reports appeared of hemorrhagic complications due to "overzealous" prescribing of dabigatran in patients with diminished kidney function. While both the 110- and 150-milligram dosing schedules were approved in some countries, only the higher dose was approved by the FDA. US physicians did not have the option of prescribing the 110-milligram dose of dabigatran that was shown to have greater major bleeding safety than warfarin. There was also concern regarding the absence of specific reversal agents should major or life-threatening hemorrhage develop in patients on DOACs. This was subsequently addressed by the development of a highly effective reversal agent for dabigatran, the monoclonal antibody idarucizumab (Praxbind, developed by Boehringer Ingelheim), which gained FDA approval in 2015. A specific reversal agent for rivaroxaban and apixaban, andexanet (Andexxa, developed by Portola and now marketed by Alexion), was approved by the FDA in 2018.

Over time, the oral factor Xa inhibitors rivaroxaban and apixaban gained favor over dabigatran for stroke prevention in atrial fibrillation. In addition to the issues cited above, there were other reasons that oral factor Xa inhibitors were preferred to dabigatran. Dabigatran was associated with an upset stomach in around 10 percent of patients in the RE-LY trial [4]. A dose-finding trial of dabigatran in patients with mechanical heart valves at high risk of stroke yielded negative results in comparison to warfarin [8]. Though dabigatran gained approval for the treatment of acute VTE, another major indication for oral anticoagulation, patients initially had to be treated with an injectable anticoagulant (i.e., low-molecular-weight heparin for at least five days) before initiating dabigatran, which was not the case for rivaroxaban and apixaban. Physicians prescribing DOACs thus became more comfortable using either rivaroxaban or apixaban for multiple clinical indications when anticoagulation was required. Given the high cost of performing large randomized clinical trials, Bayer partnered with Janssen and Bristol Myers Squibb with Pfizer in the development of rivaroxaban and apixaban, respectively; these partnerships facilitated marketing of these drugs after regulatory agency approval.

DOACs have major advantages over VKAs, including rapid onset of action, predictable anticoagulant effect, a lower bleeding risk of brain bleeds, absence of dietary interactions, and limited drug-drug interactions. Their introduction into clinical practice has resulted in an improved quality of life for patients, greater use of anticoagulation in patients with atrial fibrillation, and a decrease in the burden on the healthcare system of caring for anticoagulated patients. The higher cost of acquiring DOACs can be an issue for some patients depending on their pharmacy insurance benefits. While warfarin has been a generic medication for over two decades, making it relatively inexpensive, there are costs to healthcare systems of performing regular INR monitoring and caring for patients with treatment-related hemorrhagic complications.

Although DOACs are excellent anticoagulants, there are a number of indications for which warfarin remains the indicated anticoagulant; these include
patients with mechanical heart valves and triple-positive antiphospholipid
antibody syndrome. Warfarin therefore remains an anticoagulant option for
some patients.

NOTES AND REFERENCES

1. The development of warfarin and its evolution is discussed at length in Chapter 45.
2. Rost S, Fregin A, Ivaskevicius V, et al. Mutations in VKORC1 cause warfarin resistance
   and multiple coagulation factor deficiency type 2. *Nature* 2004;427:537–541. Li T,
   Chang CY, Jin DY, Lin PJ, Khvorova A, Stafford DW. Identification of the gene for
   vitamin K epoxide reductase. *Nature* 2004;427:541–544.
3. Akins PT, Feldman HA, Zoble RG, et al. Secondary stroke prevention with ximelagatran versus warfarin in patients with atrial fibrillation. Pooled analysis of SPORTIF III
   and V Clinical Trials. *Stroke* 2007;38:874–880.
4. Connolly SJ, Ezekowitz MD, Yusuf S, et al. and the RE-LY Steering Committee and
   Investigators. Dabigatran versus warfarin in patients with atrial fibrillation. *N. Engl.
   J. Med.* 2009;361:1139–1151.
5. Patel MR, Mahaffey KW, Garg J, Pan G, Singer DE, Hacke W, et al. Rivaroxaban
   versus warfarin in nonvalvular atrial fibrillation. *N. Engl. J. Med.* 2011;365:883–891.
6. Granger CB, Alexander JH, McMurray JJ, Lopes RD, Hylek EM, Hanna M, et al.
   Apixaban versus warfarin in patients with atrial fibrillation. *N. Engl. J. Med.*
   2011;365:981–992.
7. Giugliano RP, Ruff CT, Braunwald E, Murphy SA, Wiviott SD, Halperin JL, et al.
   Edoxaban versus warfarin in patients with atrial fibrillation. *N. Engl. J. Med.*
   2013;369:2093–2104.
8. Eikelboom JW, Connolly SJ, Brueckmann M, et al. for the RE-ALIGN Investigators.
   Dabigatran versus warfarin in patients with mechanical heart valves. *N. Engl. J. Med.*
   2013;369:1206–1214.

CHAPTER FORTY SEVEN

ASPIRIN

DOCTRINE OF SIGNATURES

Ancient medical practitioners believed in the "doctrine of signatures," which stated that natural objects that resembled parts of the body could cure diseases affecting those parts. The eyebright plant was used to cure eye diseases due to the similitude of its flowers to blue eyes. The famous Swiss physician Paracelsus was a proponent of this doctrine and stated, "Nature marks each growth, according to its curative benefit." Herbs were believed to have particular "signatures" given by God for people to identify and use. Although this doctrine had no scientific basis, it led to the discovery of a drug widely used today [1].

The ancient Egyptian Ebers Papyrus records that willow leaves were used to treat inflammatory rheumatic diseases and pain. Hippocrates administered willow leaf tea to women to ease childbirth pain [2]. The first scientific description of the beneficial effects of the bark of the willow tree was by Reverend Edward Stone and was contained in a letter to the president of the Royal Society in 1763. Stone wrote that he had accidently tasted willow tree bark and was surprised by its extreme bitterness, which was similar to the Peruvian bark (of the cinchona tree, source of quinine and used to treat malaria). He opined that the bark of the willow tree might be a potential cure for ague (malarial fever) based on the doctrine of signatures. Stone wrote:

> As the tree delights in a moist or wet soil, where agues chiefly abound, the general maxim that many natural maladies carry their cures along with them or that their remedies lie not far from their causes was so apposite to this particular case that I could not help applying it; and that this might be the intention of Providence here, I must own, it has some little weight with me. [3–5]

To appease his curiosity, he delved into various books of botany but could not find information on its medicinal properties, despite the plenitude of the trees in the region. He conducted his own experiments for which he gathered a pound of the willow bark and dried it in a bag outside a baker's oven for three months until it was reduced to a powder. He cautiously administered very small quantities of the powder every four hours to individuals with fever and found that symptoms abated. He gradually increased the dose and found that the "ague was removed." The drug was successful in curing fevers in about 50 patients, during a period of five years. To treat some obstinate cases, he added quinine (from the Peruvian bark, one-fifth by parts) and found the treatment successful. To ascertain that the effects were not confounded, he ensured that patients were never prepared by "vomiting, bleeding or purging or any other medications" before the administration of the bark. Willow bark was an important source of salicylate, the precursor of the common household drug *aspirin*.

In 1828, Johann Andreas Buchner isolated the active ingredient from willow bark in the form of bitter-tasting yellow crystals. He named the compound salicin (Latin for "willow"). Ten years later, an Italian chemist, Raffaele Piria, split the glycoside salicin to produce salicylic acid. In 1859, Hermann Kolbe, professor of chemistry at Marburg University, identified the chemical structure of salicylic acid and synthesized it. This led to industrial production of salicylic acid, and by 1874, a factory in Dresden was selling it at one-tenth the price of the material extracted naturally.

The first clinical trial on the efficacy of salicin to treat rheumatic fever (characterized by pain and inflammation) was published by Thomas John Maclagan in the *Lancet* in 1876. He too was led to willow tree bark by the doctrine of signatures, for he wrote:

> It seemed to me that a remedy for that disease would most hopefully be looked for among those plants and trees whose favourite habitat presented conditions analogous to those under which the rheumatic miasma seemed most to prevail. The bark of many species of willow contains a bitter principle called salicin. This principle was exactly what I wanted: to it, therefore, I determined to have recourse. [6,7]

Maclagan self-administered the drug and, convinced of no ill-effects, began giving it to patients. He reported its success in the treatment of eight cases of rheumatism. One of his patients developed severe throat and stomach irritation and he discontinued the drug. He urged other practitioners to report their experiences.

Six weeks later, his appeal was answered by Frederick Ensor, a South African surgeon who shared his experience with a patient who had a severe rheumatic disease. He had prescribed the patient the usual alkaline mixture, calomel and Dover's powder, at bedtime. Two months later, the patient returned cured and plainly told him that his medication hadn't helped her at all. The ameliorant was made from the shoots of the willows growing on the banks of the river, by a Hottentot "shepherd"!

PRODUCTION OF THE WORLD'S MOST SUCCESSFUL ILLEGAL DRUG

Heinrich Dreser was born in 1860, in Darmstadt. His father was a professor of physics. He received his doctorate in chemistry from Heidelberg University and became a professor at Bonn University. In 1897, he became in charge of testing the efficacy and safety of new drugs at Bayer company. The company began by manufacturing dyes, but soon became one of the world's pharmaceutical giants. During Dreser's tenure as company head, Bayer launched two drugs, the world's most successful legal drug – aspirin – and the most successful illegal drug – heroin. Diacetylmorphine (heroin) was first discovered by an English chemist, C. R. Wright, but its commercial potential was realized by Dreser [8,9].

Dreser was a pioneer in the development of various techniques for drug testing. He was the first chemist to use animal experiments on an industrial scale. While Dreser was in charge of drug testing, Arthur Eichengrün was the head of the Bayer pharmaceutical group section on new drugs. Salicylic acid was widely used to treat rheumatic fever, but it became intolerable to many patients due to severe gastric irritation and unpleasant taste. Felix Hoffmann, a chemist at Bayer, was instructed by Eichengrün to synthesize a more tolerable form of salicylic acid. Coincidently, Hoffmann's father was taking salicylic acid for his rheumatism and had severe side effects.

Hoffmann devised a process for the acetylation of the phenol group of salicylic acid to produce acetyl salicylic acid (ASA), later named aspirin. The compound was previously synthesized in 1853 by Charles Friedrich Gerhardt but it decomposed spontaneously due to instability.

Eichengrün discussed the prospect of marketing ASA with Dreser but he rejected it, opining that it would have an "enfeebling" action on the heart. Dreser's opinion was based on his interest in the other drug, heroin. He saw the potential of heroin to replace morphine as a nonaddictive painkiller for respiratory diseases. Heroin was synthesized by Hoffmann two weeks after he made ASA. Dreser was cognizant of the fact that it was originally discovered by

Wright, but he claimed it to be a Bayer invention. He gave heroin to various animals, workers, and himself and was elated by the response. The workers reported that the drug made them feel "heroic," hence the name of the drug. Heroin became popular as a "cough remedy" for tuberculosis and pneumonia, which were then prevalent. By 1899, Bayer was producing a ton of heroin annually and was exporting it to 23 countries in the form of heroin pastilles, cough lozenges, tablets, elixirs, and other products. The success of the drug was transient as researchers began reporting cases of addiction, tolerance, and "heroinism."

Bayer then shifted its focus and began testing ASA. Dreser took it himself and also gave it to rabbits. He published a paper highlighting its use for treatment of rheumatism. Dreser did not mention the contributions of Hoffmann and Eichengrün. The compound was marketed as Aspirin ("a" from "acetyl" and "spir" from *Spirea ulmania*, the plant from which salicylic acid was first isolated). The two final contenders for naming the substance had been "Euspirin" and "Aspirin." "Aspirin," some feared, would remind people of aspiration, while Eichengrün argued that a name starting with "eu" was invalid for it usually indicated an improvement of a previous version. Since the company could not market the drug directly to the public, Bayer circulated small packets to 30,000 doctors and encouraged them to prescribe it. Dreser benefited tremendously, for he received royalties for any new product introduced. Eichengrün and Hoffmann received no benefits, for they received royalties only if they invented a patentable product. By 1904, the powdered form was replaced by tablets stamped with Bayer's logo. This established a connection between Bayer and Aspirin and distinguished it from other competitors' products. Dreser was rumored to be addicted to heroin. He died of a stroke, which might have been prevented had he been addicted to the other drug, Aspirin.

One important historical figure who should not have been prescribed Aspirin was Alexei Nikolaevich, born in 1904, the heir apparent of the Russian Empire. He inherited hemophilia from his mother Alexandra, the granddaughter of Queen Victoria. Alexei was prescribed the "wonder drug" Aspirin to decrease joint pain. Aspirin made the bleeding and swelling worse. He improved when a faith healer, Rasputin, told his mother to stop all medication and rely on faith healing.

ASPIRIN PREVENTS THE BLOOD FROM CLOTTING

Lawrence L. Craven was a general practitioner at the Glendale Memorial Hospital in California posited that Aspirin might prevent myocardial infarction [10]. Myocardial infarction was due to thrombus formation at the site of atherosclerotic narrowing. He posited that Aspirin could prevent this process by prolonging the prothrombin time. In 1948, he prescribed Aspirin to 400 patients and reported in 1950 that none developed a myocardial infarct during the two-year period. He also observed recurrent hemorrhaging in post-tonsillectomy patients who chewed Aspirin gum for pain relief. In his article, published in the *Journal of Insurance Medicine*, he wrote:

> For 36 years my surgical work has been primarily removal of tonsils and adenoids. Of the hundreds of cases handled, only 5 were performed in hospitals. Surgery was performed during morning office hours and practically all patients were released to their homes by early afternoon without question of possible hemorrhage – practically none occurring until about 6 years ago, at which time an alarming number of hemorrhages were evidenced in disturbing frequency. [11]

To further support his hypothesis, he stated that men were more likely to have heart attacks than women because they were less likely to take Aspirin for common aches and pains (taking inessential medications was effeminate).

Craven continued to prescribe Aspirin to men between the ages of 45 and 65 who were overweight and led sedentary lifestyles. He reported in 1953 that none of his 1,500 patients who faithfully took Aspirin developed a myocardial infarction [12]. He acknowledged the limitations of his study but stated that his own carefully collected results gave some "preliminary impressions" that might be substantiated or refuted by subsequent research.

Craven conducted a personal experiment. He took 12 tablets of aspirin daily for five days, which resulted in spontaneous nose-bleeding. He repeated the experiment twice, with the same results. He had not previously had a nose-bleed in 50 years, adding value to the experiment. In 1956, he published another paper, updating trial results [13]. He prescribed Aspirin prophylaxis for 8,000 patients, among whom only nine later died of a heart attack. At autopsy, the cause of death in one of these patients was found to be a ruptured aortic aneurysm, not coronary thrombosis. He reported his findings with the caveat that they were not observed under controlled conditions. He also highlighted the role of Aspirin in preventing "little strokes," for none of his patients had one.

Researchers noted that "low doses" of aspirin did not prolong the prothrombin time, yet still prevented coronary thrombosis. Investigations on the process of thrombus formation established that platelet aggregates could occlude arteries. These aggregates formed white platelet-thrombin clots. During the late 1960s, Harvey J. Weiss began his experiments on the effects of aspirin on platelet aggregation. His research concluded that low doses of Aspirin prevented platelet aggregation by inhibiting ADP release. He showed that the acetyl group of aspirin was crucial for this inhibition and that the effect was irreversible [14]. In 1971, John Vane, professor of pharmacology at the University of London, published research on the inhibition of prostaglandin synthesis by aspirin [15]. Aspirin and other nonsteroidal anti-inflammatory drugs, such as indomethacin, phenylbutazone, and ibuprofen, inhibited platelet release reactions by their effects on prostaglandins and prostacyclins. He was awarded the Nobel Prize in 1982 for this work.

THERAPEUTIC TRIALS CONFIRM THE ABILITY OF ASPIRIN IN STROKE PREVENTION

During the third quarter of the twentieth century observations and treatment trials studied agents that would prevent development of white platelet-fibrin thrombi and so prevent strokes and myocardial infarction. The first agent found to alter platelet function was aspirin. The role of aspirin in reducing cardiovascular disease mortality and repeat events after acute myocardial infarction (MI) was first shown in the second International Study of Infarct Survival (ISIS-2) trial [16]. In this study, 17,187 patients from 417 hospitals were enrolled within 24 hours after onset of suspected acute MI. Aspirin use resulted in a significant reduction in nonfatal reinfarction, stroke, five-week vascular mortality, and all-cause mortality [16]. Other smaller trials had shown similar benefits for patients with a history of previous MI, but the ISIS-2 trial was the first to provide evidence of a direct effect of aspirin on acute MI. The trial showed that one month of low-dose aspirin started immediately after MI in 1,000 patients would prevent 25 deaths and 10–15 nonfatal infarcts and strokes. Additional mortality benefits were observed with longer-duration aspirin therapy.

Many other trials showed similar results when aspirin was used for secondary prevention of cardiovascular events. The Antithrombotic Trialists' Collaboration analyzed 16 trials of long-term aspirin use with doses ranging from 50 to 1,500 milligrams per day for secondary prevention of cardiovascular events, including over 17,000 subjects and 3,306 serious vascular events [17]. Aspirin use in these trials resulted in significant reductions in serious vascular events including stroke and coronary events in men and women; low-dose aspirin (75–100 mg/day) was as effective as higher doses [17]. Aspirin use for secondary prevention of serious cardiovascular events became well accepted and recommended by major organizations [18–21].

These early trial results included stroke among cardiovascular end points but were not specifically aimed at stroke prevention or treatment. Two anecdotal reports in 1971 noted the effectiveness of aspirin in treating patients who had transient loss of vision in one eye, a condition known to be related to stroke [22,23]. Aspirin was then studied in randomized therapeutic trials among large groups of patients chosen because of vascular risk factors, transient ischemic attacks, or minor strokes and shown to be effective in stroke prevention. The first such trials were the American Aspirin trial [24] and the Canadian-American trial [25]. These studies were soon followed by aspirin trials in Europe [26–28] and analyses of the results of trials by the antiplatelet trialists [29,30]. These trials and analyses lumped large groups of patients together. They did not study which patients among the large groups had which stroke mechanisms, and which vascular lesions were most likely to respond or not respond. They showed that aspirin was generally effective in stroke prevention. Chapter 43 also discusses aspirin stroke trials.

NOTES AND REFERENCES

1. Doctrine of signatures. Science Museum.org. Available at http://broughttolife .sciencemuseum.org.uk/broughttolife/techniques/doctrine.

2. A history of aspirin. *Pharmaceutical Journal*. Available at www.pharmaceutical-journal .com/news-and-analysis/infographics/a-history-of-aspirin/20066661.article.

3. Stone E. XXXII. An account of the success of the bark of the willow in the cure of agues. In a letter to the Right Honourable George Earl of Macclesfield, President of R. S. from the Rev. Mr. Edward Stone, of Chipping-Norton in Oxfordshire. *Philos. Trans.* 1763 Jan 1;53:195–200.

4. Jack DB. One hundred years of aspirin. *Lancet Lond. Engl.* 1997 Aug 9;350 (9075):437–439.

5. Pearce JMS. The controversial story of aspirin. *World Neurology*. December 2, 2014. Available at https://worldneurologyonline.com/article/controversial-story-aspirin/.

6. Buchanan WW, Kean WF. The treatment of acute rheumatism by salicin, by T. J. Maclagan – *The Lancet*, 1876. *J. Rheumatol.* 2002 Jun 1;29(6):1321–1323.

7. Snead MW, Aikawa JK. T. J. Maclagan and the treatment of rheumatic fever with salicin. *AMA Arch. Intern. Med.* 1958 May 1;101(5):997–1004.

8. Malverde J. How aspirin turned hero: Heroin, Bayer and Heinrich Dreser. Democratic Underground. Available at www.democraticunderground.com/11701737.

9. Lichterman BL. Aspirin: The story of a wonder drug. *BMJ* 2004 Dec 11;329 (7479):1408.

10. Miner J, Hoffhines A. The discovery of aspirin's antithrombotic effects. *Tex. Heart Inst. J.* 2007;34(2):179–186.

11. Craven LL. Coronary thrombosis can be prevented. *J. Insurance Med.* 1950;5:47–48.

12. Craven LL. Experiences with aspirin (acetylsalicylic acid) in the nonspecific prophylaxis of coronary thrombosis. *Miss. Valley Med. J.* 1953;75:38–44.

13. Craven LL. Prevention of coronary and cerebral thrombosis. *Miss. Valley Med. J.* 1956;78:213–215.

14. Weiss HJ, Aledort LM, Kochwa S. The effect of salicylates on the hemostatic properties of platelets in man. *J. Clin. Invest.* 1968;47:2169–2180.

15. Vane JR. Inhibition of prostaglandin synthesis as a mechanism of action for aspirin-like drugs. *Nat. New Biol.* 1971;231:232–235.

16. ISIS-2 (Second International Study of Infarct Survival) Collaborative Group. Randomised trial of intravenous streptokinase, oral aspirin, both, or neither among 17,187 cases of suspected acute myocardial infarction: ISIS-2. *Lancet* 1988;2:349–360.

17. Antithrombotic Trialists' Collaboration. Collaborative meta-analysis of randomised trials of antiplatelet therapy for prevention of death, myocardial infarction, and stroke in high risk patients. *BMJ* 2002;324:71–86.

18. Bell AD, Roussin A, Cartier R, Chan WS, Douketis JD, Gupta A, Kraw ME, Lindsay TF, Love MP, Pannu N, Rabasa-Lhoret R, Shuaib A, Teal P, Théroux P, Turpie AG, Welsh RC, Tanguay JF. The use of antiplatelet therapy in the outpatient setting: Canadian Cardiovascular Society Guidelines Executive Summary. *Can. J. Cardiol.* 2011;27:208–221.

19. Graham I, Atar D, Borch-Johnson K, et al. for the ESC Committee for Practice Guidelines. European guidelines on cardiovascular disease prevention in clinical practice: Executive summary. *Atherosclerosis* 2007;194:1–45.

20. US Preventive Services Task Force. Aspirin for the prevention of cardiovascular disease: U.S. Preventive Services Task Force recommendation statement. *Ann. Intern. Med.* 2009;150:396–404.

21. Vandvik PO, Lincoff AM, Core JM, et al. for American College of Chest Physicians. Primary and secondary prevention of cardiovascular disease: Antithrombotic Therapy and Prevention of Thrombosis, 9th ed.: American College of Chest Physicians Evidence-Based Clinical Practice Guidelines. *Chest* 2012;141:e637S–e668S.

22. Mundall J, Quintero P, von Kaulla K, et al. Transient monocular blindness and increased platelet aggregability treated with aspirin: A case report. *Neurology* 1971;21:402.

23. Harrison MJG, Marshall J, Meadows JC, et al. Effect of aspirin in amaurosis fugax. *Lancet* 1971;2:743–744.

24. Fields WS, Lemak N, Frankowski R, Hardy RJ. Controlled trial of aspirin in cerebral ischemia. *Stroke* 1977;8:301–306.

25. Canadian Cooperative Study Group. A randomized trial of aspirin and sulfinpyrazone in threatened stroke. *N. Engl. J. Med.* 1978;299:53–59.

26. UK-TIA Study Group. The UK-TIA Aspirin Trial: The interim results. *BMJ* 1988;296:316–320.

27. The SALT Collaborative Group. Swedish Aspirin Low-Dose Trial (SALT) of 75 mg aspirin as secondary prophylaxis after cerebrovascular ischemic events. *Lancet* 1991;338:1345–1349.

28. The Dutch TIA Trial Study Group. A comparison of two doses of aspirin (30 mg vs 283 mg a day) in patients after a transient ischemic attack or minor stroke. *N. Engl. J. Med.* 1991;325:1261–1266.

29. Antiplatelet Trialists' Collaboration. Collaborative overview of randomised trials of antiplatelet therapy. 1. Prevention of death, myocardial infarction, and stroke by prolonged antiplatelet therapy in various categories of patients. *BMJ* 1994;308:81–106.

30. Antithrombotic Trialists' Collaboration. Collaborative meta-analysis of randomized trials of antiplatelet therapy for prevention of death, myocardial infarction, and stroke in high risk patients. *BMJ* 2002;524:71–86.

CHAPTER FORTY EIGHT

OTHER ANTIPLATELETS

During the final years of the nineteenth century, clinicians and researchers became aware of the role that platelets played in blood clotting and bleeding. During the early 1880s in Turin, Italian physician, histologist, and researcher Giulio Bizzozero used comprehensive intravascular microscopy and in vitro flow chamber studies to identify the role of platelets in both hemostasis and thrombosis [1,2]. Sir William Osler in 1886 established that platelets contributed to human thrombotic disorders, discovering them in white thrombi in atheromatous aortic lesions and on diseased heart valves [1,3].

Research on the physiology and chemistry of platelet functions was not avidly pursued until the second half of the twentieth century, when research techniques that could analyze platelet activation, adhesion, and aggregation became available. Gustav Victor Rudolf Born introduced a method of measuring platelet aggregation in plasma in 1962 [1,4,5]. Born was born in Germany in 1921. His family left Germany, as his father and maternal grandfather were Jewish. He was educated in Götttingen in Germany and then at the University of Edinburgh. His research on platelet aggregation and functions was performed in the 1970s during his stints as the professor of pharmacology, first at Cambridge University and then at King's College London. Another very prominent researcher who advanced knowledge on platelet functions and chemistry was Barry Spencer Coller. He was born in New York City in 1945 and was educated at Columbia University and New York University Medical School. His platelet research was performed at the Rockefeller

University in New York where he was the physician-in-chief of the Rockefeller University Hospital and head of the laboratory of blood and vascular biology [1,6].

When it became apparent that aspirin and other substances could alter platelet functions and, in doing so, reduce the occurrence of coronary, cerebrovascular, and peripheral vascular ischemic events, the race was on for pharmaceutical companies to synthesize, evaluate, and market effective safe antiplatelet agents [7].

PHOSPHODIESTERASE (PDE) INHIBITORS DIPYRIDAMOLE AND CILOSTAZOLE

Dipyridamole (Aggrenox)

Dipyridamole was one of the first "antiplatelet" agents to be studied. Among other functions, cyclic guanosine monophosphate (cGMP) has an important role in vascular physiology. Dipyridamole is a phosphodiesterase (PDE) substance that inhibits cyclic guanosine monophosphate adenosine (cGAMP) functions. After many years of basic and clinical research, Boehinger-Ingelheim Pharmaceuticals, a relatively small, family-owned company, brought the drug to market as an inhibitor of platelet functions that was effective in preventing strokes. Dipyridamole (trade name Persantine) was initially tested and used clinically in patients with heart disease. It was prescribed and approved even for patients with heart transplants but was not studied in randomized therapeutic trials since this was not a requirement during the 1950s and 1960s. Dipyridamole was used to assess the ability of the coronary circulation to augment cardiac blood flow (Persantine myocardial perfusion imaging test). Although cardiologists opined that they had good results, there was no definitive information on how the drug worked.

Gustav Born convinced the company that the drug must work by inhibiting platelets. He suggested using his aggregometer in further research. Born became a long-term consultant to the chemists and pharmacologists at Boehringer-Ingelheim who were researching dipyridamole [8]. Dipyridamole alone did not inhibit platelet aggregation in vitro except in extremely high doses that were not achievable in man. Born suggested adding various quantities of aspirin. Animal studies showed that a combination of aspirin and dipyridamole protected against thrombosis induced by combined chemical and electrical stimuli when neither drug did so separately. Researchers found that 200 milligrams of dipyridamole plus 25 milligrams of aspirin attained the best effect on platelet aggregation in vitro. This combination was ultimately patented and marketed as Aggrenox [9]. Research identified issues with the metabolism of dipyridamole. Absorption of dipyridamole in the stomach required a level of acidity that was found in young individuals but was often absent in elderly patients. A modified sustained-release form of dipyridamole was synthesized that was absorbed better from the stomach and was accompanied by fewer gastrointestinal side effects.

In a study reported in 1971, there was a beneficial effect of adding dipyridamole in a dose of 400 milligrams per day to warfarin anticoagulation in preventing embolic strokes in patients who had prosthetic heart valves [10]. Two trials reported during the early 1980s showed no benefit of dipyridamole even when added to aspirin [11]. In the Canadian-American trial, dipyridamole in doses of 300 milligrams per day had no significant therapeutic effect when added to 1,300 milligrams per day of aspirin in patients with TIA or minor stroke. In a French trial, 225 milligrams of dipyridamole used with 1,000 milligrams of aspirin was not better than aspirin alone. Dipyridamole in the form given in these two trials had variable gastrointestinal absorption related to gastric acidity, and required dosing four times per day because of its pharmacokinetics. The dose of dipyridamole was low and likely did not produce adequate sustained blood levels. Two subsequent trials, the European Stroke Prevention Studies (ESPS 1 and ESPS 2), reported a beneficial effect on stroke prevention of the modified extended-release dipyridamole when used with aspirin [12]. A later trial, carried out in the Netherlands, confirmed the effectiveness of dipyridamole in stroke prevention in patients who had recent transient ischemic attacks or minor strokes [13]. A meta-analysis concluded that "the combination of aspirin and dipyridamole was more effective than aspirin alone in preventing stroke and other serious vascular events in patients with minor strokes and TIAs" [14].

The posited mechanism of action of dipyridamole (and Aggrenox) is to inhibit the attachment of platelets to perturbed endothelial lining of blood vessels as well as to directly inhibit platelet functions. Aggrenox use is accompanied by headache, cerebral vasodilatation, and increased cerebral blood flow, harkening back to the original use of the agent in cardiac patients. The PDE inhibitors are vasodilators active on vascular endothelia.

Cilostazol

Cilostazol is a phosphodiesterase inhibitor, like dipyridamole, that has both antiplatelet and vasodilator effects [15]. The Otsuka Pharmaceutical Company, a relatively small firm that began in 1921 housed on Shikoku Island, Japan, performed research on cilostazol and brought it finally to market under the trade name Pletal. Therapeutic stroke trials have been limited to Asia. The first key trial was in Japan. Cilostazol in doses of 100 milligrams twice daily reduced the frequency of recurrent strokes among more than 1,000 patients with brain infarcts acquired one to six months before entry [16]. In Korean patients with intracranial arterial stenosis, 200 milligrams of cilostazol plus 100 milligrams of aspirin was more effective than 100 milligrams of aspirin alone in reducing the frequency of progression and increasing the frequency of regression of atherostenotic vascular lesions [17]. Cilostazol increases cerebral blood flow in patients with atherosclerotic risk factors. As is the case with dipyridamole, many patients develop headache in relation to the increased blood flow. The drug is approved in the United States for use in patients with peripheral vascular occlusive disease. The effect of cilostazol on stroke prevention has been mainly studied in Asians, and the patients studied have had a high frequency of penetrating artery disease (lacunar strokes) and intracranial large artery disease. Its effect in Caucasian patients in the United States and Europe has not been studied in depth.

THIENOPYRIDINES: TICLOPIDINE, CLOPIDOGREL, PRASUGREL, TRICAGRELOR

Ticlopidine (Ticlid)

Ticlopidine was discovered during the 1970s in France by a team led by two very prominent pharmacologists and inventors, Fernand Eloy and Jean-Pierre Maffrand, at Castaigne SA, which was trying to produce a new anti-inflammatory medication. Pharmacology developers noted that this new compound had strong antiplatelet effects. Castaigne was acquired by Sanofi in 1973. Maffrad became the vice president for research at Sanofi. Unlike Boehringer-Ingelheim, the producer of dipyridamole (Aggrenox), and Otsuka, the producer of cilostazol (Pletal), which were relatively small companies active in Europe and Asia, respectively, Sanofi was a very large pharmaceutical company with global reach in mostly Europe and the United States.

The thienopyridines inhibit the adenosine diphosphate pathway of platelet aggregation; unlike aspirin, they do not inhibit the cyclooxygenase pathway [18]. Ticlopidine and later clopidogrel required metabolism by the hepatic cytochrome P450-1A enzyme system to acquire activity. Inhibition of platelet aggregation by ticlopidine was delayed until 24–48 hours after administration. Maximum inhibition occurred after three to five days, and recovery was slow after the drug was stopped [18].

Starting in 1978 the drug was marketed in France by Sanofi under the brand name Ticlid for people at high risk for thrombotic events, who had just come out of heart surgery, were undergoing hemodialysis, had peripheral vascular disease, or who were otherwise at risk for strokes and ischemic heart disease. Two large randomized therapeutic stroke trials conducted in North America showed that ticlopidine reduced the risk of stroke in patients with prior TIAs or stroke [19]. In these clinical trials, ticlopidine had an important rate of side effects, especially diarrhea and skin rash. Neutropenia and thrombotic thrombocytopenic purpura were serious but infrequent complications of ticlopidine, and patients taking ticlopidine had slight elevation of cholesterol levels. Ticlopidine was used in stroke prophylaxis during the early 1990s but recognition of serious side effects and the introduction of clopidogrel by the parent Sanofi led to the gradual disappearance of ticlopidine as a newly prescribed antiplatelet agent.

Clopidogrel (Plavix)

Clopidogrel is a thienopyridine with a closely related chemical structure that differed from ticlopidine by the addition of a carboxymethyl side group. Clopidogrel was known to be a prodrug that required activation by hepatic cytochrome P450 (CYP) enzymes to produce the active metabolite. The mechanism of platelet inactivation was attributed to specific and irreversible inhibition of the $P2Y_{12}$ subtype of the ADP receptor. Poor metabolizers of CYP2C19 had lower levels of the active metabolite and less platelet inactivation. Some common drugs, for example, proton pump inhibitors and atorvastatin, could interfere with the activation of clopidogrel. Clopidogrel was considered an agent with similar effectiveness but fewer severe side effects than ticlopidine [20]. As in the case of ticlopidine, stroke trials were performed originally mostly in North America and Europe.

The Clopidogrel versus Aspirin in Patients at Risk of Ischemic Events (CAPRIE) trial was a large (nearly 20,000 patients), randomized, double-blinded trial of clopidogrel (75 mg daily) versus aspirin (325 mg daily) in preventing ischemic events (ischemic stroke, myocardial infarction, and vascular death) [21]. Patients with myocardial infarcts and peripheral vascular disease were entered as well as those who had ischemic strokes. Clopidogrel had a relative risk reduction over aspirin of 8.7 percent, considering all end points. The frequency of myocardial infarction was more effectively reduced by clopidogrel than the frequency of stroke.

If one was good, two might be better. Reasoning that decreasing platelet activities by two different mechanisms might prove superior to single agents alone, the MATCH trial tested aspirin (75 mg/day) plus clopidogrel (75 mg/day) against clopidogrel (75 mg/day) alone in patients with brain ischemia [22]. The combination was not superior in decreasing the primary outcome measure (reduction in ischemic stroke, myocardial infarction, vascular death, and rehospitalization for acute ischemic events) and caused more life-threatening bleeding, often intracranial. In another trial of stroke prevention, the Clopidogrel and Aspirin versus Aspirin Alone for the Prevention of Atherothrombotic Events (CHARISMA) trial, clopidogrel plus aspirin was not more effective than aspirin alone in reducing the rate of myocardial infarction, stroke, or death from cardiovascular causes [23]. Moderate and severe bleeding were more common in those taking both clopidogrel and aspirin.

While long-term combined aspirin and clopidogrel treatment did not show benefit over single agents, could short-term combined therapy render benefit? Recurrent events are most common after the first few weeks of a cerebrovascular ischemic event. Researchers opined that the higher bleeding risk of double therapy could be outweighed by the added benefit of preventing ischemic events during those first few high-risk weeks. In Asian patients in the CHANCE trial, combined clopidogrel and aspirin was superior to aspirin alone in preventing stroke, and the bleeding rate was low [24]. In the POINT trial, carried out in the United States and Europe, patients with minor ischemic stroke or high-risk TIA who received a combination of clopidogrel and aspirin had a lower risk of major ischemic events but a higher risk of major hemorrhage at 90 days than those who received aspirin alone [25].

Trials in patients with coronary artery stents, especially stents that are drug-eluting, have shown that double antiplatelets are important in decreasing the frequency of in-stent thrombosis, and most often aspirin and clopidogrel are given for 6–12 months. Double antiplatelets are also routinely given for patients with carotid artery stents. Stents cover the vascular intima so they remove the contact of platelets with the endothelium; agents that effect the attachment of platelets to the endothelium (cilostazole and dipyridamole) are likely not to be effective in patients with stents. The requirement in stented patients for relatively long-term double antiplatelets is important when considering adding an anticoagulant.

Prasugrel (Efient) and Ticagrelor (Brilinta)

Other pharmaceutical companies have now brought to market newer thienopyridines. Prasugrel and ticagrelor are highly potent $P2Y_{12}$ inhibitors. Prasugrel is marketed through the Eli Lilly company and ticagrelor by AstraZeneca. These agents inhibit adenosine diphosphate–induced platelet aggregation more rapidly, more consistently, and to a greater extent than do standard and higher doses of clopidogrel. They have been studied mostly in patients with coronary artery disease. Compared with clopidogrel, both agents show more reduction in coronary events, but both have a higher rate of adverse events, including bleeding. There were two large trials of patients with minor non-cardioembolic minor strokes or TIAs who were treated with ticagrelor [26,27]. Ticagrelor was not better than aspirin in reducing the rate of stroke, myocardial infarction, or death at 90 days [26]; in another large, international trial, the risk of the composite of stroke or death within 30 days was slightly lower with ticagrelor plus aspirin than with aspirin alone, but disability did not differ significantly between the two groups, and severe bleeding was more frequent with ticagrelor [27].

In the United States and Europe there are many more cardiologists and internists than neurologists. The antiplatelet market is driven mostly by cardiologists who enthusiastically favor the thienopyridine compounds. The evidence of effectiveness of these agents in preventing cerebrovascular ischemic events is much less robust than the evidence in preventing myocardial infarction and stent thrombosis. These agents probably cause more bleeding than aspirin.

GLYCOPROTEIN IIB/IIIA ANTAGONISTS

Barry Coller of the Rockefeller University was one of the leading researchers who investigated the glycoprotein IIb/IIIa receptor [1,6,28]. Platelet aggregation is mediated by the GP IIb/IIIa receptor, a member of the integrin family of membrane-bound adhesion molecules. The platelet glycoprotein IIb/IIIa complex is the site of binding to adhesive proteins, including fibrinogen. The binding of fibrinogen to activated platelets is the final step in platelet aggregation. This step is mediated completely by GP IIb/IIIa. Expression of the GP IIb/IIIa integrin is the final common pathway for platelet aggregation by all agonists. Aspirin and the other antiplatelet agents described in this chapter tend to effect only one or some of the agonists. Binding to fibrinogen activates platelet aggregation and adhesion to blood vessels.

Abciximab, a humanized monoclonal antibody that binds to the GP IIb/IIIa complex on platelets, was the first agent used in clinical practice. Abciximab was used mostly intravenously and acutely in patients after invasive coronary and cerebral revascularization procedures [29]. This agent causes a profound impairment of the platelet functions similar to a temporary thrombasthenia, so that the rate of bleeding is potentially high. The Abciximab in Emergent Stroke Treatment Trial II (AbESTT-II), a double-blind, randomized phase III trial that compared abciximab with placebo in treatment of acute ischemic stroke patients, did not show efficacy and was terminated prematurely for safety reasons: there was excessive bleeding [30].

Some patients develop a veritable carpet of white platelet-fibrin thrombi after vascular surgery and interventional vascular treatments. In that setting abciximab may prove very useful. Abciximab has also been used during interventional procedures to accomplish reperfusion in acute stroke patients as an adjunct to thrombolytic agents.

Other parenteral small molecule, non-antibody GP IIb/IIIa antagonists, tirofiban and eptifbatide, have a shorter duration of antiplatelet activity and improved outcomes after coronary procedures and have less bleeding complications than abciximab. GP IIb/IIIa inhibiting agents that can be used orally and chronically are now being tested, but to date have been associated with excess bleeding and have not been introduced into clinical practice. Lotrafiban, an orally administered GP IIb/IIIa inhibitor, was studied in a trial (BRAVO) that included 9,190 patients admitted with coronary or cerebrovascular disease [31]. Lotrifiban in doses of 30 or 50 milligrams twice per day was compared with placebo given with aspirin. Lotrifiban administration did not show a significant decrease in the composite end point of all-cause mortality, myocardial infarction, recurrent ischemia requiring hospitalization, or urgent revascularization but had a significantly higher death rate due to vascular disease and more serious bleeding [31]. Unfortunately, oral GP IIb/IIIa inhibitors caused excess bleeding and could not yet be safely introduced into clinical practice.

Antiplatelet research and treatment was very active during the latter years of the twentieth century and first quarter of the twenty-first. The functions of various agents became clear. Aspirin and the thienopyridine drugs exerted their effect directly and irreversibly on platelets. Phosphodiesterase agents acted mostly on vascular endothelia and decreased platelet attachment to blood vessels. These drugs were given orally and were used to prevent stroke and other vascular ischemia. The GP IIb/IIIa antagonists affected attachment of platelets to fibrinogen and led to severe but temporary loss of platelet activity. They were given intravenously and were useful clinically in dealing with thrombi within vessels.

Introduction of new agents and understanding the mechanisms of their activity proved difficult for many practitioners. Users were led mostly by advertisements and marketing and by the results of therapeutic trials that involved large groups of lumped patients with diverse vascular conditions. Since cardiologists far outnumbered neurologists, the market share of the various agents was driven by them.

NOTES AND REFERENCES

1. Coller BS. Historical perspective and future directions in platelet research. *J. Thromb. Haemost.* 2011;9(suppl 1):374–395.

2. Bizzozero G. Su di un nuovo elemento morfologico del sangue dei mammiferi e della sua importanza nella trombosi e nella coagulazione. *L'Osservatore* 1881;17:785–787. Bizzozero J. Uber einen neuen formbestandteil des blutes und dessen rolle bei der thrombose und blutgerinnung. *Virchows Archiv* 1882;90:261–332.

3. Osler W. On certain problems in the physiology of the blood corpuscles. *Med. News* 1886;48:421–425. The stroke contributions of Sir William Osler and his medical textbooks are discussed further in Chapter 14.

4. Gustav Victor Rudolf Born. Wikipedia. Available at https://en.wikipedia.org/wiki/Gustav_Victor_Rudolf_Born.

5. Born GV. Aggregation of blood platelets by adenosine diphosphate and its reversal. *Nature* 1962;194:927–929. Born GVR, Cross MJ. The aggregation of blood platelets. *J. Physiol.* 1963;168(1):178–195.

6. Brownlee C. Biography of Barry S. Coller. *Proc. Natl. Acad. Sci. U.S.A* 2004 Sep 7;101 (36):13111–13113.

7. The history and evolution of the antiplatelet introduction of aspirin by Bayer is discussed in detail in Chapter 46.

8. Personal communication from Wolfgang Eisert, who directed dipyridamole research at Boehringer-Ingelheim.

9. Eisert W, Gruber P. Pharmaceutical compositions containing dipyridamole or mopidamol and acetylsalicylic acid or the physiologically acceptable salts thereof, processes for preparing them and their use in treating clot formation. US Patent 6015577A. https://patents.google.com/patent/US6015577A/en.

10. Sullivan J, Harken D, Gorlin R. Pharmacologic control of thromboembolic complications of aortic valve replacement. *N. Engl. J. Med.* 1971;284:1391–1394.

11. Fields WS, Yatsu F, Conomy J, et al. Persantine-aspirin trial in cerebral ischemia: The American-Canadian Cooperative Study group. *Stroke* 1983;14:97–103. Bousser MG, Eschwege E, Hagenah M, et al. "AICLA" controlled trial of aspirin and dipyridamole in the secondary prevention of athero-thrombotic cerebral ischemia. *Stroke* 1983;14:5–14.

12. ESPS Group. European Stroke Prevention Study (ESPS): Principal endpoints. *Lancet* 1987; 2:1351–1354. Diener HC, Cunha L, Forbes C, et al. European Stroke Prevention Study 2. Dipyridamole and acetylsalicylic acid in the secondary prevention of stroke. *J. Neurol. Sci.* 1996;143:1–13.

13. The ESPRIT Study group. Aspirin plus dipyridamole versus aspirin alone after cerebral ischaemia of arterial origin (ESPRIT): Randomized controlled trial. *Lancet* 2006;367:1665–1673.

14. Verro P, Gorelick PB, Nguyen D. Aspirin plus dipyridamole versus aspirin for prevention of vascular events after stroke or TIA: A meta-analysis. *Stroke* 2008;39 (4):1358–1363.

15. Ikeda Y, Kikuchi M, Murakami H. Comparison of the inhibitory effects of cilostazole, acetylsalicylic acid, and ticlopidine on platelet function ex vivo: Randomized, double-blind cross-over study. *Drug Res.* 1987;37:563–566. Tanaka K, Ishikawa T, Hagiwara M, et al. Effects of cilostazole, a selective camp phosphodiesterase inhibitor, on the contraction of vascular smooth muscle. *Pharmacology* 1988;36:313–320.

16. Gotoh F, Tohgi H, Hirai S, et al. Cilostazole stroke prevention study: A placebo-controlled double-blind trial for secondary prevention of cerebral infarction. *J. Stroke Cerebrovasc. Dis.* 2000;9:147–157.

17. Kwon SU, Cho Y-J, Koo J-S, et al. Cilostazole prevents the progression of the symptomatic intracranial stenosis: The multicenter double-blind placebo-controlled trial of cilostazole in symptomatic intracranial arterial stenosis. *Stroke* 2005;36:782–786.

18. Quinn MJ, Fitzgerald DJ. Ticlopidine and clopidogrel. *Circulation* 1999;100:1667–1672. Sharis PJ, Cannon CP, Loscalzo J. The antiplatelet effects of ticlopidine and clopidogrel. *Ann. Intern. Med.* 1998;129:394–405.

19. Hass WK, Easton JD, Adams HP Jr, Pryse-Phillips W, Molony BA, Anderson S, et al. A randomized trial comparing ticlopidine hydrochloride with aspirin for the prevention of stroke in high-risk patients. Ticlopidine Aspirin Stroke study group. *N. Engl. J. Med.* 1989;321:501–507. Gent M, Blakely JA, Easton JD, Ellis DJ, Hachinski VC, Harbison JW, et al. The Canadian American Ticlopidine Study (CATS) in thromboembolic stroke. *Lancet* 1989;1:1215–1220.

20. Maffrand JP. The story of clopidogrel and its predecessor, ticlopidine: Could these major antiplatelet and antithrombotic drugs be discovered and developed today? *C. R. Chim.* 2012;15(8):737–743.

21. A randomised, blinded, trial of clopidogrel versus aspirin in patients at risk of ischaemic events (CAPRIE). CAPRIE steering committee. *Lancet* 1996;348:1329–1339.

22. Diener HC, Bogousslavsky J, Brass LM, Cimminiello C, Csiba L, Kaste M, et al. Aspirin and clopidogrel compared with clopidogrel alone after recent ischaemic stroke or transient ischaemic attack in high-risk patients (MATCH): Randomised, double-blind, placebo-controlled trial. *Lancet* 2004;364:331–337. Hankey GJ, Eikelboom JW. Adding aspirin to clopidogrel after TIA and ischemic stroke: Benefits do not match risks. *Neurology* 2005;64:1117–1121.

23. Bhatt DL, Fox KA, Hacke W, Berger PB, Black HR, Boden WE, et al. Clopidogrel and aspirin versus aspirin alone for the prevention of atherothrombotic events. *N. Engl. J. Med.* 2006;354:1706–1717.

24. Wang Y, Wang Y, Zhao X, et al. and Johnston SC for the CHANCE Investigators. Clopidogrel with aspirin in acute minor stroke or transient ischemic attack. *N. Engl. J. Med.* 2013;369:1–13.

25. Johnston SC, Easton JD, Farrant M, et al. for the Clinical Research Collaboration, Neurological Emergencies Treatment Trials Network, and the POINT Investigators. Clopidogrel and aspirin in acute ischemic stroke and high-risk TIA. *N. Engl. J. Med.* 2018;379:215–225.

26. Johnston SC, Amarenco P, Albers GW, et al. for the SOCRATES Steering Committee and Investigators. Ticagrelor versus aspirin in acute stroke or transient ischemic attack. *N. Engl. J. Med.* 2016;375:35–43.

27. Johnston SC, Amarenco P, Denison H, et al. for the THALES Investigators. Ticagrelor and aspirin or aspirin alone in acute ischemic stroke or TIA. *N. Engl. J. Med.* 2020;383:207–217.

28. Coller BS. Anti-GPIIb/IIIa drugs: Current strategies and future directions. *Thromb. Haemost.* 2001;86(1):427–443.

29. Lefkovits J, Plow EF, Topol EJ. Platelet glycoprotein IIb/IIIa receptors in cardiovascular medicine. *N. Engl. J. Med.* 1995;332:1553–1559.

30. Adams HP Jr, Effron MB, Torner J, Davalos A, Frayne J, Teal P, et al. Emergency administration of abciximab for treatment of patients with acute ischemic stroke: Results of an international phase III trial: Abciximab in emergency treatment of stroke trial (AbESTT-II). *Stroke* 2008;39:87–99.

31. Topol EJ, Easton D, Harrington RA, Amarenco P, Califf RM, Graffagnino C, et al. Randomized, double-blind, placebo-controlled, international trial of the oral IIb/IIIa antagonist lotrafiban in coronary and cerebrovascular disease. *Circulation* 2003;108:399–406.

CHAPTER FORTY NINE

OTHER MEDICAL TREATMENTS

Advances in stroke prevention and improvement in the care and management of stroke patients can, in a large measure, be attributed to advances in knowledge about various medical conditions and their treatment. These stories of stroke could not be written without some attention to the medical risk factors and comorbidities prevalent in stroke patients. Many books would be needed to cover all the medical history. Some information is covered in Chapter 38 on epidemiology and stroke prevention. This chapter includes brief clips about the development of knowledge and ideas concerning major important medical conditions and their management.

HYPERTENSION

Measurement of Blood Pressure

Physicians of the nineteenth and preceding centuries customarily studied the pulse of their patients and estimated cardiac function by the size of the heart and its pulsitivity. Adolph Wallenberg recognized that his famous patient, a 38-year-old rope-maker, had important cardiovascular disease because of his pounding pulse, dyspnea, and enlarged heart. He was not surprised that the patient developed a medullary brain infarct in 1893 [1]. Richard Bright and his Guy's Hospital colleagues recognized that nephritis could lead to increased blood pressure, cardiac enlargement, and chronic degenerative changes in systemic arteries. During the later years of the nineteenth century, Frederick Akbar Mahomed (1849–1884), an Irish-Indian physician who also worked at Guy's Hospital in London, recognized that high blood pressure (BP) could develop without preceding kidney disease [2]. He showed that hypertension could develop in apparently healthy individuals, was more likely in older patients, and that the heart, kidneys, and brain could be affected by high arterial tension. Akbar's clinical studies were aided by a quantitative sphygmogram that measured pulse waves that he developed while a medical student. He described characteristic features of the pressure pulse in patients with high blood pressure and in older persons with arteriosclerosis [2].

The first modern blood pressure meter (sphygmomanometer, from the Greek *sphygmos*, pulse, and French *manomètre*, pressure meter) was developed by the Austrian-Jewish physician Samuel Siegfried Karl Ritter von Basch (1837–1905) [3]. Basch was educated at Karl University in Prague and at the University of Vienna. He then studied chemistry in a laboratory in Vienna, and five years later began the practice of medicine. In 1864, he became chief surgeon of the military hospital at Puebla Mexico. Soon after that, he was appointed as Maximilian's personal physician. Basch remained with Maximilian until the emperor's execution by firing squad in 1867. In 1878 he was appointed extraordinary professor in experimental pathology. His BP measuring device used a small bulb with a balloon-like diaphragm stretched across the bottom that connected to a manometer, an instrument for measuring the pressure of gases and liquids. The diaphragm pressed on the artery until the pulse stopped and indicated the systolic blood pressure. He authored many publications, but his chief work was "The Physiology and Pathology of the Circulation" published in1892 [3].

Surgical and Medical Treatment

Treatment of hypertension lagged behind recognition of its importance in contributing to cardiac disease and stroke. Franklin D. Roosevelt, the US president during World War II, developed severe hypertension during the last years of the war [4]. One BP was recorded at 240/130. His hypertension led to congestive heart failure. His doctors had no effective agent to lower blood pressure. He died in 1945 after a massive intracerebral hemorrhage attributed directly to his uncontrolled hypertension [4].

Based on the presumption that high BP was attributable to overaction of sympathetic nerves, surgical sympathectomies were undertaken and the results were reported in the late 1940s and early 1950s [5]. The effect of the surgery on BP lowering was temporary. Pharmacological treatments were designed during the later years of the twentieth century based on basic physiological research [6]. Beginning in 1967, Arthur Guyton, a renal physiologist and professor of physiology at the University of Mississippi, developed his theory of pressure natriuresis [7]. He posited that long-term control of BP was vested almost entirely in the control of body fluid volumes, primarily by the kidney. This idea led to development during the middle years of the twentieth century of thiazides and thiazide-like compounds from the sulfa molecule that were found to have natriuretic properties. Chlorothiazide was the first to be marketed, followed by hydrochlorothiazide, and then chlorthalidone a few years later. These drugs showed potent hypotensive effects. Small studies showed thiazides' tolerability and effectiveness of this new group of drugs in lowering BP [8].

Sir James Black made important contributions to pharmacology by showing that new major classes of drugs could be developed by applying basic knowledge of receptor-driven cell-signaling systems to clinical problems [9]. He developed beta-blockers for cardiovascular disease. In 1964, he synthesized the first clinically significant beta-blockers: propranolol and pronethalol. They were initially used to treat angina pectoris and coronary artery disease. They were later introduced into the treatment of hypertension [9]. During the latter years of the twentieth century and the beginning of the twenty-first century, an armamentarium of effective antihypertensive treatments were marketed, including diuretics, beta-blockers, angiotensin converting enzyme (ACE) inhibitors, angiotensin 2 receptor blockers, calcium channel blockers, alpha-blockers, alpha-2 receptor agonists, and combined alpha- and beta-blockers. Organizations periodically reviewed the relative effectiveness and safety of these agents.

DIABETES AND THE METABOLIC SYNDROME

Diabetes circa 1920s: Minot and Joslin

The state of medical care for diabetes mellitus during the first quarter of the twentieth century can be captured in the lives and careers of two very important physicians, George Minot and Elliott Joslin.

George Richards Minot (1885–1950) was born in Boston, Massachusetts. His father was a physician; his father's cousin was an anatomist; and a great-grandfather was a cofounder of Massachusetts General Hospital (MGH). Minot became interested in the natural sciences, and then, in medicine. He graduated from Harvard College and Harvard Medical School. Between 1913 and 1915, he worked in a laboratory at Johns Hopkins, studying blood proteins. In 1915, he secured a junior position on the medical staff at MGH where he began research on anemia, and in 1917, he began working at Huntington Memorial Hospital, a clinical and research cancer center in Boston. And then a personal disaster struck [10].

In October 1921, at age 36, he developed fatigue, general weakness, and increased thirst. He tested his own urine and found sugar. He contacted Elliott Joslin, who confirmed the diagnosis of severe diabetes mellitus. Minot was six feet one inch tall and weighed 135 pounds. Joslin put him on a diet of only 530 calories per day. Minot, like most every diabetes patient at the time, would probably die within a year. During the next years, despite dietary restriction and continued weight loss, Minot managed to struggle to appear at the hospital each day. Joslin was able to obtain small amounts of insulin from Banting and Best, who had discovered insulin in Canada in 1922, and delivered them to Minot. For the remainder of his life, Minot ate no food at home that was not weighed, measured, and recorded. When dining out, advanced knowledge of the menu aided him in estimating the caloric and carbohydrate content so that he could adjust his insulin requirement [10].

In 1922 Minot became physician-in-chief of the Huntington Memorial Hospital of Harvard University, and later was appointed to the staff of the Peter Bent Brigham Hospital. In 1928 he was appointed professor of medicine at Harvard University, director of the Thorndike Memorial Laboratory, and visiting physician to the Boston City Hospital. Minot shared the 1934 Nobel Prize in Physiology or Medicine with William Murphy and George Whipple for work on the treatment of anemia. They had discovered an effective treatment for pernicious anemia, which was a terminal disease at that time, with liver concentrate high in vitamin B_{12} later identified as the critical compound in the treatment. Minot began developing complications associated with diabetes in 1940 and had a serious stroke in 1947, which partially paralyzed him.

Elliott Proctor Joslin was born in 1869 in Oxford, Massachusetts, to wealthy parents. His father was a mill owner. He matriculated at Yale College. While in college, Joslin's Aunt Helen was diagnosed with diabetes. He studied her disease. After graduating from Yale, he extended his time at the university by enrolling in a master's degree in physiological chemistry. This interest in chemistry, along with his aunt's recent diagnosis of diabetes, led him to an interest in glucose metabolism and metabolic diseases. He attended Harvard Medical School and graduated first in his class. (Harvey Cushing was number 2 in the same class.) In 1893, while a medical student, Joslin was assigned to examine a frail young girl who had diabetes. He entered her data in a ledger similar to the one he maintained throughout his medical career. Long before he became one of the world's leading authorities on diabetes, he understood the importance of careful documentation. Thorough and very detailed observation of his patients helped him develop his approach to the treatment of diabetes. He prescribed a strict diet that regulated blood sugar levels. He wanted patients to be able to manage their own care. Joslin helped his mother, who had been diagnosed with diabetes in 1899, to live 10 years after her diagnosis through a combination of meal planning, exercise, and food management [11].

In 1921 in an editorial, Joslin told the story about three adjacent houses in a peaceful New England village that housed seven individuals [12]. All but one succumbed to diabetes mellitus. He warned of an epidemic and wrote about diagnosis and prevention of this important condition.

Joslin saw his first patient in 1898 at his parents' townhouse at 517 Beacon Street. He practiced there until 1905 when he moved his office to 81 Bay State Road. His townhouse and the adjacent building served as his practice for the next 50 years. In 1956 the office was moved to its current location at 1 Joslin Place. Joslin Diabetes Center was the world's first diabetes care facility.

He was challenged by the outcomes of diabetes patients and began creating a list of his patients in large accounting books, complete with all the facts, progress, and outcomes. This was the first diabetes registry in the world. He compared his data with public statistics. The field of diabetes epidemiology was launched. Joslin carried out extensive metabolic balance studies, examining fasting and feeding in patients with varying severities of diabetes. Elliott Joslin saw 15 patients per day until a week before his death in 1962, at age 93.

Insulin

Frederick Banting, a young Ontario, Canada, orthopedic surgeon, was given laboratory space by J. J. R. Macleod, the head of physiology at the University of Toronto, to investigate the function of the pancreatic islets. McLeod provided a student assistant, Charles Best, and an allotment of dogs to test Banting's hypothesis that ligation of the pancreatic ducts before extraction of the pancreas could destroy the enzyme-secreting cells, but the islets of Langerhans, which produced an internal secretion regulating sugar metabolism, would remained intact [13]. The name "insuline" had been introduced in 1909 for this posited endocrine substance. Best's experiments produced an extract of pancreas that reduced the hyperglycemia and glycosuria in dogs made diabetic after pancreatic removal. By August 1921, Banting and Best had prepared an effective extract from a canine pancreas. James B. Collip then isolated insulin sufficiently pure for human use [13].

In October 1923, Banting and Macleod received the Nobel Prize in Physiology or Medicine for the discovery of insulin. Banting was outraged that Macleod and not Best was selected, and he briefly threatened to refuse the award. He announced that he was giving half of his share of the prize money to Best and publicly acknowledged Best's contribution to the discovery of insulin. Macleod also gave half of his money award to Collip. Years later, the official history of the Nobel Committee admitted that Best should have been awarded a share of the prize [13].

Newer Insulins and Oral Agents

The first patient to receive insulin was a 14-year-old pale, dying boy who smelled of acetone and weighed only 65 pounds. Seven and a half cubic centimeters of the extract made by Banting and Best were injected into each buttock. Banting's team made an agreement with the Ely Lilly Company, and by 1923 insulin was commercially available in the United States. In 1936 the first extended-action insulin (protamine zinc insulin) became available. In 1946, the Nordisk Insulkin laboratory in Denmark synthesized and released the second extended-release formulation (neutral protamine Hagedorn (NPH)) insulin. In 1956 lente, semilente, and ultralente forms became available. All of these preparations before 1983 came from animal sources, mostly pork and beef. In 1996 the first rapid-acting human insulin analog was approved [14].

Oral antihyperglycemics began to enter the market in 1959 mostly for treatment of adult onset type II diabetes. Phenformin was first studied but found to often cause lactic acidosis. Metformin was introduced in 1959. Sulfonylureas were the next oral agents to be described; first tolbutamide followed by glipizide and glyburide in 1984 and glimepride in 1995. Glitazones followed in 1996. These agents were posited to enhance skeletal muscle insulin sensitivity and to reduce glucose production in the liver. Pioglitazone and rosiglitazone became available early in the twenty-first century. Other agents with different mechanisms continue to be tested and marketed [14]. Modern diabetologists have a full armamentarium of potential insulins and oral agents to treat their diabetic patients.

Insulin Resistance and the Metabolic Syndrome

In 1988, Gerald Reaven, during his American Diabetes Association Banting award lecture, introduced the concept of the link between insulin resistance and other metabolic abnormalities [15]. He called the entity "Syndrome X." The "X" was used to emphasize the fact that the importance of insulin resistance as a cardiovascular risk factor was relatively unknown. This constellation of conditions included increased blood pressure, high blood sugar, and abnormal high-density lipid (HDL) cholesterol and triglyceride levels. This entity later became known as the *metabolic syndrome*. The presence of the syndrome became an important indicator of increased risk for heart disease, stroke, and diabetes.

Gerald Reaven was born in Gary, Indiana, in 1928 but grew up in Cleveland, Ohio. He earned his undergraduate and medical school degrees at the University of Chicago and completed his medical residency training at the University of Michigan. He joined the Stanford University faculty in

1960 and worked first in the endocrinology division and then, after semi-retirement, in the cardiovascular division. His wife, Eve Reaven, was an electron microscopist. His son, Peter Reaven, became an endocrinologist and director of the diabetes research program at the Phoenix Veterans Affairs Health Care System in Arizona. Peter said, "Both my dad and mom were academics; often dinner conversations were about academics and science. Somehow that became comfortable." Gerald Reaven won many awards, including the William S. Middleton Award for outstanding achievement in medical research from the Veterans Affairs Administration, the Banting Medal for Scientific Achievement from the American Diabetes Association, the Fred Conrad Koch Award from the Endocrine Society, the Distinction in Clinical Endocrinology Award from the American Association of Clinical Endocrinologists, and the National Lipid Association Honorary Lifetime Member Award [15].

The metabolic syndrome included a constellation of interrelated metabolic risk factors that promoted the development of atherosclerotic cardiovascular disease. The predominant underlying risk factors for the syndrome were identified as abdominal obesity and insulin resistance. Physical inactivity, aging, and hormonal imbalances also contributed to the adverse cardiovascular effects of the syndrome. The history of the metabolic syndrome is rooted in the recognition of adipose tissue as a heterogeneous, biologically active organ, as well as in the concepts of insulin resistance and its consequences [15]. Later developments targeted recognition and management of the components of the syndrome.

HYPERLIPIDEMIA AND THE STATINS

Blood Lipids and Atherosclerosis

The original observation of the relationship of elevated blood cholesterol to future cardiovascular disease came from epidemiological studies during the middle of the twentieth century, such as the Framingham Heart Study [16]. Later research, using epidemiological, genetic, basic science, and subclinical atherosclerosis imaging methodology, consistently showed the relationship of cholesterol levels to atherosclerosis development and regression [17].

Early work that highlighted the importance of cholesterol in the body was performed by Konrad Bloch, a German-American biochemist who was awarded the Nobel Prize in Physiology or Medicine in 1964 for his work in clarifying the metabolism of cholesterol. His discoveries centered on how cholesterol was formed and converted in the body and its functions. He was born in January 1912, in Upper Silesia, then Germany (later Poland). He studied in Munich at the Technical High School where he became attracted to organic chemistry, especially the structure of natural products. Because he was Jewish, his studies in Munich were ended in 1934 after he had obtained the degree of Diplom-Ingenieur in Chemistry. This was the highest nondoctoral degree in science, business, or engineering in Germany.

He went to Switzerland and in 1936 Bloch was able to immigrate to the United States. He first studied at Columbia University. His later appointments and discoveries were made at the University of Chicago and Harvard University where he was chairman of the department of chemistry. He died in 2000. His studies were the forerunner of research regarding cholesterol subdivisions and treatment of increased blood cholesterol levels.

Knowledge about Lipoproteins and Their Metabolism

Cholesterol is one of three major classes of lipids that all animal cells make and use to construct membranes. Cholesterol is a precursor of steroid hormones and bile acids and is an important component of the central nervous system. It is synthesized by astrocytes, oligodendrocytes, microglia, and, to a lesser extent, neurons. Cholesterol is insoluble in water. It is transported in the blood plasma within protein particles called lipoproteins. Lipoproteins are classified by their density: high-density lipoproteins (HDL) are cholesterol-rich particles that transport cholesterol to the liver for disposal or recycling; very low-density lipoproteins (VLDL) are triglyceride-rich carriers of hepatic synthesized triglycerides; and intermediate and low-density lipoproteins (IDL and LDL) are cholesterol-rich remnant particles derived from lipolysis of triglycerides in VLDL. Chylomicra are triglyceride-rich carriers of dietary fats. Elevated levels of the lipoproteins other than HDL (termed non-HDL cholesterol), particularly LDL cholesterol, were shown to be associated with an increased risk of atherosclerosis and coronary heart disease [17,18]. Higher levels of HDL cholesterol were shown to be protective [17,18]. Low HDL was identified as a component of the metabolic syndrome.

Treatment of Hyperlipidemia

Three individuals, Joseph Goldstein, Michael Brown, and Akiro Endo, were most instrumental in furthering knowledge about cholesterol and its genetic control and in the subsequent development of statins, the first very effective treatment of hypercholesterolemia.

Joseph L. Goldstein was born in April 1940. He grew up in a small town in South Carolina. He earned a BS degree in chemistry summa cum laude from Washington and Lee College in 1962 [19]. He then attended Southwestern Medical School in Dallas, Texas. Goldstein was an intern and resident in medicine at the Massachusetts General Hospital during 1966–1968 in Boston where he first met Michael S. Brown, his long-term scientific collaborator. Goldstein spent the next two years at the National Institutes of Health (NIH), where he worked in the laboratory of Marshall Nirenberg, who had been awarded a Nobel prize for his genetic studies. Goldstein also served as a clinical associate at the National Heart Institute. He cared for patients with homozygous familial hypercholesterolemia, which piqued his interest in blood lipids and their genetic control. While at NIH, Goldstein and Brown (who was a fellow in gastrointestinal diseases) became avid duplicate bridge players. Their successful bridge partnership proved to be a valid testing ground for their future scientific partnership.

Goldstein spent the next two years as a Special NIH Fellow in medical genetics with Arno G. Motulsky at the University of Washington. Motulsky was one of the creators of human genetics as a medical specialty. In Seattle, Goldstein initiated and completed a genetic population study that determined the frequency of the various hereditary lipid disorders in an unselected population of heart attack survivors. He and his colleagues showed that 20 percent of all heart attack survivors had one of three single gene–determined types of hereditary hyperlipidemia. He then returned to his medical school where he remained the remainder of his academic career.

In 1973, Goldstein and Brown discovered the LDL receptor in cells that take in cholesterol and clarified how the conversion of cholesterol is regulated by genes and other substances [20]. Their research became the basis for statins, medications that reduce blood cholesterol levels.

Michael S. Brown was born in 1941, in Brooklyn, New York. His family moved to Elkins Park, Pennsylvania, when Brown was 11 years old [21]. He graduated in 1962 from the University of Pennsylvania, majoring in chemistry.

He earned his MD degree from the University of Pennsylvania School of Medicine in 1966. The next two years were spent as intern and resident in internal medicine at Massachusetts General Hospital in Boston where he met Goldstein. The years 1968–1971 were spent at NIH Health where Brown served initially as clinical associate in gastroenterology and hereditary disease. He then joined the laboratory of biochemistry. In 1971 Brown joined the division of gastroenterology in the department of internal medicine at the University of Texas Southwestern Medical School in Dallas.

Soon after his arrival in Dallas, Brown succeeded in solubilizing and partially purifying 3-hydroxy-3-methylglutaryl coenzyme A reductase, a previously enigmatic enzyme that catalyzes the rate-controlling enzyme in cholesterol biosynthesis. He and Goldstein had developed the hypothesis that abnormalities in the regulation of this enzyme were the cause of familial hypercholesterolemia, a genetic disease in which excess cholesterol accumulates in blood and tissues. The formal scientific collaboration with Goldstein began one year later, in 1972. In 1977 he was appointed Paul J. Thomas Professor of Medicine and

Genetics, and director of the Center for Genetic Disease at the same institution. In 1985, Brown was appointed Regental Professor of the University of Texas and shared the Nobel Prize in Physiology or Medicine with Goldstein that same year [21].

Two boys from very different parts of the country and different backgrounds and initial directions of research – genetics and gastroenterology – somehow joined together to make very important discoveries in lipidology.

The third key individual came from Japan and from a very different family and educational background and a different original topic of study, bacteriology. Akira Endo was born into a rural farming family in northern Japan. He lived in Akita for 17 years with his extended family, including grandparents. He became fascinated with mushrooms and other molds, and at the age of 10 dreamt of becoming a scientist. He entered Tohoku University's College of Agriculture in Sendai, where he recalls being inspired by the biography of Alexander Fleming, who discovered penicillin [22]. At that time, many Japanese drug companies and universities were conducting active research and development in finding effective antibiotics. He was impressed by the knowledge that antibiotics had saved the lives of many patients with infectious diseases. Endo's early scientific work began in the applied microbiology group of Sankyo, a Tokyo pharmaceutical company. In the mid-1960s, still focused on developing antibacterial substances, he became interested in cholesterol biosynthesis. He spent two years at the Albert Einstein College of Medicine where he researched the role of phospholipids in an enzyme system required for building bacterial cell walls.

In 1968, Endo returned to Sankyo where he was allowed to develop his own project. He hoped to isolate an enzyme that would rob bacteria of the cholesterol they needed to build their cell walls, and use that enzyme to inhibit production of cholesterol in humans [22]. In 1972, after a year spent combing through thousands of culture broths from 3,800 strains of fungi, Endo found his potent 3-hydroxy-3-methylglutaryl-coenzyme A (HMG-CoA) reductase inhibitor, a molecule called citrinin. Unfortunately, it was toxic to rat kidneys. By 1973, he had isolated another HMG-CoA reductase inhibitor produced by a blue-green mold he found at a rice shop. These chemical reductase inhibitors were, for simplicity, later referred to as "statins." That substance, known as compactin, was later given to eight test patients, in whom it dropped their cholesterol by 30 percent with no severe side effects. Subsequent clinical trials had similar success, but when a trial in dogs (using doses 200 times what had been given to humans) appeared to cause lymphoma, Endo's pharmaceutical employer Sankyo shelved the drug. Endo left the company for a university post in 1978.

A year later, Endo and Merck separately isolated similar compounds from fungi. Endo's came from *Monascus ruber* and Merck's from *Aspergillus terreus*. Merck had confidentially purchased compactin samples and related research information from Sankyo in 1976. In 1979, monacolin K and mevinolin were found to be the same compound (later both changed to lovastatin). In 1981, Brown and Goldstein reported that lovastatin could raise liver LDL receptors in dogs, and this led to a profound fall in plasma LDL levels. Lovastatin was then tested in humans, and shown to produce a profound fall in plasma LDL levels.

Statins and Other Agents That Lower High Lipid Levels

Many vascular disease experts rate statins as the most important class of agents introduced into medicine during the last half century. After lovastatin was commercialized, six statins, including two semi-synthetic statins (simvastatin and pravastatin) and four synthetic statins (fluvastatin, atorvastatin, rosuvastatin, and pitavastatin), were introduced to the market. Statins were tested in many large-scale clinical trials. The results in all these studies have been consistent: treatment with statins lowers plasma LDL levels by 25–35 percent and reduces the frequency of heart attacks by 25–30 percent. A large international study, the Stroke Prevention by Aggressive Reduction in Cholesterol Levels (SPARCL) trial led by Pierre Amarenco of France, showed the effectiveness of statins in stroke prevention [23].

Other agents were often prescribed, especially to lower triglycerides and chylomicra levels: fibric acid derivatives called fibrates; bile acid sequestrants, also called bile acid resins; nicotinic acid; selective cholesterol absorption inhibitors; ezetimibe, which lowers LDL by inhibiting the absorption of cholesterol in the intestines; and omega 3 fatty acids and fatty acid esters.

More recently, two other classes of agents have been introduced into clinical medicine and shown to be effective even in patients already treated with statins. Proprotein convertase subtilisin/kexin type 9 (PCSK9), a serine protease enzyme encoded by the PCSK9 gene, binds to the low-density lipoprotein receptor on the surface of liver cells. This leads to the degradation of the receptor and subsequently to higher plasma LDLcholesterol levels. Antibodies to PCSK9 interfere with binding of the receptor, leading to higher hepatic receptor expression and lower plasma LDL cholesterol levels. Two FDA-approved medications, the monoclonal antibodies alirocumab and evolocumab, have a powerful effect on LDL cholesterol levels and can prevent heart attacks and strokes [24]. The other new class of agents inhibits the enzyme adenosine triphosphate-citrate lyase (ACL). The enzyme's action can be inhibited by the coenzyme A-conjugate of bempedoic acid (Nexletol), a compound that also effectively lowers LDL cholesterol in humans [25].

Doctors caring for patients with hypertension, diabetes, and high cholesterol and lipid levels had by the end of the first quarter of the twenty-first century an extensive array of agents that could effectively treat these important precursors and risks for stroke.

NOTES AND REFERENCES

1. Caplan LR. *Vertebrobasilar Ischemia and Hemorrhage: Clinical Findings, Diagnosis, and Management of Posterior Circulation Disease*. Cambridge: Cambridge University Press, 2014, pp. 215–216.

2. O'Rourke MF. Frederic Akbar Mahomed. *Hypertension* 1992;19:212–217. Saklayen MG, Deshpande N. Timeline of history of hypertension treatment. *Front. Cardiovasc. Med.* 2016;3:3. doi: 10.3389/fcvm.2016.00003.

3. Samuel Siegfried Karl von Basch (1837–1905). *Nature* 1937;140:393–394.

4. Bruenn HG. Clinical notes on the illness and death of president Franklin D. Roosevelt. *Ann. Intern. Med.* 1970;72:579–591.

5 Smithwick, R. H. Hypertensive cardiovascular disease: Effect of thoracolumbar splanchnicectomy on mortality and survival rates. *JAMA* 1951;147:1611–1615.

6 Saklayen MG, Deshpande N. Timeline of history of hypertension treatment. *Front. Cardiovasc. Med.* 2016;3:3. doi: 10.3389/fcvm.2016.00003. Kotchen TA. Historical trends and milestones in hypertension research. *Hypertension* 2011;58:522–538.

7 Guyton AC. Blood pressure control: Special role of kidneys and body fluid. *Science* 1991;252:1813–1816.

8 Freis ED, Wanko A, Wilson IM, Parrish AE. Treatment of essential hypertension with chlorothiazide (diuril); its use alone and combined with other antihypertensive agents. *JAMA* 1958;166:137–140.

9. Prof. Sir James W. Black. Lindau Nobel Laureate Meetings. Available at www.mediatheque.lindau-nobel.org/laureates/black.

10 Castle WB. George Richards Minot. *Biographical Memoirs of the National Academy of Sciences* 1974;45:337–383.

11 Obituary. Elliott P. Joslin. *Br. Med. J.* 1962;1:729.

12 Joslin EP. The prevention of diabetes mellitus. *JAMA* 1921;76(2):79–84.

13 Rosenfeld L. Insulin: Discovery and controversy. *Clin. Chem.* 2002;48:2270–2288. Hegele RA, Maltman GM. Insulin's centenary: The birth of an idea. *Lancet Diabetes Endocrinol.* 2020;8(12):971–977.

14 White JR Jr. A brief history of the development of diabetes medications. *Diabetes Spectr.* 2014;27(2):82–86.

15 Reaven G. Syndrome X, a short history. *Ochsner J.* 2001;3(3):124–125. Reaven GM. Banting lecture 1988. Role of insulin resistance in human disease. *Diabetes* 1988;37:1595–1607. Ferrannini E, Haffner SM, Mitchell BD, Stern MP. Hyperinsulinemia: The key feature of a cardiovascular and metabolic syndrome. *Diabetologia* 1991;34:416–422.

16 Kannel WB, Dawber TR, Friedman GD, Glennon WE, McNamara PM. Risk factors in coronary heart disease: An evaluation of several serum lipids as predictors of coronary heart disease; the Framingham Study. *Ann. Intern. Med.* 1964;61:888–899.

17 Golding SS, Allen NB. Cholesterol and atherosclerotic cardiovascular disease: A lifelong problem. *J. Am. Heart Assoc.* 2019;8(11):e012924.

18 Duncan MS, Vasan RS, Xanthakis V. Trajectories of blood lipid concentrations over the adult life course and risk of cardiovascular disease and all-cause mortality: Observations from the Framingham Study over 35 years. *J. Am. Heart Assoc.* 2019;8: e011433.

19 Joseph L. Goldstein, biographical. The Nobel Prize. Available at www.nobelprize.org/prizes/medicine/1985/goldstein/biographical/.

20 Goldstein JL, Brown MS. The LDL receptor. *Arterioscler. Thromb. Vasc. Biol.* 2009;29 (4):431–438.

21 Michael S. Brown, biographical. The Nobel Prize. Available at www.nobelprize.org/ prizes/medicine/1985/brown/biographical/.

22. Endo A. A historical perspective on the discovery of statins. *Proc. Japan Academy Ser. B Phys. Biol. Sci.* 2010;86(5):484–493. Endo A. The discovery and development of HMG-CoA reductase inhibitors. *J. Lipid Res.* 1992;33:1569–1582. Brown MS, Goldstein JL. A tribute to Akira Endo, discoverer of a "penicillin" for cholesterol. *Atheroscler. Suppl.* 2004;5:13–16.

23. Amarenco P, Goldstein LB, Szarek M, et al. Effects of intense low-density lipoprotein cholesterol reduction in patients with stroke or transient ischemic attack: The Stroke Prevention by Aggressive Reduction in Cholesterol Levels (SPARCL) trial. *Stroke* 2007;38:3198–3204. Amarenco P, Labreuche J. Lipid management in the prevention of stroke: Review and updated meta-analysis of statins for stroke prevention. *Lancet Neurol.* 2009;8:453–463.

24. Karatasakis A, Danek B, Karacsonyi J, et al. Effect of PCSK9 inhibitors on clinical outcomes in patients with hypercholesterolemia: A meta-analysis of 35 randomized controlled trials. *J. Am. Heart Assoc.* 2017;6(12):e006910. doi: 10.1161/ JAHA.117.006910. Cholesterol Treatment Trialists' (CTT) Collaboration, Baigent C, Blackwell L, Emberson J, et al. Efficacy and safety of more intensive lowering of LDL cholesterol: A meta-analysis of data from 170,000 participants in 26 randomised trials. *Lancet* 2010 Nov;376(9753):1670–1681. doi: 10.1016/S0140-6736(10)61350-5. Epub 2010 Nov 8.

25. Banach M, Duell PB, Gotto AM Jr, et al. Association of bempedoic acid administration with atherogenic lipid levels in phase 3 randomized clinical trials of patients with hypercholesterolemia. *JAMA Cardiol.* 2020 Jul 1. doi: 10.1001/jamacardio.2020.2314 (Epub ahead of print).

CHAPTER FIFTY

NEUROPROTECTION

Lives of great men all remind us
We can make our lives sublime,
And, departing, leave behind us
Footprints on the sands of time.
—Henry Wadsworth Longfellow

The history of neuroprotection might start on a cold winter day with the tale of Ann Green, a young serving girl found guilty of having a child out of wedlock, allegedly fathered by a member of the English aristocracy. She was hanged at Carfax, Oxford, one December morning in 1650 [1]. At the execution she was clearly hypothermic, and likely hypoglycemic. Rendered unconscious, the body was taken down and conveyed from the site of public execution to the lodgings of Thomas Willis. In preparation for her dissection, and to confirm she was dead, Willis's technician stomped on her chest and unexpectedly revived her. She recovered over several hours, leaving no discernible neurological damage. Despite a period of anoxia and a transient global ischemic insult, her recovery was because of prompt reperfusion assisted by the then unknown but later discovered neuroprotective properties of hypothermia and hypoglycemia, accounting for her impressive neurological outcome.

For almost 400 years, but particularly over the last half century of intensive preclinical and clinical investigation with innumerable agents and protocols, no treatment strategy has yet proven to be clinically beneficial in focal stroke. The oldest and most intriguing neuroprotective agent is therapeutic hypothermia (TH), first described in an Egyptian papyrus from 5,000 years ago. Hippocrates used it to reduce hemorrhage in wounded soldiers, and Napoleon's chief surgeon used it to reduce the pain of amputation. TH was rediscovered in the 1930s for analgesia, and in the 1950s and 1960s for intraoperative neuroprotection during cardiac and brain surgery [2]. The complications of moderate systemic hypothermia (28–32°C) initially limited clinical applications. By the 1980s, the benefits of even mild cooling following cardiac arrest became apparent. The publication of two trials in 2002 definitively established TH as an effective neuroprotectant following cardiac arrest [3]. Over the last two decades investigators have tried to extend this to focal stroke paradigms.

Beyond hypothermia, the most promising targets in acute ischemia were and remain excitotoxicity, calcium channels, glutamate production, oxidative and nitrosative stress, inflammation, and cellular apoptosis. While small animal models have repeatedly shown promise using multiple drugs targeting individual steps in the ischemic cascade, none has been translated into humans. Since the 1990s, over 12,000 acute stroke patients have been enrolled in trials targeting free radicals, ion channels, excitotoxicity, immune modulation, and inflammation, all of which failed or at best shown marginal benefit [4]. The failure to translate benefit to humans is multifactorial, including poor trial design and methodological weaknesses of many preclinical studies, publication bias, small sample sizes, and models that differ from the typical human condition in mostly elderly patients with comorbidities. In clinical trials, neuroprotection was often started too late, and only a minority received concurrent endovascular therapy (EVT) or thrombolysis.

GLOBAL VERSUS FOCAL ISCHEMIA STROKE MODELS, WINDOWS FOR EVALUATING NEUROPROTECTION

A central aim is to extend the ischemic time window for thrombolysis and EVT and thereby increase the overall number of patients treated. With the demonstration of an ischemic penumbra electrophysiologically and then through positron emission tomography (PET) imaging and later by magnetic resonance imaging (MRI) perfusion/diffusion mismatch, the goal moved from a time window to an imaging-based tissue window allowing study of longer time intervals. A more modern, nuanced approach moved into the concept of a *brain-time continuum*, seeking windows of opportunity with different cells having different time courses. Precise target windows for each heterogeneous cell type need to be defined. These cell specific target windows might be susceptible to temperature, glucose levels, and circadian influences. They need to be combined with rational approaches to different physiological situations, including different durations and severities of ischemia.

To understand target windows and the cellular basis of selective neuronal injury, we must go back to 1925 and Spielmeyer's original observations following transient global ischemia that demonstrated selective neuronal vulnerability of hippocampal CA-1 cells [5]. The slow death of these cells was initially reported by Russian physiologists during the 1950s, and later brought to attention in the West through the use of novel global ischemia models such as the four-vessel occlusion model of Pulsinelli [6] and the two- vessel occlusion models used by Siesjo and Diemer for rodents [7] and by Ito and Kirino for gerbils [8]. These contributors demonstrated selective loss of specific neurons in the cortex, striatum, and the hippocampus. The initial demonstration of the time course or maturation of this differential regional vulnerability was in rodents. Carol Petito later extended this observation to humans, in patients who had briefly survived cardiac arrest but then died at the New York Hospital [9].

Early research on brain cellular metabolism took place in Sweden under the leadership of Bo Siesjö and in New York in Fred Plum's group. Bo K. Siesjö was born in Sweden in 1930. He graduated from Lund University medical school in 1958 and defended his PhD thesis there in 1962 [10]. His postgraduate training was in Sweden and Cambridge. In the late 1980s he was a visiting scientist in Nice and then held academic appointments at Lund University and its University Hospital until his retirement in 1995. He created the Laboratory for Experimental Brain Research in Lund, which trained and housed many important contributors, such as David and Martin Ingvar and Tadeus Wieloch. The Swedish Research Council established a special professorship for him in 1974. After his retirement he went to Hawaii to build a neuroscience research department at Queen's Medical Center in Honolulu. He died in 2013. Siesjö's research focus was on cerebral metabolism in the normal and injured brain [10].

Fred Plum was born in Atlantic City, New Jersey, in 1924. His motivation for medicine and neurology was prompted by the death of a sister from poliomyelitis [11]. He attended Dartmouth College and Dartmouth Medical School, and graduated from Cornell University Medical College in 1947. He served first as an intern and then as a resident in neurology at the New York Hospital. At age 29, he was recruited to head the neurology division of the department of medicine at the University of Washington. He returned to the New York Hospital as chief of neurology and professor and chair of neurology at Cornell University. His research focused on coma and the study of cerebral blood flow and metabolism [11]. Plum's research group at Cornell included Bill Pulsinelli, Carol Petito, Richard Kraig, Costantino Iadecola, and Alastair Buchan, all of whom contributed to knowledge about brain and neuronal metabolism and blood flow.

While the global models showed a way of assessing delayed post-ischemic neuronal injury, focal models of cortical and subcortical infarction were developed to mimic arterial infarction in thromboembolic strokes. Initially, this utilized large animals such as nonhuman primates [12]. Lindsay Symon's team at Queen Square London showed in the 1970s that two to three hours of transient occlusion in a nonhuman primate model would induce an infarct similar in size to a permanent occlusion in humans [13]. Shorter intervals of ischemia reduced injury as measured by infarct volumes, showing for the first time a time window of somewhere between one and three hours for successful reperfusion while hypoperfused tissue remained viable. These experiments were pivotal in positing the concept of a core and a potentially reversible penumbra. This concept was confirmed by PET studies, particularly those of Jean-Claude Baron in France, Robert Ackerman in Boston, Wolf-Dieter Heiss in Germany, and Antoine Hakim in Canada [14]. Using this novel imaging approach, they showed that reduced blood flow increased oxygen extraction. Ultimately, inadequate oxygen utilization led to a dynamic penumbra that was similar in humans and nonhuman primates, underlining the translational potential of pharmacological studies in focal animal models. PET scan research is discussed in Chapter 35.

Rodent models necessary to study the penumbra and infarct core for both transient and permanent focal ischemia were developed in the 1980s by several labs, including those of Myron Ginsberg, Bill Pulsinelli, and Alastair Buchan. Their time-course studies showed that a striatal core together with a cortical penumbra could be achieved in the rat and mouse. Their penumbras followed the same time course as in humans, making it an important target for those studying neuroprotection [15]. The availability of these models allowed for a vastly expanded repertoire of tools for studying specific molecular targets, through transgenic studies in murine models and scalable in vivo pharmacological studies. These studies paved the way for mechanistic insights into processes of ischemic cell death.

Cellular Targets

Neuroprotective interventions, while ultimately defined by their ability to improve neurological recovery, must have a cellular mechanistic basis through which this is achieved. Initially, cells were thought to die from necrosis. Observations of selective neuronal vulnerability led to the concept that cells may die more slowly through apoptosis. This was shown in hippocampal neurons following global ischemia, and penumbral neurons in focal ischemia [16]. The idea of apoptotic neuronal cell death following ischemia gave rise to the suggestion that caspase inhibition could provide neuroprotection. This concept proceeded to clinical trials relatively quickly, but these were found wanting.

Related approaches included mitochondrial pore inhibitors as antiapoptotic agents [17]. To date, these have not been translated to the clinic.

Preventing neuronal apoptosis remains an appealing idea and has had a renaissance through mechanisms such as productive autophagy and mTOR suppression such as with rapamycin, replicating mechanisms seen intrinsically in regions of selective resistance to ischemia, a concept termed "endogenous neuroprotection," as exemplified by the upregulation of the Tsc1 gene product (hamartin) [18].

Cellular injury was thought of initially as the need to protect neurons from direct hypoxic damage. Understanding the mechanism of the injury and its impacts on the wider neurovascular unit – a term encompassing neurons, astrocytes, microglia, pericytes, endothelial cells, and vascular smooth muscle cells – has expanded. There is now a greater appreciation of the close interconnections between cell types and indirect mechanisms of injury. The tissue-window concept provides opportunities for protection of different cell types, each at different times with different molecular targets. Neuronal injury may occur very early following reperfusion, while injury of the microvasculature may come next, followed by a breakdown of the blood-brain barrier. Glial protection and stimulating glia to help with recovery occurs considerably later. Understanding the varied opportunities and targets in different epochs of time became the focus for cellular-based interventions that recognized the heterogeneity of the different cell targets at different ischemic and post-ischemic time points [19].

Targeting neurons specifically had proven insufficient under conditions of widespread multicellular dysfunction such as hyperacute neuroinflammation and post-ischemic inflammation and a compromised blood-brain barrier due to matrix metalloprotease activity. Inflammation was a particularly appealing target as its prolonged duration after the ischemic incident provided a promising window for cellular protection. The ASTIN trial failed to show that inhibition of neuroinflammation led to a significantly improved stroke outcome [20]. The microvasculature has been the subject of extensive study in ischemia, to ensure that capillary constriction does not limit the benefits of large-vessel recanalization. One example is ensuring the relaxation of pericytes, which, under hypoxic conditions, constrict and eventually die in rigor [21].

Excitotoxicity and Channel Targets

Neuronal excitotoxicity was shown to be driven by glutamate-mediated influx of calcium [22]. Subsequent investigations showed that the NMDA receptor gated calcium into neurons, causing excitotoxicity. This mechanism was posited to be the underpinning of selective hippocampal CA-1 loss and the process in which a potential salvageable penumbra became core ischemic tissue over time [23].

Research during the late 1980s used agents that blocked excitotoxicity given before or during ischemia, or after reperfusion. Studies in a model of global ischemia showed that an early competitive NMDA antagonist was effective at preventing loss of CA-1 cells [24]. Merck's noncompetitive NMDA antagonist MK-801 became the prototypic neuroprotectant. Studies in gerbils suggested that even delayed administration of MK-801 might prevent selective neuronal death [25]. Extensive studies at Cornell that used the correct physiological controls and appropriate sample sizes found no discernible neuroprotection with MK-801 in global ischemia in gerbils and other rodents. A surprise finding was that the drop in temperature following administration of MK-801, in association with transient global ischemia, resulted in hypothermic neuroprotection. If the core temperature was maintained after administration, no neuroprotection from MK-801 was discerned [26]. Hypothermia alone at temperatures similar to that observed with ischemia and MK-801, but without MK-801, resulted in more robust neuroprotection. MK-801 was shown to be effective at preventing hypoglycemic neuronal injury [27].

Clinical trials were taken forward with NMDA antagonists, such as CGS19755 and MK-801, with the hope that improvements seen in focal rodent models might translate into effective treatment for patients in the early days before the availability of reperfusion therapies. Autoradiographic cerebral blood flow studies for both CGS-19755 and MK-801 showed that the reduced volume of infarcted tissue with NMDA antagonists given during focal ischemia probably related to the ability of NMDA antagonists to enhance intra-ischemic regional cerebral blood flow [28].

On the heels of the NMDA failure, a breakthrough appeared promising in the early 1990s when AMPA antagonists developed from aniline dyes by Novo-Nordisk suggested that blocking the AMPA receptor, particularly the gluR-2 subunit, was important in preventing calcium fluxes in post-global ischemia CA1 injury. Neuroprotection was achieved in both global and focal animal ischemia models [29]. Early promise was tempered by the observation that much of the neuroprotection was a postponement of injury rather than long-term reductions in cell death or tissue preservation, leading to the concept that indefatigable cell survival was a necessary hallmark [29].

Treatments to prevent calcium influx during nearly four decades with agents such as nimodipine and then agents blocking NMDA or AMPA receptors have proven wanting, largely because of the effects seen in animal models that were probably related to coincidental improvement providing protection through inadvertent physiological rather than direct and lasting pharmacological protection.

FREE RADICALS

Bo Siesjö pursued the free radical hypothesis. The early interventions used free radical scavenging agents [30]. Initially, N-tert-butyl-α-phenylnitrone (PBN), previously used to measure the accumulation of free radicals, was repurposed into use as a therapeutic scavenger in animal models and later in clinical trials. Early studies of PBN appeared very promising. Centaur with AstraZeneca developed a derivative compound that improved blood-brain barrier penetration. In a series of important clinical trials in the early 2000s, the SAINT 1 trial investigated the effects of NXY-059 treatment in ischemic stroke patients, more than 40 percent of whom received rtPA, and showed strong evidence of efficacy [31]. The confirmatory SAINT 2 trial was brought to an early conclusion on the basis of a futility analysis, famously causing a precipitous drop in the AstraZeneca stock price [32]. Many other compounds have been tested for free radicals and oxidative stress, including inhibitors of lipid peroxidation such as Upjohn's 21-aminosteroids, for example, tirilazad/U-74006F, collectively termed "lazaroids" in reference to the biblical resurrection of Lazarus. The only one that has found significant clinical use is edaravone, which is used clinically in East Asia, although there is no clear evidence base for a clinically meaningful benefit.

Cellular and Vascular Intervention

Following the unsuccessful CHANT and SAINT trials, attention shifted from the excitotoxicity theory and free radicals toward improving blood flow and metabolism. Extensive studies by Myron Ginsberg and colleagues in Miami showed that improving cerebral blood flow by increasing volume with infusions of albumin could reduce injury in a variety of models in both temporary and focal middle cerebral artery territory ischemia [33]. Early proof-of-concept studies in humans suggested that this could translate to useful protection in embolic stroke. The NINDS ALIAS phase 3 trials, clinically led by Michael Hill as part of the Calgary clinical trial group, administered albumin infusions, but issues with volume overload in elderly patients led the trial to be stopped on the basis of futility analysis despite excellent preclinical data [34]. Efforts to improve blood flow with nimodipine, which had been shown to improve outcome following SAH, or using a more interventional approach by partially occluding the aorta with the NeuroFlo device in the Sentis Trial, sponsored by CoAxia, did not result in successful clinical adoption [35].

One potential reason for the many unsuccessful neuroprotection trials might be that patients were not enrolled on the basis of brain imaging that used standard stratification. Neuroprotection trials were based on evidence from rodent studies when the putative neuroprotective drug was administered while there was still a large penumbra or even before the initial occlusion. Clinical trials could not pretreat in anticipation of a stroke. Infarction may have been well on the way or might have already reached its full extent before the start of treatment. Had the trials of NMDA or AMPA antagonists or NXY-059 and the like focused on patients most likely to show protection, had albumin been used in patients with more robust cardiovascular systems, and had stratification with imaging been the road map into the clinic, successful translation might have been achieved.

Because of the frequent failures of clinical trials, guidelines for preclinical studies, envisaged by the STAIR collaborators to improve translational success, were published [36]. To date they have not prevented further setbacks. The most recent and very prominent example is the ESCAPE NA-1 trial in which the eicosapeptide nerinetide, which targets neuronal excitotoxicity by preventing downstream nitric oxide production, had shown extremely promising rodent and primate results adhering to the STAIR guidelines [37]. A phase I/II proof-of-concept trial in patients being coiled for aneurysms showed reduced brain injury after coiling when pretreated with nerinetide [38]. This might have been evidence for direct neuroprotection or improved flow, perhaps through vasodilation as with MK-801. The ESCAPE NA-1 trial, in which reperfusion with endovascular treatment was combined with nerinetide, showed no overall benefit compared to those who received placebo, although there was the tantalizing suggestion of benefit in the subgroup of those not concurrently receiving tPA [37].

HYPOTHERMIA

Therapeutic hypothermia (TH) is the only intervention so far that targets the multiple aspects of acute ischemic brain injury. TH reduces oxygen demand. The cerebral metabolic rate decreases by 5 percent for every 1°C cooling. TH reduces enzymatic degradation, neurotransmitter uptake, and intracellular acidosis, and stabilizes membranes. It decreases hyperemia after reperfusion, reduces the production of excitatory amino acids, and prevents release of oxidative and nitrosative agents. TH reduces astrocyte and microglial activation, preserves the blood-brain barrier, and attenuates the release of pro-apoptotic mediators, even in late stages of ischemia. TH can even assist post-ischemic neurogenesis [39].

The application of TH as a neuroprotectant during surgery dates back to Canada in the 1950s. Bigelow in Toronto used systemic TH in dogs to explore possible use in human cardiac surgery [40]. He reported a 50 percent reduction in cerebral metabolic rate at 28°C and a 75 percent reduction at 25°C. Experiments with selective cerebral TH in dogs led to the use of adjunctive TH for the surgical management of cerebral aneurysms.

Numerous preclinical studies have shown the benefits of TH in acute stroke models. A systematic review and meta-analysis analyzed the results in over 100 publications dating back to 1957, including 3,353 animals in focal ischemic models [41]. TH reduced infarct volumes by up to 44 percent and improved functional outcomes by up to 33 percent. TH was most effective with lower temperatures, treatment starting before or at the onset of ischemia, and temporary rather than prolonged hypothermia. There was also benefit with mild cooling to 35°C, initiation between 90 and 180 minutes of onset for both transient and permanent ischemia [41].

Translation to the bedside has remained problematic. Humans do not tolerate systemic cooling below 32°C without major cardiac complications. Whole-body cooling by external methods takes hours to induce. Several trials have studied the benefit of TH in human acute stroke. The COOLAID trial was the first to show the feasibility of endovascular cooling with delivery of ice-cold saline via a catheter in the inferior vena cava [42]. A target temperature of 33°C was reached in 77 minutes in 13 of 18 patients. The ICTuS-L trial was the first to investigate endovascular TH with the use of intravenous alteplase [43]. The mean time to achieve target temperature was 67 minutes in 26 of 28 patients. ReCCLAIM in 2014 used TH cooling to 33°C in association with mechanical thrombectomy, achieving target temperature in 64 minutes [44]. None of these studies showed any significant clinical benefit. Both Pat Lyden's ambitious ICTuS 2 trial [45] and the ReCCLAIM II Trial were stopped early due to recruitment problems. A pioneering group in the Netherlands led by Bart van der Worp organized the most ambitious trial of TH in acute stroke, EuroHYP-1, in 2014. This study aimed to enroll 1,500 patients and randomize patients to endovascular cooling to 34–35°C within six hours of stroke onset and maintained for 12–14 hours. Only 98 patients were enrolled over four and a half years. Only 31 percent achieved the target temperature, and 38 percent had adverse events. There was no difference in the primary outcome (mRS at 90 days) between TH and control groups [46].

Selective TH, whereby the brain alone is cooled, has always been a more attractive but technically more challenging option. The advantages include a much faster time to reach target temperature and avoidance of systemic complications. The methods to achieve selective TH include ice-cold saline infusion, extracorporeal blood cooling, and intracarotid closed-loop cooling. Animal investigations with selective TH date back to the 1950s when a focal brain temperature of 20°C was reached in 20 minutes in dogs, with maintenance of the systemic temperature of 35°C [47]. Later work in primates achieved a temperature of 25°C in one carotid artery in 12 minutes that was maintained for three hours while keeping the systemic temperature at 34°C [48].

Translation of selective TH for neuroprotection in humans has been fraught with clinical and logistical difficulties. It has been utilized in refractory cardiac arrest and during cerebral aneurysm surgery, but setup times for extracorporeal blood cooling and selective carotid catheterization can take up to 40 minutes, a serious disadvantage for use in acute stroke patients. Superselective TH through microcatheters with infusion of ice-cold saline has the advantages of speed and incorporation into standard endovascular treatment protocols. Pilot studies have shown the safety and feasibility of this approach, but as yet no clinical efficacy has been shown.

TH is the only neuroprotectant to withstand the test of time and to show efficacy in both small and large animal models of acute stroke. The logistics of clinical monitoring during and after TH and the organization of a meaningful clinical trial of selective TH remain challenging. TH is also discussed in Chapter 42.

No matter which neuroprotectant strategy is investigated, the ground-breaking results from interventional trials make it clear that neuroprotection must be integrated with reperfusion. Collaboration between experimentalists, acute stroke neurologists, and neurointerventionalists is essential. Many drugs that were initially ineffective may be more potent post-thrombectomy or when delivered directly into a reperfused brain. As interventional treatment matures and becomes widespread, neuroprotection remains the next frontier of acute stroke care. Despite all the science, all the evidence of efficacy in animal models, and the successful proof-of-concept studies in man, there have to date been no successful phase III trials.

NOTES AND REFERENCES

1. Breathnach CS, Moynihan JB. Intensive care 1650: The revival of Anne Greene (c. 1628–59). *J. Med. Biogr.* 2009;17:35–38.

2. Drake CG, Barr HW, Coles JC, Gergely NF. The use of extracorporeal circulation and profound hypothermia in the treatment of ruptured intracranial aneurysm. *J. Neurosurg.* 1964;21:575–581. Karnatovskaia LV, Wartenberg KE, Freeman WD. Therapeutic hypothermia for neuroprotection: History, mechanisms, risks, and clinical applications. *Neurohospitalist* 2014;4:153–163.

3. Bernard SA, Gray TW, Buist MD, et al. Treatment of comatose survivors of out-of-hospital cardiac arrest with induced hypothermia. *N. Engl. J. Med.* 2002;346:557–563. Hypothermia after Cardiac Arrest Study Group. Mild therapeutic hypothermia to improve the neurologic outcome after cardiac arrest. *N. Engl. J. Med.* 2002;346:549–556.

4. van der Worp HB, de Haan P, Morrema E, Kalkman CJ. Methodological quality of animal studies on neuroprotection in focal cerebral ischaemia. *J. Neurol.* 2005;252:1108–1114.

5. Spielmeyer W. Zur pathogenese örtlich elektiver grehirnveränderungen. *Zeitschrift für die gesamte Neurologie und Psychiatrie* 1925;99:756–776.

6. Pulsinelli WA, Brierley JB, Plum F. Temporal profile of neuronal damage in a model of transient forebrain ischemia. *Ann. Neurol.* 1982;11:491–498.

7. Diemer NH, Jorgensen MB, Johansen FF, Sheardown M, Honore T. Protection against ischemic hippocampal CA1 damage in the rat with a new non-NMDA antagonist, NBQX. *Acta Neurol. Scand.* 1992;86:45–49. Eklof B, Siesjo BK. The effect of bilateral carotid artery ligation upon the blood flow and the energy state of the rat brain. *Acta Physiol. Scand.* 1972;86:155–165.

8. Ito U, Spatz M, Walker JT Jr, Klatzo I. Experimental cerebral ischemia in Mongolian gerbils. I. Light microscopic observations. *Acta Neuropathol.* 1975;32:209–223. Kirino T. Delayed neuronal death in the gerbil hippocampus following ischemia. *Brain Res.* 1982;239:57–69.

9. Petito CK, Feldmann E, Pulsinelli WA, Plum F. Delayed hippocampal damage in humans following cardiorespiratory arrest. *Neurology* 1987;37:1281–1286.

10. Paulson OB, Hossman K-A, Ingvar M, Sokoloff L. In memoriam: Bo K. Siesjö, 1930–2013. *J. Cereb. Blood Flow Metab.* 2014;34(1):1. Siesjö BK. Cell-damage in the brain: A speculative synthesis. *J. Cereb. Blood Flow Metab.* 1981;1:155–185.

11. Posner JB. Fred Plum, MD (1924–2010). *Arch. Neurol.* 2010;67(11):1409–1410.

12. Branston NM, Symon L, Crockard HA, Pasztor E. Relationship between the cortical evoked potential and local cortical blood flow following acute middle cerebral artery occlusion in the baboon. *Exp. Neurol.* 1974;45:195–208. Jones TH, Morawetz RB, Crowell RM, et al. Thresholds of focal cerebral ischemia in awake monkeys. *J. Neurosurg.* 1981;54:773–782.

13. Symon LN, Branston M, Strong AJ, Hope TD. The concepts of thresholds of ischaemia in relation to brain structure and function. *J. Clin. Pathol. Suppl. (R. Coll. Pathol.)* 1977;11:149–154.

14. Baron JC. Mapping the ischaemic penumbra with PET: Implications for acute stroke treatment. *Cerebrovasc. Dis.* 1999;9:193–201. Heiss WD, Graf R, Wienhard K, et al. Dynamic penumbra demonstrated by sequential multitracer PET after middle cerebral artery occlusion in cats. *J. Cereb. Blood Flow Metab.* 1994;14:892–902. Hakim AM. The cerebral ischemic penumbra. *Can. J. Neurol. Sci.* 1987;14:557–559.

15. Ginsberg MD, Busto R. Rodent models of cerebral ischemia. *Stroke* 1989;20:1627–1642. Buchan AM, Xue D, Slivka A. A new model of temporary focal neocortical ischemia in the rat. *Stroke* 1992;23:273–279.

16. Brown AW, Brierley JB. The earliest alterations in rat neurones and astrocytes after anoxia-ischaemia. *Acta Neuropathol.* 1973;23:9–22. MacManus JP, Hill IE, Huang ZG, Rasquinha I, Xue D, Buchan AM. DNA damage consistent with apoptosis in transient focal ischaemic neocortex. *Neuroreport* 1994;5:493–496.

17. Abe K, Aoki M, Kawagoe J, et al. Ischemic delayed neuronal death: A mitochondrial hypothesis. *Stroke* 1995;26:1478–1489.

18. Dirnagl U, Simon RP, Hallenbeck JM. Ischemic tolerance and endogenous neuro-protection. *Trends Neurosci.* 2003;26:248–254. Papadakis M, Hadley G, et al. Tsc1 (hamartin) confers neuroprotection against ischemia by inducing autophagy. *Nature Medicine* 2013;19(3):351–357.

19. Chamorro A, Lo EH, Renù A, van Leyden K, Lyden P. The future of neuroprotection in stroke. *J. Neurol. Neurosurg. Psychiatry* 2021;92(2):129–135.

20. Krams MK, Lees R, Hacke W, Grieve AP, Orgogozo JM, Ford GA, and ASTIN study investigators. Acute Stroke Therapy by Inhibition of Neutrophils (ASTIN): An adaptive dose-response study of UK-279,276 in acute ischemic stroke. *Stroke* 2003;34:2543–2548.

21. Hall CN, Reynell C, Gesslein B, et al. Capillary pericytes regulate cerebral blood flow in health and disease. *Nature* 2014;508:55–60.

22. Rothman SM, Olney JW. Glutamate and the pathophysiology of hypoxic-ischemic brain damage. *Ann. Neurol.* 1986;19:105–111.

23. Choi DW, Rothman SM. The role of glutamate neurotoxicity in hypoxic-ischemic neuronal death. *Annu. Rev. Neurosci.* 1990;13:171–182.

24. Simon RP, Swan JH, Griffiths T, Meldrum BS. Blockade of N-methyl-D-aspartate receptors may protect against ischemic damage in the brain. *Science* 1984;226:850–852.

25. Gill R, Foster AC, Woodruff GN. Systemic administration of MK-801 protects against ischemia-induced hippocampal neurodegeneration in the gerbil. *J. Neurosci.* 1987;7:3343–3349.

26. Buchan A, Pulsinelli WA. Hypothermia but not the N-methyl-D-aspartate antagonist, MK-801, attenuates neuronal damage in gerbils subjected to transient global ischemia. *J. Neurosci.* 1990;10:311–316.

27. Nellgard B, Wieloch T. Cerebral protection by AMPA- and NMDA-receptor antagonists administered after severe insulin-induced hypoglycemia. *Exp. Brain Res.* 1992;92:259–266.

28. Takizawa S, Hogan M, Hakim AM. The effects of a competitive NMDA receptor antagonist (CGS-19755) on cerebral blood flow and pH in focal ischemia. *J. Cereb. Blood Flow Metab.* 1991;11:786–793. Buchan AM, Slivka A, Xue D. The effect of the NMDA receptor antagonist MK-801 on cerebral blood flow and infarct volume in experimental focal stroke. *Brain Res.* 1992;574:171–177.

29. Sheardown, MJ, Suzdak PD, Nordholm L. AMPA, but not NMDA, receptor antagonism is neuroprotective in gerbil global ischaemia, even when delayed 24 h. *Eur. J. Pharmacol.* 1993;236:347–353. Colbourne F, Li H, Buchan AM. Continuing post-ischemic neuronal death in CA1: Influence of ischemia duration and cytoprotective doses of NBQX and SNX-111 in rats. *Stroke* 1999;30:662–668.

30. Siesjo BK, Agardh CD, Bengtsson F. Free radicals and brain damage. *Cerebrovasc. Brain Metab. Rev.* 1989;1:165–211.

31. Lees KR, Zivin JA, Ashwood T, et al. for the Stroke-Acute Ischemic NXY Treatment (SAINT I) Trial Investigators. NXY-059 for acute ischemic stroke. *N. Engl. J. Med.* 2006;354:588–600.

32. Shuaib, A, Lees KR, Lyden P et al., and Saint Il Trial Investigators. NXY-059 for the treatment of acute ischemic stroke. *N. Engl. J. Med.* 2007;357:562–571.

33. Belayev L, Liu Y, Zhao W, Busto R, Ginsberg MD. Human albumin therapy of acute ischemic stroke: Marked neuroprotective efficacy at moderate doses and with a broad therapeutic window. *Stroke* 2001;32:553–560.

34. Martin RH, Yeatts SD, Hill MD, et al. and ALIAS Parts 1 and 2 and Nett Investigators. ALIAS (Albumin in Acute Ischemic Stroke) trials: Analysis of the combined data from parts 1 and 2. *Stroke* 2016;47:2355–2359.

35. Shuaib A, Bornstein NM, Diener HC, et al. and Sentis trial investigators. Partial aortic occlusion for cerebral perfusion augmentation: Safety and efficacy of NeuroFlo in Acute Ischemic Stroke trial. *Stroke* 2011;42:1680–1690.

36. Fisher M, Feuerstein G, Howells DW, et al. STAIR Group. Update of the stroke therapy academic industry roundtable preclinical recommendations. *Stroke* 2009;40 (6):2244–2250.

37. Hill MD, Goyal M, Menon BK, et al. and Escape-Na Investigators. Efficacy and safety of nerinetide for the treatment of acute ischaemic stroke (ESCAPE-NA1): A multicentre, double-blind, randomised controlled trial. *Lancet* 2020;395:878–887.

38. Hill MD, Martin RH, Mikulis D, et al. and ENACT trial investigators. Safety and efficacy of NA-1 in patients with iatrogenic stroke after endovascular aneurysm repair (ENACT): A phase 2, randomised, double-blind, placebo-controlled trial. *Lancet Neurol.* 2012;11:942–950.

39. Karnatovskaia LV, Wartenberg KE, Freeman WD. Therapeutic hypothermia for neuroprotection: History, mechanisms, risks, and clinical applications. *Neurohospitalist* 2014;4:153–163.

40. Bigelow WG, Lindsay WK, Greenwood WF. Hypothermia, its possible role in cardiac surgery: An investigation of factors governing survival in dogs at low body temperatures. *Ann. Surg.* 1950;132:849–866.

41. van der Worp HB, Sena ES, Donnan GA, Howells DW, Macleod MR. Hypothermia in animal models of acute ischaemic stroke: A systematic review and meta-analysis. *Brain* 2007;130:3063–3074.

42. De Georgia MA, Krieger DW, Abou-Chebl A, et al. Cooling for Acute Ischemic Brain Damage (COOL AID): A feasibility trial of endovascular cooling. *Neurology* 2004;63:312–317.

43. Hemmen TM, Raman R, Guluma KZ, et al. and ICTuS-L Investigators. Intravenous thrombolysis plus hypothermia for acute treatment of ischemic stroke (ICTuS-L): Final results. *Stroke* 2010;41:2265–2270.

44. Horn CM, Sun CH, Nogueira RG, et al. Endovascular Reperfusion and Cooling in Cerebral Acute Ischemia (ReCCLAIM I). *J. Neurointerv. Surg.* 2014;6:91–95.

45. Lyden P, Hemmen T, Grotta J, et al. and collaborators. Results of the ICTuS 2 Trial (Intravascular Cooling in the Treatment of Stroke 2). *Stroke* 2016;47:2888–2895.

46. van der Worp HB, Macleod MR, Bath PMW, et al. and the EuroHYP-1 Investigators. Therapeutic hypothermia for acute ischaemic stroke: Results of a European multicentre, randomised, phase III clinical trial. *Eur. Stroke J.* 2019;4:254–262.

47. Lougheed WM, Kahn DS. Circumvention of anoxia during arrest of cerebral circulation for intracranial surgery. *J. Neurosurg.* 1955;12:226–239.

48. Schwartz AE, Stone JG, Finck AD, et al. Isolated cerebral hypothermia by single carotid artery perfusion of extracorporeally cooled blood in baboons. *Neurosurgery* 1996;39:577–581; discussion 81–82.

CHAPTER FIFTY ONE

THROMBOLYSIS

Knowledge about thrombosis, the formation of clots, dates back to Virchow, who is discussed in Chapter 13. Perturbation of a vessel leads to release of a thrombokinase that catalyzes the transformation of a precursor protein *prothrombin* to *thrombin*. Thrombin, a clot-promoting protein, catalyzes the transformation of *fibrinogen* (another precursor protein) into *fibrin*. Fibrin provides the scaffolding that holds clots together. Clots are necessary for survival since they stem bleeding. Equally necessary are chemical reactions that dissolve clots. An "activator" converts plasminogen (another precursor protein) to *plasmin*, a powerful fibrin-dissolving, clot-dissolving enzyme. Tissue plasminogen activator (tPA) is the molecule in question. It has the special property of acting upon plasminogen only in the presence of fibrin, only where there is a clot. The process of breaking up clots is referred to as thrombolysis. Thrombolytic agents act by breaking up fibrin bridges within thrombi and, in doing so, allow blood to flow. The process is often referred to as fibrinolysis since fibrin is the main target. Fibrinolytic drugs degrade the fibrin network mesh of red erythrocyte-fibrin clots. The formation of thrombi in the body stimulates a natural fibrinolytic mechanism for thrombolysis. Plasmin is formed and its activity is concentrated at the sites of fibrin deposition. The ideal thrombolytic agent would adhere specifically to fibrin in clots and would not affect circulating fibrinogen. Lowering circulating fibrinogen levels excessively could promote bleeding.

Physicians began to explore the use of thrombolytic agents during the 1950s for a variety of systemic thromboembolic conditions, including pulmonary embolism and myocardial infarction due to coronary artery thrombosis [1,2].

STREPTOKINASE

Early attempts used cow-derived or human thrombolysins or streptokinase. Another natural activator of plasminogen, called urokinase, was extracted from urine and also tested as a fibrinolytic agent. The body confines infections by surrounding them with a fibrin-like substance. This prevents spread to deeper and deeper layers of tissue. Some bacteria, for example, streptococci, have mechanisms to break down that barrier, causing conditions such as cellulitis. In 1933, William Smith Tillett, a microbiologist, observed that clots dissolved in test tubes that contained certain strains of streptococcus [2,3]. He concluded that bacteria produced a substance called "fibrinolysin" (later named strepto-kinase) that dissolved the clots. First at Johns Hopkins, then as chief of medicine at New York University School of Medicine, Tillett helped inaugurate a whole school of fibrinolytics research in the United States [1–3]. Tillett and his colleagues isolated streptokinase in its stable form. In 1946 Tillett put Sol Sherry in charge of investigating streptokinase for its therapeutic potential. Sherry had been a student of Tillett. Sherry's clinical research proceeded, initially in New York at Bellevue Hospital and later at Washington University in St. Louis [3]. Study patients were chosen who had a hemothorax and empyema. In those individuals the effects could be easily seen on radiographs, and the fluid could be drawn for analysis. They injected streptokinase into the chest of a patient with loculated hemothorax and found that all the loculations dissolved after six hours. After extraction of the lysed coagulum, a chest X-ray showed the pleural space drained of its previous contents [1–4].

Their streptokinase preparation was only 10 percent pure. It contained other enzymes, elicited severe febrile reactions, and was not suitable for intravenous administration. In 1957, Lederle Laboratories successfully developed purified preparations of streptokinase that were well tolerated by patients. In 1958, Sherry and his colleagues reported the first study of intravenously administered streptokinase in patients with acute myocardial infarction [4]. Patients treated within 14 hours had lower in-hospital mortality rates, while the ones treated anywhere between 20 and 72 hours had mortality rates like untreated patients, thus highlighting the need for early intervention. The role of thrombolytic therapy for coronary artery disease was debated for decades because some cardiologists suggested that coronary thrombosis was a "result" rather than the cause of myocardial necrosis. Some patients with heart attacks were thought to have heart muscle or coronary artery spasms, and about one third had no postmortem clots (the body's natural fibrinolytic system may have dissolved them) [1–3].

The perception changed in 1980 when Marcus DeWood and colleagues in Spokane, Washington, published a landmark paper [5]. They performed coronary angiography (previously considered a dangerous procedure) in live patients within 24 hours of onset of symptoms and found coronary blockage in 110 of 126 patients. They managed to retrieve clots in half of the patients with the use of a Fogarty catheter [5]. This report led to the resurgence of thrombolytic therapy for myocardial infarction. Similarly, with the advent of pulmonary angiography, urokinase (isolated from human urine) and streptokinase were used for clot lysis of pulmonary emboli.

During the early 1960s, John Sterling Meyer and colleagues performed therapeutic studies of streptokinase in stroke patients [6]. They randomized 73 patients with worsening strokes to receive streptokinase intravenously and/or concomitant anticoagulants within three days of stroke onset. The clots did lyse in some patients, but 10 patients died, and some had brain hemorrhages [6]. More modern clinical studies using streptokinase were performed in Australia [7] and Europe [8]. Streptokinase was given intravenously during the first four hours after stroke onset in Australia and within six hours in the European MAST-E study. The Australian study was led by Geofrey Donnan, who later became the first editor of the *International Journal of Stroke*, and by Steve Davis, who later served as the president of the World Stroke Organization. In each study streptokinase use was associated with increased bleeding. Streptokinase not only activated the plasminogen bound to the fibrin clot but activated it systemically, producing plasmin that degraded various molecules involved in the coagulation cascade and predisposed other organs to bleeding. The conclusion of the Australian study was "the administration of streptokinase within 4 hours of acute ischemic stroke increased morbidity and mortality at 3 months. While treatment within 3 hours of stroke was safer and associated with significantly better outcomes than later treatment, it showed no significant benefit over placebo" [7]. The European study similarly concluded that the administration of streptokinase resulted in an increase in mortality. After these studies, streptokinase was considered too dangerous to use for stroke, and the use of streptokinase for systemic and cardiac thromboembolism was considered contraindicated in the presence of brain lesions or past strokes. A small pilot study in 1976 of urokinase infusions in 31 patients with acute brain infarcts also led to hemorrhagic complications and did not show any favorable results [9].

TISSUE PLASMINOGEN ACTIVATOR

Much of the credit for discovering tissue plasminogen activator (tPA) and introducing it into clinical medicine goes to Désiré Collen. He was born in 1943 in the Flemish town of Sint-Truiden, Belgium. He began his studies in medicine at the University of Leuven. After his third year of the seven-year curriculum, he combined his studies with research: first in the physiology laboratory and then in the blood coagulation laboratory [10,11]. He studied the rate at which the coagulation proteins fibrinogen and plasminogen were cleared from the circulation. This early experience drew him to seek a career in full-time research rather than as a practicing physician. He combined his education in medicine with academic studies in chemistry. He graduated from the University of Leuven as doctor in medicine in 1968 and master in chemistry in 1969. His major research career was spent at the university where he was professor of the faculty of medicine and director of the Center for Thrombosis and Vascular Research. Considered brilliant and original, competitive but also highly collaborative, Collen ran a multidisciplinary laboratory and forged close relationships with researchers in many fields, in both Europe and the United States [2,10,11].

While on vacation in the Netherlands, Daniel Rifkin, a cell biologist then at Rockefeller University, stopped by the University of Leuven to meet with Collen. They both were performing cancer research and shared ideas and materials. Collen gave Rifkin antiplasmin and Rifkin gave Collen a cancer cell line: the Bowes melanoma cells. On February 13, 1979, Collen performed an experiment in which he combined fibrin and fibrinogen in test tubes to form clots. Then to one test tube he added the exudate produced by the Bowes cell line; in the other, he added urokinase. He centrifuged the contents of each tube separately. The result was a concentrated clot substance and a clear liquid supernatant from which Collen could recover urokinase. In contrast, not a trace of the Bowes cell exudate was found in the liquid. It was instead embedded in the clot. Affinity for fibrin was its salient property. Collen deduced that if plasminogen had been present, the clot would have dissolved. Further experiments confirmed this deduction [2].

The challenge was to produce a pure derivative of the plasminogen activator from the Bowes melanoma cell line. During October 1979 Dingeman Rijken, a biochemist who had previously worked with tPA, arrived in Collen's laboratory. Within a month, Collen and Rijken avowed that the substance they variously called melanoma plasminogen activator or human extrinsic plasminogen activator (HEPA) was homogenous and could not be distinguished by any known assay from tPA [2,11].

At a medical conference reception on April 21, 1981, Alfons Billau, a cell biologist, met a physician and friend Willem Weimar. Weimar had a patient who had a complication after a kidney transplant: a thrombus in the main vein leading from the graft. The large blood clot was visible on X-ray, floating within the inferior vena cava, and obstructing circulation. If nothing was done, the patient, a 30-year-old woman, could be expected to lose her new kidney. Weimar knew about HEPA because he had helped Désiré Collen grow the cells that produced it. He remembered when Collen showed up with a flask of the cells, just arrived from the United States, requesting he grow them in Billau's laboratory. He collected from Collen a vial of the purified material they were calling HEPA, packed it in ice, and drove back to Rotterdam. When Weimar injected his patient, the clot completely dissolved. There were no side effects. Twenty-eight years later the patient was still alive [2,11]. HEPA was soon recognized to be identical to endogenous tPA, the body's own clot-dissolving molecule.

In June 1980, Collen presented his findings at a European congress on fibrinolysis in Sweden. After the conference he was approached by Diane Pennica, a young PhD working for Genentech, a then small biotech company that was started in San Francisco in 1976. Genentech's decision to find out more about tPA was due to Herb Heynecker, a Dutch biochemist, one of the original Genentech scientists [2]. Reading the literature on urokinase, which Genentech had contracted to clone, he learned about tPA, which along with urokinase had been extracted and purified. Heynecker recognized the potential of tPA and told colleagues that it was even more interesting than urokinase. Heynecker had sent Diane Pennica to the congress on fibrinolysis. Pennica had arrived early in Malmo, Sweden, introduced herself to Collen, and explained why she was there. Collen invited her to join him and other investigators at dinner. On the spot, since the mammalian gene that produced tPA had been identified, Pennica brashly suggested that Genentech would clone it. Once cloned, it could be produced in large quantities and tested as a possible clot-busting drug. In about a year Pennica cloned tPA using tissue culture of Chinese hamster ovary cells and produced rt-PA (recombinant tPA). Genentech was able to produce large quantities of rt-PA. Trials of tPA were performed in the 1980s and the agent came into wide clinical use for acute myocardial infarction [12].

During the 1980s and early 1990s, stimulated by success in treating coronary artery thrombosis, clinicians turned again to thrombolytics to treat cerebrovascular thromboembolism. A consortium of investigators – Werner Hacke, Herman Zeumer, Klaus Poeck, Berndt Ringelstein, Andreas Ferbert, and Helmet Bruckmann in Achen Germany; Greg del Zoppo and Shirley Otis from Scripps Clinic, La Jolla California; Mike Pessin and Louis Caplan from the New England Medical Center, Tufts University in Boston; Tony Furlan from the Cleveland Clinic, in Ohio; and Etsuo Mori, from Japan – met in Germany and the United States to plan investigations with thrombolytic drugs in stroke patients. Streptokinase, urokinase, and rt-PA were the most common agents used. In these early studies, acute stroke patients were screened clinically and by CT scans, and then catheter angiography was performed [13]. If an intracranial arterial occlusion was shown, thrombolytic drugs were given either intra-arterially into the clots or intravenously. Follow-up angiography was performed after treatment to assess recanalization. These studies showed that thrombolytic agents often could open blocked arteries. Opening of the arteries correlated with better outcomes than when the arteries remained occluded. Intracranial branch arteries opened more often after use of the thrombolytic agent than larger arteries (the neck and intracranial carotid arteries and the basilar artery). These studies were not randomized trials, but were observational to show the potential effectiveness of thrombolysis and its safety.

In the mid-1980s a consortium of investigators supported by the National Institute of Neurological Diseases and Stroke (NINDS) began to plan studies and randomized therapeutic trials to test the safety and effectiveness of rt-PA (alteplase) in patients with acute ischemic strokes. Alteplase was the name given to Genentech's agent. These investigators included Clark Haley, David Levy, Tom Brott, Tom Kwiatkowski, Mike Frankel, Pat Lyden, Jim Grotta, Steve Levine, Joe Broderick, Bill Barsan, and Ken Gaines. The initial trials were dose-finding safety studies of alteplase given within 90 minutes and then at 90–180 minutes [14]. The first patient was treated in Cincinnati in April 1987. In later trials acute stroke patients were treated within three hours using the rt-PA dose of 0.9 milligrams per kilogram selected via the dose-finding studies. The researchers investigated factors that correlated with effectiveness and with development of brain hemorrhages after treatment [15].

The major results of the NINDS tPA trial were published in the *New England Journal of Medicine* in 1995 [16]. Among the 624 patients randomized to receive either placebo or alteplase, patients treated with t-PA were 30 percent more likely to have minimal or no disability at three months on the scales used to assess outcomes. Symptomatic intracerebral hemorrhage within 36 hours after the onset of stroke developed in 6.4 percent of patients given t-PA compared to 0.6 percent of patients given placebo. Mortality at three months was 17 percent in the t-PA group and 21 percent in the placebo group. The authors concluded that "despite an increased incidence of symptomatic intracerebral hemorrhage, treatment with intravenous t-PA within three hours of the onset of ischemic stroke improved clinical outcome at three months" [16].

During the summer of 1996, about half a year after the publication of the NINDS trial, the US Food and Drug Administration (FDA) approved the use of t-PA for the treatment of stroke patients when the drug was given within the first three hours. Caplan had urged the FDA committee to delay approval. He argued that the NINDS trial was preliminary and did not study which patients would be most likely to be helped and which might be harmed. He urged further research before approval. Under pressure from the NINDS, the committee voted to approve release of alteplase. The American Heart Association and American Academy of Neurology published treatment recommendations that adopted the inclusions and exclusions and the treatment protocols of the NINDS trial. The recommendations suggested that a CT scan done before thrombolysis should not show major infarction, mass effect, or hemorrhage.

These NINDS-sponsored trials were the very first randomized therapeutic trials concerning intravenously administered tPA in acute ischemic stroke. These studies showed that tPA was effective and reasonably safe when administered within three hours after stroke symptom onset in patients in whom a CT scan had not shown brain bleeding. A follow-up study showed that the treatment was durable in that effectiveness was still present when analyzed a year after treatment [17]. Two other important accomplishments of these investigators were the establishment of the dose of tPA that was used worldwide and the creation and later multicenter validation of a scoring system for quantifying the severity of neurological abnormalities, dubbed the NINDS stroke scale (NIHSS) [18]. The NIHSS scoring scale was adopted by nearly all later investigators worldwide as a uniform scoring system that allowed comparison of the results of different treatment protocols.

A consortium of investigators carried out trials of intravenous tPA in Europe and Australia that overlapped in time with the US studies. The leaders of these studies included Hacke, Hennerici, and von Kummer in Germany; Boysen and Waldron in Sweden; Kaste in Finland, Fieschi and Toni in Italy; Davalos in Spain; and Donnan and Davis in Australia [19]. These European Cooperative Acute Stroke Studies (ECASS) led to additional information about the effectiveness and safety of tPA at various time intervals after the onset of acute stroke symptoms. ECASS I concluded that rt-PA was effective in some patients but that "intravenous thrombolysis cannot currently be recommended for use in an unselected population of acute ischemic stroke patients" [19]. ECASS II concluded that the results did not show a statistical benefit for alteplase. "However, we believe the trend towards efficacy should be interpreted in the light of evidence from previous trials. Despite the increased risk of intracranial hemorrhage, thrombolysis with alteplase at a dose of 0.9 mg/kg in selected patients may lead to a clinically relevant improvement in outcome" [19]. ECASS III was an observational study that showed that rt-PA was effective if given between 3 and 4.5 hours after stroke onset. The results of the European-Australian studies were much less positive than the US NINDS study.

The US and European-Australian studies were widely reported and commented on in the public media. There was a potential treatment for stroke, but it had to be administered very soon after symptom onset. Stroke was an emergency and individuals suspected of having an acute stroke must get to a hospital emergency room as soon as possible, bypassing their regular physicians. Neurologists trained and experienced in stroke care should be ready to see the patients rapidly in the emergency room. "Time is brain" algorithms were developed for stroke patients, for every step in the treatment process, beginning at stroke symptom onset and culminating with initiation of treatment. An emergency transport culture was developed with transport personnel for stroke patients resembling those already in place for patients with acute myocardial infarction (MI), including prearrival notifications to the destination hospital. For the first time, stroke in the United States became "911-stroke" for paramedics and emergency medical technicians. In emergency departments, pathways for urgent care were put in place for the stroke patient, for the first time, to allow for rapid diagnosis and treatment. On the investigator side, a 24/7 on-call system came into use, also new for stroke. Emerging cell-phone technology was also developed at all the NINDS centers, to expedite and coordinate investigator notification and investigator communications (e.g., telephoned calls to emergency departments, radiology, the hospital laboratory, the pharmacy, the intensive care unit). This new urgent care culture and the methods developed in the United States were widely emulated internationally. In the United States, the urgent-care model is the model needed for hospitals to be designated as stroke centers by certifying agencies.

Approval of t-PA for acute stroke came much later in Europe and other countries. The European Medicines Evaluation Agency (EMEA) conditionally approved alteplase (rt-PA) in 2002 for treatment of ischemic stroke by experienced clinicians within three hours of symptom onset. A condition required by the European Union regulatory authorities was that treatment safety would be monitored during a three-year period by entering all treated patients in a web register. Physicians performing thrombolysis in Europe were urged to enter all of their cases in the SITS Monitoring Study's SITS-MOST Registry [20]. The registry results showed that intravenous tPA use was safe and effective in routine clinical practice.

When tPA was first approved for treatment in the United States, most hospitals were unprepared to adopt the treatment guidelines. There were too few trained stroke doctors, and protocols for taking and reading CT scans quickly were not in place. Many emergency physicians were skeptical about the effectiveness and especially the safety of tPA and had little experience in treating acute stroke patients. Less than 2 percent of those patients eligible according to the guidelines were treated within the first years after approval. With time, education, and publication of post-marketing results in the United States and in Europe and Asia, and with development of experienced stroke centers, more and more patients during the ensuing decades were given IV thrombolysis throughout the world.

In the NINDS-sponsored studies and in the ECASS studies, the imaging requirement was a CT scan. No vascular studies were performed to show if there was an occluded artery and, if so, where. In 1995 many hospitals did not have technology available to perform screening vascular imaging with either

CT or MRI. Some experienced stroke clinicians including Caplan, Mohr, Kistler, and Koroshetz argued during the early years after tPA approval that vascular imaging would be very useful in selecting patients for treatment and should accompany brain imaging. They urged more investigation to determine which patients with which brain lesions and which vascular lesions would benefit from thrombolytic treatment. In which situations would thrombolysis not be beneficial and might cause harm [21]?

Knowledge accumulated from observational studies that included vascular imaging on what factors correlated with good outcomes and about which arterial blockages opened up after intravenous tPA. Small clots in branch arteries opened well but major blockages in the largest arteries opened less than a third of the time [22]. The carotid artery ending in the cranium and the basilar artery opened less than 5 percent of the time [22]. Clearly, a different strategy was needed to open these major arterial blockages. Studies using modern brain imaging at large, usually academic, medical centers were able to show whether a brain infarct was present and where it was located and its size; whether an artery was blocked and what the clot burden was (the composition and the length and width of the clot); the extent of brain supplied by the blocked artery that was threatened with further stroke damage; and the reserve capability of the brain vascular system to supply the threatened region.

Many patients did not arrive early after stroke onset to medical centers that had the personnel and technology for up-to-date treatment. Clinicians and researchers sought more effective ways to accelerate arrival at capable stroke treatment centers. They also explored three approaches to treat patients who arrived later than four and a half hours after symptom onset and patients with unknown time of onset (e.g., on awakening). One approach was to use "image-based" treatment rather than time-based. Perfusion-diffusion MRI or CT perfusion testing was used to screen eligible patients who were given alteplase or placebo in randomized trials. Eligible patients had to have small or no brain infarcts and the size of their perfusion deficiency had to considerably exceed their diffusion lesion (a so-called diffusion-perfusion mismatch). Software that automatically and quickly showed treating doctors the important results greatly facilitated the performance of trials and clinical management. These studies showed that the window for use of alteplase could be extended to at least nine hours and potentially up to 24 hours in patients selected by modern imaging criteria [23].

The second strategy was to explore the use of thrombolytic agents that might be more effective and easier to deliver than tPA. The third strategy was to apply more aggressive treatment of stroke patients, especially those who arrived after the time of effectiveness of intravenous tPA or in those in whom intravenous thrombolytics were contraindicated. In late-arriving patients, those with favorable results of advanced brain and vascular imaging (no large infarct already present, large area of threatened brain, and a blocked artery reachable by catheter), trained interventionalists used a variety of ways to unblock arteries. They could inject a thrombolytic agent directly into the clot, aspirate the clot using a simple syringe, or use a stent-retriever to pull out the clot. Several trials showed definitively that some patients with favorable results of advanced imaging who were treated by experienced interventionalists as long as 24 hours after stroke onset had favorable outcomes when blocked arteries were opened [24]. Clot extraction is discussed in more detail in Chapter 56.

TENECTEPLASE

Tenecteplase (TNK) is a recombinant plasminogen activator derived from native t-PA by modifying its protein structure. It binds to the fibrin component of thrombi and selectively converts thrombus-bound plasminogen to plasmin, which degrades the fibrin matrix of the thrombus. Tenecteplase has a higher fibrin specificity and greater resistance to inactivation by its endogenous inhibitor PAI-1 compared to native t-PA. TNK has practical delivery advantages over alteplase. Its pharmacokinetic profile allows TNK to be administered as a single bolus. Hemorrhagic complications are posited to be less common than with alteplase. TNK is used to treat patients who have acute myocardial infarctions. In head-to-head trials against alteplase it has shown equal therapeutic efficacy and fewer major bleeding complications [25]. Comparisons of treatment with TNK and alteplase in acute stroke patients have shown that TNK is equally or more effective and may be safer than alteplase [26]. The agent is clearly easier to use; it need not be premixed and can be given in a single bolus.

INTRA-ARTERIAL THROMBOLYSIS

Doctors using intravenously administered thrombolytic agents were always concerned about the possibility of severe lowering of fibrinogen levels in the blood, leading to serious bleeding complications. Beginning during the last years of the twentieth century, studies and trials explored the use of thrombolytics injected directly into thrombi within cranial arteries. Preliminary research in observational studies had shown the potential utility and safety of this approach [13].

Werner Hacke, Herman Zeumer, and their colleagues in Aachen, Germany, were among the first to study the use of intra-arterial thrombolysis in acute stroke patients. In 1998, they reported their results in patients with basilar artery occlusion, a condition known to have a high mortality. They treated 65 consecutive patients with clinical signs of severe brainstem ischemia with angiographically confirmed thrombotic vertebrobasilar artery occlusions. Local intra-arterial thrombolytic therapy (urokinase or streptokinase) was administered to 43 patients. Recanalization was shown angiographically in 19 of the 43, while in 24 patients the occlusion persisted. All patients without recanalization died, but 14 of the 19 patients who recanalized survived, 10 with a favorable clinical outcome. Only three of the 22 patients who received conventional therapy survived, all with a moderate clinical deficit [27]. This report gave considerable impetus to try intra-arterial treatment especially in situations in which intravenous treatment was not indicated or unlikely to be effective.

In the United States at about the same time, clinicians and researchers performed two related trials of intra-arterial (IA) thrombolysis. They studied the effectiveness of intra-arterially administered recombinant pro-urokinase (r-proUK) in patients who had middle cerebral artery (MCA) occlusions [28,29]. The Prolyse in Acute Cerebral Thromboembolism I trial (PROACT I) compared the recanalization rate of locally injected, IA r-proUK versus heparin within six hours of onset in patients with a radiographically proven MCA occlusion [28]. The interventionalist was not allowed to mechanically disturb the clot (contrary to the usual practice in the community) and was to inject r-proUK at the proximal end of the thrombus. There was successful recanalization in 15 out of 26 (58%) of patients treated with the thrombolytic agent, while 2 out of 14 (14%) recanalized with heparin alone [28].

PROACT II was more extensive [29]. Although it was an open-label study, the follow-up was blinded to medication versus placebo. The study showed favorable recanalization rates in the intra-arterial treatment group (66%) versus 18% in the control group (P < 0.001). The symptomatic hemorrhage rate was 10 percent in the treatment group versus 2 percent in the placebo group. Patients benefited from intra-arterial thrombolysis despite the excess hemorrhage rate, and there was no excess mortality. Although intra-arterial thrombolytic treatment was effective and met the pre-trial guidelines discussed with the FDA, the drug was not approved, partly because the composition of the pro-urokinase was not defined. The company stopped synthesizing the agent.

Studies of intra-arterial thrombolysis used a variety of thrombolytic agents (streptokinase, urokinase, alteplase), sometimes with glycoprotein IIb/IIIa inhibitors or other antithrombotic agents that were given with or after thrombolytic injections [30]. Basilar artery occlusions were a common target for these intra-arterial thrombolytic studies [31]. When clot retraction devices, suctioning of thrombi, and stent retrievers came into use, intra-arterial use of thrombolytics became less prevalent. Intra-arterial instillation was often performed by interventionalists as part of a multifaceted clot retraction procedure. Clot retraction and arterial recanalization by interventionalists is the topic of Chapter 53.

NOTES AND REFERENCES

1. The early history of thrombolysis, streptokinase, and tPA is discussed in Maroo A, Topol EJ. The early history and development of thrombolysis in acute myocardial infarction. *J. Thromb. Haemostasis* 2004;2:1867–1870. Gruppo Italiano per lo Studio della Streptochinasi nell'Infarto Miocardico (GISSI). Effectiveness of intravenous thrombolytic treatment in acute myocardial infarction. *Lancet* 1986;8478:397–402. Sloan MA. Thrombolysis and stroke. *Arch. Neurol.* 1987;44:748–768. Gray D. Thrombolysis: Past, present, and future. *Postgrad. Med. J.* 2006;82(968):372–375.

2. Zivin JA, Simmons JG. *tPA for Stroke: The Story of a Controversial Drug.* New York: Oxford University Press, 2011.

3. Bryan TPJ. The rise and fall of the clot buster: A review on the history of streptokinase. *Pharm. J.* 2014. Available at www.pharmaceutical-journal.com/news-and-analysis/features/the-rise-and-fall-of-the-clot-buster-a-review-on-the-history-of-streptokinase/20065679.article.

4. Sherry S. The origin of thrombolytic therapy. *J. Am. Coll. Cardiol.* 1989 Oct 1;14(4):1085–1092.

5. DeWood MA, Spores J, Notske R, et al. Prevalence of total coronary occlusion during the early hours of transmural myocardial infarction. *N. Engl. J. Med.* 1980;303:897–902.

6. Meyer JS, Gilroy J, Barnhart MI, Johnson JF. Therapeutic thrombolysis in cerebral thromboembolism. *Neurology* 1963;13:927–937. Meyer JS, Gilroy J, Barnhart MI, et al. Anticoagulants plus streptokinase therapy in progressive stroke. *JAMA* 1964;189(5):373. Meyer JS, Gilroy J, Barnhart ME, Johnson JF. Therapeutic thrombolysis in cerebral thromboembolism: Randomized evaluation of intravenous streptokinase. In Millikan CH, Siekert W, Whisnant JP (eds.), *Cerebral Vascular Diseases.* New York: Grune & Stratton, 1964, pp. 200–213.

7. Donnan GA, Davis SM, Chambers BR, et al. Streptokinase for acute ischemic stroke with relationship to time of administration: Australian Streptokinase (ASK) Trial Study Group. *JAMA* 1996;276(12):961–966.

8. Multicenter Acute Stroke Trial-Europe Study Group: Hommel M, Cornu C, Boutitie F, Boissel JP. Thrombolytic therapy with streptokinase in acute ischemic stroke. *N. Engl. J. Med.* 1996;335(3):145–150.

9. Fletcher AP, Alkjersig N, Lewis M, Tulevski V, Davies A, Brooks JE, Hardin WB, Landau WM, Raichle ME. A pilot study of urokinase therapy in cerebral infarction. *Stroke* 1976;7:135–142.

10. Desiree Collen. Wikipedia. Available at https://en.wikipedia.org/wiki/D%C3%A9sir%C3%A9_Collen.

11. Collen D, Lijnen HR. Tissue-type plasminogen activator: A historical perspective and personal account. *J. Thromb. Haemostasis* 2004;2(4):541–546.

12. Van de Werf F, Ludbrook PA, Bergmann SR, et al. Coronary thrombolysis with tissue-type plasminogen activator in patients with evolving myocardial infarction. *N. Engl. J. Med.* 1984;310:609–613. Collen D, Topol EJ, Tiefenbrunn AJ, et al. Coronary thrombolysis with recombinant human tissue-type plasminogen activator: A prospective, randomized, placebo-controlled trial. *Circulation* 1984;70:1012–1017.

13. The early investigations of thrombolytic therapy are reviewed in del Zoppo GJ, Poeck K, Pessin MS, et al. Recombinant tissue plasminogen activator in acute thrombotic and embolic stroke. *Ann. Neurol.* 1992;32:78–86. Wolpert SM, Bruckmann H,

Greenlee R, Wechsler L, Pessin MS, del Zoppo GJ Neuroradiologic evaluation of patients with acute stroke treated with recombinant tissue plasminogen activator. The rt-PA Acute Stroke Study Group. *AJNR Am. J. Neuroradiol.* 1993;14:3–13. Pessin MS, del Zoppo GJ, Furlan AJ. Thrombolytic treatment in acute stroke: Review and update of selected topics. In *Cerebrovascular Diseases, 19th Princeton Conference, 1994.* Boston: Butterworth-Heinemann, 1995, pp. 409–418.

14. Brott T, Haley EC, Levy DE, et al. Urgent therapy for stroke: Pilot study of tissue plasminogen activator administered within 90 minutes. *Stroke* 1992;23:632–640. Haley EC, Levy DE, Brott TG, et al. Urgent therapy for stroke, part II: Pilot study of tissue plasminogen activator administered 90–180 minutes from onset. *Stroke* 1992;23:641–645.

15. Levy DE, Brott TG, Haley EC, et al. Factors related to intracranial hematoma formation in patients receiving t-PA for acute, ischemic stroke. *Stroke* 1994;25:291–297.

16. The National Institute of Neurological Disorders and Stroke rt-PA Stroke Study group. Tissue plasminogen activator for acute ischemic stroke. *N. Engl. J. Med.* 1995;333:1581–1587.

17. Kwatkowski TG, Libman RB, Frankel M, et al. Effects of tissue plasminogen activator for acute ischemic stroke at one year. *N. Engl. J. Med.* 1999;340(23):1781–1787.

18. Brott T, Adams HP Jr, Olinger CP, et al. Measurements of acute cerebral infarction: A clinical examination scale. *Stroke* 1989;20(7):864–870. Lyden P, Brott T, Tilley B, et al. and the NINDS tPA study group. Improved reliability of the NIH Stroke Scale using video training. *Stroke* 1994;25:2220–2226.

19. The European Investigators published the results of the European Cooperative Acute Stroke Study (ECASS). Hacke W, Kaste M, Fieschi C, et al. Intravenous thrombolysis with recombinant tissue plasminogen activator for acute hemispheric stroke. The European Cooperative Acute Stroke Study (ECASS). *JAMA* 1995;274:1017–1025. Hacke W, Kaste M, Fieschi C, et al. Randomised double-blind placebo-controlled trial of thrombolytic therapy with intravenous alteplase in acute ischaemic stroke (ECASS II). *Lancet* 1998;352:1245–1251. Hacke W, Kaste M, Bluhmki E, et al. for the ECASS Investigators. Thrombolysis with alteplase 3 to 4.5 hours after acute ischemic stroke. *N. Engl. J. Med.* 2008;359:1317–1329.

20. Toni D, Lorenzano S, Puca E, Prencipe M. The SITS-MOST registry. *Neurol. Sci.* 2006;27(suppl 3):S260–S262. Wahlgren N, Ahmed N, Dávalos A, et al. for the SITS-MOST investigators. Thrombolysis with alteplase for acute ischaemic stroke in the Safe Implementation of Thrombolysis in Stroke-Monitoring Study (SITS-MOST): An observational study. *Lancet* 2007;369(9558):275–282.

21. Caplan LR, Mohr JP, Kistler JP, Koroshetz W. Thrombolysis: Not a panacea for ischemic stroke. *N. Engl. J. Med.* 1997;337:1309–1310, 1313. Caplan LR. The case against the present guidelines for stroke thrombolysis. In Lyden P (ed.), *Thrombolytic Therapy for Stroke.* Totowa, NJ: Humana Press, 2001, pp. 223–235.

22. Bhatia R, Hill MD, Shobha N, Menon B, Bal S, Kochar P, Watson T, Goyal M, Demchuk AM. Low rates of acute recanalization with intravenous recombinant tissue plasminogen activator in ischemic stroke: Real-world experience and a call for action. *Stroke* 2010;41:2254–2258.

23. Thomalla G, Simonsen CZ, Boutitie F, et al. WAKE-UP Investigators. MRI-guided thrombolysis for stroke with unknown time of onset. *N. Engl. J. Med.* 2018;379 (7):611–622. Campbell BCV, Ma H, Ringleb PA, et al. EXTEND, ECASS-4, and EPITHET Investigators. Extending thrombolysis to 4.5–9h and wake-up stroke using

perfusion imaging: A systematic review and meta-analysis of individual patient data. *Lancet* 2019;394(10193):139–147.

24. Nogueira RG, Jadhay AP, Hausen DG, et al. for the DAWN Trial Investigators. Thrombectomy 6 to 24 hours after stroke with a mismatch between deficit and infarct. *N. Engl. J. Med.* 2018;378:11–21. Albers GW, Marks MP, Kemp S, et al. for the DEFUSE 3 Investigators. Thrombectomy for stroke at 6 to 16 hours with selection by perfusion imaging. *N. Engl. J. Med.* 2018;378:708–718.

25. Van de Werf F, Cannon CP, Luyten A, et al. Safety assessment of single bolus administration of TNK-tPA in acute myocardial infarction: The ASSENT-1 trial. *Am. Heart J.* 1999;137:786–791. Guillermin A, Yan DJ, Perrier A, Marti C. Safety and efficacy of tenecteplase versus alteplase in acute coronary syndrome: A systematic review and meta-analysis of randomized trials. *Arch. Med. Sci.* 2016;12:1181–1187.

26. Huang X, MacIsaac R, Thompson JL, Levin B, Buchsbaum R, Haley EC, et al. Tenecteplase versus alteplase in stroke thrombolysis: An individual patient data meta-analysis of randomized controlled trials. *Int. J. Stroke* 2016 11:534–543. Campbell BCV, Mitchell PJ, Churilov L, et al. for the EXTEND-IA TNK Investigators. Tenecteplase versus alteplase before thrombectomy for ischemic stroke. *N. Engl. J. Med.* 2018;378:1573–1582. Burgos AM, Saver JL. Evidence that tenecteplase is noninferior to alteplase for acute ischemic stroke: Meta-analysis of 5 randomized trials. *Stroke* 2019;50:2156–2162.

27. Hacke W, Zeumer H, Ferbert A, Bruckman H. Intra-arterial thrombolytic therapy improves outcome in patients with acute vertebrobasilar occlusive disease. *Stroke* 1998;29:1216–1222.

28. del Zoppo GJ, Higashida RT, Furlan AJ, et al. PROACT: A phase II randomized trial of recombinant pro-urokinase by direct arterial delivery in acute middle cerebral artery stroke. PROACT Investigators. Prolyse in Acute Cerebral Thromboembolism. *Stroke* 1998;29:4–11.

29. Furlan AJ, Higashida RT, Wechsler L, et al. PROACT II. Intra-arterial pro-urokinase for acute ischemic stroke: A randomized controlled trial. *JAMA* 1999;282;2003–2011.

30. Furlan AJ, Higashida R, Katzan I, Abou-Chebl A, Russman A. Intra-arterial thrombolysis in acute ischemic stroke. In Lyden PD (ed.), *Thrombolytic Therapy for Acute Stroke*, 2nd ed. Totowa, NJ: Humana Press, 2005, pp. 159–184.

31. Lindberg PJ, Mattle HP. Therapy of basilar artery occlusion: A systematic analysis comparing intra-aerterial and intravenous thrombolysis. *Stroke* 2006;37:922–928. Schoneville W, Wijman, CAC, Michel P, et al. on behalf of the BASICS Study Group. Treatment and outcomes of acute basilar artery occlusion in the Basilar Artery International Cooperation Study (BASICS), a prospective registry study. *Lancet Neurol.* 2009;8:724–730.

CHAPTER FIFTY TWO

TREATMENT OF CEREBRAL VENOUS THROMBOSIS

TO TREAT OR NOT TO TREAT

Although thrombotic cerebral complications were reported as early as 1825, it was almost 120 years later when the first scientific record of a treatment attempt was published [1]. This record, written by a British gynecologist, Frederick Ross Stansfield, included two case reports and started a discussion that continued during the decades that followed.

Frederick Ross Stansfield was born in 1904 at Ilkley, Yorkshire, the son of a cotton manufacturer. After studies at the University of Leeds and St. Bartholomew's Hospital, he served as a house surgeon at Queen Charlotte's Hospital and worked at the Chelsea Hospital for Women as a resident medical officer. In 1932, he became a general practitioner in Ipswich and practiced as a visiting gynecologist at the local hospital. He became a consultant gynecologist and obstetrician after World War II. Stansfield was a proud sailor. He was particularly proud of winning the Harwich to Hook of Holland race in 1958. In the scientific world he is mainly remembered because of his gynecological articles [2].

In 1942 Stansfield published an article entitled "Puerperal Cerebral Thrombophlebitis Treated by Heparin" in which he described two different treatment approaches in two similar clinical cases. Both cases concerned a twenty-five-year-old woman with acute neurological symptoms in the post-partum period. The first patient developed numbness, hemiplegia, and convulsions eight days after delivery. She was diagnosed with longitudinal sinus thrombosis and treated with glucose and magnesium sulfate and repeated lumbar punctures to reduce intracranial pressure. Despite these efforts she died. The second patient presented two months later. She developed numbness, hemianopia, dysarthria, headache, and convulsions nine days after an otherwise uneventful delivery. With the experiences of the previous case fresh in his mind, the diagnosis of cerebral venous thrombosis – then called cerebral thrombophlebitis – was quickly established. Stansfield opined that this condition was caused by a thrombus formed in the pelvic veins that, due to increased pressure in the inferior vena cava, passed through the vertebral venous plexuses into the cerebral veins to cause the neurological symptoms. Stansfield, as a treating physician, sought consultation from Ronald Jones, an honorary physician in the Ipswich hospital, to discuss treatment options [3].

Jones, educated at the Queens' College at University of Cambridge and London Hospital, became a consultant physician at age 29. He was younger than Stansfield, yet in 1940 he was already a consultant with a couple years of experience [4]. With his extensive interests in cardiology and internal medicine, he must have been aware of recent scientific developments and the increasing importance of heparin in prophylaxis and treatment of venous thrombosis [5]. Heparin, as a new anticoagulant, had already cautiously been used as prophylaxis to prevent thrombosis in the pelvis and lower extremities in gynecological patients. After discussions, Stansfield and Jones initiated an experimental heparin treatment. The patient, having received a pint (equivalent to 200 mg) of heparin every four hours for four days (which at the time was well above the recommended dose), fully recovered [3].

Stansfield concluded: "The introduction of heparin gives us an effective weapon to treat what has invariably been a fatal complication of the puerperium, and the clinician's reward for an early diagnosis will be the survival of the patient rather than the sterile pleasure of making an accurate diagnosis and confirming it in the postmortem room" [3]. This successful treatment of a disease that until then was fatal in more than in half of recorded cases, was unprecedented.

HEPARIN CONTROVERSY

After publication of Stansfield's paper, there were several other reports of successful heparin treatment in cerebral venous thrombosis (CVT) [6,7]. With growing optimism came a wave of criticism. It was argued that CVT in the puerperium sometimes resolved spontaneously and that the reported cases merely showed the unpredictability of the disease, rather than the effectiveness of anticoagulation [8]. Even more importantly, administering anticoagulants in a condition that in almost half of the cases was accompanied by an intracranial hemorrhage might do more harm than good. Forty years later, the results of the first randomized controlled trial (RCT) on anticoagulation in CVT were published.

The report of the RCT, published in the *Lancet* in 1991, was authored by Karl Max Einhäupl, a highly regarded professor of neurology at the Ludwig Maximilians University in Munich, and later chairman of the board at the Charité Hospital in Berlin [9,10]. The study, based on only 20 patients, clearly showed a benefit of heparin treatment. The trial also included patients with an intracerebral hemorrhage at baseline. Much to the surprise of critics, these patients recovered completely. No new intracerebral hemorrhages, or any other major bleeding, occurred in the heparin group. In the placebo group, two patients developed new intracerebral hemorrhages; one patient had a fatal pulmonary embolism; and two patients who already had an intracerebral hemorrhage at baseline died [10]. This trial, for the first time, provided unbiased evidence in favor of heparin to treat CVT.

The study methodology drew criticism. "We do not agree," wrote Jan Stam and colleagues in a letter to the *Lancet*, "with their conclusion that heparin can now be regarded as a proven effective and safe treatment for Cerebral Venous Sinus Thrombosis" [11]. The Dutch researchers from the Academic Medical Center in Amsterdam argued that the primary outcome measure used in the trial had low validity and that there was a risk of bias due to unblinding. If the trial results were dichotomized into good versus poor outcome, the difference was not statistically significant.

Jan Stam, who would later become one of the leading researchers in the field of CVT, was at that time an aspiring professor of neurology at the Academic Medical Center in Amsterdam. During his medical studies at the University of Utrecht, he had a particular interest in psychology, and specifically in the methodology and statistical analysis used in this field. He became interested in medicine in its broadest sense. He decided to train in tropical medicine at the Dutch Royal Tropical Institute. He then worked as a district medical officer at the Ministry of Health in Angola, setting up basic rural health care in Angola, which had recently become an independent state. After returning to the Netherlands, he worked at an addiction center in Amsterdam, before starting his neurology residency training at the Academic Medical Center in Amsterdam. During his residency, he started writing his PhD thesis under supervision of Prof. dr. Hans van Crevel. Van Crevel, a prominent neurologist, later became known for setting up the first neurological clinical trials in the Netherlands and revolutionizing stroke care in the country. Van Crevel had recently moved from Rotterdam to work in the Amsterdam clinic. He was particularly interested in clinimetrics, a field focusing on the reliability of clinical measurements. His work and his novel approach sparked the interest of Stam and led him to pursue research on the value of tendon reflexes in the neurological examination [12,13].

After his PhD, Stam's interest in CVT research was sparked by a single case. Despite extensive discussions and review of the available literature, neurologists could not agree on what treatment should be given. This triggered Stam to take matters into his own hands. As a seasoned neurologist and talented researcher – with a novel methodological basis learned from Van Crevel – he began his own research on CVT. Following the *Lancet* publication, he visited Einhäupl in Munich with colleagues from Amsterdam. He concluded that a new trial with a larger sample size, using modern methodological standards, was required. A contributing factor was the introduction of low-molecular-weight-heparin, which could be given subcutaneously instead of intravenously, and was easier to dose than unfractionated heparin.

The results of this double-blinded placebo-controlled multicenter trial containing 60 patients was published in 1999 [14]. The results were promising. Patients with CVT, also with intracranial hemorrhages, treated with low-molecular-weight heparin seemed to have better outcomes. There were no new intracranial hemorrhages in the anticoagulation arm, again showing safety of anticoagulation in these patients. The difference in outcome between the placebo and heparin arm, however, was not statistically significant [14,15].

Given the rarity of CVT, performing a new trial would have been extremely challenging [16]. Cerebral venous thrombosis became recognized more and more often after the advent of modern brain and vascular imaging. There was a need for practical guidelines for treating physicians. One of the most vocal and respected researchers on CVT at the time was Marie-Germaine Bousser. She referred to Stam's trial as unnecessary and "unethical," because in her opinion, it was already proven beyond doubt that heparin was the optimal therapy for CVT [13,17].

Bousser, the head of the neurology department and professor of neurology at Lariboisère hospital in Paris, was born in 1943 and graduated from Paris-Sorbonne University in neuropsychiatry in 1972. She spent a year at "the mecca for neurologists" – the National Hospital for Neurology and Neurosurgery at Queen Square in London – before returning to Paris. She had identified a new monogenetic hereditary cause of stroke: cerebral autosomal dominant arteriopathy with subcortical infarcts and leukoencephalopathy (CADASIL) [18]. She raised awareness about the problem of neurovascular diseases among women. Having served as the personal physician of Jacques Chirac during his stroke treatment in 2005, she was dubbed "the queen of neurology" and given many awards, including the French Legion of Honour [19,20]. Her long-term mentee

Valérie Biousse said that "she could be as helpful and kind, and spend as much time attending to the homeless who came in after an accident at Gare du Nord, as to the celebrities who came to seek her professional opinion" [19].

Bousser became interested in cerebral venous thrombosis. She wrote in 1999:

> Cerebral venous thrombosis is ... an infrequent condition that is extremely variable in its clinical presentation, mode of onset, imaging appearance, and outcome.... Its prognosis, although much better than classically thought, remains largely unpredictable.... It is thus not surprising that neurologists – many of whom have little experience with this condition – have not reached a consensus about treatment, particularly regarding the use of antithrombotic drugs. [17]

She clearly articulated her opinion on the heparin controversy:

> The new randomized trial of heparin has shown once again that heparin is safe and the benefit, although statistically not significant, is clinically relevant, particularly when combined with the results of the previous randomized trial. This indicates that as long as we are unable to predict which cerebral venous thrombosis patient will recover spontaneously, first, heparin is indicated whatever the clinical or neuroimaging pattern, and second, no placebo group should be included in further randomized trials. [17]

It had become clear that CVT research required larger numbers of patients in future studies to allow for more robust conclusions. This was achieved by the establishment of an International Study on Cerebral Vein and Dural Sinus Thrombosis (ISCVT) in which 89 centers from 21 participating countries participated, collecting data on more than 624 patients. ISCVT was led by the Portuguese neurologist José Ferro, and this study added supporting evidence for the efficacy and safety of heparin for the treatment of cerebral venous thrombosis [21]. Patients without anticoagulation had a higher frequency of thromboembolic complications; anticoagulated patients rarely had hemorrhagic complications.

In 2006, the joined forces of Einhäupl, Bousser, Stam, and Ferro, among others, produced the first treatment guidelines on cerebral venous thrombosis. Based on the available evidence, anticoagulation therapy was safe and outcomes were consistent and clinically relevant. The European Federation of the Neurological Sciences recommended use of either adjusted-dose unfractionated heparin or low-molecular-weight heparin to treat patients with cerebral vein thrombosis in the acute phase, regardless of presence of intracerebral hemorrhage [22].

LOW-MOLECULAR-WEIGHT HEPARIN VERSUS UNFRACTIONATED HEPARIN

Was there a superiority of low-molecular-weight heparin over unfractionated heparin? Although studies in deep vein thrombosis and pulmonary embolism had shown superiority of low-molecular-weight heparin in terms of safety and effectiveness in preventing complications, there was insufficient evidence of its use in cerebral venous thrombosis [23]. Heparin, although it required intravenous access, continuous laboratory monitoring, and dose adjustments, was quickly reversible, making it useful in unstable patients who might require surgery. Low-molecular-weight heparin was a new agent not often used by neurologists in clinical practice.

In a 2011 survey among treating physicians about their treatment preferences in cerebral venous thrombosis, 64 percent of physicians favored unfractionated heparin, as opposed to 36 percent who favored low-molecular-weight heparin. The ratio of low-molecular-weight heparin versus unfractionated heparin in this survey was the same as in the ISCVT study performed 10 years previously [24]. The ultimate choice was ultimately left to treating physicians.

THROMBOLYTIC AND ENDOVASCULAR TREATMENT

Anticoagulants, although safe and effective in preventing growth and formation of blood clots, could not dissolve blood clots already present in the venous system. Researchers began experimenting with thrombolytic therapies that could potentially rapidly recanalize affected veins and achieve better outcome. The first mention of thrombolytic treatments for cerebral venous thrombosis was in 1971 [25], followed by a study in 1988 that also showed promising results of intravenous thrombolytics [26]. Studies on systemic thrombolytics showed a high risk of intracranial hemorrhage. Given the safety concerns, a new solution was sought.

A small breakthrough occurred when a previously healthy 33-year-old with a progressive headache and transient syncopal episodes was admitted to a local hospital in Indiana in 1988. As his consciousness declined, he was transferred to the Indiana University Medical Center Hospital in Indianapolis. While in the helicopter, he became unresponsive. Cerebral arteriography revealed thrombosis of the superior sagittal, straight, and both lateral sinuses. In the operating room, an infusion catheter was inserted into the cerebral venous system and local urokinase infusion was administered. After eight hours, patency of the superior sagittal and left lateral sinuses was achieved. Although this treatment was complicated by an intracranial hemorrhage, the previously severely affected patient was discharged with only minor functional impairment [27]. During the ensuing years urokinase and recombinant tissue plasminogen activator (rt-PA) were infused into thrombosed dural sinuses [28]. Local thrombolysis recanalized clots and restored blood flow better than heparin. It was unclear whether these results translated into better clinical outcomes. For which patients was this treatment appropriate?

The next step was combining local thrombolysis with a mechanical technique of removing the clot [29]. Although this approach allowed for a decrease in the dose of fibrinolytic agents, it had a risk of damaging vessel walls [30]. This complex approach, initially tested in patients who did not respond adequately to anticoagulant therapy, had mixed results. The treatment was effective in some patients, but the risk of intracerebral hemorrhage remained an important concern [31]. The evidence, based on case series and retrospective studies, was not sufficient to justify the use of systemic or local thrombolysis with or without mechanical thrombectomy.

The TO-ACT trial was the first prospective randomized study that researched the effect of endovascular treatment in CVT. It included 67 patients, was terminated prematurely, and did not show an improved outcome in patients in the intervention group (mechanical thrombectomy, local infusion of urokinase or alteplase, or a combination of both) compared to standard care [32].

DECOMPRESSIVE HEMICRANIECTOMY

The most feared complication of cerebral venous thrombosis is transtentorial herniation, caused by mass effect from large venous infarctions and hemorrhages. If untreated, it ultimately results in brainstem compression and death. Although rare, it is the most fatal and the most common cause of death in CVT patients [33]. Patients with severely increased intracranial pressure should be treated quickly and aggressively. Decompressive hemicraniectomy, as an emergency procedure, has shown excellent results in reducing intracranial pressure and preventing brain herniation. Although no randomized clinical trial has been performed, it quickly became standard procedure in patients showing signs of transtentorial herniation [34].

ORAL ANTICOAGULATION IN THE SUBACUTE AND CHRONIC PHASE

In early reports of cerebral venous thrombosis, the main focus was on treatment during the acute phase. Stansfield wrote in his 1942 article, after four days of heparin treatment, that "the patient had apparently fully recovered." This same patient developed thrombophlebitis and cerebral symptoms less than a month later, which resolved with a second heparin treatment [3]. A 1989 report noted "mild or severe sequelae after discharge" in four out of 20 patients

[35]. Stam and Einhäupl also observed fatal pulmonary embolism in their trials. CVT patients are at increased risk of recurrent venous thrombotic events (VTEs) in the cerebral veins and dural sinuses, veins of the limbs, and splanchnic veins, and pulmonary embolism [21]. To prevent these complications, physicians agreed that anticoagulation treatment should be continued after the acute phase.

The guideline by Einhäupl, Stam, Bousser, et al. extrapolated the recommendation developed for deep vein thrombosis patients [22]. The length of oral anticoagulation depended on the cause of thrombosis. Patients with CVT due to trauma, infection, or other transient risk factors would receive oral anticoagulants for three months; patients with unknown causes would receive it for six months; while "severe" thrombophilia patients were recommended lifelong anticoagulant treatment [22].

The first widely used oral anticoagulants were vitamin K antagonists. After administration of heparin in the acute phase, warfarin and acenocoumarol were the most commonly chosen anticoagulants in the post-acute phase. This practice continued for more than 50 years. The introduction of direct non–vitamin K oral anticoagulants (DOAC) changed clinical practice. Their superior safety profile and ease of use without need for laboratory measurements made DOACs a study target. In a survey performed between 2018 and 2019, 23 percent of physicians reported that they used DOAC in CVT patients with transient risk factors [36]. Although underpowered, the first randomized trial on dabigatran in cerebral venous thrombosis indicated that dabigatran was a safe and effective alternative to warfarin [37]. Studies performed with other DOACs have also shown promising results [38].

NOTES AND REFERENCES

1. Ribes MF. Des recherches faites sur la phlebite. In *Revue Médicale Francaise et Etrangere et Journal de Clinique de l'Hotel-Dieu et de la Charité de Paris.* 1825, vol. 3, pp. 5–41.

2. Plarr's Lives of the Fellows. Frederick Ross Stansfield. The Royal College of Surgeons of England. Available at https://livesonline.rcseng.ac.uk/client/en_GB/lives/search/detailnonmodal/ent:$002f$002fSD_ASSET$002f0$002fSD_ASSET:379868/one.

3. Stansfield FR. Puerperal cerebral thrombophlebitis treated by heparin. *Br. Med. J.* 1942;1(4239):436–438.

4. Ronald Arthur Jones. Royal College of Physicians. Available at https://history.rcplondon.ac.uk/inspiring-physicians/ronald-arthur-jones.

5. Crafoord C. Preliminary report on post-operative treatment with heparin as a preventive of thrombosis. *Acta Chir. Scand.* 1937(79):407–426.

6. Van Creveld S, De Bruyne JI, Stronk MG. [Thrombosis of the superior sinus longitudinalis in an infant treated with heparin and intravenous fluid supply]. *Ned. Tijdschr. Geneeskd.* 1949;93(15):1144–1148.

7. Holub K. [Intracranial venous thrombosis and thrombophlebitis]. *Wien Klin. Wochenschr.* 1953;65(26):540–541.

8. Cairns DR, Melton G. Thrombosis of cerebral veins in the puerperium. *Br. Med. J.* 1942;1(4239):439.

9. Ehrenmitgliedschaft Prof. Dr. Karl Max Einhäupl. Charite – Universitätsmedizin Berlin. Available at https://alumni.charite.de/start_unterseiten/prof_dr_k_m_ein haeupl_ehrenmitglied/.

10. Einhäupl KM, Villringer A, Meister W, Mehraein S, Garner C, Pellkofer M, et al. Heparin treatment in sinus venous thrombosis. *Lancet* 1991;338(8767):597–600.

11. Stam J, Lensing AWA, Vermeulen M, Tijssen JGP. Heparin treatment for cerebral venous and sinus thrombosis. *Lancet* 1991;338(8775):1154.

12. Vermeulen M, Stam J, Hijdra A, van Gijn J. In memoriam Prof. Dr. H. van Crevel. August 26, 2002. Available at www.ntvg.nl/artikelen/memoriam-profdrhvan-crevel/volledig.

13. Based on an interview with Prof. dr. Jan Stam.

14. de Bruijn SF, Stam J. Randomized, placebo-controlled trial of anticoagulant treatment with low-molecular-weight heparin for cerebral sinus thrombosis. *Stroke* 1999;30 (3):484–488.

15. Coutinho JM, Stam J. How to treat cerebral venous and sinus thrombosis. *J. Thromb. Haemost.* 2010;8(5):877–883.

16. Stam J, De Bruijn SF, DeVeber G. Anticoagulation for cerebral sinus thrombosis. *Cochrane Database Syst Rev.* 2002(4):Cd002005. Stam J. Thrombosis of the cerebral veins and sinuses. *N. Engl. J. Med.* 2005;352(17):1791–1798. Stam J, de Bruijn S, deVeber G. Anticoagulation for cerebral sinus thrombosis. *Stroke* 2003;34 (4):1054–1055.

17. Bousser MG. Cerebral venous thrombosis: Nothing, heparin, or local thrombolysis? *Stroke* 1999;30(3):481–483.

18. Bousser MG, Eschwege E, Haguenau M. Aspirin and stroke prevention. *Lancet* 1988;1 (8578):179.

19. Cabut S. Marie-Germaine Bousser, reine de la neurologie. *Le Monde*, January 3, 2013. Available at www.lemonde.fr/sciences/article/2013/01/03/marie-germaine-bousser-reine-de-la-neurologie_1812632_1650684.html.

20. The Brain Prize: Marie-Germaine Bousser. Lundbeckfonden. Available at https://lundbeckfonden.com/marie-germaine-bousser. The education and career of Dr. Bousser is also included in Chapter 21.

21. Ferro JM, Canhão P, Stam J, Bousser MG, Barinagarrementeria F. Prognosis of cerebral vein and dural sinus thrombosis: Results of the International Study on Cerebral Vein and Dural Sinus Thrombosis (ISCVT). *Stroke* 2004;35(3):664–670.

22. Einhäupl K, Stam J, Bousser MG, De Bruijn SF, Ferro JM, Martinelli I, et al. EFNS guideline on the treatment of cerebral venous and sinus thrombosis in adult patients. *Eur. J. Neurol.* 2010;17(10):1229–1235.

23. The Columbus Investigators. Low-molecular-weight heparin in the treatment of patients with venous thromboembolism. *N. Engl. J. Med.* 1997;337(10):657–662. van den Belt AGM, Prins MH, Lensing AWA, Castro AA, Clark OAC, Atallah AN, et al. Fixed dose subcutaneous low molecular weight heparins versus adjusted dose unfractionated heparin for venous thromboembolism. *Cochrane Database of Systematic Reviews* 1999;4.

24. Coutinho JM, Seelig R, Bousser MG, Canhão P, Ferro JM, Stam J. Treatment variations in cerebral venous thrombosis: An international survey. *Cerebrovasc. Dis.* 2011;32(3):298–300.

25. Vines FS, Davis DO. Clinical-radiological correlation in cerebral venous occlusive disease. *Radiology* 1971;98(1):9–22.

26. Di Rocco C, Iannelli A, Leone G, Moschini M, Valori VM. Heparin-urokinase treatment in aseptic dural sinus thrombosis. *Arch. Neurol.* 1981;38(7):431–435.

27. Scott JA, Pascuzzi RM, Hall PV, Becker GJ. Treatment of dural sinus thrombosis with local urokinase infusion: Case report. *J. Neurosurg.* 1988;68(2):284–287.

28. Kim SY, Suh JH. Direct endovascular thrombolytic therapy for dural sinus thrombosis: Infusion of alteplase. *AJNR Am. J. Neuroradiol.* 1997;18(4):639–645.

29. Caso V, Billeci AM, Leys D. Interventional neuroradiology in the treatment of cerebral venous thrombosis. *Front. Neurol. Neurosci.* 2008;23:144–160.

30. Coutinho JM, van den Berg R, Zuurbier SM, Majoie CB, Stam J. Mechanical thrombectomy cannot be considered as first-line treatment for cerebral venous thrombosis. *J. Neurointerv. Surg.* 2013;5(6):621–622.

31. Stam J, Majoie CB, van Delden OM, van Lienden KP, Reekers JA. Endovascular thrombectomy and thrombolysis for severe cerebral sinus thrombosis: A prospective study. *Stroke* 2008;39(5):1487–1490.

32. Coutinho JM, Zuurbier SM, Bousser MG, Ji X, Canhão P, Roos YB, et al. Effect of endovascular treatment with medical management vs standard care on severe cerebral venous thrombosis: The TO-ACT randomized clinical trial. *JAMA Neurol.* 2020;77 (8):966–973.

33. Canhão P, Ferro JM, Lindgren AG, Bousser MG, Stam J, Barinagarrementeria F. Causes and predictors of death in cerebral venous thrombosis. *Stroke* 2005;36 (8):1720–1725.

34. Ferro JM, Bousser M-G, Canhão P, Coutinho JM, Crassard I, Dentali F, et al. European Stroke Organization guideline for the diagnosis and treatment of cerebral venous thrombosis – Endorsed by the European Academy of Neurology. *European J. Neurol.* 2017;24(10):1203–1213.

35. Milandre L, Gueriot C, Girard N, Ali Cherif A, Khalil R. [Cerebral venous thrombosis in adults. Diagnostic and therapeutic aspects in 20 cases]. *Ann. Med. Interne (Paris)* 1989;139(8):544–554.

36. Riva N, Carrier M, Gatt A, Ageno W. Anticoagulation in splanchnic and cerebral vein thrombosis: An international vignette-based survey. *Res. Pract. Thromb. Haemost.* 2020;4(7):1192–1202.

37. Ferro JM, Coutinho JM, Dentali F, Kobayashi A, Alasheev A, Canhão P, et al. Safety and efficacy of dabigatran etexilate vs dose-adjusted warfarin in patients with cerebral venous thrombosis: A randomized clinical trial. *JAMA Neurol.* 2019;76(12):1457–1465.

38. Lurkin A, Derex L, Fambrini A, Bertoletti L, Epinat M, Mismetti P, et al. Direct oral anticoagulants for the treatment of cerebral venous thrombosis. *Cerebrovasc. Dis.* 2019;48(1–2):32–37.

CHAPTER FIFTY THREE

RECOVERY AND REHABILITATION

Physical medicine and rehabilitation emerged as a specialty during the first half of the twentieth century. Significant growth and development was stimulated by two world wars and epidemics of paralytic poliomyelitis. Physicians and therapists were needed to treat soldiers returning from war with serious injuries and chronic disabling conditions. The availability of antibiotics and improved surgical techniques during World War II allowed more injured soldiers to survive, albeit with significant disabilities. Among civilians, severe epidemics of polio and industrial and motor vehicle accidents were major causes of disability. These events necessitated the development of new restorative treatment programs incorporating new physical and rehabilitative techniques, and establishment of training programs for physicians and therapists to administer treatments [1].

The Father of Physical Medicine

Frank Hammond Krusen (1898–1973) is widely regarded as the "Father of Physical Medicine." He influenced this developing field in the United States and internationally during the 1930s and 1940s. Krusen graduated from Jefferson Medical College in Philadelphia in 1921. His planned surgical career was interrupted when he developed pulmonary tuberculosis in 1924. He became interested in physical medicine during convalescence in a sanatorium. He realized that physical deconditioning increased dependence and eroded self-esteem. Krusen believed that self-esteem and independence could be restored in patients with disabilities with appropriate physical reconditioning, vocational rehabilitation, and reintegration into society [1].

Krusen returned to Philadelphia in 1926 and was appointed associate dean at Temple Medical School, where he started the first academic department of physical medicine in 1929. In 1930, Krusen published an undergraduate curriculum in physical medicine. Krusen moved to the Mayo Clinic in Rochester, Minnesota, in 1935, where he founded the department of physical medicine, developed the first three-year residency program in physical medicine, and opened a school of physical therapy. During World War II, he helped train a large cadre of medical officers from the US Armed Forces with 90-day intensive courses in physical medicine at Mayo Graduate School of Medicine. Trainees were labeled "90-day wonders" [1].

Krusen served as an organizational leader for the specialty during the late 1930s and through the 1940s. With William Bierman and John S. Coulter, Krusen established the American Registry of Physical Therapy Technicians. Krusen and Coulter founded the Society of Physical Therapy Physicians, and Krusen was elected its first president. Krusen wrote the first widely used textbook of physical medicine, *Physical Medicine: The Employment of Physical Agents for Diagnosis and Therapy*. Krusen played a critical role in the founding and initial leadership of the Baruch Committee of Physical Medicine, the American Board of Physical Medicine and Rehabilitation (1947), and the International Federation of Physical Medicine (1952) [1].

The Polio Epidemic and Rehabilitation

The first epidemic of poliomyelitis in the United States in 1916 involved 27,000 cases nationwide and around 6,000 deaths. Many survivors were left with lifelong disabilities. Epidemics progressively increased during the 1940s and early 1950s. The worst epidemic in 1952 resulted in about 58,000 cases of paralytic poliomyelitis. Polio epidemics led to major advances in respiratory management (such as development of the "iron lung") and physical therapy. It established the role of physicians in managing neuromuscular conditions, especially limb and respiratory weakness, contractures, and gait disorders [1].

Franklin Delano Roosevelt (1882–1945), the most famous polio victim, played an important role in the development of rehabilitation medicine. He contracted the disease in the summer of 1921 and was paralyzed from the waist down. Despite his disability, he was elected president of the United States in 1932. He helped remove some of the social stigma of physical disability, provided inspiration and hope, promoted the idea that polio victims should be seen as equal to those without disabilities, and provided a mechanism for widespread supportive social action and philanthropy. In 1927, Roosevelt founded the Georgia Warm Springs Foundation, which helped develop physical therapy and rehabilitation approaches for polio patients. In 1937, the foundation was reorganized as the National Foundation for Infantile Paralysis and was directed by Roosevelt's former law partner, D. Basil O'Connor. This foundation organized a highly successful fundraising campaign utilizing an annual "President's Birthday Ball." This campaign was labeled "The March of Dimes." It generated extraordinary interest and raised an unprecedented $268,000 in 1938. The National Foundation led the "first large-scale, nationwide biomedical initiative" by a charitable organization and was instrumental in subsidizing hospital and rehabilitation costs of polio patients, funding basic and applied research concerning the causes and prevention of polio in the 1940s and early 1950s, training nurses and physical therapists, sponsoring pilot programs to improve the teaching of rehabilitation medicine in medical schools, and ultimately underwriting the Salk vaccine field trial in 1954 [1].

The Father of Comprehensive Rehabilitation Medicine

The Association of Academic Physiatrists designated Howard Rusk the "Father of Rehabilitation Medicine" and Krusen the "Father of Physical Medicine." In 1942, Rusk left his well-established private internal medicine practice in St. Louis to join the Army Air Corps, as chief of Medical services at the 1,000-bed Jefferson Barracks in St. Louis. There he observed much boredom among patients, and a high rate of readmission because patients were not physically fit enough to return to active duty after hospital discharge, even though they no longer needed hospitalization. Rusk engaged patients in mental and physical restorative and training activities that used their time efficiently, increased their fitness, and decreased recidivism. Rusk's approach to rehabilitation emphasized treating the "whole person," including their emotional, psychological, and social needs and not only the illness or specific disability. His experience with rehabilitation of wounded soldiers during World War II established the concept of comprehensive rehabilitation [1].

Rehabilitation programs were limited before World War II. Many believed that people with disabilities could not become productive. Individuals with strokes and other brain and spinal cord injuries received at best custodial care and often died within a short time [1]. "The old wives' tale was that you had one stroke, and then you sat around waiting for a second one, or a third one, or however many it took to kill you. If you had any kind of brain injury affecting your locomotive functions, everyone assumed your life was finished" [1,2].

In 1945, Rusk joined New York University Medical School, and combined the two separate programs of physical and occupational therapy into a new department of rehabilitation medicine. He hired George Deaver from New York's Institute of Crippled and Disabled Men as the medical director. By 1947, Rusk and Deaver had established the "first comprehensive, total medical rehabilitation program in any community hospital" at New York's Bellevue Hospital. Rusk gained the support of prominent philanthropists and founded the Institute of Physical Medicine and Rehabilitation at NYU Medical Center in 1951. This institute is now the largest university-affiliated center for treatment of civilians with disabilities and for research and training in rehabilitation medicine [1].

Rusk worked tirelessly to promote the nascent field of rehabilitation and to increase public awareness of the need for rehabilitation through numerous speeches and consultations across the country and around the world. Rusk received many awards and honors for his work, including three Lasker Awards.

Evolution of Stroke Rehabilitation

During the late nineteenth and early twentieth century, most medical investigations concerning stroke dealt with clinical phenomenology, pathology, clinicopathologic correlation, and pathophysiology. Very little was attempted to rehabilitate stroke patients. The antecedents of rehabilitation available in the early twentieth century included, for example, the tedious repetition of reading, spelling, repeated words for aphasia; passive movement of severely paralyzed limbs and programs of exercises for less severe paralysis; various orthotic and assistive devices, such as splints to prevent contractures, light braces for support, canes, crutches, and wheelchairs; use of electrical stimulation to facilitate recovery or prevent muscle wasting; and various surgical procedures to limit contractures or spasticity [1].

Rehabilitation of stroke patients was not systematically developed until the second half of the twentieth century. In the 1970s and 1980s, the stroke rehabilitation team approach began to develop and spread. Stroke units sometimes allowed a seamless transition between acute care and rehabilitation. They were developed in larger hospitals in urban areas. Outpatient rehabilitation resources were developed, including services provided by health departments, visiting nurse associations, freestanding day care centers, and hospital-associated and independent physical therapy practices [1].

NEUROPLASTICITY AND NEUROREHABILITATION

Views about the plasticity of the mature mammalian central nervous system (CNS) and the possibility of improvement in functional impairments in the chronic phase following substantial damage to the CNS were fixed and rarely questioned for most of the twentieth century. Potential for CNS recovery was thought to be confined to immature organisms. In adults, the structure of the brain and spinal cord was considered hard-wired and unchanging, no matter what rehabilitation or environmental influence was applied after CNS damage. This belief originated after the work of Broca on anatomic localization of motor function in the brain and was most prominently stated by Santiago Ramon y Cajal. Alternate views were periodically expressed but were a minority. An important challenge to the standard view was discovery of collateral intraspinal sprouting of dorsal root axons after spinal cord damage. The establishment of synaptic connections in the brain by similar sprouted fibers was shown later. For a quarter of a century after the discovery of collateral intraspinal sprouting, there was no clear demonstration that its occurrence in the brain had important significance for recovery of motor or sensory function of adult mammals. There was no compelling evidence-based reason to change the prevailing view of an anatomically fixed brain [3].

The classic views on the lack of modifiability of the CNS after damage and the persistence of functional deficits were overturned by the experiments of Edward Taub [3]. As Taub worked toward transforming stroke rehabilitation at his lab at Silver Spring, his animals became the most famous lab animals in the history of research.

The Silver Spring Monkeys, Constraint-Induced Movement Therapy, and the Animal Rights Movement

Edward Taub was born in 1931 in Brooklyn. He studied behaviorism under Fred Keller at Columbia University. He became a research assistant in a neurology lab and became involved in primate deafferentation experiments.. Deafferentation involves opening the spinal cord and cutting sensory afferent nerves [4–6].

With the help of a neurosurgeon, Taub deafferented limbs of monkeys on one side, while keeping the other side intact. After deafferenting limbs on one side, monkeys were unable to perceive pain, touch, or temperature sensations in those limbs. They began treating the deafferented limbs as if they were detached from their bodies and were foreign objects. Since monkeys did not feel pain, they injured their arms and even tried biting them. The monkeys used only their good arms for feeding and other purposes. Taub described it as the "learned non-use" of the deafferented arm, for it developed during conditioned suppression of movement [4,7].

Although the procedure involved severing only sensory nerves, afterward both the sensory and motor neurons in the spinal cord were unable to fire for about a period of two to six months while the spinal cord was in a state of shock. Recovery from "spinal shock" required considerable time. Use of the affected extremity during this time led to incoordination and falling, loss of food items, and failure of all activities. Monkeys gradually learned to balance on three limbs and used the intact arm for eating. Poor function associated with using the deafferented limb and positive enforcement when using the unaffected good limb led to learned non-use of the deafferented limb. Even when motor function returned in the deafferented limb after a few months, monkeys were not able to learn that the limb was again potentially useful [4,7].

Taub conducted a series of deafferentation experiments. In one experiment, he constrained the use of the unaffected limb by applying a sling. The monkey was forced to use the deafferented limb to reach for food. In another experiment, he deafferented both arms of a monkey and to his surprise the monkey used both limbs. In another experiment, instead of constraining the good limb, he constrained the deafferented limb during the period of spinal shock. When he removed the sling three months later, the monkey was able to learn to use the limb. He applied the concept of learned non-use to stroke patients and developed Constraint-Induced Movement Therapy (CIMT) [4,7].

While undergoing CIMT therapy the unaffected upper extremity is restricted using a mitt or sling. The individual is encouraged to perform various task-based activities with the affected arm. The unaffected arm is restricted for about 90 percent of waking hours for two weeks. Task-related activity using the affected arm is encouraged for six hours daily. Therapy begins with single-joint movement and then gradually proceeds to more complex movements involving multiple joints, such as reaching to grasp a cup of coffee. Repetitive use of the affected arm is more important than restraining the unaffected arm. Steve Wolf at Emory University and Carolee Winstein of the University of Southern California later showed the effectiveness of CIMT in helping stroke patients regain movement [8]. Besides overcoming learned non-use, use stimulates the brain to reorganize [7,8].

While Taub worked toward transforming stroke rehabilitation at his Silver Spring, Maryland, lab, the "Silver Spring monkeys" in his lab became the prime target of the People for Ethical Treatment of Animals (PETA) activist group [4,9]. In May 1981, Taub was approached by Alex Pacheco, a graduate student at George Washington University, to volunteer in his lab. Pacheco, the son of a doctor, was raised in Mexico and initially wanted to become a priest. He underwent a major transformation after visiting a slaughterhouse and reading Peter Singer's *Animal Liberation*. He stopped eating meat and collaborated with Ingrid Newkirk, a local poundmaster, to form PETA in 1980. To gain experience in an animal research lab, he decided to work in one. He chose Taub's lab as it was nearest to his home and was government funded. Taub offered him an unpaid lab position. Norman Doidge wrote, "When Pacheco volunteered to work with Taub, his goal was to free the seventeen

Silver Spring Monkeys and make them a rallying cry for an animal rights campaign" [4,9].

During the summer of 1981 when Taub was away for three weeks, Pacheco grabbed the opportunity and took pictures of the lab depicting filthy living conditions of the animals. He alleged that the monkey cages had not been cleaned for ages and that they were filled with feces and urine. He said that the monkeys were underfed. Since the monkeys could not feel their limbs, they were severely injured. Most injuries were self-inflicted as the animals tried to bite their arms, now foreign to them. He said that no one bandaged them or applied antibiotics. He persuaded Maryland authorities and the local police to raid the lab and seize the monkeys. The raid received extensive media coverage and presented Taub as atrocious and barbaric [4,9].

When Taub returned, he was arrested and charged with 119 counts. The NIH, fearful of being PETA's next target, turned against Taub and suspended his $115,000 research grant. Taub faced many consequences, including life threats to him and his wife [4,9]. Taub argued that he was framed and that his lab had been clean when he left for vacation and that Pacheco himself had failed to clean the cages in his absence, neglected the animals, and presented false reports. He said that during his vacation, two employees who cleaned the lab and fed the animals were absent. On three of those absentee days, Pacheco brought people to view the monkeys [4,9].

The police gave custody of the monkeys to Lori Kenealy, of the local humane society, who kept them in her basement. The monkeys were official evidence and Taub and his lawyers demanded the monkeys' return, a request granted by the court. The monkeys suddenly disappeared from Kenealy's home. PETA was informed that Taub could not be prosecuted without the monkeys. The monkeys suddenly returned after a holiday in Florida, and were returned to Taub. After Taub's first trial, 113 out of 119 charges against him were dismissed. He secured a second trial and was exculpated when the court ruled that Maryland's Prevention of Cruelty to Animals law did not apply to federally funded laboratories. Some 67 American professional societies made representations on his behalf to the NIH, which reversed its decision and supported him. Taub was hired by the University of Alabama and received a grant to study stroke. He opened a clinic where he developed and practiced his Constraint-Induced Movement Therapy [4,5].

During the early 1980s, animal rights organizations also targeted head injury research at the University of Pennsylvania. PETA produced a film that showed a hydraulic device striking the heads of unanesthetized but sedated baboons whose wrists and ankles were tied and strapped to a table. Their heads were secured inside helmets [10]. The experiments were conducted by neurosurgeons as part of a research project into head injuries such as were caused in vehicle accidents. The footage was edited down to 26 minutes by Alex

Pacheco and narrated by Ingrid Newkirk, and was then distributed to the media and Congress. After a four-day sit-in by animal rights activists at NIH, the Secretary of Health and Human Services ordered suspension of the annual $1 million NIH grant supporting the baboon research [10].

Following Taub, many scientists began exploring the concept of neuroplasticity. The concept of neuroplasticity states that the brain has the ability to reorganize itself based on the stimuli it receives. Blind individuals have increased sensitivity to touch. Deaf dancers are still able to dance on beat, sensing vibrations produced by speakers. When visual stimuli from the eyes cease, visual areas in the occipital lobe can assume other functions by changing neuronal connections. When a brain region is damaged by stroke, the surrounding areas of the brain have the potential to reorganize by forming new connections that assume the function of a damaged segment [4].

The Silver Spring monkeys were viewed as a valuable resource to prove this concept. Scientists wanted to study neuroplastic changes that might have developed in the brains of the monkeys after they were deprived of sensory inputs from their limbs for 12 years after deafferentation. The monkeys were in custody at the NIH. As the monkeys grew old, they became sick and were dying. NIH scientists proposed a final set of experiments under deep anesthesia, which were to be followed by euthanization. One of the monkeys was anesthetized, a part of his skull was removed, and electrodes were inserted in the sensory cortex arm area. When scientists stroked the monkey's arm, as expected, no signals were sent to the electrodes. But when they stroked the monkey's face, the neurons in the monkey's deafferented arm began to fire, confirming that the facial map had supplanted the arm map. This brain reorganization developed over an area of 14 millimeters, the largest that was ever mapped [4].

Cortical reorganization could be achieved by providing continual stimuli to the brain by exercising damaged limbs and restraining unaffected limbs. Many people benefited from CIMT at Taub's clinic. Taub developed a computerized version of his therapy called AutoCITE for those who could not visit his clinic. His therapy showed some effect even in individuals who enrolled years after their debilitating stroke [4].

EMERGING THERAPIES FOR STROKE REHABILITATION

Noninvasive Brain Stimulation

Noninvasive brain stimulation (NIBS) involves applying weak electrical or magnetic fields to the brain via the surface of the scalp with the goal of changing or normalizing brain activity. The aim is to modify cortical activity through an increase in ipsilateral cortical excitability and/or a decrease in contralesional cortical excitability [11]. This approach is based on the inter-hemispheric competition model wherein functional recovery in stroke patients is hindered due to reduced output from the affected hemisphere and excessive transcallosal inhibition from the unaffected hemisphere [12].

The two most common forms of stimulation are transcranial magnetic stimulation (TMS) and transcranial direct current stimulation (tDCS). Transcranial magnetic stimulation uses a rapidly changing magnetic field to induce electric currents in the brain, causing neuronal depolarization and action potentials. Transcranial direct current stimulation uses a small, battery-powered device to deliver weak electric currents (usually 1–2 milliamps) to the brain via saline-soaked sponges placed over stimulation sites. Depending on the technique used, the direction of the neuromodulatory effect (i.e., increase or decrease in cortical excitability) is achieved by altering the stimulus frequency, changing the pattern of stimulation, or reversing the polarity of the electrodes. In recent years, the feasibility and effectiveness of NIBS in modulating cortical excitability and in facilitating motor recovery after stroke has been studied. TMS and tDCS are safe and effective in modulating cortical excitability and can enhance motor adaptation and learning and influence motor memory consolidation in healthy adults and stroke patients [11].

Mirror Neurons and Mirror Box Therapy

A relatively new concept that has stimulated rehabilitative strategies relates to discovery and popularization of "mirror neurons" by Rizzolatti and colleagues [13]. These nerve cells located in one cerebral hemisphere discharge during activity of their contralateral cerebral hemisphere counterparts during various physical actions and also while observing performance of actions. This system is used during learning to imitate novel complex actions and in internal rehearsal of actions. Mental practice of doing actions and tasks and observing others performing tasks can be combined with physical activity to enhance recovery.

The concept of "learned paralysis" states that visual feedback of immobility after a stroke reinforces acquired knowledge that the limb cannot move. As the brain constantly sees that the limb does not move with the motor output sent to it, the representation of that limb in the sensory cortex progressively shrinks. The spared neurons for that region gradually reorganize, leading to further impairment of that limb. This concept is different from Taub's "learned non-use," which postulated that it was simply the non-use that led to cortical reorganization. His therapeutic intervention was based on restricting the good arm. Therapy for learned paralysis, however, involves sending false visual feedback to the brain. The brain is shown and made to believe that the paralyzed arm is functional again. This is achieved by using a mirror and a box [11,14,15].

Mirror box therapy or mirror visual feedback was developed by V. S. Ramachandran, originally to help people with phantom limb pain, where the patient would feel constant pain from an amputated limb. A mirror box has two mirrors in the center, one facing each way. The patient places the good limb into one side and the affected limb into the other. The patient looks into the mirror on the side with the good limb and performs symmetric movements of both limbs, such as trying to lift both hands up. As the patient sees the reflection of the good hand moving, it appears as if the paralyzed hand is also moving. Using this artificial feedback, the patient regains some control over the paralyzed limb and may be able, for example, to unclench it from uncomfortable positions [14].

The reflection of the working limb stimulates movement in a weak or paralyzed limb after stroke. By watching the mirror image of the good arm, the brain begins to form neural connections and new pathways that help in recovery of function of the paralyzed limb. The major advantage of this therapy is that it is easy to establish and can be practiced at home. Various trials have shown that this therapy is a useful adjunct to conventional therapy [11,15].

Melodic Intonation Therapy

Physicians observed that patients with nonfluent aphasia often can sing words that they cannot speak. Melodic Intonation Therapy (MIT) is a music-based treatment that uses melody and rhythm to improve aphasic patients' fluency. It capitalizes on preserved function (singing) and engaging language-capable regions in the undamaged right cerebral hemisphere. Aphasic individuals intone or sing two- to three-syllable phrases and progress to speaking more than five syllables during three levels of treatment. Each level consists of 20 high probability words or social phrases presented with visual cues. The therapist begins by humming a phrase while tapping the patient's hand. The therapist then sings the phrase while tapping the patient's hand. This is followed by the therapist and the patient singing the phrase together along with hand tapping, The therapist next fades away while the patient continues to sing the phrase; hand tapping is continued. Next, the therapist sings the phrase and then the patient repeats it, assisted only by hand tapping. Finally, the therapist intones a question, and the patient answers by intoning the target phrase. Hand tapping is the only form of assistance, without any facial or visual cues [16].

As the therapy progresses from elementary to advanced level the phrases become more complex. For instance, the individual would start by singing, "I love you," will then progress to singing, "I love my children," and finally to "I love my son and daughter" in the advanced level [16].

Stroke a Chord is a choir in Melbourne, Australia, comprised of stroke patients who have lost the ability to talk but can sing. Research exploring the impact of participation in musical activities showed that music enhances general mobility, social interaction, and social stability and decreases depression and anxiety [17].

Pharmacological Agents

Researchers have explored the use of pharmacological agents to enhance recovery [18]. The most frequently tried agents were noradrenergic or dopaminergic, including amphetamine, methylphenidate, amantidine, memantine, bromcriptine, and carbidopa/levodopa. The most favorable results have come from the use of selective serotonin reuptake inhibitors (SSRI). Fluoxetine, an SSRI developed in 1974, was approved by the FDA in 1987 for use in treating depression. Early animal studies indicated that drugs that modulate brain amine concentrations influence the rate and degree of recovery from cortical lesions. Many trials showed that SSRIs were effective in treating or preventing post-stroke depression. Some studies of SSRIs after stroke also reported outcomes such as neurologic recovery, functional recovery, and independence with daily activities, with mixed results [11].

Researchers have also explored administration of various growth factors. Growth factors are polypeptide proteins that influence cell growth, maturation, and division and have an important role in the response to stroke [18]. Brain levels of many growth factors increase after stroke. Basic fibroblastic growth factor (bFGF), brain-derived neurotrophic factor (BDNF), vascular endothelial growth factor (VEGF), erythropoietin (EPO), and granulocyte colony-stimulating factor (GCSF) have all shown promise in experimental studies of brain ischemia [18]. The challenge has been when and how to introduce these factors into brain ischemic regions.

Robotics

Robot-assisted therapy has been shown to enhance motor recovery. A robot is a mechanical device, guided by a computer, that senses or moves within its environment. Robots are devices that perform repetitive movements and measurements according to design and programming. Robotic devices have potential advantages such as consistent output, programmability, ability to precisely measure patient behavior, and reducing the requirement for constant therapist supervision. Many different robotic devices have been designed [18]. Potential applications include lower extremity, gait, and sensory deficits.

Stem Cell Therapy

Stem cell therapy is an exciting emerging area of research in the clinical arena of stroke therapy. Animal studies have shown promising results in induced models of stroke, although transition to the bedside is still in infancy. The definitive methods and guidelines pertaining to the choice of cell type to be used, cell numbers to be given, optimum timing of treatment, and optimum route of delivery are yet to be established [19].

Clinical approaches to stem cell therapy in stroke can be broadly divided into endogenous and exogenous approaches. The endogenous approach aims to stimulate mobilization of primitive cells already present within the individual. Examples of this approach include the use of granulocyte colony-stimulating factor (GCSF), which is routinely used to mobilize stem cells for transplantation in hematological malignancies. GCSF has been shown to be beneficial in rodent models of stroke (exhibiting neuroprotective and neuroregenerative activities) and to be safe in phase I clinical trials of human stroke when used within 7 days, or 7–30 days poststroke. A number of phase II trials are currently underway to investigate its efficacy in patients with ischemic stroke [19].

The exogenous approach involves transplantation of stem cells delivered locally (e.g., direct intracerebral implantation) or systemically (e.g., intravenous). This may involve in vitro culture of cells for the expansion of cell numbers before admission. Stem cells are classified into two major types based on their source: embryonic stem (ES) cells and adult stem cells. Human ES cells are pluripotent and isolated from five-day-old human blastocysts. The major limiting factors to their widespread use are ethical concerns regarding the use of unwanted embryos and the ability of ES cells to form teratomas [19].

Adult stem cells are multipotent stem cells found in developed organisms that are used to replace cells that have died or lost function. They have been identified within many different organ systems, including bone marrow, brain, heart, skin, and bone. They are usually quiescent and held in an undifferentiated state until they receive a stimulus to differentiate [19].

Stem cell therapy for ischemic stroke focuses on a regenerative strategy to restore not only neural elements but also supporting structures such as blood vessels. A variety of stem cell types from humans have been tested in stroke, in both experimental and clinical studies. Some of these are neural stem cells (NSCs), which occur in discrete areas of mammalian adult brain throughout life, giving rise to new population of neurons and glia; the NT2 cell line, an immortalized cell line derived from a human teratocarcinoma; and bone marrow–derived stem cells, which consist of both hematopoietic stem cells (HSCs) and mesenchymal stem cells (MSCs) [19]. Douglas Kondziolka, Gary Steinberg, Larry Wechsler, Sean Savitz, and Steve Cramer have led research into applying stem cell treatment to stroke care and recovery.

NOTES AND REFERENCES

1. Lanska DJ. The historical origins of stroke rehabilitation. In Stein J, Harvey RL, Macko RF, Winstein CJ, Zorowitz RD (eds.), *Stroke Recovery and Rehabilitation*. New York: Demos Medical Publishing, 2009, pp. 3–30.

2. Rusk HA. *A World to Care For: The Autobiography of Howard A. Rusk, M.D.* Random House, 1972.

3. Taub E. Foreword for neuroplasticity and neurorehabilitation. *Front. Hum. Neurosci.* 2014 Jul 24;8. Available at www.ncbi.nlm.nih.gov/pmc/articles/PMC4109562/.

4. Doidge N. *The Brain That Changes Itself: Stories of Personal Triumph from the Frontiers of Brain Science.* Penguin UK, 2008.

5. Edward Taub. Wikipedia. Available at https://en.wikipedia.org/w/index.php?title=Edward_Taub&oldid=85886212.

6. Over the Horizon. The Brain That Changes Itself – Full documentary. YouTube. May 26, 2013. Available at www.youtube.com/watch?v=bFCOm1P_cQQ.

7. Taub E, Uswatte G. Constraint-induced movement therapy: Bridging from the primate laboratory to the stroke rehabilitation laboratory. *J. Rehabil. Med.* 2003 May; (41 Suppl):34–40.

8. Kwakkel G, Veerbeek JM, van Wegen EEH, Wolf SL. Constraint-induced movement therapy after stroke. *Lancet Neurol.* 2015 Feb;14(2):224–234. Wolf SL, Lecraw DE, Barton LA, Jann BB. Forced use of hemiplegic upper extremities to reverse the effect of learned nonuse among chronic stroke and head-injured patients. *Experimental Neurology* 1989;104:125–132. Wolf SE, Winstein CJ, Miller JP, et al. Effect of constraint-induced movement therapy on upper extremity function 3 to 9 months after stroke: The EXCITE randomized clinical trial. *JAMA* 2006;296 (17):2095–2104.

9. Silver Spring monkeys. Wikipedia. Available at https://en.wikipedia.org/w/index .php?title=Silver_Spring_monkeys&oldid=880337663.

10. *Unnecessary Fuss.* Wikipedia. Available at https://en.wikipedia.org/wiki/Unnecessary_Fuss.

11. Claflin ES, Krishnan C, Khot SP. Emerging treatments for motor rehabilitation after stroke. *Neurohospitalist* 2015 Apr;5(2):77–88.

12. Boonzaier J, van Tilborg GAF, Neggers SFW, Dijkhuizen RM. Noninvasive brain stimulation to enhance functional recovery after stroke: Studies in animal models. *Neurorehabil. Neural Repair* 2018 Nov;32(11):927–940.

13. Gallese V, Fadiga L, Fogassi L, Rizzolatti G. Action recognition in the premotor cortex. *Brain* 1996;119(2):593–609.

14. Ramachandran VS, Altschuler EL. The use of visual feedback, in particular mirror visual feedback, in restoring brain function. *Brain* 2009 Jul 1;132(7):1693–1710.

15. Tosi G, Romano D, Maravita A. Mirror box training in hemiplegic stroke patients affects body representation. *Front. Hum. Neurosci.* 2018 Jan 4;11. Available at www.ncbi .nlm.nih.gov/pmc/articles/PMC5758498/.

16. Norton A, Zipse L, Marchina S, Schlaug G. Melodic intonation therapy: Shared insights on how it is done and why it might help. *Ann. N Y Acad. Sci.* 2009 Jul;1169:431–436.

17. Tamplin J, Baker FA, Jones B, Way A, Lee S. "Stroke a Chord": The effect of singing in a community choir on mood and social engagement for people living with aphasia following a stroke. *NeuroRehabilitation* 2013;32. Available at https://pubmed.ncbi.nlm .nih.gov/23867418/.

18. Cramer SC, Caplan LR. Recovery, rehabilitation and repair. In Caplan L (ed.), *Caplan's Stroke: A Clinical Approach*, 5th ed. New York: Cambridge University Press, 2016, pp. 608–626.

19. Kondziolka D, Steinberg GK, Wechsler L, Meltzer CC, Elder E, Gebel J, et al. Neurotransplantation for patients with subcortical motor stroke: A phase 2 randomized trial. *J. Neurosurg.* 2005;103:38–45. Savitz SI, Dinsmore JH, Wechsler LR, Rosenbaum DM, Caplan LR. Cell therapy for stroke. *NeuroRx* 2004;1:406–414. Savitz S, Rosenbaum D, Dinsmore J, Wechsler L, Caplan L. Cell transplantation for stroke. *Ann. Neurol.* 2002;52:266–275.

CHAPTER FIFTY FOUR

CAROTID ARTERY SURGERY

It is even conceivable that someday vascular surgery will find a way to bypass the occluded portion of the artery during the period of ominous fleeting symptoms. —C. Miller Fisher [1]

Ambroise Paré performed the first carotid artery ligation to control bleeding in a wounded French soldier in 1552 [2]. Although life-saving, the ligation rendered him aphasic and hemiplegic. In 1793, Hebenstreit of Germany accidently injured a carotid artery while excising a tumor. Bleeding was controlled by ligating the carotid; the patient survived for many years [2]. In 1798, John Abernathy ligated the common carotid artery to control bleeding in a man who was gouged by the horn of a cow [2]. In 1803, David Fleming, a naval surgeon, performed successful carotid ligation in a servant who had attempted suicide by cutting his throat [2]. Sir Astley Cooper was the first to perform carotid artery ligation to treat an aneurysm in 1808 [3]. He wrote:

> Mary Edwards, aged 44 was brought to my house by Mr. Robert Pugh of Gracechurch Street, that I might examine a tumor in the neck which was obviously an aneurysm of the right carotid artery. When the swelling was examined at the hospital, great doubts were entertained if there were sufficient space between the clavicle and the tumor for the application of a ligature. [3]

Although the artery was successfully ligated, the patient died a week later; inflammation and sepsis caused the wound to swell, choking the patient.

Cooper improved his technique and made yet another attempt to ligate a carotid artery three years later. He succeeded this time, and the patient lived for the next 13 years [3].

In 1809, Benjamin Travers performed the first carotid artery ligation in a patient with a carotid cavernous fistula [2]. Hans Chiari, a physician born in Vienna Austria, was a professor of pathology in Prague when he drew attention to carotid artery disease in 1905 [4]. Chiari's attention to the carotid artery was stimulated by one case. Chiari found at postmortem a brain infarct in this patient and searched unsuccessfully for a cause in the usual places: the heart and aorta. He then examined the neck arteries and was surprised to find severe arteriosclerosis of the carotid artery on the side of the brain infarct. A long thrombus that blocked the common carotid artery and extended into the internal carotid artery (ICA) was found. Chiari observed occlusive carotid artery disease in a series of similar patients and was the first to propose that "thrombus in the area of the carotid bifurcation may embolize to the cerebral arteries" [4].

Diagnosis of carotid artery disease became feasible during life after introduction of angiography, first by Egaz Moniz in Lisbon in 1927 [5]. Modern cerebral angiography began with the work of Seldinger in Sweden, who devised a technique during the 1950s in which a small catheter could be inserted into an artery over a flexible guide wire [6]. Catheter angiography of selected vessels in the carotid and vertebral artery circulations was then possible without surgical incisions. Introduction of MR and CT angiography and duplex ultrasound of the neck arteries further improved clinical detection of carotid artery disease. Chapters 15, 29, and 31 also discuss the history of the diagnosis of carotid artery disease.

EARLY CAROTID ARTERY SURGERY

During the 1930s and 1940s surgical treatment for carotid artery disease was excision of the occluded segment and artery ligation to prevent embolization of thrombus fragments. In 1938, Chao et al. at the medical college in Beijing performed an arterectomy of an occluded ICA in a patient with transient ischemic attacks. Their intention was to confirm the diagnosis. He treated a second patient, a 48-year-old Russian man who had a stroke one year before and was pseudobulbar [7]. Chao's rationale was to control the patient's severe hypertension by arterectomy, which denervated the excised carotid sinus.

Some advancement in carotid artery surgical techniques came from oncologists who noted that ligation of a carotid artery that was displaced or infiltrated by tumor often resulted in neurological symptoms. Led by a New York oncology surgeon, John Conley, innovative techniques including saphenous vein and contralateral external carotid artery anastomosis were attempted [8].

Miller Fisher established the link between occlusion of the ICA and stroke through his landmark papers published in 1951 and 1954 [1,9]. The attempts to restore cerebral circulation by reconstruction of the carotid arteries began soon after.

The first carotid artery reconstruction was performed by Raul Carrea and his colleagues at the Institute of Experimental Medicine in Buenos Aires, Argentina, in 1951 [10]. The patient was a 41-year-old businessman who had difficulty speaking, left eye blindness, and right hemiparesis. He lived 1,200 kilometers from Buenos Aires. His neurologist, Guillermo Murphy, called Carrea, who had just returned from the Neurological Institute in New York and had read Fisher's article on carotid artery disease. After two percutaneous angiographic studies, Carrea and Mahels Molins, a thoracic surgeon, operated on the patient two weeks after admission. The diseased portion of the ICA was resected, and an anastomosis was made between the external carotid artery and the distal portion of the ICA. Angiography confirmed that blood flow was reestablished. Except for left eye blindness, the patient had a normal neurological examination 39 months later and was followed for another 27 years. Carrea published the report in 1955 in the *Acta Neurologica Latinoamericana*, a journal with a limited audience [10].

The operation that gave the greatest impetus to the development of surgery for carotid occlusive disease was that of Harry (Felix) Eastcott, George Pickering, and Charles Rob, performed on May 19, 1954, at St. Mary's Hospital in London and published in November 1954, a year before the Argentine report [11]. The patient was a 66-year-old woman who had had about 33 transient episodes of right hemiparesis, aphasia, and left amaurosis during a five-month period. A percutaneous left carotid arteriogram showed a severe stenosis of the left carotid bifurcation. With the patient under general anesthesia with hypothermia to 28°C (82.4°F) by means of ice bags for cerebral protection, the bifurcation was resected and blood flow restored by end-to-end anastomosis between the common carotid and distal ICA. The carotid artery was occluded for 28 minutes. The patient was completely relieved of her symptoms and was alive and well at the age of 86 [11].

Cid Dos Santos, a Portuguese surgeon, had shown in 1947 that it was possible to remove a long occluding thrombus along with the underlying plaque from the femoral artery by using a "loop stripper." The artery was incised, and the thrombus was separated from the wall and removed. He had introduced "thromboendarterectomy" [12].

Strully and colleagues performed the first carotid endarterectomy in 1953 at Montefiore Hospital in New York in a 52-year-old man who had a stroke 16 days before surgery [13]. Angiography showed an ICA stenosis with a superimposed thrombus. They could not restore flow despite extraction of a seven-centimeter clot fragment and had to resect the artery. They emphasized the importance of an early diagnosis to increase the possibility of reopening an occluded vessel.

The first successful carotid endarterectomy was performed by Michael DeBakey in 1953 [14]. The case was reported 19 years later in 1975 [13]. The surgery was performed on a 52-year-old man who had intermittent episodes of weakness in the right arm and leg, hesitancy and difficulty in speaking, and difficulty in writing. The pulsations in the left carotid artery were extremely weak, while they were normal on the right side. A diagnosis of occlusion of the left ICA was made clinically without an angiogram. On August 7, 1953, the patient had general anesthesia and his left common, internal, and external carotid arteries were exposed through a neck incision. An occluding clamp was placed two and a half centimeters below the bifurcation of the common carotid artery, to stop blood flow through the artery during the procedure. A longitudinal incision was made in the ICA and a yellowish-brown atherosclerotic plaque was removed. Good retrograde flow was obtained. About 15 milligrams of heparin was injected into the origin of the artery to prevent clot formation. The arterial wall was then closed using silk sutures. An arteriogram was obtained while the patient was on the operating table, which ascertained the patency of the artery as the radiopaque material moved from the ICA to the middle cerebral artery in the brain. Good pulsations were felt in the common, internal, and external carotid arteries, and the wound was closed in layers. The patient was discharged after eight days. The patient was followed for 19 years until his death due to heart disease [14].

A similar procedure was performed by Denton Cooley in March 1956 at the Methodist Hospital in Houston, on a 71-year-old man who had heard a "swishing" noise in his left ear for four months [15]. Carotid stenosis at the bifurcation was shown on an arteriogram. The unique aspect of this procedure was that the patient's head was immersed in crushed ice to prevent brain damage during temporary interruption of blood supply during the procedure. A polyvinyl shunt with needles was inserted at both the ends to bypass the carotid bifurcation. An endarterectomy was performed. The total period of occlusion was nine minutes. The patient reported that the noises were gone after the procedure, but he developed aphasia and right hemiparesis, which improved over time [15].

DeBakey and Cooley were cardiovascular surgeons in Houston, Texas. Each had an ego as big as Texas, and they became bitter rivals. William S. Fields was the neurologist at the hospital where DeBakey operated. Fields was a pioneer and a very active and influential stroke neurologist. He would customarily see and examine DeBakey's carotid surgery patients after their operations, many of whom Fields had originally referred. When he began to find neurological abnormalities, DeBakey told him not to examine his patients after surgery. It became clear in Texas and elsewhere that the major risk factor for neurological complications from surgery was being examined by a neurologist.

Various surgical strategies for carotid revascularization were attempted until the early 1960s, such as subclavian to common carotid artery bypass, aortic arch to carotid artery bypass, and side-to-side anastomosis from the external to the internal carotid artery [16].

CAROTID SURGERY: 1960–2020

Growing interest in cardiovascular surgery and in operations on the carotid artery and other branches of the aortic arch gave impetus to a national study of occlusive disease of the arteries in the neck. The Joint Study of Extracranial Arterial Occlusion, planned and organized under the supervision of Michael DeBakey and Bill Fields in 1959, included 6,535 patients randomized to surgery or medical care in 24 centers, mostly in the United States [17]. The study was supported by the National Heart Institute. The results showed no difference in the occurrence of stroke or death between the surgical and medical groups. Surgical morbidity and mortality were significantly different for the same group of surgeons at the beginning and at the end of the study due to improvements in surgical technique and perioperative care over the years (mortality in 1961 was 9.5% and by 1969 it had decreased to 2.8%). Patients selected for surgery had the most severely stenotic lesions. Other degrees of stenosis and ulcerations with embolic potential were excluded from randomization. There was a high immediate postsurgical cardiac mortality [17].

The availability of a rather simple neck procedure to potentially save brains and lives led to a dramatic increase in the number of carotid surgeries performed, especially in the United States. In 1971, 15,000 surgeries were performed; this number reached 180,000 in 1989 following enthusiasm caused by the apparent treatment benefits [18]. Should surgery be performed only on patients with related symptoms or be done as a preventive procedure in patients with carotid artery disease but no related symptoms?

Controversy about carotid surgeries reached the point that three very prominent neurologists, Henry Barnett from Canada, Fred Plum from Cornell University in New York, and John Walton from the United Kingdom, published an editorial in the journal *Stroke* entitled "An Expression of Concern" [19]. They wrote:

> Those interested in stroke prevention must face the serious responsibility of evaluating the benefits of endarterectomy for symptomatic patients by deploying all the scientific resources at our disposal. We cannot pretend to patients with carotid disease that we yet have any final answers.... The undersigned neurologists represent different clinical backgrounds, different patterns of socio-economic circumstances governing the practice of

medicine, and different ways of looking at technological advances in relation to the quality of life. We share a common concern about the status of endarterectomy in stroke prophylaxis. [19]

Henry Barnett, one of the cosigners of this editorial, proceeded to lead and conduct major trials of carotid surgery. Henry J. M. Barnett (Barney) was born in February 1922 in Newcastle-upon-Tyne, England, and died in Toronto, Canada, in October 2016 [20]. An apocryphal story recounts that as a boy rambling around the marshes at Ashbridge's Bay in Toronto, he chanced upon two ornithologists who showed him through binoculars a hoary redpoll. From then on, birds, natural science, and eventually medical science captivated him. He remained a birder all of his life as a hobby. In 1944, he graduated from the University of Toronto Medical School in 1944 at age 22. He continued his studies in Toronto, then Queen Square, London, and Oxford. At Oxford, he worked with Charles Symonds, Hugh Cairns, and Richard Doll. He was a member of Toronto's neurology faculty from 1952 to 1969; in 1967 he founded the department of neurosciences at Sunnybrook Hospital and two years later cofounded the world's first multidisciplinary department of clinical neurological sciences at the University of Western Ontario. He was chairman of the department from 1974 until 1986 when he cofounded with neurosurgeon Charles Drake the Robarts Research Institute, which he led for eight years [20]. At midcareer, his emphasis changed from meticulous clinical neurology to an emphasis on randomized therapeutic stroke trials. He devised and led many trials of both medical and surgical treatments, including influential trials of carotid surgery.

Many questions were unsettled. Which patients, with which vascular lesions and severity of stenosis, with which symptoms, with which comorbidities, previously treated with which medicines, should be operated on by which surgeons at which medical centers, using which anesthesia? Trials conducted during the remainder of the twentieth and first decades of the twenty-first century sought to answer these questions. Trials proved to be a moving target since technology and surgical and interventional experience and trial methodology evolved rapidly and consistently.

Surgery on Patients with Relevant Symptoms

Barnett was the guiding force behind the North American Symptomatic Carotid Endarterectomy Trial (NASCET) [21]. Specific instructions for grading the severity of ICA stenosis were used; results were analyzed according to the severity of the stenosis. The relative risk reduction attributable to surgery was 12 percent in the 70–80 percent stenosis subgroup, 18 percent for the 80–90 percent group, and 26 percent for patients with 90–99 percent stenosis.

Surgical benefit was not significant in patients with 50–69 percent stenosis. Surgery was judged to be not indicated for patients with less than 50 percent stenosis. In this latter group, the incidence of stroke in the medically managed group was lower than the surgical morbidity and mortality [21].

In Europe, Charles Warlow and colleagues used a different strategy to enter patients with ICA disease [22]. They planned a "pragmatic" trial; it was hoped that the directions were simple enough that any physician could enter a patient and the entry sheet be short and easy to fill out. They introduced the "uncertainty" principal, which was later used in other randomized trials. Physicians could choose in which patients they felt that surgical benefit was uncertain. Some might be certain that patients with greater than 90 percent stenosis required and would benefit from surgery, and patients with less than 25 percent stenosis would not benefit. So their 25–90 percent stenosis patients would be randomized. Another physician might be uncertain about all but less than 10 percent stenosis so that 10–99 percent would be randomized. Analysis was performed on all the uncertain patients according to the severity of ICA stenosis.

Charles Picton Warlow was born in September 1943 in Nottingham, England [23]. He matriculated at Cambridge University for both his bachelor and his doctor of medicine degrees. He then became a house officer at the National Hospital, Queen Square London, and the University College Hospital, London, from 1974 to 1976. He was a staff neurologist and stroke researcher in Oxford from 1976 to 1986. In 1987 Warlow took up the chair of neurology in Edinburgh and organized there a very effective stroke research consortium.

In the Medical Research Council European Carotid Surgery Trial (ECST), organized and led by Charles Warlow, eligible patients had to have had one or more carotid-territory ischemic events involving the brain or eye during the previous six months [22]. Patients who likely had cardiac-origin embolism were excluded. After contrast angiography of the symptomatic ICA, physicians and surgeons enrolled patients for randomization when they were "substantially uncertain" whether or not to recommend endarterectomy of the affected artery. The results showed that "on average, the immediate risk of surgery was worth trading off against the long-term risk of stroke without surgery when the stenosis was greater than about 80% diameter" [22].

The results of these carotid surgery trials and published results in series of carotid surgery patients led to a general consensus that patients with an ICA stenosis between 70 and 99 percent who had related ocular or hemispheric symptoms benefited from carotid endarterectomy. The reduction with surgery in the five-year risk of developing an ipsilateral ischemic stroke and in any perioperative stroke or death was greater in men and less evident in women [24]. To achieve beneficial results, the surgical complication rate had to be

6 percent or less. The greater the stenosis, the greater the benefit. Patients with "near" occlusion had good results when medically managed and surgery did not show any definite benefit. Endarterectomy should be performed early (within the first two weeks) following development of symptoms. The benefit of surgery was lost after months had elapsed from symptom onset.

Carotid Artery Surgery in Patients with No Relevant Symptoms

Concurrent with the so-called *symptomatic* trials were studies of so-called *asymptomatic* patients. The latter were defined as not having neurological symptoms that could be attributed to ICA disease in the neck. James Toole was instrumental in leading a large trial in the United States of carotid surgery in these asymptomatic patients. After graduating from Princeton University, Toole spent his early career at the University of Pennsylvania. He came to the Bowman Gray School of Medicine in Winston-Salem, North Carolina, in 1962 when he was appointed the Walter C. Teagle Professor of Neurology and chairman of the department of neurology, a position he held until 1983. Toole helped launch a stroke research unit and was active in research on ultrasound. He promoted the diagnostic use of ultrasound in vascular disease in the neck. He was a consummate politician who became the president of the International Stroke Society, president of the American Neurological Association, and president of the World Federation of Neurology. He authored a popular textbook on cerebrovascular disorders that has had six editions. He was very skillful in attracting researchers and participants to various research projects and trials.

The Asymptomatic Carotid Atherosclerosis Study (ACAS), led by Toole, allowed entry if ICA stenosis was diagnosed by ultrasound as well as angiography [25]. Previous studies had required cerebral dye contrast angiography. There was a central adjudication center that qualified the ultrasound diagnostic equipment and interpreters. In this study, 1,662 patients were randomized to surgery or medical treatment Surgical treatment was judged to be superior to medical treatment in patients with ICA stenosis greater than 60 percent [25].

The results proved controversial. Results were extrapolated at five years, although the study was interrupted after a median follow-up of 2.7 years. A benefit was shown for a combined end point, but it was not significant for individual events (major stroke prevention, major cardiovascular event, or death). The absolute risk reduction was from 2 to 1 percent (50% relative risk reduction). Risk reduction in men was 66 percent but only 17 percent for women. The difference was due to a greater surgical risk and lower overall stroke risk in women. There was no benefit associated with an increase in deciles for stenosis as had been found in NASCET. Finally, 40 percent of surgeons considered for ACAS were rejected, suggesting that results could not be extrapolated into general medical practice in the community. ACAS also showed that endarterectomy was not beneficial in patients with contralateral carotid occlusion [25].

The Asymptomatic Carotid Surgery Trial (ACST), led by Allison Halliday, a professor of vascular surgery at Oxford University, was published nearly a decade later in 2004 [26]. This study included 3,120 patients with greater than 60 percent ICA stenosis. Half of the patients were operated on more than one month after randomization. In asymptomatic patients younger than 75 years of age with carotid diameter reduction about 70 percent or more on ultrasound, carotid endarterectomy soon after diagnosis halved the net five-year stroke risk from about 12 to about 6 percent. Half of this five-year benefit involved disabling or fatal strokes. The benefit in women was questionable. Benefits in patients older than 74 years were uncertain and small. There was no increasing benefit with greater degree of stenosis [26].

A published meta-analysis reviewed the results among five randomized trials that studied 2,440 asymptomatic patients [27]. The risk of developing an ipsilateral stroke or a perioperative stroke or death was clearly reduced, with no significant heterogeneity across the five trials. The adjusted rate of these outcomes was 6.4 percent for the medically treated patients and 4.4 percent for the surgical group, yielding an absolute reduction after carotid endarterectomy of about 2 percent during a mean follow-up of about three years. With three years of follow-up, about 50 patients would have to undergo surgery to prevent one stroke event. The authors concluded:

> Carotid endarterectomy in patients with asymptomatic carotid stenosis unequivocally reduces the incidence of ipsilateral stroke, although the absolute benefit is relatively small. Given the modest benefit of surgery for unselected patients with asymptomatic ICA stenosis, carotid endarterectomy cannot be routinely recommended for these patients pending reliable identification of high risk subgroups. Medical management is a sensible alternative for most patients. [27]

Carotid Artery Endarterectomy versus Stenting

The advent of angioplasty and stenting of cervical arteries (the topic of Chapter 55) eventually led to a number of trials that evaluated the procedure and compared the results with carotid endarterectomy. Angioplasty was rapidly replaced by stenting. Stenting had obvious benefits since it avoided surgical risk, did not require anesthesia, and involved a shorter hospital stay. Thousands of patients were treated. Most early reports were patient registries without controls, and most procedures were performed on low-risk, asymptomatic patients, and none had independent audits. The technology rapidly evolved and used different devices and different systems of protection devices.

An editorial review published in 2011 [28] commented on the past surgery versus stenting trials, reports of results in patients not entered in trials, the results of the Carotid Revascularization Endarterectomy versus Stenting Trial (CREST) [29], and a meta-analysis of trials [30].

Both carotid endarterectomy and carotid artery stenting were effective. Both procedures showed a relatively low rate of serious complications. Surgery was superior concerning some outcomes; stenting seemed to have advantages in others. Each has its own frequency of complications. Stenting was complicated by more acute strokes, more incidences of restenosis, and more blood pressure fluctuations during the procedure. Diffusion-weighted MRI shortly after the procedure had shown small regions of infarction undoubtedly caused by microembolism during angioplasty/stent insertion [28]. Stenting was preferred by some patients because there was no incision and there was a short recovery period if no stroke developed. Surgery was associated with fewer strokes but more cranial nerve injuries and more periprocedural myocardial infarcts. Both surgery and stenting could affect the carotid artery sinus, so blood pressure monitoring was considered mandatory after both types of intervention. Age made a difference because stenting seemed to show better outcomes in younger patients, while surgical results were better in older patients; the inflection point varied but was around age 70 [28].

The advent of carotid artery surgery focused attention on carotid artery disease. Two thirds of the patients diagnosed with carotid artery atherosclerosis were men. Women had less carotid disease; those women who had severe atherosclerotic disease had more risk factors than men. Women had more complications of carotid surgery, especially early restenosis. Medical therapy of carotid disease and atherosclerosis became more effective over time and the advantage of carotid surgery over medical treatment diminished in those patients who had no related symptoms..

NOTES AND REFERENCES

1. Fisher CM. Occlusion of the internal carotid artery. *AMA Arch. Neurol. Psychiatry* 1951;65:346–377.

2. Pearce JMS. Historical note on carotid disease and ligation. *Eur. Neurol.* 2014;72:26–29.

3. Cooper A. Account of the first successful operation performed on the common carotid artery for aneurysm in the year 1808, with post-mortem examination in 1821. *Guy's Hosp. Rep.* 1836;1:53–59.

4. Chiari H. Uber das Verhalten des Tielungswinkels der Carotis communis bei der Endarteritis chronica deformans. *Verhandl. deutschpath. Gesellsch.* 1905;9:326–330. Chapter 15 includes more information about Hans Chiari and his work.

5. The work of Moniz and the later evolution of cerebral angiography is discussed in detail in Chapter 31.

6. Seldinger SI. Catheter replacement of the needle in percutaneous arteriography. *Acta Radiol.* 1953;39:368–376.

7. Chao WH, Kwan ST, Lyman RS, et al. Thrombosis of the left internal carotid artery. *Arch. Surg.* 1938:37:100–111.

8. Conley J, Pack G. Surgical procedure for lessening the hazard of carotid bulb excision. *Surgery* 1952;31:845–858.

9. Fisher CM. Occlusion of the carotid arteries: Further experiences. *AMA Arch. Neurol. Psychiatry* 1954;72;187–204. The life and contributions of Miller Fisher are captured in Chapter 29 and in a biography: Caplan LR. *C. Miller Fisher: Stroke in the 20th Century.* Oxford: Oxford University Press, 2020. Chapter 15 also recounts Fisher's role in the recognition of the importance of carotid artery disease.

10. Carrea R, Molins M, Murphy G. Surgical treatment of spontaneous thrombosis of the internal carotid artery in the neck: Carotid carotideal anastomosis. *Acta Neurol. Latinoamer.* 1955;1:71–78.

11. Eastcott H, Pickering G, Rob C. Reconstruction of internal carotid artery in a patient with intermittent attacks of hemiplegia. *Lancet* 1954;267(2):994–996. Thompson JE. The Willis Lecture: The evolution of surgery for the treatment and prevention of stroke. *Stroke* 1996;27:1427–1434.

12. Dos Santos JC. From embolectomy to endarterectomy or the fall of a myth. *J. Cardiovasc. Surg.* 1976;17:113–128.

13. Strully KJ, Hurwitt ES, Blankenberg HW. Thromboendarterectomy for thrombosis of the internal carotid artery in the neck. *J. Neurosurg.* 1953;10:474–482.

14. DeBakey M. Successful carotid endarterectomy for cerebrovascular insufficiency: Nineteen-year follow-up. *JAMA* 1975;233:1083–1085.

15. Cooley D, Al-Naaman Y, Carton C. Surgical treatment of arteriosclerotic occlusion of common carotid artery. *J. Neurosurg.* 1956;13:500–506.

16. Bahnson H, Spencer F, Quattlebaum JJ. Surgical treatment of occlusive disease of the carotid artery. *Ann. Surg.* 1959;149:711–720.

17. Fields WS, Maslenikov V, Meyer JS, et al. Joint Study of Extracranial Artery Occlusion: V. Progress report of prognosis following surgery or non- surgery treatment for transient ischemic attacks and cervical carotid artery lesions. *JAMA* 1970;211:1993–2003.

18. National Center for Health Statistics. *Detailed Diagnosis and Procedures, National Hospital Discharge Survey.* Vital and Health Statistics. Series 13. Washington, DC: Government Printing Office, 1992–1997.

19. Barnett HJM, Plum F, Walton JN. An expression of concern. *Stroke* 1984;15 (6):942–943.

20. Spence JD, Hachinski V. In memoriam. Henry J. M. Barnett, 1922–2016. *Stroke* 2017;48(1):2–4.

21. North American Symptomatic Carotid Endarterectomy Trial Collaborators. Beneficial effect of carotid endarterectomy in symptomatic patients with high-grade carotid stenosis. *N. Engl. J. Med.* 1991;325:445–453. Barnett HJM, Taylor DW, Eliasziw M, et al. Benefit of carotid endarterectomy in patients with symptomatic moderate or severe stenosis. *N. Engl. J. Med.* 1998;339:1415–1425.

22. European Carotid Surgery Trialists' Collaborative Group. Randomised trial of endarterectomy for recently symptomatic carotid stenosis: Final results of the MRC European Carotid Surgery Trial (ECST). *Lancet* 1998;351(9113):1371–1387.

23. Charles Picton Warlow. Prabook. Available at https://prabook.com/web/charles_picton.warlow/315427.

24. DeRango P, Brown MM, Didier L, et al. Management of carotid stenosis in women: Consensus document. *Neurology* 2013;80(24):2258–2268.

25. Executive Committee for the Asymptomatic Carotid Atherosclerosis Study. Endarterectomy for asymptomatic carotid artery stenosis. *JAMA* 1995;273:1421–1428.

26. Halliday A, Mansfield A, Marro J, et al. Prevention of disabling and fatal strokes by successful carotid endarterectomy in patients without recent neurological symptoms: Randomised controlled trial. *Lancet* 2004;363(9420):1491–1502.

27. Benavente O, Moher D, Pham B. Carotid endarterectomy for asymptomatic carotid stenosis: A meta-analysis. *BMJ* 1998;317:1477–1480.

28. Caplan LR, Brott TG. Of horse races, trials, meta-analyses, and carotid artery stenosis (Editorial). *Arch. Neurol.* 2011;68:157–159.

29. Brott TG, Hobson RW II, Howard G, et al. CREST Investigators. Stenting vs endarterectomy for treatment of carotid-artery stenosis. *N. Engl. J. Med.* 2010;363:11–23.

30. Bangalore S, Kumar S, Wetterslev J, et al. Carotid artery stenting vs carotid endarterectomy: Meta-analysis and diversity-adjusted trial sequential analysis of randomized trials. *Arch. Neurol.* 2011;68(2):172–184.

CHAPTER FIFTY FIVE

ANGIOPLASTY AND STENTING

CAROTID ARTERY STENTING IN THE NECK

Carotid revascularization includes all procedures that open clogged carotid arteries to restore blood flow to the brain. While the first traditional carotid surgery (carotid endarterectomy) was reported in 1951, it was not until 1977 that percutaneous transluminal angioplasty of the internal carotid artery (ICA) was attempted by Andreas Gruentzig.

Andreas Gruentzig, a German radiologist, performed pioneering work on coronary balloon angioplasty. In 1984, while at Emory University, Gruentzig invited Gary Roubin, an Australian cardiologist, to pursue an interventional cardiology fellowship with him. Roubin had had rigorous training in Australia, starting his career with a veterinary medical degree, and then proceeding to medical school, internal medicine residency, and cardiovascular medicine fellowship, followed by a PhD in impaired left ventricular hemodynamics. Coronary angiography was at that time considered a radiological procedure with mostly radiologists performing or overseeing it, while peripheral vascular surgeries were performed by cardiologists. Roubin had interdisciplinary collaborations with other fields while training with Gruentzig. He left Emory University after his fellowship to join the University of Alabama at Birmingham (UAB).

In 1992, while at an international meeting, Roubin met radiologist Robert Ferguson. During an informal discussion at the meeting, Ferguson wondered about the utility of balloon angioplasty in the carotid arteries. On returning to UAB, Roubin assembled a team of diverse, curious-minded individuals like him who would help accomplish this daunting task.

The first individual was Jiri Vitek, a neurosurgeon who then pursued interventional radiology. Vitek was known to be far ahead of his time. He had published a case series of 2,000 cerebral angiography cases in 1972 with an emphasis on strokes in the elderly. He also performed the first subclavian/brachiocephalic angioplasty in 1979. His first carotid bifurcation angioplasty was in 1980 in a patient who developed a hemiparesis and concerning cortical signs. This man had an occluded ICA and a large external carotid artery that was supplying collateral circulation to the brain. Vitek also pioneered innominate artery angioplasty in 1984 [1].

The second individual was Sriram Iyer, an interventional cardiology fellow in training with Roubin. Iyer had experience in carotid surgeries during a fellowship in Milwaukee, Wisconsin.

The third individual was Jay Yadav, a neurologist who approached Roubin mentioning that he wanted to offer secondary stroke prevention with interventional procedures. Roubin offered him an interventional fellowship at UAB.

Together, this team, a Czechoslovakian, an Australian, and two Indians, made a request to the Institutional Review Board (IRB) at UAB for a prospective study of carotid angioplasty as an alternative to the already well-established practice of carotid endarterectomy. While this enthusiastic team had support from the IRB and their neurosurgery colleagues, vascular surgeons were pessimistic about the study.

In March 1994, the first patient was enrolled (Figure 55.1). The fifth patient enrolled, a 54-year-old woman who presented with symptomatic carotid

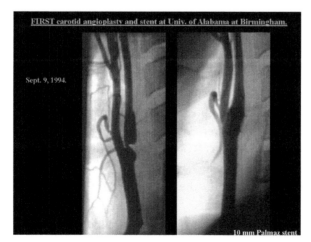

55.1. First carotid angioplasty and stent at the University of Alabama. Courtesy Dr. G. Roubin.

stenosis, was the first to show complications. She continued to have recurrent transient ischemic attacks due to distal embolization during and after surgery. The team decided to intervene again, ballooned the lesion, and administered more antiplatelets. The patient worsened, and imaging showed an intracranial hemorrhage into the stroke bed. She eventually died.

This development made the team question some techniques that were being used for carotid angioplasty. They stopped recruiting patients in the trial. Stenting of the iliac and femoral arteries including the coronary arteries had already taken over the field of cardiology and vascular surgery, but using the same stents for carotid and brachiocephalic arteries posed significant challenges. The only stent long enough at that time was the Palmaz stent, a stainless steel insertable mesh stent recently approved for use in peripheral arteries. Roubin applied for an IRB revision at UAB that was approved. The new protocol included an examination by Yadav with NIHS scores recorded. Enrollment quickly occurred. After 30 successful Palmaz stent cases, they noticed that, in three patients, the balloon-expandable stent had succumbed to pressure and caused compression and restenosis on follow-up imaging [2].

The group was convinced that stenting was safer than angioplasty, but a better stent was needed. The only known self-expandable, flexible stent long enough to extend from the groin access site to the ICA was the 300-centimeter-long tracheobronchial Wallstent, which was not approved for use in blood vessels. The team found a company that created a guide wire for the stent. They were then successfully able to treat another 100 patients with the Wallstent without major complications or deaths. A few patients had minor, nondisabling strokes.

A coronary version of the Wallstent soon became commercially available and was also used in the trial with success. The Wallstent continued to yield excellent results by skilled operators in the angiography suite, with a small downside of increased rates of restenosis.

Roubin started to teach carotid stenting to others in the United States and internationally via live case demonstrations. He knew that pursuing carotid stenting as an alternative to endarterectomy required acceptance by key opinion leaders. He wanted to validate this innovation in the most rigorous ways that would lead to acceptance of the procedure by the greater medical community. Carotid endarterectomy had taken 40 years to mature.

The first group of surgeons who visited UAB to learn from Roubin were from the University of Louisville in Kentucky. They returned to their institute and started using the Wallstent for carotid artery stenting. They published a single-center randomized trial that showed no difference in major stroke or death rates between carotid artery stenting and carotid endarterectomy [3]. Roubin knew that neurologists examining each trial patient would lead to recognizing more strokes after treatment and so he urged including that requirement in subsequent trials.

Transcranial Doppler ultrasound (TCD) helped Roubin's team identify phases in the procedure where embolization was occurring. In many patients, Vitek pursued detailed intracranial angiography and intraoperative TCD studies. While large-artery occlusions were rare, occlusions of small ascending parietal branches were often found that caused hemispheric symptoms. Roubin realized that the focus of teaching the procedure had to be on careful, facile operation that avoided distal embolization of clot.

The first embolic device filters were approved by the FDA in 1994. These were regarded as the first line of defense. Operators had to be taught a facile way of deploying a sheath into the ICA and then manipulating catheters through the lesion. In complicated cases such as difficult aortic arches, distal embolization should be minimized before an embolic filter was placed. When stenotic lesions were very severe, expansion of the lumen by balloon stretching was needed to advance the filter device past the stenotic area, adding further risk for embolization. The embolic protection devices could also irritate or denude the intima above the stent placement, making it a potential nidus for thrombus formation in the hours and days after the procedure. Roubin placed extreme significance on patient selection and an experienced neat technique, often relating it to driving: "If you drive dangerously, seat belts don't help you."

Yadav completed his fellowship and left UAB for a position at the Cleveland Clinic. He developed the Precise stent and participated in the SAPPHIRE trial, the first randomized control trial that compared carotid artery stenting with embolic protection to carotid endarterectomy in patients at high risk for carotid surgery [4]. The results showed that among patients with severe carotid artery stenosis and coexisting conditions, carotid stenting using an emboli protection device was not inferior to carotid endarterectomy. The trial was criticized by some for having a poor randomization process and unclear end points.

During nearly 4,000 carotid stentings, Roubin noted that elderly patients and long complex lesions raised potential complications [5]. Patients under the age of 55 years did better with carotid stenting. Between 55 and 75 years of age, the difference between carotid endarterectomy and carotid artery stenting remained equivocal. The biological age rather than the numerical age of these patients mattered the most.

Elderly patients who had significant microangiopathic disease or cognitive dysfunction would not benefit from a procedure where the injection of contrast and microbubbles would pose risks for distal particulate embolization. A younger patient with the same procedure and risks might avoid clinical manifestations of a neurological event despite embolization, making them reasonable candidates. Another factor was the tortuosity of calcified arteries in older patients, which meant more manipulation with microcatheters during carotid stenting. Tortuous and misshapen aortic arches were difficult to navigate.

The first-generation Wallstent resulted in most examples of restenosis as its non-expandability limited its use. Patients who had neck radiation seemed more susceptible to restenosis, which was attributed to an exaggerated endothelial response to the stent. The advent of drug-eluted stents and improved instrumentation reduced the complication and restenosis rates.

CAVATAS, a relatively small trial that included 504 patients recruited between 1992 and 1997, showed no significant difference between carotid endarterectomy and endovascular therapy for disabling stroke or death [6]. This reassured Roubin, although he realized that trials still did not have rigorous patient follow-up by certified neurologists.

By the turn of the century enough experience with stenting had been accrued that a larger trial could be conducted. Tom Brott, a neurologist, and Robert Hobson, a surgeon, were the major movers in designing the Carotid Revascularization Endarterectomy versus Stenting Trial (CREST) and bringing it to completion. Thomas G. Brott grew up in the Chicago area and received his undergraduate degree at Harvard and his MD from the University of Chicago. He was an intern in medicine at the Beth Israel Hospital in Boston, and his neurology residency was in the Harvard Longwood Avenue program. During this training he was mentored by Lou Caplan and decided to develop a career as a stroke neurologist. During his tenure at the University of Cincinnati, he was a leader in the NINDS thrombolytic study and was the developer of the NIHSS scale. He moved to the Mayo Clinic in Jacksonville, Florida, where he is the Eugene and Marcia Applebaum Professor of Neurosciences, and the James C. and Sarah K. Kennedy Dean for Research.

Robert Hobson grew up in Illinois. He received his BS in chemistry and his medical degree from the George Washington University and its School of Medicine in 1963. He trained in surgery at Walter Reed Hospital in Washington and served with the US Army 5th Special Forces Group in Vietnam. He became a leader in the Vascular Surgery Society. He was professor of surgery at the Rutgers University of New Jersey Medical School. Hobson recruited qualified surgeons for the trial. He died before final tabulation of the CREST results.

The CREST results showed that carotid stenting was comparable to carotid surgery [7]. An editorial summarized the findings in this and other surgery versus stenting trials [8]. Both carotid endarterectomy and carotid artery stenting were effective. Both procedures showed a relatively low rate of serious complications. Surgery was superior concerning some outcomes; stenting had advantages in others. Stenting was complicated by more acute strokes, more incidences of restenosis, and more blood pressure fluctuations during the procedure. Diffusion-weighted MRI shortly after stenting showed small regions of infarction undoubtedly caused by microembolism during angio-plasty/stent insertion [8]. Stenting was preferred by some patients because there was no incision and there was a short recovery period if no stroke developed. Surgery was associated with fewer strokes but more cranial nerve injuries and more periprocedural myocardial infarcts. Both surgery and stent-ing could affect the carotid artery sinus, so blood pressure monitoring was considered mandatory after both types of intervention. Age made a difference because stenting seemed to show better outcomes in younger patients, while surgical results were better in older patients; the inflection point varied but was about age 70 [8].

Carotid artery stenting continued to evolve. Embolic protection devices were improved. Covered stents began to be employed. A multicenter publi-cation that included 700 patients showed a cumulative stroke rate of 0.54 percent with the CGuard covered stent, showing the superiority of this third-generation technology [9]. A new trial (CREST-2) that included more vigor-ous monitored medical treatment was begun [10]. Newer strategies for avoiding the aortic arch for catheter entry were explored. Both carotid stenting and carotid surgery continued to evolve.

EVOLUTION OF INTRACRANIAL ANGIOPLASTY AND STENTING

Treatment of stenosing lesions that involved intracranial vessels lagged behind treatment of carotid artery neck lesions. The terrain was quite different. The diameter of intracranial arteries was much smaller. Access through small, tortuous vessels was more difficult. The media and adventitia of intracranial arteries differed from neck arteries. The large intracranial basal arteries, espe-cially the basilar and middle cerebral arteries, gave off multiple penetrating arteries at right angles from the parent artery, while the carotid artery had no branches in the neck. Carotid artery lesions were prevalent in white men of European extraction, while intracranial atherosclerotic lesions were more prevalent in Asian people (Chinese, Korean, Japanese, Thai), in Black people, and in women.

The cadre of physicians who dealt with intracranial arterial conditions was also very different. Carotid stenting was often performed by cardiologists and vascular surgeons. Neuroradiologists, neurosurgeons, and, later, neurology-trained physicians dealt more with intracranial vascular lesions. During the 1980s and 1990s most vascular neurosurgeons were trained to treat intracranial vascular disease through an intravascular approach. These interventionalists obliterated aneurysms and arteriovenous malformations intravascularly. They began to open recently occluded intracranial arteries using thrombolytics and clot retrievers [11]. These physicians, especially neurosurgeons and interventional neuroradiologists, were the physicians who began to do angioplasty and stent intracranial arteries that were narrowed by plaques and fibrotic lesions.

The first balloon angioplasties for intracranial occlusive disease were reported in the mid-1980s. Most patients who were treated had TIAs that preceded strokes. The introduction of improved microballoon catheters and smaller balloon-expandable stents led to a major increase in intracranial interventions. Many reports of small series of anecdotal experiences were published. The reported technical success rate exceeded 90 percent, but the complication rate was significant, varying between 0 and 20 percent [12]. In 1999, Buddy Connors and Joan Wojak described changes in their technique during a four-year period during which they treated 70 patients with intracranial disease [13]. They had learned to use slow inflation of an undersized balloon and aimed at moderate reduction of the luminal stenosis rather than complete opening.

Revascularization by balloon angioplasty was sometimes complicated by recoiling and dissection in the absence of mechanical support by a stent. The first off-label use of a coronary balloon-expandable stent for stenosis in the intracranial ICA was in 1996 [14]. Many case reports and single-center series of stenting were published [15]. Experience with the balloon-expandable stents showed shortcomings that included plaque dislodgement, dissections, and poor stent-to-wall apposition due to vascular curvature. The self-expandable Wingspan stent system was designed to overcome these shortcomings and soon became popular [15]. Interventional deployment consisted of initial angioplasty followed by deployment of the self-expanding stent by unsheathing it, then withdrawing the balloon. With the warmth of the blood, the stent (usually chosen with a diameter slightly greater than the vessel wall diameter) immediately sprang out and assumed the shape of the vessel wall and exerted radial force on the wall.

When it became clear that medical treatment of intracranial atherosclerosis was followed by a relatively high rate of recurrences, and sufficient experience was gained with the Wingspan stent, Mark Chimowitz, Colin Derdeyn, and colleagues designed a randomized trial to compare stenting of intracranial severe stenotic lesions and medical treatment: the Stenting versus Aggressive Medical Management for Preventing Recurrent Stroke in Intracranial Stenosis (SAMMPRIS) trial [16].

Mark Ivor Chimowitz was born in South Africa. He graduated from the University of Capetown Medical School in 1981 and then emigrated to the United States. His neurology residency was at Tufts–New England Medical Center in 1985–1988 where he was mentored by Lou Caplan and Michael Pessin. It was there that he decided to pursue vascular neurology as a career. He then had a Stroke Fellowship at the Cleveland Clinic under the tutelage of Tony Furlan and Cathy Sila. Mark then had leadership stroke academic staff positions at the University of Michigan, Emory, and the Medical University of South Carolina in Charleston. An early and persistent passion was in mathematics and quantitative analysis. He centered his career on developing and carrying out randomized trials involving intracranial atherosclerosis. Prior to the SAMMPRIS trial he had led trials (WASID) of medical therapy of intracranial atherosclerotic lesions [17].

Colin Derdeyn matriculated at the University of Virginia for his undergraduate and medical degrees. He became professor of radiology, neurology, and neurological surgery at Washington University and director of the Washington University/Barnes Jewish Hospital Stroke and Cerebrovascular Center. He then moved to Iowa where he is the Krabbenhoft Professor and chair of the department of radiology at the University of Iowa Hospitals and Clinics, and director of the Iowa Institute for Biomedical Imaging. He has been the chair of the American Heart Association Stroke Council and is a past president of the Society of Neurointerventional Surgery.

Derdeyn commented on progress that led up to SAMMPRIS:

> As coronary balloons got increasingly flexible and able to navigate the bony channels that constrain passage to the intracranial vasculature, they became increasingly used for intracranial angioplasty. There was still a great deal of difficulty as those devices were not optimized for the intracranial cavity. It was even harder for balloon-mounted stents because of the right angle turns within the petrous bone. Over the years, these technical barriers were overcome through device optimization.

In SAMMPRIS, patients with symptomatic intracranial atherosclerotic disease (ICAD) who had 70–99 percent stenosis were randomized to either aggressive medical therapy alone or aggressive medical therapy with interventional deployment of the Wingspan stent. Aggressive medical management consisted of dual antiplatelet therapy for 90 days (followed by aspirin monotherapy), statins with goal LDL of less than 70, blood pressure reduction, effective management of diabetes, and lifestyle modification that included a nutritionist and monitoring of exercise and cessation of smoking. The intracranial angioplasty and stent arm patients had angioplasty followed by insertion of a self-expanding stent. On the medical side, there were surprisingly much lower rates of stroke than expected from WASID. A subgroup analysis of patients with posterior circulation ICAD had the best outcome on medical therapy but the worst outcome and highest complication rate with angioplasty and stenting [16].

The NINDS stopped recruitment in the SAMMPRIS trial after 451 of the planned 764 patients had been enrolled from 50 US centers. Among patients in the stent arm, 14 percent had a stroke or died within 30 days after entry compared to 5.8 percent of patients in the medical treatment arm. Those patients who met the exercise requirement had the least number of strokes [16,18]. A major complication in the stent arm of SAMMPRIS were perforator artery strokes. These occurred predominantly in patients with stenotic lesions in the intracranial vertebral, basilar, and M1 portion of the MCAs. This was attributed to the so-called snow-plowing effect in which the procedure pushed atheromatous debris into the perforator origins and the stents held the debris in place [18].

A concurrent trial, the Vitesse Intracranial Stent Study for Ischemic Stroke Therapy (VISSIT), was an international, multicenter trial that enrolled 112 patients, including 59 who were randomized to receive balloon-expandable stent plus medical therapy and 53 who received only medical treatment [19] Enrollment was halted after the SAMMPRIS trial results were released. The use of the stent compared with medical therapy resulted in an increased 12-month risk of stroke (ischemic and hemorrhagic) or TIA in the same vascular territory, and increased the 30-day risk of any stroke or TIA [19].

The results of these two trials severely diminished enthusiasm for intracranial stenting. There was continued interest in identifying a subgroup of patients who might benefit from angioplasty and stenting. The WEAVE registry trial was born out of this quest. The registry enrolled 22 80-year-old patients who had symptomatic ICAD of 70–99 percent, modified Rankin score less than 4, recurrent stroke with at least one representing a failure of medical therapy, and stenting after seven days from the last stroke. The WEAVE investigators found a low (2.6%) rate of periprocedural stroke, bleeding, or death when stents were deployed by experienced interventionalists [20].

One of the legacies of the SAMMPRIS trial was the aggressive medical treatment protocol. In most prior surgical and procedural trials "best medical treatment" consisted of doctors issuing prescriptions and directions for treatment. The effects of these prescribed treatments were not monitored nor was attention directed to lifestyle management. Subsequent therapeutic trials adopted many of the aspects of aggressive medical treatment outlined in SAMMPRIS.

NOTES AND REFERENCES

1. Vitek JJ, Raymon BC, Oh SJ. Innominate artery angioplasty. *AJNR* 1984;5:113–114.
2. Roubin GS, Yadav S, Iyer SS, Vitek J. Carotid stent-supported angioplasty: A neurovascular intervention to prevent stroke. *Am. J. Cardiol.* 1996 Aug 14;78(3A):8–12.
3. Brooks WH, McClure RR, Jones MR, et al. Carotid angioplasty and stenting versus carotid endarterectomy: Randomized trial in a community hospital. *J. Am. Coll. Cardiol.* 2001;38:1589–1595.
4. Yadav JS, Wholey MH, Kuntz RE, et al. Protected carotid-artery stenting versus endarterectomy in high-risk patients. *N. Engl. J. Med.* 2004;351:1493–1501.
5. Roubin GS, New G, Iyer SS, Vitek JJ, et al. Immediate and late clinical outcomes of carotid artery stenting in patients with symptomatic and asymptomatic carotid artery stenosis: A 5-year prospective analysis. *Circulation* 2001;103(4):532–537.

6. Ederle J, Bonati LH, Dobson J, et al. CAVATAS Investigators. Endovascular treatment with angioplasty or stenting versus endarterectomy in patients with carotid artery stenosis in the Carotid and Vertebral Artery Transluminal Angioplasty Study (CAVATAS): Long-term follow-up of a randomised trial. *Lancet Neurol.* 2009;8(10):898–907.

7. Brott TG, Hobson RW II, Howard G, Roubin GS, et al. CREST Investigators. Stenting versus endarterectomy for treatment of carotid-artery stenosis. *N. Engl. J. Med.* 2010;363(1):11–23.

8. Caplan LR, Brott TG. Of horse races, trials, meta-analyses, and carotid artery stenosis (Editorial). *Arch. Neurol.* 2011;68:157–159.

9. Sirignano P, Stabile E, Mansour W, et al. 1-month results from a prospective experience on CAS using CGuard stent system: The IRONGUARD 2 study. *JACC Cardiovasc. Interv.* 2020;13(18):2170–2177.

10. Lal BK, Meschia JF, Brott TG. Clinical need, design, and goals for the Carotid Revascularization and Medical Management for Asymptomatic Carotid Stenosis trial. *Semin. Vasc. Surg.* 2017;30(1):2–7. Epub April 27, 2017.

11. Interventional treatment of aneurysms is discussed in Chapter 57, interventional treatment of AVMs in Chapter 59, and clot extraction in Chapter 56.

12. Higashida RT, Myers PM, Connors JJ III, et al. Intracranial angioplasty and stenting for cerebral atherosclerosis: A position statement of the American Society of Interventional and Therapeutic Neuroradiology, Society of Interventional Radiology, and the American Society of Neuroradiology. *AJNR Am. J. Neuroradiol.* 2005;26:2323–2327.

13. Connors JJ III, Wojak JC. Percutaneous transluminal angioplasty for intracranial atherosclerotic lesions: Evolution of technique and short-term results. *J. Neurosurgery* 1999;91:415–423.

14. Feldman RL, Trigg L, Gaudier J, Galat J. Use of coroanry Palmaz-Schatz stent in the percutaneous treatment of an intracranial carotid artery stenosis. *Cathet. Cardiovasc. Diagn.* 1996;38:316–319.

15. Leung TW, Wabnitz AM, Miao Z, Chimowitz M. Agioplasty and stenting. In Kim J, Caplan LR, Wong KS (eds.), *Intracranial Atherosclerosis: Pathophysiology, Diagnosis and Treatment.* Front. Neurol. Neurosci. Basel: Karger, 2016, vol. 40, pp. 152–163.

16. Chimowitz MI, Lynn MJ, Derdeyn CP, et al. for the SAMMPRIS Trial Investigators. Stenting versus aggressive medical therapy for intracranial arterial stenosis. *N. Engl. J. Med.* 2011;365(11):993–1003.

17. Chimowitz MI, Kokkinos J, Strong J, et al. The Warfarin-Aspirin Symptomatic Intracranial Disease Study. *Neurology* 1995;45:1488–1493. Chimowitz MI, et al. Comparison of warfarin and aspirin for symptomatic intracranial arterial stenosis. *N. Engl. J. Med.* 2005;352(13):1305–1316.

18. Derdeyn CP, Chimowitz MI, Lynn MJ, et al. for the for the SAMMPRIS Trial Investigators. Aggressive medical treatment with or without stenting in high risk patients with intracranial arterial stenosis (SAMMPRIS): The final trial results. *Lancet* 2014;383:333–341.

19. Zaidat OO, Fitzsimmons BF, Woodward BK, for the VISSIT Trial Investigators. Effect of a balloon expandable intracranial stent vs medical therapy on risk of stroke in patients with symptomatic intracranial stenosis: The VISSIT randomized clinical trial. *JAMA* 2015;313:1240–1248.

20. Alexander, M.J., Zauner A, Chaloupka JC, et al. WEAVE Trial: Final results in 152 on-label patients. *Stroke* 2019;50(4):889–894.

CHAPTER FIFTY SIX

ENDOVASCULAR TREATMENT OF ACUTE ISCHEMIC STROKE

EARLY HISTORY

The interventional treatment of acute ischemic stroke (AIS) began in the 1950s, when surgical approaches for cervical carotid disease (thrombendarteriectomy, bypass with vascular bridging graft, and diseased arterial segment resections) were first reported. In 1958, Bernard Sussman and Tom Fitch reported the first three cases of intraarterial (IA) infusion of fibrinolytics (fibrinolysin) to treat cerebral arterial occlusions [1]. The results were angiographically and clinically suboptimal but paved the way for future endovascular therapy investigations. In 1983, Herman Zeumer and his German colleagues reported the feasibility of IA fibrinolytic infusion (streptokinase) in five patients who had basilar artery occlusions (BAO) through 3F catheters placed in the distal cervical vertebral artery [2]. Zeumer was an early neuroradiologist who often thought "outside the box" and was an important innovator. Successful recanalization with clinical improvement occurred in three patients. A year later, the same authors reported the first two cases of IA infusion of urokinase into the internal carotid artery (ICA) to treat ICA occlusions [3].

In the late 1980s, interventional stroke treatment extended to middle cerebral artery (MCA) occlusions when Etsuo Mori and colleagues reported rapid improvement of symptoms following recanalization in 10 of 22 patients with MCA occlusion after intracarotid urokinase infusions [4]. A case-control series of 65 consecutive patients with vertebrobasilar occlusions was reported, including 43 patients treated with local IA thrombolytic therapy (urokinase or streptokinase) and 22 patients treated with conventional therapy (antiplatelet agents or anticoagulants). The interventional group had higher rates of recanalization, fewer neurological deficits, and lower mortality rates [5].

THE TRANSITION TO RANDOMIZED CLINICAL TRIALS

The first randomized clinical trial that evaluated the safety and efficacy of IA thrombolytic infusion in patients with proximal MCA occlusion was PROACT: A Phase II Randomized Trial of Recombinant Pro-Urokinase by Direct Arterial Delivery in Acute Middle Cerebral Artery Stroke [6]. Patients with ischemic stroke due to MCA-M1 or M2 occlusions presenting within six hours of symptom onset were randomized at a 2:1 ratio to receive either an IA infusion of recombinant pro-urokinase (rpro-UK) (n = 26) or placebo (n = 14) over 120 minutes into the proximal thrombus face. All patients also received intravenous heparin. The infused group had significantly higher rates of recanalization compared to placebo (58% vs. 14.%) and higher rates of symptomatic intracranial hemorrhage (sICH) within 24 hours of treatment (15% vs. 7%), which were both found to be heparin dose–dependent.

The PROACT II trial was designed to improve recanalization while limiting sICH [7]. The investigators increased the total dose of rpro-UK from six to nine milligrams given over two hours while using the "low heparin" dose used in PROACT I. Patients were randomized to receive IA rpro-UK plus heparin (n = 121) or heparin only (n = 59) with functional independence "defined as 90-day modified Rankin score (mRS) 0–2" as the primary outcome. The rpro-UK group had higher rates of 90-day functional independence (40% vs. 25%) and arterial recanalization (66% vs. 18%) compared to controls. Mortality rates were similar. The magnitude of clinical effects was substantial and never previously observed in any stroke study. The FDA failed to approve the agent. The components of rpro-UK were not fully known and a second trial was requested but not performed.

The Middle Cerebral Artery Embolism Local Fibrinolytic Intervention Trial (MELT) in Japan randomized stroke patients with MCA-M1 or M2 segments occlusion presenting within six hours of symptom onset to receive IA urokinase (UK) or conventional treatment [8]. The trial was discontinued in 2005 after the approval of intravenous recombinant tissue plasminogen activator (IV-tPA) in Japan. Excellent functional outcome at 90 days (mRS 0–1) was significantly higher in the UK group than in controls. There was no difference in 90-day mortality.

After IV-tPA approval for acute ischemic stroke treatment in 1996, tPA was given intravenously and intraarterially. Several trials studied the safety and effectiveness of combined IV and IA tPA [9]. The results were not definitive but better than placebo without excessive bleeding. No conclusion could be reached about whether IV tPA given before IA infusion was beneficial.

In 2013, three trials represented a major effort to evaluate endovascular treatment (EVT) versus standard medical management that included IV–tPA [10]. These trials had limitations, including suboptimal patient selection (some patients did not have documented large artery occlusions) and delayed and inadequate endovascular reperfusion. These trials did not show a significant difference between EVT and standard medical management.

THE EVOLUTION OF ENDOVASCULAR DEVICES

Infusion of thrombolytic agents evolved. Different agents were used. Technical improvements included mechanical clot disruption (thrombor-rhexis) with micro-guidewire or balloon maceration of the thrombus and development of adjuvant techniques [11]. The low rates of complete reperfusion and relatively high hemorrhagic complication rate seen with the use of IAT led to development of devices to mechanically remove thrombi. The Mechanical Embolus Removal in Cerebral Ischemia (MERCI) trial was a prospective, single-arm, nonrandomized, multicenter study that enrolled patients from 25 US centers. The trial was designed to test the safety and efficacy of the MERCI retrieval device (a corkscrew-shaped tapered wire with five helical loops of decreasing diameter at its distal end that resembled a wine bottle cork removal device) in recanalizing occluded intracranial blood vessels within the first eight hours of symptom onset or within three hours of symptom onset with a contraindication to IV–tPA [12]. Patients were enrolled if their baseline NIHSS score was 10 or more and a diagnostic angiogram showed occlusion of the ICA, MCA-M1 or MCA-M2 segment, BA, or vertebral artery. Recanalization was achieved in only 48 percent of the 141 patients in whom the device was deployed. Significant procedural complications occurred in 7 percent, and sICH occurred in 8 percent of patients. Patients with successful recanalization had higher rates of independence and lower mortality at 90 days compared to those with unsuccessful recanalization. In 2005, the MERCI retriever became the first device to be approved for endovascular treatment (EVT) of AIS.

In 2008 the safety and efficacy of the second generation of MERCI retrieval devices (L5 Retriever) were evaluated in the Multi MERCI trial [13]. The trial extended the eligibility to include those with persistent large vessel occlusion (LVO) after IV–tPA. The rates of successful recanalization were not significantly higher with the novel L5 Retriever than with the previous technology.

The Penumbra Pivotal Stroke Trial aimed to prove "substantial equivalence" in the safety and effectiveness of a new-generation device, the

Penumbra System, which debulked thrombi and aspirated through the Penumbra reperfusion catheter and Penumbra separator (a wire with an olive-shaped component used to fragment thrombi) [13]. Among 125 patients, 82 percent were successfully recanalized with 2 percent serious procedural events and 11 percent sICH. Only a quarter of the patients achieved an mRS score of 2 or less. The Penumbra System was the second device to receive FDA approval for neurothrombectomy.

THE STENT-RETRIEVER ERA

The Solitaire stent was originally developed as an alternative to balloon remodeling in the treatment of cerebral aneurysms. The system allowed immediate restoration of flow upon deployment in patients with large vessel occlusions (LVOs). Clot extraction could be accomplished without permanent stent implantation. This category of device was labeled stent retriever (SR). The safety and effectiveness of the Solitaire AB was studied in revascularization of 20 patients with ICA and MCA occlusion who presented within eight hours of symptom onset [14]. Successful revascularization was achieved in 90 percent of patients. Other studies subsequently reported the safety and efficacy of the Solitaire AB and the nondetachable Solitaire FR (flow restoration) along with other SR, for example, the Trevo and the Revive retriever devices, as the exclusive device, in combination with IV and IA thrombolytics, or as rescue treatment after other devices [15]. Two randomized clinical trials showed the superiority of stent retrievers compared to the MERCI retriever in terms of both revascularization success and safety profile [16].

These early stent retriever trials were led and the results later analyzed by Jeff Saver, Greg Albers, Tudor Jovin, Mayank Goyal, and Raul Nogueira, among others. These leaders were also movers and shakers in many of the subsequent interventional trials.

Jeff Saver received his undergraduate and medical degrees from Harvard University and trained in internal medicine at Brigham and Women's Hospital in Boston and in neurology at the Harvard-Longwood Neurological Training Program. Saver had subspecialty fellowship training in cognitive neuroscience at the University of Iowa and in cerebrovascular disease at Brown University. He then moved to UCLA where he has led the stroke clinical and research program for decades. He made many innovations in the design and statistical evaluation of stroke trials.

Greg Albers received his MD from the University of California San Diego School of Medicine in 1984. He then went to Stanford for his neurology residency and stayed on as a faculty member. He was appointed as the director of the Stanford Stroke Center shortly after arriving at Stanford and is the Coyote Foundation Professor of Neurology and Neurological Sciences at

Stanford. Greg has been instrumental in helping to design and study novel imaging assessment techniques and stroke trials in patients with AIS.

Tudor Jovin grew up in a family of physicians. Both parents and his paternal grandfather were physicians. He received his medical degree from Heinrich Heine University Medical School in Dusseldorf, Germany, and completed an internship and residency in neurology at the University of Pennsylvania Health System in Philadelphia. He completed a cerebrovascular fellowship followed by a fellowship in interventional vascular neurology at the Presbyterian Hospital in Pittsburgh, Pennsylvania. Jovin served as professor of neurology and neurosurgery at the University of Pittsburgh School of Medicine and director of the Center for Neuroendovascular Therapy. He was the director of the Stroke Institute. He then moved to New Jersey as the chair of the Cooper Neurological Institute. He influenced the rapid evaluation and technical details of EVT.

Mayank Goyal received his MD degree from the All India Institute of Medical Sciences in Delhi, India, where he also fulfilled a radiology residency. He then moved to Canada and trained in diagnostic and interventional neuroradiology at the University of Toronto. He was recruited to Alberta as professor of radiology and clinical neurosciences at the University of Calgary. He is the director of imaging and endovascular treatment at the Calgary Stroke Program. Goyal's main research interest is acute stroke imaging, workflow, and intervention.

Raul Nogueira completed his medical school training at the Federal University of Ceará in Fortaleza, Brazil, where he also had a residency in internal medicine. After an internal medicine internship at the University of Miami, he completed his neurology residency at the Massachusetts General Hospital (MGH) and Brigham and Women's Hospital/Harvard Medical School in 2002. He then had fellowships in vascular and critical care neurology as well as interventional neuroradiology at MGH. He moved to Atlanta in September 2010 to help build the Marcus Stroke and Neuroscience Center at the Grady Memorial Hospital where he is the director of the neuroendovascular service. He is professor of neurology and radiology at the Emory University School of Medicine, the former editor-in-chief for the *Interventional Neurology* journal and a former president of the Society of Vascular and Interventional Neurology. He has been instrumental in the design and interpretation of interventional stroke trials.

MODERN ERA MECHANICAL THROMBECTOMY TRIALS

Early Time Window Trials

In 2015, randomized controlled trials reported the overwhelming superiority of EVT over standard medical care alone (including intravenous alteplase for eligible patients) in patients with anterior circulation LVOs treated within the time windows approved at the time of the studies [17]. Two later trials showed similar results. These trials overcame limitations of the previous negative trials by optimizing work flow and patient selection (e.g., requiring imaging to identify patients with proximal occlusion and parenchymal viability) as well as by using stent retrievers as the primary device.

The first positive trial was the Multicenter Randomized Clinical Trial of Endovascular Treatment for Acute Ischemic Stroke in the Netherlands (MR CLEAN) [18]. The Netherlands proved to be an ideal site for this pivotal study. It was a relatively small country with an excellent primary care system and rapid referral to large stroke centers in Amsterdam, Rotterdam, and Utrecht. The trial studied 500 patients (233 in the EVT arm and 267 in the standard medical management arm) with baseline NIHSS score greater than 2 and proximal anterior circulation occlusions who presented within six hours of onset. The results showed a clear benefit of EVT in terms of its primary end point, the adjusted common odds ratio for a shift in the direction of lower disability on the mRS at 90 days. The rate of 90-day functional independence was also significantly higher in the intervention group (33% vs. 19%). The rates of sICH and 90-day mortality were comparable. Following early interim analyses prompted by the positive MR CLEAN results, the five other ongoing trials stopped recruitment.

Five other trials performed in different countries and sites confirmed the positive results of the MR CLEAN trial [19-24]. The Endovascular Treatment for Small Core and Anterior Circulation Proximal Occlusion with Emphasis on Minimizing CT to Recanalization Times (ESCAPE) trial was conducted among 22 sites in Canada, United States, Ireland, and South Korea [19]. The trial recruited 316 patients (165 EVT, 150 controls). Functional independence (90-day mRS 0–2) was increased with the intervention (53% vs. 29%) There was a significant reduction in mortality in EVT (10% vs. 19%). The five other confirmatory trials were (1) the Solitaire with the Intention for Thrombectomy as Primary Endovascular Treatment for Acute Ischemic Stroke (SWIFT PRIME) trial, conducted in 39 United States and European sites [20]; (2) the Revascularization with Solitaire FR® Device vs. Best Medical Therapy in the Treatment of Acute Stroke Due to Anterior Circulation Large Vessel Occlusion Presenting within Eight Hours of Symptom Onset (REVASCAT) trial, conducted in four centers in Catalunya, Spain [21]; (3) the Extending the Time for Thrombolysis in Emergency Neurological Deficits with Intra-Arterial Therapy (EXTEND-IA) trial, conducted among 10 sites in Australia and New Zealand [22]; (4) the THRACE (Thrombectomie des artères cérébrales) trial recruited 414 patients across 26 centers in France [23]; and (5) the Pragmatic Ischemic Thrombectomy Evaluation (PISTE) trial, which enrolled 65 IV-tPA eligible patients with proximal anterior circulation occlusions to combined treatment with thrombectomy or IVT alone among 10 UK centers [24].

The data of the MR CLEAN, ESCAPE, SWIFT-Prime, REVASCAT, and EXTEND-IA trials was combined in a patient-level meta-analysis. The Highly Effective Reperfusion Evaluated in Multiple Endovascular Stroke Trials (HERMES) collaboration included a total of 1,287 patients (634 endovascular thrombectomy, 653 controls) out of which approximately 85 percent received intravenous alteplase [25]. This analysis confirmed the large benefit of thrombectomy for anterior circulation proximal arterial occlusion strokes presenting within the first 6–12 hours from stroke onset in terms of the degree of overall disability, the number needed to treat (2.6), and the chance of achieving functional independence. Thrombectomy was not associated with any significant added risks of parenchymal hematoma, sICH, or 90-day mortality. Prespecified subgroup analysis showed that the benefits extended across broad patient populations with no heterogeneity of treatment effect across differences in age, sex, baseline NIHSS score, baseline ASPECTS, use of intravenous alteplase, occlusion site, and time to randomization.

These trials were performed in high-resource countries with healthcare environments configured to easily incorporate technological advances. It was uncertain whether thrombectomy would be viable and beneficial under less than ideal conditions typically found in developing countries. The Randomization of Endovascular Treatment with Stent-Retriever and/or Thromboaspiration versus Best Medical Therapy in Acute Ischemic Stroke due to Large Vessel Occlusion Trial (RESILIENT) was conducted in the public health care system of Brazil [26]. The trial design was similar to the REVASCAT trial [21]. RESILIENT was stopped early because of efficacy after 221 of a planned 690 patients were randomized. Distribution on the 90-day mRS scores favored the thrombectomy group. The rates of 90-day functional independence were 35 percent in the thrombectomy versus 20 percent in the control group. sICH occurred in 4.5 percent of the patients in each group.

Extension of the Time Window

Stimulated by trials that showed the effectiveness of EVT administered within approved time windows, trials began to explore extending the treatment time windows.

The DWI or CTP Assessment with Clinical Mismatch in the Triage of Wake-Up and Late Presenting Strokes Undergoing Neurointervention with Trevo (DAWN) trial enrolled patients with baseline NIHSS of 10 or greater and occlusion of the ICA or MCA-M1 who were last known well from 6 to 24 hours and had a mismatch between the stroke severity score and infarct volume [27]. The trial stopped after the results of a prespecified interim analysis after enrollment of 206 patients: EVT ($n = 107$) and control group ($n = 99$). The EVT group had a significantly higher mean of 90-day utility-weighted mRS scores and higher rates of 90-day functional independence (49% vs. 13%). The rates of sICH and 90-day mortality were comparable [27].

The DEFUSE 3 trial assessed the efficacy and safety of EVT in patients with baseline NIHSS of 6 or greater and intracranial ICA or MCA-M1 occlusion who presented 6–16 hours after last known well, who had infarct size of less than 70 milliliters, and a mismatch ratio of 1.8 or more [28]. The trial was stopped prematurely due to the results of the DAWN trial after randomizing 182 (92 EVT, 90 control) patients. EVT plus medical therapy was associated with a favorable shift in the distribution of functional outcomes on mRS and a higher rate of functional independence at 90 days (45% vs. 17%) compared with medical therapy alone. There was a trend toward lower rates of 90-day mortality in the EVT group (14% vs. 26%). The frequencies of sICH were similar between both groups [28].

A pooled analysis of data from trial patients who were treated beyond six hours from time last seen well confirmed a strong benefit of thrombectomy [29].

Other EVT Queries

Clinicians and interventionalists have begun to launch studies that seek to refine various aspects of EVT. They have studied aspirating clots versus stent retrievers [30], general anesthesia versus local anesthesia and/or conscious sedation [31], taking the patient directly for angiography rather than performing advanced CT or MRI studies [32], basilar artery occlusion (prior trials were mostly limited to the anterior circulation) [33], and EVT alone or preceded by IV thrombolysis [34]. Future issues will likely consider improving protocols for delivering patients to tertiary stroke centers capable of EVT and enhancing the clot removal and reperfusion process by using neuroprotective and anticlotting agents.

NOTES AND REFERENCES

1. Sussman BJ, Fitch TS. Thrombolysis with fibrinolysin in cerebral arterial occlusion. *J. Am. Med. Assoc.* 1958;167:1705–1709.
2. Zeumer H, Hacke W, Ringelstein EB. Local intraarterial thrombolysis in vertebrobasilar thromboembolic disease. *AJNR Am. J. Neuroradiol.* 1983;4:401–404.
3. Zeumer H, Hündgen R, Ferbert A, Ringelstein EB. Local intraarterial fibrinolytic therapy in inaccessible internal carotid occlusion. *Neuroradiology* 1984;26:315–317.
4. Mori E, Tabuchi M, Yoshida T, Yamadori A. Intracarotid urokinase with thromboembolic occlusion of the middle cerebral artery. *Stroke* 1988;19:802–812.

5. Hacke W, Zeumer H, Ferbert A, Brückmann H, del Zoppo GJ. Intra-arterial thrombolytic therapy improves outcome in patients with acute vertebrobasilar occlusive disease. *Stroke* 1988;19:1216–1222.

6. del Zoppo GJd, Higashida RT, Furlan AJ. PROACT: A phase II randomized trial of recombinant pro-urokinase by direct arterial delivery in acute middle cerebral artery stroke. *Stroke* 1998;29:4–11.

7. Furlan A, Higashida R, Wechsler L, Gent M, Rowley H, Kase C, et al. Intra-arterial prourokinase for acute ischemic stroke. The PROACT II study: A randomized controlled trial. Prolyse in acute cerebral thromboembolism. *JAMA* 1999;282:2003–2011.

8. Ogawa A, Mori E, Minematsu K, et al. Randomized trial of intraarterial infusion of urokinase within 6 hours of middle cerebral artery stroke: The Middle Cerebral Artery Embolism Local Fibrinolytic Intervention Trial (MELT) Japan. *Stroke* 2007;38: 2633–2639.

9. Lewandowski CA, Frankel M, Tomsick TA, et al. Combined intravenous and intra-arterial r-tPA versus intra-arterial therapy of acute ischemic stroke: Emergency Management of Stroke (EMS) bridging trial. *Stroke* 1999;30:2598–2605. Combined intravenous and intra-arterial recanalization for acute ischemic stroke: The Interventional Management of Stroke Study. *Stroke* 2004;35:904–911. The Interventional Management of Stroke (IMS) II Study. *Stroke* 2007;38:2127–2135.

10. Broderick JP, Palesch YY, Demchuk AM, et al. Endovascular therapy after intravenous t-PA versus t-PA alone for stroke. *N. Engl. J. Med.* 2013;368:893–903. Kidwell CS, Jahan R, Gornbein J, et al. A trial of imaging selection and endovascular treatment for ischemic stroke. *N. Engl. J. Med.* 2013;368:914–923. Ciccone A, Valvassori L, Nichelatti M, et al. Endovascular treatment for acute ischemic stroke. *N. Engl. J. Med.* 2013;368:904–913.

11. Nogueira RG, Schwamm LH, Hirsch JA. Endovascular approaches to acute stroke, part 1: Drugs, devices, and data. *AJNR Am. J. Neuroradiol.* 2009;30:649–661.

12. Smith WS, Sung G, Saver J, Budzik R, Duckwiler G, Liebeskind DS, et al. Mechanical thrombectomy for acute ischemic stroke: Final results of the Multi MERCI trial. *Stroke* 2008;39:1205–1212.

13. The Penumbra Pivotal Stroke Trial: Safety and effectiveness of a new generation of mechanical devices for clot removal in intracranial large vessel occlusive disease. *Stroke* 2009;40:2761–2768.

14. Castaño C, Dorado L, Guerrero C, et al. Mechanical thrombectomy with the Solitaire AB device in large artery occlusions of the anterior circulation: A pilot study. *Stroke* 2010;41:1836–1840.

15. Roth C, Papanagiotou P, Behnke S, et al. Stent-assisted mechanical recanalization for treatment of acute intracerebral artery occlusions. *Stroke* 2010;41:2559–2567.

16. Saver JL, Jahan R, Levy EI, et al. Solitaire flow restoration device versus the Merci retriever in patients with acute ischaemic stroke (SWIFT): A randomised, parallel-group, non-inferiority trial. *Lancet* 2012;380:1241–1249. Nogueira RG, Lutsep HL, Gupta R, et al. Trevo versus Merci retrievers for thrombectomy revascularisation of large vessel occlusions in acute ischaemic stroke (Trevo 2): A randomised trial. *Lancet* 2012;380:1231–1240.

17. Examples include Goyal M, Demchuk AM, Menon BK, et al. Randomized assessment of rapid endovascular treatment of ischemic stroke. *N. Engl. J. Med.* 2015;372:1019–1030. Saver JL, Goyal M, Bonafe A, et al. Stent-retriever thrombectomy after intravenous t-PA vs. t-PA alone in stroke. *N. Engl. J. Med.*

2015;372:2285–2295. Jovin TG, Chamorro A, Cobo E, de Miquel MA, Molina CA, Rovira A, et al. Thrombectomy within 8 hours after symptom onset in ischemic stroke. *N. Engl. J. Med.* 2015;372:2296–2306.

18. Berkhemer OA, Fransen PS, Beumer D, et al. for the MR CLEAN Investigators. A randomized trial of intraarterial treatment for acute ischemic stroke. *N. Engl. J. Med.* 2015;372:11–20.

19. Goyal M, Demchuk AM, Menon BK, et al. Randomized assessment of rapid endovascular treatment of ischemic stroke. *N. Engl. J. Med.* 2015;372:1019–1030.

20. Saver JL, Goyal M, Bonafe A, et al. Stent-retriever thrombectomy after intravenous t-PA vs. T-PA alone in stroke. *N. Engl. J. Med.* 2015;372:2285–2295.

21. Jovin TG, Chamorro A, Cobo E, et al. Thrombectomy within 8 hours after symptom onset in ischemic stroke. *N. Engl. J. Med.* 2015;372:2296–2306.

22. Campbell BC, Mitchell PJ, Kleinig TJ, et al. Endovascular therapy for ischemic stroke with perfusion-imaging selection. *N. Engl. J. Med.* 2015;372:1009–1018.

23. Bracard S, Ducrocq X, Mas JL, et al. Mechanical thrombectomy after intravenous alteplase versus alteplase alone after stroke (THRACE): A randomised controlled trial. *Lancet Neurol.* 2016;15:1138–1147.

24. Muir KW, Ford GA, Messow CM, et al. Endovascular therapy for acute ischaemic stroke: The Pragmatic Ischaemic Stroke Thrombectomy Evaluation (PISTE) randomised, controlled trial. *J. Neurol. Neurosurg. Psychiatry* 2017;88:38–44.

25. Goyal M, Menon BK, van Zwam WH, et al. Endovascular thrombectomy after large-vessel ischaemic stroke: A meta-analysis of individual patient data from five randomised trials. *Lancet* 2016;387:1723–1731.

26. Martins SO, Mont'Alverne F, Rebello LC, et al. Thrombectomy for stroke in the public health care system of Brazil. *N. Engl. J. Med.* 2020;382:2316–2326.

27. Nogueira RG, Jadhav AP, Haussen DC, et al. Thrombectomy 6 to 24 hours after stroke with a mismatch between deficit and infarct. *N. Engl. J. Med.* 2017;378:11–21.

28. Albers GW, Marks MP, Kemp S, et al. Thrombectomy for stroke at 6 to 16 hours with selection by perfusion imaging. *N. Engl. J. Med.* 2018;378:708–718.

29. Jovin T, Nogueira RG, Lansberg M, et al. Thrombectomy for anterior circulation stroke beyond 6 hours from time last known well: The AURORA (analysis of pooled data from randomized studies of thrombectomy more than 6 hours after last known well) collaboration. Lancet 2021, in press.

30. Lapergue B, Blanc R, Gory B, et al. Effect of endovascular contact aspiration vs stent retriever on revascularization in patients with acute ischemic stroke and large vessel occlusion: The ASTER randomized clinical trial. *JAMA* 2017;318:443–452. Turk AS III, Siddiqui A, Fifi JT, et al. Aspiration thrombectomy versus stent retriever thrombectomy as first-line approach for large vessel occlusion (COMPASS): A multicentre, randomised, open label, blinded outcome, non-inferiority trial. *Lancet* 2019;393:998–1008.

31. Schönenberger S, Hendén PL, Simonsen CZ, et al. Association of general anesthesia vs procedural sedation with functional outcome among patients with acute ischemic stroke undergoing thrombectomy: A systematic review and meta-analysis. *JAMA* 2019;322:1283–1293.

32. Mendez B, Requena M, Aires A, et al. Direct transfer to angio-suite to reduce workflow times and increase favorable clinical outcome. *Stroke* 2018;49:2723–2727.

33. Liu X, Dai Q, Ye R, et al. Endovascular treatment versus standard medical treatment for vertebrobasilar artery occlusion (BEST): An open-label, randomised controlled

trial. *Lancet Neurol.* 2020;19:115–122. Langezaal LCM, van der Hoeven EJRJ, Mont'Alverne FJA, et al. Endovascular therapy for stroke due to basilar-artery occlusion. *N. Engl. J. Med.* 2021;384:1910–1920.

34. Yang P, Zhang Y, Zhang L, et al. Endovascular thrombectomy with or without intravenous alteplase in acute stroke. *N. Engl. J. Med.* 2020;382:1981–1993.

CHAPTER FIFTY SEVEN

BRAIN ANEURYSM TREATMENT

A brain aneurysm can remain unruptured or create a devastating intracranial hemorrhage. Throughout history, neurosurgeons have tried to understand its pathology in order to devise optimal treatment. Despite many procedures and surgical approaches, aneurysms continue to confound management. Treatments gradually progressed from ligation of proximal arteries to surgical clip placement to endovascular occlusion and to modern blood flow diversion techniques.

RECOGNITION OF ANEURYSMS

In 2725 BCE, the Egyptian physician Imhotep used a fire-glazed instrument to cauterize a bulging peripheral artery aneurysm. As the father of Egyptian medicine, he is believed to have said the following in the Ebers Papyrus about aneurysm treatment [1]: "This is a vessel swelling, a disorder I will treat. It is the vessels that cause it. It originates from an injury upon the vessel. Then thou shalt apply to it treatment with the knife; this [the knife] is heated in fire; the bleeding will not be considerable" [1].

Despite this early intervention and observation, understanding of aneurysms was almost nonexistent for centuries due to religious, cultural, and superstitious hindrances. It wasn't until 2,000 years later when the next scientific account of an aneurysm was made when the Ephesian physician Flaenius Rufus of Alexandria (117 BCE) suggested that an aneurysm may be the result of injury sustained by an artery [1]. Many years later, the Greek physician Galen of Perganon (129–210 CE) coined the term "aneurysm" (Greek *aneurysma*, a widening; from *anu*, across, and *eurys*, broad) [2]: "An artery having become anastomosed (i.e., dilated) the affection is called aneurysm; it also arises from the wound of the same, when the skin lies over it is cicatrized, but the wound in the artery remains, and neither unites nor is blocked by flesh" [3].

During the next few hundred years understanding and management of peripheral artery aneurysms grew. The first intracranial aneurysm, an unruptured postmortem aneurysm of the posterior carotid artery branches, was described by Morgagni of Padua (1682–1771 CE) in 1764 [4]. Four years later, Francisci Biumi published another account of a ruptured cavernous carotid artery aneurysm found at postmortem [2]. No diagnostic tools existed during this period to diagnose an intracranial aneurysm during life. Alert clinicians identified clinical signs such as a third nerve palsy, bruits on auscultation, and pulsations seen at the patient's head that suggested the presence of a brain aneurysm. A method of treatment would not be offered until the late nineteenth century.

EARLY RECOGNITION AND TREATMENT

The first treatment of intracranial aneurysm was based on the work of Scottish scientist and surgeon John Hunter (1728–1793) when he ligated the proximal femoral artery from feeding a popliteal aneurysm and induced thrombosis within the aneurysm [5]. Despite its effectiveness, it would not become a method of treatment for intracranial aneurysms until the nineteenth century. Jean Louis Petit (1674–1750) observed that the brain could survive on a single carotid artery supply after following a patient who had a completely occluded carotid artery for seven years [2]. Encouraged by this observation, Mason Cogswell (1761–1830) pioneered carotid ligation for carotid aneurysms, but the results and success of this procedure were widely unpredictable and variable [2]. Sir Astley Cooper (1768–1841), a surgeon at Guy's Hospital in London, applied the principles of Hunterian ligation and recorded the treatment and results in two cervical aneurysm patients [6]. First in 1805, he ligated the carotid artery in a patient with a massive carotid aneurysm consuming two thirds of her neck, but the patient became hemiplegic and died soon after. Cooper persisted and in 1808, he successfully ligated a smaller aneurysm at the angle of the jaw, and the patient returned to work months after the procedure [6]. The first intracranial aneurysms were found only by chance and during the treatment of other intracranial diseases.

In 1885, Victor Horsley (1857–1916), recorded a massive internal carotid artery (ICA) aneurysm that compressed the optic chiasm, which he treated with bilateral cervical artery occlusion [7]. In February 1886, the Board of

Governors of the National Hospital for the Paralysed and Epileptic in Queen Square, London, appointed Horsley to take forward cranial surgery. This was the first neurosurgical post in history. Victor Horsley was only 28, but he had already made a name for himself as an outstanding research scientist. In 1902, Horsley uncovered a massive middle cranial fossa ICA aneurysm while operating on a patient for a suspected brain tumor and performed a cervical carotid artery ligation [7]. According to reports, the patient was doing well five years later.

Although proximal carotid artery ligations provided early neurosurgeons with a treatment option, many remained doubtful about the safety and therapeutics of carotid ligations as a treatment for intracranial aneurysms. Harvey Cushing (1869–1939), for one, expressed his own skepticism: "A lesion having such remote surgical bearings . . . whether there are surgical indications such as ligation of the internal carotid, further experience alone can tell" [8].

During exploratory craniotomies Cushing documented nine patients in his "little black book" who were initially suspected to harbor brain tumors, but were found to have a pulsating mass instead (Figure 57.1) [8]. Cushing would confirm the diagnosis of an aneurysm by puncturing the mass and observing a gush of blood. He would then wrap the mass with muscle to promote thrombosis. On occasion, Cushing would treat the aneurysm by ligating the carotid artery. This was a procedure he hated due to its postoperative complications [8].

To prevent the postoperative complications of carotid ligation, the idea of gradually occluding the carotid artery was tested. The invention of the Selverstone clamp changed aneurysm treatment. Various other similar clamps

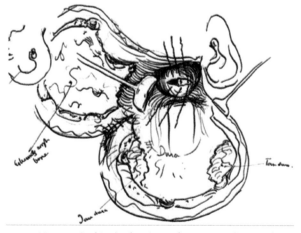

57.1. Harvey Cushing's drawing of an internal carotid aneurysm found on craniotomy. Reprinted from Cohen-Gadol AA, Spencer DD. Harvey W. Cushing and cerebrovascular surgery: Part I, aneurysms. *J. Neurosurg.* 2004;101:547–552, with permission of the publisher. Copyright © 2004, American Association of Neurological Surgeons.

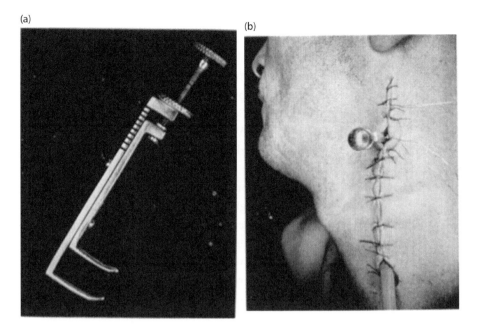

57.2. (a) Poppen-Blalock clamp. Calibration along shaft indicates degree of occlusion. (b) Head of the clamp and tentative wire ligatures, showing relation to the wound. From Fager CA, Poppen JL. Observations on controlled ligation of the internal carotid artery. *Surg. Clin. North Am.* 1956 Jun;36 (3):567–582.

were also designed and used. The Poppin–Blalock clamp and its positioning in the neck of a patient is shown in Figure 57.2. The clamp was designed to be placed around the internal carotid artery. During 72 hours the artery would be gradually tightened to reduce the blood pressure to promote wall thickening and clot formation within the sac, while simultaneously allowing for the development of collateral cerebral circulation [9]. This tool provided surgeons with the ability to control the degree of occlusion postoperatively, since the tool used to tighten the device extended from the clamp to the surface of the neck, allowing for reopening at the first sign of persistent brain ischemia. This approach reduced the incidence of carotid ischemic complications. As an intern, Lou Caplan was instructed to manipulate the clamp after it was inserted into the neck of a patient with a large left intracranial carotid aneurysm. He was told "if the patient stops talking and goes weak on the right, then loosen the clamp and wait until the next day to tighten it further."

Due to technological limitations, the primary treatments available to treat cerebral aneurysms during the early twentieth century were ligatures and clamps. Frustrated by the outcomes of these methods, Sir Norman Dott (1897–1973) began to explore a more direct approach to treat this fatal disease [10]. Dott was a Scottish neurosurgeon. He was born in Edinburgh in 1897, the third of five children. He intended a career in engineering, but a serious motorcycle accident hospitalized him and left him with a permanent leg injury. The long in-hospital spell changed his career plan and he focused on medicine rather than engineering [10]. He studied medicine at the University of Edinburgh, graduating with an MB in 1919 and PhD in 1922. He received a Rockefeller Traveling Scholarship that allowed him to travel to America to study in Boston under Harvey Cushing. In 1932 he began lecturing at the University of Edinburgh. During World War II, Dott created a specialist brain injuries unit. In 1947, he received the professorship in neurosurgery (one of the first in the world). He was made a Commander of the Order of the British Empire (CBE) for his wartime work in 1948. In 1960 he created a department of neurosurgery at the Edinburgh Royal Infirmary, one of the first such facilities in the National Health Service of the United Kingdom.

In 1931, Dott successfully treated a ruptured internal carotid aneurysm by directly exposing and wrapping it with muscle taken from the patient's thigh, a technique he acquired from Harvey Cushing during his mentorship [10]. Expanding on this approach, Dott perfected the complicated technique of ligating the neck of an aneurysm with a suture. Placement of the suture was difficult and could instantly rupture the friable aneurysm wall.

Years before Dott's efforts, Harvey Cushing had designed a silver clip in 1911 to occlude and control deep blood vessels from hemorrhaging during intracranial tumor resection [11]. Cushing never used his silver clip to treat aneurysms. Walter Dandy (1886–1946) used the Cushing clip after it was modified by Kenneth McKenzie to successfully clip the first intracranial aneurysm in a 43-year-old man with a right third nerve palsy in 1937 [12].

Dandy grew up in Sedalia, Missouri, and graduated from the University of Missouri in 1907 [13]. He graduated from the Johns Hopkins School of Medicine in 1910 at the age of 24, and became the sixth appointee to the Hunterian Laboratory of Experimental Medicine under Harvey Cushing. He then joined the Johns Hopkins Hospital surgical house staff for one year as Cushing's assistant resident (1911–1912). Dandy's personal style clashed with Cushing's, and they later became bitter rivals and enemies [13]. Pioneering these efforts, Walter Dandy, as a resident at Johns Hopkins, diagnostically injected air into the ventricles (ventriculography). After numerous successful trials of ventriculography used in the treatment of hydrocephalus in adults and children, Dandy published a case series in which he commented: "Even in the few cases here reported, ventriculography has proven of great practical value. For the first time, we have a means of diagnosing internal hydrocephalus in the early stages ... before a considerable amount of cortical destruction has resulted" [13].

Dandy noticed that air leaked out of the ventricular system and traversed to the surface of the brain. From these observations, wishing to be able to visualize intracranial structures at the brain base and around the brain surface,

Dandy introduced the pneumoencephalogram in 1918, which, although painful, potentially allowed for visualization of intracranial tumors and aneurysms. Dandy made many other neurosurgical discoveries and innovations, including the description of the cranial circulation of cerebrospinal fluid, surgical treatment of hydrocephalus, description of brain endoscopy, and the first clipping of an intracranial aneurysm. Dandy joined the staff of the Johns Hopkins Hospital in 1918 and immediately focused his energies on the surgical treatment of disorders of the brain and spinal cord. Dandy was the only neurosurgeon at the Johns Hopkins Hospital from 1922 until his death there in 1946.

Despite Dandy completing the aneurysm surgery in 1937, it was not published in the *Annals of Surgery* until 1938 [12]. The patient was a 43-year-old man with a past medical history of chronic alcohol use and gastric disorder who was referred to Dandy due to complaints of six days of worsening right frontal headache, diplopia, and right cranial nerve III palsy. After initial assessment and diagnosis of an aneurysm by a neurologist, Dandy posited that the aneurysm was likely located at the right internal carotid artery or the posterior communicating artery due to the third nerve palsy. On March 23, 1937, the patient was taken to surgery, and Dandy approached the aneurysm by performing a right frontotemporal craniotomy for a "hypophyseal approach." There was marked cortical atrophy due to the patient's alcohol use. After retraction of the frontal and temporal lobes and exposure of the optic chiasm, a "pea-sized aneurysm" was spotted originating from the ICA adjacent to the posterior communicating artery (PComA). The aneurysm did not involve the PComA and was firmly attached to the dura. The third nerve coursed behind the aneurysm in its regular anatomical position. Once the small neck of the aneurysm was identified, the Cushing-McKenzie silver clip was placed around it (Figure 57.3). After the clip was placed, the aneurysm obliterated completely and the dome was cauterized. Dandy then watched as the dome softened and stopped pulsating, permanently leaving the clip in place to fulfill its purpose. Postoperatively, other than an episode of delirium tremens, the patient made a good recovery and left the hospital two weeks after the procedure. Extraocular movements were normal seven months later.

INTRACRANIAL ANEURYSM SURGERY AND CLIPPING

The practice of aneurysm clipping spread worldwide as Dandy continued his direct approach to aneurysm treatment and collected a large patient series, which he published in 1944 [14]. Valentine Logue (1913–2000), an Australian-born London neurosurgeon, clipped the A1 segment to trap an anterior communicating artery aneurysm in 1956 and developed techniques for direct management of anterior communicating artery aneurysms [15].

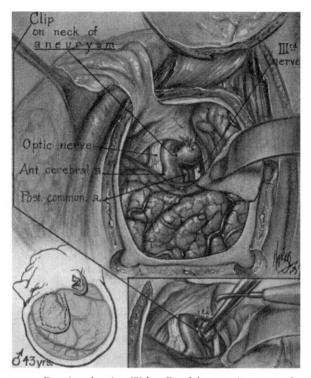

57.3. Drawing showing Walter Dandy's operative approach to an aneurysm. From Dandy W. Intracranial aneurysms of the internal carotid artery cured by operation. *Ann. Surg.* 1938;107:654–659.

Intracranial direct aneurysm surgery and clipping took great talent, visualization, and dexterity because it was performed before introduction of the operating microscope and microsurgery. The advent of angiography by Egas Moniz in 1927 and the ability to visualize an aneurysm before and after surgery encouraged neurosurgeons to more confidently approach intracranial aneurysms [16]. Intracranial surgery had its risks. Due to suboptimal magnification, morbidity with the direct approach remained high, leading many neurosurgeons to continue practicing the indirect method of proximal artery ligation and bed rest up until the 1970s.

The V-shaped Cushing-Mackenzie clip proceeded through a myriad of variations and modifications. Hebert Olivecrona modified this malleable silver clip by adding winged blades to the side, allowing the clip to be adjusted and reopened in order to secure the grip around the neck of the aneurysm [17]. These clips could crush the neck of an aneurysm while shearing and tearing it. In order to avoid these complications, Frank Mayfield and George Kees slimmed down the size of the applicator and made clips with variable sizes, improving the ergonomics of clip placement [18]. The Mayfield-Kees clip was the predominant choice during the 1950s and 1960s. During the following decades, significant modifications and improvements were made to the

Mayfield-Kees clip. Better biocompatible metals were used, blade openings were widened, and the shape of the clip was modified to allow better visualization during placement. While preparing to treat a basilar artery aneurysm, Charles Drake (1920–1998) recognized the need for a clip that would allow him to access the neck of an aneurysm without compromising the other arteries and nerves surrounding it. The night prior to the procedure, Kees modified the Mayfield-Kees clip with a fenestration and delivered it to Drake just in time to treat a basilar artery aneurysm without compromising the posterior cerebral artery [19]. These clips became known as "fenestrated clips," and variations of them are still in use today. Later, newer, modified clips had to become compatible with the new magnetic resonance imaging. Concurrent with development, modifications to aneurysm clips were based on metallurgy and design configurations that helped improve surgical efficacy and safety in aneurysm treatment.

Charley Drake, professor of neurosurgery in London, Ontario, was a pioneer in surgery on posterior fossa aneurysms [20]. He was known to tackle large vertebral and basilar artery aneurysms considered inoperable by other physicians. He used a variety of techniques, including sacrificing feeding arteries and clipping. He was made a Companion of the Order of Canada, and also became president of the Royal College of Physicians and Surgeons of Canada (1971–1973), the American Association of Neurological Surgeons (1977), the American College of Surgeons (1984–1985), and the World Federation of Neurological Societies (1977–1981). Drake was one of the only neurosurgeons to be honored as the president of the American College of Surgeons.

MICRONEUROSURGERY AND GAZI YAŞARGIL

Introduction of the surgical microscope challenged surgeons to navigate through surgical corridors previously considered unreachable. In the early 1970s, ear, nose, and throat surgeons were beginning to use the operating microscope for various procedures. Raymond M. P. (Pete) Donaghy was working at the University of Vermont on the use of the operating microscope in neurosurgery [21]. He developed a cadaver dissection lab and began using it for human surgeries. Word of his innovative work began to spread, and the history of neurosurgery changed when Gazi Yaşargil came to Vermont.

Mahmut Gazi Yaşargil was born in Lice, a small Kurdish-populated town in Turkey, in 1925 [22]. He moved with his family to Ankara when three months old. During his childhood, he lost his brother Ihsan to abdominal typhus, an event that inspired him and his brothers to study medicine. He matriculated at Ankara University in Turkey and then went to Germany to study medicine at the Friedrich Schiller University of Jena. He left Jena in April 1945 near the end of World War II. He was accepted at the University of Basel, Switzerland, where he had his first contact with microsurgery. In January 1953, he began his training in neurosurgery in Zurich under the mentorship of Hugo Krayenbül, studying neuroanatomy. He spent many years in the department of neurosurgery in Zurich studying, watching, and being mentored by Krayenbül. In 1965 Yaşargil came to the United States, first to Massachusetts General Hospital and then to be trained in vascular microsurgery under the tutelage of Raymond Donaghy in Burlington, Vermont. He was at that time 40 years old and already had had 13 years of experience in classical neurosurgical procedures. Yaşargil stayed in Vermont for two years where he was mentored in microneurosurgical techniques. He worked with Donaghy on microdissection under the microscope to reach various structures and aneurysms in particular. He then returned to Zurich where he further enthusiastically and skillfully developed microsurgery. In 1973 Yaşargil was appointed professor and chairman of the department of neurosurgery in Zurich, succeeding his mentor, Prof. Krayenbül. Over the next 20 years, he carried out laboratory work and clinical applications of microneurosurgical techniques, performing 7,500 intracranial operations in Zurich until his retirement from there in 1993. He later moved to Arkansas where he continued to expand microneurosurgy in the United States [22,23].

Yaşargil and Donaghy pioneered the technique of extracranial to intracranial artery bypass (EC-IC bypass) for ischemia by anastomosing the superficial temporal artery to the middle cerebral artery. They taught the technique to many young vascular neurosurgeons. Yaşargil refined techniques of aneurysmal dissection and clipping using the operating microscope. He and his colleagues invented a cross-section spring clip with strong closing pressures and a narrow base, which increased the visibility of the aneurysm neck [22,23].

ENDOVASCULAR TREATMENT

The endovascular approach to treat aneurysms did not take place until the 1960s. As a basis for endovascular approach, Alfred Velpeau (1795–1867), a French surgeon, is credited with noting the formation of thrombosis within an aneurysm and its exclusion from the systemic circulation after inserting foreign materials into the aneurysm itself [2]. Building on this observation, Barney Brooks (1884–1952) introduced a strap of muscle into the internal carotid artery and thrombosed a carotid-cavernous fistula in 1930 [2]. During the next decades, various materials such as horse hair and copper wire were introduced experimentally to induce thrombosis within an aneurysm.

Endovascular catheter treatment and technology progressed with the work of two Georgetown University neurosurgeons, Alfred J. Luessenhop and William T. Spence, who successfully deposited silastic spheres into the internal carotid artery to treat an arteriovenous malformation in 1960 [24]

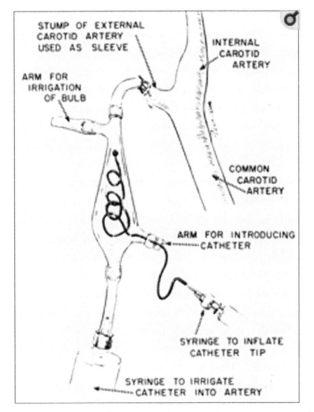

57.4. Schematic illustration showing the report on the first catheterization of intracranial arteries. From Luessenhop AJ, Velasquez AC, Observations on the tolerance of the intracranial arteries to catheterization. *J. Neurosurg.* 1964;21:85–91.

(Figure 57.4). Two years later, Steven Rothenberg introduced an angiotactic balloon via a 4-French delivery system, demonstrating the use of balloons for the treatment of intracranial endovascular disease [25]. In 1964, Luessenhop and Alfredo Velaquez safely deployed a balloon into the internal carotid artery, demonstrating the exclusion of an aneurysm from systemic circulation after balloon inflation [24]. Magnets were also employed to direct material into aneurysms. E. H. Frei and colleagues developed the Para-Operational Device (POD) in 1966 [26], which was further modified when Shyam Yodh and colleagues developed a method of endovascular techniques using metal filings and external magnets [27].

Neurosurgeons continued to modify balloon treatment and catheterization when they were able to place nondetachable balloons within the aneurysm, resulting in persistent thrombosis. Serbinenko further revolutionized endovascular treatment during the second half of the twentieth century. Fiódor Andreevitch Serbinenko was born in 1928 in a small village in the Northern Caucasus portion of the Soviet Union [28]. His father worked as a mechanic in the local flour mill, and his mother was a homemaker. His schooling was interrupted by World War II, during which his older brother was killed. Serbinenko, at age 14, worked as an apprentice machinist from 1941 to 1945 to support his family. After the war, he continued working as a machinist but studied at night. Economic hard times in postwar Russia compelled him to often work during medical school at extracurricular jobs that involved hard physical labor. When he graduated from medical school in 1954, he received an appointment as an Academy of Medical Sciences intern at the N. N. Burdenko Neurosurgery Institute in Moscow where he worked for the next 44 years.

Serbinenko first became skilled at percutaneous cerebral angiography, performed by direct carotid and vertebral artery puncture. In 1957, he became a neurosciences doctoral candidate, and part of his thesis concerned cerebrovascular fistulae. A perhaps apocryphal story is told that in 1959, at a May Day celebration in Moscow's Red Square, Serbinenko's attention was attracted to helium-filled balloons held by children. These balloons were easily maneuvered by manipulating their tether lines. He wondered whether a tiny balloon at the end of a long catheter could be similarly maneuvered and navigated intravascularly for diagnostic or therapeutic blockage of a vessel [28].

Serbinenko organized a small laboratory to investigate potential materials for the creation of a balloon catheter. After much trial and error, he created prototype silicone and latex balloon catheters. With improved design and with careful balloon inflation and deflation, the balloon-tipped microcatheter had excellent flow directional capabilities that allowed navigation of the tortuous vascular anatomy at the cranial base. This made possible the first effective intracranial catheterization. Flow directional characteristics allowed the balloon tip to preferentially seek high-flow arteriovenous fistulae and major AVM feeding arteries. With the use of multiple balloon devices, superselective intracranial catheterization became possible.

On February 8, 1964, the first selective external carotid angiogram was performed with the assistance of temporary internal carotid artery balloon occlusion. Temporary balloon occlusion became an important adjunct to direct puncture carotid angiography at the Burdenko Institute. From 1969 to 1972, Serbinenko performed 304 such procedures with only two recorded deaths. Permanent therapeutic occlusion of cervical and intracranial arteries and vascular lesions was accomplished using a different balloon device. This device was inflated at a target site with a mixture of silicone polymer and tantalum powder to create a radiopaque material that quickly become a stable gel within the balloon and distal catheter lumen. The catheter could be severed without risking polymer leakage from the distal catheter segment. He later developed a balloon with a valve mechanism that allowed balloon detachment from its delivery microcatheter by placing traction on the catheter. From 1970 to 1973, Serbinenko performed 162 therapeutic cerebral vascular occlusions, treating aneurysms, carotid-cavernous fistulas, and major feeding vessels to AVMs, with only two reported deaths. He later adopted the transfemoral Seldinger technique for his endovascular procedures [28].

In 1974, Serbinenko reported and published the use of selective catheterization to deliver and deploy detachable balloons filled with liquid silicone for the treatment of arteriovenous malformations and cerebral aneurysms in 300 patients [29]. This marked the beginning of balloons that could be detached and deployed to occlude the neck of an aneurysm. Results in large series of patients of balloon occlusion included significant complications such as intraoperative and delayed rupture, with recurrent recanalization of an aneurysm at rates as high as 20 percent [30]. While balloon deployment was being perfected, Guido Guglielmi began to work on techniques that would combine the concepts of electrothrombosis and endovascular approaches in his laboratory at the University of Rome [31].

A urologist's son, Guido Guglielmi was born in Rome, Italy, in 1948 [31]. He studied engineering at the University of Rome, but changed to medicine. As his particular interest was neurology, he entered as a neurosurgery resident at the University of Rome. Guglielmi took a great interest in electronics and engineering, and began studying the concept of electrothrombosis of intracranial aneurysms in 1974. That same year, Guido's father had an aneurysmal subarachnoid hemorrhage. In 1976, as a junior physician at the University of Rome, Guglielmi started his neurosurgical practice. During the next three years he read and thought about the possibility of using electrothrombosis for aneurysm treatment, and, in 1979, he conducted a series of in vivo experiments by using electrothrombosis for obliteration of experimental aneurysms in rabbits [31]. In 1983, Guglielmi met with Fernando Viñuela, who was then a junior staff physician at the University of Western Ontario in London, Ontario. When Fernando moved to Los Angeles, they began to collaborate on research efforts directed toward development of new techniques for the treatment of aneurysms. Guglielmi and his family came to Los Angeles, and in January 1989, a research project involving treatment of aneurysms using a combination of metallic microspheres and micromagnets delivered using an endovascular approach was begun at UCLA [31].

Guglielmi initially built a microwire with a magnet that would be introduced endovascularly within an aneurysm. He then injected iron microspheres into the circulation, which would be attracted to the small magnet within the aneurysm and induce thrombosis. Observing the electrolytic capabilities of stainless steel, he attached an electrolysis-resistant platinum coil to the stainless steel wire and invented the concept of a detachable coil [32]. In 1990, the first coil was deployed in a patient with a traumatic carotid cavernous fistula who failed balloon occlusion. A month later, Guglielmi, along with the help of Ivan Sepetka, treated the first aneurysm with an electrolytic detachable coil successfully [32]. Coiling ensured more complete occlusion of aneurysms than balloon deployment and reduced the risk of distal embolization.

Observations and reports found that although endovascular surgery using coils had excellent long-term results with small aneurysms, the large aneurysms had a significant recanalization rate. To address this issue, balloons would be placed across the neck of an aneurysm, while the coil would be deployed with a second microcatheter into the aneurysm. By using this technique, better packing was achieved with less protrusion of the coil into the parent artery. Bioactive coatings were used with coils in the hope that such technology might improve healing at the aneurysm neck and reduce aneurysm recurrence. Later, stents were introduced to help ensure that the detachable coils would be directed only into aneurysmal sacs. Endovascular coiling was performed after stent deployment through a microcatheter; the coils were advanced through the stent struts or had been placed inside the aneurysm sac before the stents were introduced and impacted between the stent and the vessel wall [33].

During the first decade of the twenty-first century, flow-diverting stents were introduced to treat large intracranial aneurysms. These flow diverters disrupted flow near the neck of aneurysms, inducing thrombosis in the aneurysmal sac while preserving blood flow in the parent vessel and in adjacent branches [34]. These were mostly used to treat large aneurysms.

Observational studies and trials showed that interventional treatment of aneurysms was at least as effective as surgery and was associated with less mortality and morbidity. Neurosurgeons began to train in interventional treatment as the twentieth century ended. The number of neurosurgeons, neurologists, and neuroradiologists trained to provide interventional treatments through the vascular system grew dramatically after the onset of the twenty-first century. More than two thirds of intracranial aneurysms are treated in the United States and Europe through an endovascular approach.

Chapter 18 on recognition of aneurysms and Chapter 59 on treatment of arteriovenous malformations cover some similar topics.

NOTES AND REFERENCES

1 Moulin D. Ebers Papyrus. *Arch. Chir. Neerl.* 1961;12:49–63.

2 Milinis K, Thapar A, O'Neill K, Davies AH. History of aneurysmal spontaneous subarachnoid hemorrhage. *Stroke* 2017;48:e280–e283.

3 Magnus V. Aneurysm of the internal carotid artery. *JAMA* 1927;88:1721–1713.

4 Morgagni J. *Sedibus et causis morborum per anatomen indagatis. Venetis, ex typog. Remodiniana.* New York: Hafner, 1960, p. 1. The career of Morgagnis is the topic of Chapter 7, and Morgagni's description of an intracranial aneurysm is described also in Chapter 17.

5 Pool JL. The development of modern intracranial aneurysm surgery. *Neurosurgery* 1977;1:233–237.

6 Hunter J, Ottley D, Bell T, Home E, Babington GG, Owen R. *The Works of John Hunter, FRS with Notes*. London: Longman, Rees, Orme, Brown, Green, and Longman, 1837.

7 Cooper B. *Lectures on the Principles and Practices of Surgery*, 2nd ed. Philadelphia: Blanchard & Lee, 1852. Cooper A. A case of aneurism of the carotid artery. *Med. Chir. Trans.* 1809;1:1–121. Cooper A. A second case of aneurism of the carotid artery. *Med. Chir. Trans.* 1809;1:224–235.

8 Powell MP. Sir Victor Horsley at the birth of neurosurgery. *Brain* 2016;139(2):631–634. Keen W. Intracranial lesions. *Med. News NY* 1890;57:443.

9 Cohen-Gadol AA, Spencer DD, Harvey W. Cushing and cerebrovascular surgery: Part I, aneurysms. *J. Neurosurg.* 2004;101:547–552. doi:10.317/jns.2004.101.3.0547. Sir Charles Symonds's account of the inadvertent discovery of an intracranial aneurysm by Cushing is recounted in detail in Chapter 18.

10 Mount LA. Results of treatment of intracranial aneurysms using the Selverstone clamp. *J. Neurosurg.* 1959;16:611–618.

11 Dott N. Intracranial aneurysms: Cerebral arterioradiography: Surgical treatment. *Edinb. Med. J.* 1933;40(12):T219–T240. Todd NV, Howie JE, Miller JD. Norman Dott's contribution to aneurysm surgery. *J. Neurol. Neurosurg. Psychiatry* 1990;53:455–458. Norman Dott. Wikipedia. Available at https://en.wikipedia.org/wiki/Norman_Dott.

12 Cushing HI. The control of bleeding in operations for brain tumors: With the description of silver "clips" for the occlusion of vessels inaccessible to the ligature. *Ann. Surg.* 1911;54:1–19.

13 Dandy W. Intracranial aneurysms of the internal carotid artery cured by operation. *Ann. Surg.* 1938;107:654–659.

14 Fox, WL. *Dandy of Johns Hopkins*. Baltimore, MD: Williams and Wilkins, 1984. Bliss M. *Harvey Cushing: A Life in Surgery*. Oxford: Oxford University Press, 2005. Dandy WE. Ventriculography following injection of air into the cerebral ventricles. *Ann. Surg.* 1918;68:5–11.

15 Dandy WE. *Intracranial Arterial Aneurysms*. Ithaca, NY: Comstock, 1944.

16 Logue, V. Surgery in spontaneous subarachnoid haemorrhage: Operative treatment of aneurysms on the anterior cerebral and anterior communicating artery. *Brit. Med. J.* 1956 4965:473–479.

17 Moniz's introduction of brain angiography and the evolution of angiography is the topic of Chapter 31.

18 Fox JL (ed.). *Intracranial Aneurysms*. New York: Springer-Verlag, 1983, vols. 1–7. Norlén G, Olivecrona H. The treatment of aneurysms of the circle of Willis. *J. Neurosurg.* 1953;10:404–415.

19 Mayfield FH, Kees G Jr. A brief history of the development of the Mayfield clip. Technical note. *J. Neurosurg.* 1971;35:97–100.

20 Del Maestro RF: Origin of the Drake fenestrated aneurysm clip. *J. Neurosurg.* 2000;92:1056–1064.

21 Kassell, NF. George Charles Drake MD 1920–1998, an Obituary. *J. Neurosurg.* 1999;90:797–801.

22 Link TE, Bisson E, Horgan MA, Tanner BI. Raymond MP. Donaghy: A pioneer in microneurosurgery. *J. Neurosurg.* 2010;112(6):1176–1181.

23 Stienen MN, Serra, C, Stieglitz LH, Krayenbühl N, Bozinov O, Regli L. UniversitätsSpital Zürich: 80 years of neurosurgical care in Switzerland. *Acta Neurochir. (Wien)* 2018;160(1):3–22. Tew JM. M. Gazi Yaşargil: Neurosurgery's man

of the century. *Neurosurgery* 1999;45:1010–1014. Yasargil MG, Vise WM, Bader DC. Technical adjuncts in neurosurgery. *Surg. Neurol.* 1977;8:331–336.

24 Lussenhop AJ, Velaquez AC. Artificial embolization of cerebral arteries: Report of use in a case of arteriovenous malformation. *JAMA* 1960;172:1153–1155. Lussenhop AJ, Velaquez AC. Observations on the tolerance of the intracranial arteries to catherization. *J. Neurosurg.* 1964;21:85–91.

25 Rothenberg SF, Penka EJ, Conway LW. Angiotactic surgery: Preliminary studies. *J. Neurol. Neurosurg. Psychiatry* 1962;19:877–883.

26 Frei EH, Driller J, Neufeld HN, Barr I, Bieiden L, Askeray HN. The POD and its application. *Med. Res. Eng.* 1966;5:11–18.

27 Yodh SB, Pierce NT, Weggel RJ, Montgomery DB. A new magnet system for intravascular navigation. *Med. Biol. Eng.* 1968;6:143–147.

28 Teitelbaum GP, Larsen DW, Zelman V, Lysachev AG, Likhterman LB. A tribute to Dr. Fedor A. Serbinenko, founder of endovascular neurosurgery. *Neurosurgery* 2000;46 (2):462–469.

29 Serbinenko FA. Balloon catheterization and occlusion of major cerebral vessels. *J. Neurosurg.* 1974;41:125–145.

30 Higashida RT, Halbach VV, Barnwell SL, Dowd C, Dormandy B, Bell J, Hieshima GB. Treatment of intracranial aneurysms with preservation of the parent vessel: Result of percutaneous balloon embolization in 84 patients. *AJNR Am. J. Neuroradiol.* 1990;11:633–640.

31 Guido Guglielmi. Whonamedit? Available at www.whonamedit.com/doctor.cfm/ 3137.html.

32 Guglielmi G. Endovascular treatment of intracranial aneurysms. *Neuroimag. Clin. N. Am.* 1992;2:269–278. Guglielmi G, Viñuela F, Dion J, Duckwiler G. Electrothrombosis of saccular aneurysms via endovascular approach. Part 2: Clinical experience. *J. Neurosurg.* 1991;75:8–14.

33 Fiorella D, Albuquerque FC, Deshmukh VR, McDougall CG. Usefulness of the Neuroform stent for the treatment of cerebral aneurysms: Results at initial (3–6-mo) follow-up. *Neurosurgery* 2005;56:1191–1201, discussion 1201–1202. Geyik S, Yavuz N, Yurttutan N, Saatci I, Cekirge HS. Stent-assisted coiling in endovascular treatment of 500 consecutive cerebral aneurysms with long-term follow-up. *AJNR Am. J. Neuroradiol.* 2013;34:1–6.

34 D'Urso PI, Lanzino G, Cloft HJ, Kallmes DF. Flow diversion for intracranial aneurysms: A review. *Stroke* 2011;42:2363–2368. Chalouhi N, Tjoumakaris S, Starke RM, Gonzalez LF, Randazzo C, Hasan D, McMahon JF, Sunghal S, Moukarzel LA, Dumont AS, Rosenwasser R, Jabbour P. Comparison of flow diversion and coiling in large unruptured intracranial saccular aneurysms. *Stroke* 2013;44:2150–2154.

CHAPTER FIFTY EIGHT

MEDICAL AND SURGICAL TREATMENTS OF INTRACEREBRAL HEMORRHAGE

The history of treatment approaches to intracerebral hemorrhage (ICH) involved testing various strategies based on the understanding and perceived importance of the components of ICH pathophysiology. These included attempts at (1) limiting the deleterious effects of ICH on surrounding brain parenchyma, (2) accelerating ICH and intraventricular hemorrhage (IVH) resolution, and (3) controlling the effects of hematoma expansion. The chronological sequence in which these approaches were applied reflects, in part, the timing of new advances in the understanding of the various factors that contributed to the morbidity and mortality of ICH. These approaches include both medical and surgical interventions. Treatment of ICH has required collaboration between neurologists and vascular neurosurgeons. The dramatic events at onset of ICH present clinicians with the option of early surgical intervention as a lifesaving approach for a condition of high mortality, along with nonsurgical measures that may contribute to improved outcomes.

TREATMENT MEASURES AIMED AT LIMITING THE DELETERIOUS EFFECTS OF ICH IN THE SURROUNDING BRAIN PARENCHYMA

Several local factors contribute to the morbidity and mortality of ICH. Effective ways of limiting them should lead to improved outcomes. One factor that was initially addressed was peri-hematoma edema, a known component of acute ICH that adds to the mass effect and increased intracranial pressure (ICP) that characterize medium-sized and large ICHs [1]. The concept that peri-hematoma edema played an important role in the outcome of ICH led some during the 1960s through the mid-1980s to use corticosteroids during the acute stage to minimize edema formation. This practice was supported by seminal observations on the local effects of ICH, especially the effect of peri-hematoma edema on adjacent brain parenchyma in experimental ICH [2]. These experiments were conducted in the laboratory of Julian (Buz) Hoff (1936–2007), a neurosurgeon who obtained his MD degree from Cornell University and trained in neurosurgery at New York Hospital, where he became interested in brain edema and stroke research. He first pursued his cerebrovascular research as a junior faculty member at the University of California at San Francisco, where he was recruited by Charles Wilson, a pioneer vascular neurosurgeon. Hoff's research interest in brain edema and ICH remained for his entire academic career, which continued at the University of Michigan, where he was chair of neurosurgery for 25 years until his retirement in 2006.

The potential value of corticosteroid therapy in ICH was first formally tested in a clinical trial conducted by Niphon Poungvarin et al. in Thailand and published in 1987 [3]. The theoretical value of this approach was further supported by more recent data suggesting that inflammation plays a significant role in the occurrence of neuronal injury at the margins of an ICH [4]. The trial involved the use of dexamethasone in decreasing daily doses for nine days, compared with placebo. The study was terminated early because of lack of benefit, but also harm from dexamethasone because of an increased rate of complications in the active treatment arm. As a result, specific recommendations against the use of this agent in acute ICH became part of the American Heart Association/American Stroke Association [5] and Canadian [6] guidelines for the management of acute ICH.

More recent attempts at testing potential treatments in the acute phase of ICH were based on additional observations about the pathophysiology of ICH. Among these, the pivotal role of local toxicity from hemoglobin-derived iron in the brain parenchyma with development of brain edema was recognized [7]. This led to testing of the iron-chelating agent deferoxamine in a multicenter phase II futility-design randomized clinical trial in the United States and Canada, led by Magdy Selim of the Beth Israel-Deaconess Medical Center in Boston. The trial showed the safety of deferoxamine, but did not reveal a signal of significant benefit that would justify progression into a larger, definitive phase III trial [8].

Although the data was limited, these two clinical trials, separated by more than 30 years, failed to show promise for strategies aimed at altering the processes that lead to peri-hematoma edema via either inflammation or local toxicity of blood-derived products.

TREATMENT MEASURES AIMED AT ENHANCING HEMATOMA RESOLUTION

The history of this approach to ICH treatment is extensive. Surgical hematoma evacuation by craniotomy spans more than 135 years, since the first operation attributed to Sir William Macewen in 1883 at the Royal infirmary in Glasgow, Scotland [9]. This eminent surgeon, born on the Island of Bute in Scotland in 1848, a disciple of Lister, was credited with the first use of endotracheal intubation (initially as part of the treatment of diphtheria, subsequently during anesthesia), the implementation of many techniques of asepsis and sterilization in the operating room, and the successful surgical treatment of brain abscesses. Harvey Cushing regarded Macewen as the founder of neurosurgery. His pioneer contributions included the management of brain abscesses, drainage of intracranial hematomas, removal of brain tumors, and correction of spinal pathology due to Pott's disease [9]. During subsequent decades, the results of the surgical treatment of ICH were mainly evaluated in clinical series, mostly retrospectively analyzed, not always with a nonsurgical comparison group. This resulted in the unscientific implementation of treatment protocols that varied across institutions and among surgeons, with expected local variability in surgical techniques (open craniotomy vs. endoscopic vs. stereotactic aspiration), timing of surgery from onset of symptoms (ultra-early vs. early vs. delayed), and use of concomitant measures (such as lytic agents to promote hematoma liquefaction and drainage).

The era of randomized clinical trials for the surgical treatment of ICH started with the publication of Wylie McKissock et al. in 1961 [10]. This pre-CT-era study was the first randomized trial of surgical ($n = 89$) versus nonsurgical ($n = 91$) treatment of supratentorial ICH. Despite the lack of imaging confirmation of the hematoma, it was a well-designed and well-conducted study that showed no difference in outcome between treatment groups. The results suggested that patients with lobar hematomas had better outcomes than those with basal ganglia or thalamic hematomas, a difference noted in several subsequent trials of ICH treatment. Sir Wylie McKissock (1906–1994), born in Staines, Surrey, England, studied neurosurgery in Stockholm with Herbert Olivecrona, and later practiced the specialty at St. George's Hospital and at the National Hospital for Neurology and Neurosurgery at Queen Square, in London. He developed an extensive experience in psychosurgery, performing over 1,800 "rostral" leucotomies in "mental hospitals" in southern England and Wales [11]. He also made contributions to the treatment of brain aneurysms, promoting the use of angiography to locate and obliterate the lesions, as well as hypothermia as a means of reducing operative mortality.

During the following decades, several randomized trials addressed the surgical evacuation of intracerebral hematomas, with overall results generally showing no benefit for surgery (see Table 58.1) [10,12–27]. In the modern area, the measures aimed at enhancing hematoma resolution have included open craniotomy and a variety of less invasive procedures. The largest randomized trial of open craniotomy versus medical management, the Surgical Trial in Intracerebral Haemorrhage (STICH), was conducted between 1995 and 2003 in 27 countries [21]. The design included early surgery (within 24 hours from randomization), mostly by open craniotomy, versus medical management. The trial was a major accomplishment, implementing the protocol throughout a varied group of institutions in multiple countries. The study leader was Alexander David Mendelow, professor of neurosurgery at the University of Newcastle-upon-Tyne and previous head of the department of neurosurgery at Newcastle General Hospital. He was a prominent clinical trialist in the United Kingdom, with interest and expertise in vascular neurosurgery. Born in South Africa, he attended medical school at the Witwatersrand University in Johannesburg, followed by training in neurosurgery at Edinburgh University in Scotland. He developed an early interest in brain circulation, head trauma, intracranial pressure measurements, and intracranial hemorrhage. During that time his mentor, W. Brian Jennett, the first professor of neurosurgery at the University of Glasgow, was involved in pioneering work in these fields, along with contemporaneous researchers such as Graham Teasdale, a collaboration that resulted in developing the Glasgow Coma Scale. Mendelow is credited with implementation of a methodical series of operating room checklists, in part based on his experience with his other passion in life, airplane flying. An enthusiast of flying and aerobatics and used to the routine of checklists required for safe flying, he promoted a similar approach to preparation for and conduction of neurosurgical procedures. The results of the STICH trial were neutral, without evidence of benefit of surgical evacuation of the hematoma. Similarly, the subsequent STICH II trial [25], which only included patients with superficial lobar hematomas located within one centimeter of the cortical surface, did not show benefit from surgery.

These disappointing results with conventional craniotomy led to the search for less invasive techniques of hematoma drainage, based on the idea that minimizing surgical trauma could lead to improved outcomes. The techniques of minimally invasive surgery (MIS) were developed at several institutions, and consisted of the stereotactic insertion of a catheter into the center of the hematoma, with repeated aspiration facilitated by local instillation of lytic agents to liquefy portions of the hematoma. This technique was used in the Minimally Invasive Surgery plus Alteplase for Intracerebral Hemorrhage Evacuation (MISTIE) trials, which documented the safety of this approach for hematoma removal [28]. This led to the phase III trial MISTIE III, an international multicenter trial of MIS with local instillation of alteplase versus medical management of supratentorial ICH [27]. The study was led by Daniel

F. Hanley, a graduate of Williams College and Cornell University Medical College in New York, with subsequent training in neurology and research fellowship in critical care at Johns Hopkins University, where he was the founding director of the Division of Brain Injury Outcomes and professor of neurology, neurosurgery, and anesthesiology and critical care. His long-standing interest and expertise in managing neurologic emergencies led him to address the unmet needs of safe and effective drainage of ICH in the acute phase. The process that eventually made possible the testing of MIS in ICH was the result of Hanley's collaboration with neurological and neurosurgical colleagues throughout the world, including Mario Zuccarello (University of Cincinnati), who pioneered these novel techniques in animal models, and Issam A. Awad (University of Chicago), who was instrumental in the refinement, standardization, and implementation of these techniques throughout the institutions participating in the MISTIE trials worldwide.

Although the evidence for significant clinical benefit from MIS in the surgical management of ICH remains elusive, its reported safety suggests that further technical improvements and large-scale randomized trials of selected ICH populations will eventually clarify its role in the acute management of ICH [29].

TREATMENTS TO CONTROL THE EFFECTS OF HEMATOMA EXPANSION

Understanding the time course during the initial hours after ICH onset evolved. Until the late 1980s, the prevailing view was that of a relatively brief process of blood extravasation into brain parenchyma, based on a study of premortem injection of $^{[51]}$Cr-labeled red blood cells in 11 patients with ICH between one to two and four to five hours from onset [30]. The absence of postmortem detection of the radioactive tracer in the hematoma was taken as indication that blood extravasation was essentially completed by at least two to five hours after ICH onset. This observation contrasted with reported instances of active arteriographic visualization of contrast extravasation in patients with ICH in whom arteriography was performed within a few hours after symptom onset [31]. When CT became available, serial scans were obtained that showed a dynamic early course of ICH. Some of these observations occurred when IV thrombolytic agents were given within 90 minutes from onset of neurological symptoms. Investigators assessed some patients before CT scans, sometimes revealing ICH rather than ischemic stroke as the presenting event. This led to the observation of early hematoma growth between the baseline CT and later ones, at times performed because of neurological deterioration observed after hospital presentation [32]. Additional observations established the dynamic course of the early stages of ICH with growth of lesions for hours [33].

Hematoma expansion became a therapeutic target in subsequent clinical trials based on its close correlation with early neurological deterioration and poor clinical outcome.

Among the variables potentially associated with promotion of hematoma expansion, persistent hypertension and anticoagulant effect were main targets in clinical therapeutic trials in ICH, along with the use of procoagulant agents such as recombinant activated factor VII (rFVIIa) and tranexamic acid, and decompressive craniectomy, treatments intended to minimize hematoma expansion and its effects.

Blood Pressure Control

Two trials addressed the potential benefit of blood pressure control in the acute phase of ICH: the Intensive Blood Pressure Reduction in Acute Cerebral Hemorrhage (INTERACT-2) trial [34] and the Antihypertensive Treatment of Acute Cerebral Hemorrhage (ATACH 2) trial [35]. They were conducted virtually in parallel, and reported in the early 2000s. They were led by Craig Anderson and Adnan Qureshi, respectively, and both trials addressed reduction in hematoma expansion in the two treatment groups, which lowered systolic blood pressure (SBP) to conventional/standard levels (SBP < 180 mmHg) versus intensive (SBP < 140 mmHg) blood pressure control. Although in INTERACT-2 there was a nonsignificant trend toward benefit with intensive BP control, in ATACH 2 there was not only lack of a signal of benefit, but evidence of harm due to kidney dysfunction in the intensive BP control group. Neither study showed a significant effect of intensive BP control on hematoma expansion.

Hemostatic Agents

The use of hemostatic agents to control hematoma expansion during the acute phase of ICH began in the early 2000s, with the use of rFVIIa, an FDA-approved agent used to treat bleeding episodes and perioperative management of patients with hemophilia A and B. Due to its ability to bind to tissue factor at sites of vascular injury, pharmacological doses of rFVIIa generate large amounts of thrombin (a "thrombin burst"), which activates platelets and the coagulation cascade, leading to the formation of a hemostatic plug at the vessel injury site [36]. Clinical trials conducted by Stephan Mayer et al. showed a consistent effect of rFVIIa in significantly reducing hematoma expansion in comparison with the control group, but the effect did not translate into clinical benefit [37]. There was also a significant increase in thrombotic complications. Further attempts at testing rFVIIa in the acute stage of ICH involved its use in specific subgroups of ICH patients at high risk of hematoma expansion, such as those with evidence of the "spot sign" on initial CTA, a sign of ongoing bleeding within hematomas, shown to predict a high likelihood of hematoma expansion [38]. The simultaneous Spot Sign for Predicting and Treating ICH Growth (STOP-IT) and "Spot Sign" Selection of Intracerebral Hemorrhage to Guide Hemostatic Therapy (SPOTLIGHT) trials, conducted in the United States and Canada, respectively, compared rFVIIa with placebo in patients with ICH with a positive "spot sign" on initial CTA evaluation, treated within six and a half hours from onset. The joint publication of the results among 69 patients in both studies combined revealed that hematoma expansion was very small (about 2.5 ml) and not significantly different in the active agent and placebo groups. Clinical outcomes, including mortality, were no different between the treatment groups [39].

The hemostatic agent tranexamic acid is an antifibrinolytic drug that is safe and effective in reducing mortality from traumatic and postpartum hemorrhage. Tranexamic acid was tested in the Tranexamic Acid for Hyperacute Primary Intracerebral Hemorrhage (TICH-2) trial [40]. It reduced hematoma expansion in comparison with placebo, but without a difference in clinical outcomes, including mortality at 90 days. A later study (STOP-AUST) that tested tranexamic acid against placebo in patients with ICH treated within four and a half hours from onset failed to prevent hematoma expansion, while mortality and thromboembolic complications were no different between the two treatment groups [41].

Reversal of Anticoagulant and Antiplatelet Effect

Intracranial bleeding is the most feared complication of warfarin use. It carries high rates of hematoma expansion, progressive neurological deterioration, and mortality [42]. Reversal of warfarin anticoagulant effect in the setting of ICH is standard-of-care. Reversal was traditionally achieved in the United States with fresh frozen plasma (FFP), which restitutes all four coagulation factors (II, VII, IX, X) inhibited by warfarin. Disadvantages include the need for ABO group compatibility, thawing for 30–60 minutes, and a requirement of large infusion volumes (15 ml/kg, about 1 liter in a 70-kg person) that put patients with poor cardiac function at risk of developing congestive heart failure [43]. FFP took between 13 and 48 hours to fully reverse the coagulopathy, at a time when hematoma expansion was most likely to continue. These many disadvantages of FFP stimulated development of better strategies, among them the introduction of prothrombin complex concentrates (PCCs). These contain factors II, VII, IX, and X ("four-factor" PCC), as well as the procoagulant proteins C and S. PCCs were used earlier and more widely in Europe than in the United States. Underuse prevailed for years, likely as a result of lack of familiarity with its advantages, low availability in hospital formularies, and reliance on off-label use of rFVIIa for warfarin anticoagulation reversal [44]. The latter agent was shown to normalize the international normalized ratio (INR), a test heavily dependent on the levels of factors VII and X (but not of factors II and IX), resulting in persistence of coagulopathy and increased risk of bleeding, despite INR normalization [45].

Subsequent studies compared FFP and PCC for the correction of warfarin anticoagulation, including the randomized INCH trial [46]. Faster correction of the INR with PCC correlated with reduced hematoma expansion, although 90-day mortality (19% with PCC, 35% with FFP) and other measures of clinical outcomes were not significantly different in this study with small numbers of patients (n = 50; 23 FFP, 27 PCC). As a result of these observations, current guidelines in Canada recommend PCC as the agent of choice to reverse warfarin anticoagulation in patients with ICH [6].

Direct oral anticoagulants (DOACs), including the factor II inhibitor dabigatran and the factor Xa inhibitors rivaroxaban, apixaban, and edoxaban, were recently introduced into clinical use. DOACs were studied between 2009 and 2013 for stroke prevention in patients with atrial fibrillation. Data on DOAC-related ICH is relatively scanty, most from two German registries [47]. The ICH profiles included observation of hematoma expansion in about one third of patients, mortality of 28–30 percent at 90 days, and high levels of disability in two thirds of survivors. The widespread use of PCCs for anticoagulation reversal (in 57–64% of cases) had no impact on hematoma expansion or unfavorable outcomes, although the combination of PCC with SBP reduction below 160 mmHg resulted in significant benefit regarding hematoma expansion. The recently developed antidotes idarucizumab for dabigatran and andenaxet alpha for the anti-Xa agents could play an important role in the emergency treatment of DOAC-related ICH.

The data on prior treatment with *antiplatelet agents* in patients with ICH have been inconsistent, resulting in lack of clarity about the value of platelet transfusions in the setting of pre-ICH treatment with antiplatelet agents. This issue was addressed in the PATCH trial in which platelet transfusions within 90 minutes from imaging diagnosis of ICH resulted in a detrimental effect regarding clinical outcomes, without differences in hematoma expansion [48]. Canadian guidelines for the management of spontaneous ICH recommended against using platelet transfusions [6].

Decompressive Craniectomy

Decompressive craniectomy, with or without concomitant surgical drainage of ICH, is among treatment options intended to reduce the effects of increased ICP in patients with ICH. The basis for this approach was the benefit of the procedure in experimental animals [49] and in patients with hemorrhagic

TABLE 58.1. *Randomized trials comparing hematoma evacuation with conservative management*[a]

Authors, year [ref.]	Technique	N (med./surgical)	Timing (hours)	Findings
McKissock et al., 1961 [10]	Craniotomy	180 (91/89)	48	No difference in outcomes
Auer et al., 1989 [13]	Endoscopic evacuation	100 (50/50)	48	Decreased mortality, favorable outcome in lobar hematomas
Juvela et al., 1989 [14]	Craniotomy	52 (26/26)	48	No difference in outcomes
Batjer et al., 1990 [15]	Craniotomy	21 (13/8)	24	No difference in outcomes
Morgenstern et al., 1998 [16]	Craniotomy	41 (34/7)	12	Better outcomes in conservative group
Zuccarello et al., 1999 [17]	Craniotomy[b]	20 (11/9)	24	No difference in outcomes
Morgenstern et al., 2001 [18]	Craniotomy	11 (all surgical)	4	Interrupted because of high rates of rebleeding
Teernstra et al., 2003 [19]	Stereotactic evacuation[c]	71 (35/36)	22	No difference in outcomes
Hattori et al., 2004 [20]	Stereotactic evacuation	242 (121/121)	ND	Better outcomes with surgery
Mendelow et al., 2005 [21]	Craniotomy > others[d]	1,033 (530/503)	72	No difference in outcomes
Pantazis et al., 2006 [22]	Craniotomy	108 (54/54)	8	No difference in outcomes
Kim et al., 2009 [23]	Stereotactic evacuation	387 (183/204)	12–120	Better outcomes with surgery
Wang et al., 2009 [24]	MIS with urokinase	377 (182/195)	21.1	No difference in outcomes
Mendelow et al., 2013 [25]	Craniotomy	601 (294/307)	48	No difference in outcomes
Vespa et al., 2016 [26]	Stereotactic endoscopic	24 (all surgical)	48	Better outcomes with surgery
Hanley et al., 2019 [27]	MIS with alteplase	506 (251/255)	72	No difference in outcomes

[a] Modified from reference [12].
[b] Craniotomy with CT-guided stereotactic placement of catheter.
[c] Stereotactic aspiration with urokinase instillation.
[d] Craniotomy in 75% of cases, the rest by a variety of techniques, including stereotactic and endoscopic.
Note: MIS, minimally invasive surgery; ref., reference number..

infarction due to cerebral venous thrombosis [50]. The human experience in ICH patients is limited to small clinical series, which were reviewed in a meta-analysis of eight studies by Yao et al. [51]. The overall conclusion was that decompressive craniectomy plus hematoma evacuation in comparison with hematoma evacuation alone was effective in reducing mortality, with uncertain benefit with regard to functional status of survivors.

REFERENCES

1. Xi G, Keep RF, Hoff JT. Mechanisms of brain injury after intracerebral haemorrhage. *Lancet Neurol.* 2006;5:53–63.

2. Xi G, Keep RF, Hoff JT. Erythrocytes and delayed brain edema formation following intracerebral hemorrhage in rats. *J. Neurosurg.* 1998;89:991–996. Xi G, Wagner KR, Keep RF, et al. The role of blood clot formation on early edema development following experimental intracerebral hemorrhage. *Stroke* 1998;29:2580–2586. Yang GY, Betz AL, Chenevert TL, Brunberg JA, Hoff JT. Experimental intracerebral hemorrhage: Relationship between brain edema, blood flow, and blood-brain barrier permeability in rats. *J. Neurosurg.* 1994;81:93–102.

3. Poungvarin N, Bhoopat W, Viriyavejakul A, et al. Effects of dexamethasone in primary supratentorial intracerebral hemorrhage. *N. Engl. J. Med.* 1987;316:1229–1233.

4. Aronowski J, Zhao X. Molecular pathophysiology of cerebral hemorrhage: Secondary brain injury. *Stroke* 2011;42:1781–1786.

5. Hemphill JC, Greenberg SM, Anderson CS, et al. Guidelines for the management of spontaneous intracerebral hemorrhage: A guideline for healthcare professionals from the American Heart Association/American Stroke Association. *Stroke* 2015;46:2032–2060.

6. Shoamanesh A, Lindsay MP, Castellucci LA, et al. Canadian stroke best practice recommendations: Management of spontaneous intracerebral hemorrhage, 7th edition update 2020. *Int. J. Stroke* 2021;16:321–341.

7. Wagner KR, Sharp FR, Ardizzone TD, Lu A, Clark JF. Heme and iron metabolism: Role in cerebral haemorrhage. *J. Cereb. Blood Flow Metab.* 2003;23:629–652.

8. Selim M, Foster LD, Moy CS, et al. Deferoxamine mesylate in patients with intracerebral hemorrhage (i-DEF): A multicentre, randomized, placebo- controlled, double-blind phase 2 trial. *Lancet Neurol.* 2019;18:428–438.

9. James CDT. Sir William Macewen. *Proc. Roy. Soc. Med.* 1974;67:237–242. Horwitz NH. William Macewen. *Neurosurgery* 1995;37:352–355.

10. McKissock W, Richardson A, Taylor J. Primary intracerebral haemorrhage: A controlled trial of surgical and conservative treatment in 180 unselected cases. *Lancet* 1961;2:221–226.

11. McKissock W. Rostral leucotomy. *Lancet* 1951;258:91–94. Wylie McKissock (obituary). *The Times,* May 11, 1994.

12. de Oliveira Manoel AL. Surgery for spontaneous intracerebral hemorrhage. *Critical Care* 2020;24:45. https://doi.org./10.1186/s13054-020-2749-2.

13. Auer LM, Deinsberger W, Niederkorn K, et al. Endoscopic surgery versus medical treatment for spontaneous intracerebral hematoma: A randomized study. *J. Neurosurg.* 1989;70:530–535.

14. Juvela S, Heiskanen O, Poranen A, et al. The treatment of spontaneous intracerebral hemorrhage: A prospective randomized trial of surgical and conservative treatment. *J. Neurosurg.* 1989;70:755–758.

15. Batjer HH, Reisch JS, Allen BC, Plaizier LJ, Su CJ. Failure of surgery to improve outcome in hypertensive putaminal hemorrhage: A prospective randomized trial. *Arch. Neurol.* 1990;47:1103–1106.

16. Morgenstern LB, Frankowski RF, Shedden P, Pasteur W, Grotta JC. Surgical treatment for intracerebral hemorrhage (STICH): A single-center, randomized clinical trial. *Neurology* 1998;51:1359–1363.

17. Zuccarello M, Brott T, Derex L, et al. Early surgical treatment for supratentorial intracerebral hemorrhage: A randomized feasibility study. *Stroke* 1999;30:1833–1839.

18. Morgenstern LB, Demchuk AM, Kim DH, Frankowski RF, Grotta JC. Rebleeding leads to poor outcome in ultra-early craniotomy for intracerebral hemorrhage. *Neurology* 2001;56:1294–1299.

19. Teernstra OPM, Evers SMAA, Lodder J, et al. Stereotactic treatment of intracerebral hematoma by means of a plasminogen activator: A multicenter randomized controlled trial (SICHPA). *Stroke* 2003;34:968–974.

20. Hattori N, Katayama Y, Maya Y, Gatherer A. Impact of stereotactic hematoma evacuation on activities of daily living during the chronic period following spontaneous putaminal hemorrhage: A randomized study. *J. Neurosurg.* 2004;101:417–420.

21. Mendelow AD, Gregson BA, Fernandes HM, et al. Early surgery versus initial conservative treatment in patients with spontaneous supratentorial intracerebral haematomas in the International Surgical Trial in Intracerebral Haemorrhage (STICH): A randomised trial. *Lancet* 2005;365:387–397.

22. Pantazis G, Tsitsopoulos P, Mihas C et al. Early surgical treatment vs conservative management for spontaneous supratentorial intracerebral hematomas: A prospective randomized study. *Surg. Neurol.* 2006;66:492– 501.

23. Kim YZ, Kim KH. Even in patients with a small hemorrhagic volume, stereotactic-guided evacuation of spontaneous intracerebral hemorrhage improves functional outcome. *J. Korean Neurosurg. Soc.* 2009;46:109–115.

24. Wang W-Z, Jiang B, Liu H-M, et al. Minimally invasive craniopuncture therapy vs. conservative treatment for spontaneous intracerebral hemorrhage: Results from a randomized clinical trial in China. *Int. J. Stroke* 2009;4:11–16.

25. Mendelow AD, Gregson BA, Rowan EN, et al. Early surgery versus initial conservative treatment in patients with spontaneous supratentorial lobar intracerebral haematomas (STICH II): A randomised trial. *Lancet* 2013;382:397–408.

26. Vespa P, Hanley D, Betz J, et al. ICES (intraoperative stereotactic computed tomography-guided endoscopic surgery) for brain hemorrhage: A multicenter randomized controlled trial. *Stroke* 2016;47:2749–2755.

27. Hanley DF, Thompson RE, Rosenblum M, et al. Efficacy and safety of minimally invasive surgery with thrombolysis in intracerebral haemorrhage evacuation (MISTIE III): A randomised, controlled, open-label, blinded endpoint phase 3 trial. *Lancet* 2019;393:1021–1032.

28. Hanley DF, Thompson RE, Muschelli J, et al. Safety and efficacy of minimally invasive surgery plus alteplase in intracerebral haemorrhage evacuation (MISTIE): A randomised, controlled, open-label, phase 2 trial. *Lancet Neurol.* 2016;15:1228–1237.

29. Kase CS, Hanley DF. Intracerebral hemorrhage: Advances in emergency care. *Neurol. Clin.* 2021;39:405–418.

30. Herbstein DJ, Schaumburg HH. Hypertensive intracerebral hemorrhage: An investigation of the initial hemorrhage and rebleeding using chromium Cr 51-labelled erythrocytes. *Arch. Neurol.* 1974;30:412–414.

31. Mizukami M, Araki G, Mihara H, Tomita T, Fuginaga R. Arteriographically visualized extravasation in hypertensive intracerebral hemorrhage; report of seven cases. *Stroke* 1972;3:527–537.

32. Broderick JP, Brott TG, Tomsick T, Barsan W, Spilker J. Ultra-early evaluation of intracerebral hemorrhage. *J. Neurosurg.* 1990;72:195–199.

33. Kazui S, Naritomi H, Yamamoto H, Sawada T, Yamaguchi T. Enlargement of spontaneous intracerebral hemorrhage: Incidence and time course. *Stroke* 1996;27:1783–1787. Brott T, Broderick J, Kothari R, et al. Early hemorrhage growth in patients with intracerebral hemorrhage. *Stroke* 1997;28:1–5.

34. Anderson CS, Huang Y, Wang JG, et al., INTERACT Investigators. Intensive blood pressure reduction in acute cerebral haemorrhage trial (INTERACT): A randomised pilot trial. *Lancet Neurol.* 2008;7(5):391–399. Anderson CS, Heeley E, Huang Y, et al., INTERACT2 Investigators. Rapid blood-pressure lowering in patients with acute intracerebral hemorrhage. *N. Engl. J. Med.* 2013;368:2355–2365.

35. Qureshi AI, Palesch YY, Barsan WG, et al., ATACH-2 Trial Investigators and the Neurological Emergency Treatment Trials Network. Intensive blood-pressure lowering in patients with acute cerebral hemorrhage. *N. Engl. J. Med.* 2016;375:1033–1043. Qureshi AI, Palesch YY, Foster LD, et al. Blood pressure-attained analysis of ATACH 2 Trial. *Stroke* 2018;49:1412–1418.

36. Hoffman M, Monroe DM. A cell-based model of hemostasis. *Thromb. Haemost.* 2001;85:958–965.

37. Mayer SA, Brun NC, Begtrup K, et al. Recombinant activated factor VII for acute intracerebral hemorrhage. *N. Engl. J. Med.* 2005;352:777–785. Mayer SA, Brun NC, Begtrup K, et al. Efficacy and safety of recombinant activated factor VII for acute intracerebral hemorrhage. *N. Engl. J. Med.* 2008;358:2127–2137.

38. Demchuk AM, Dowlatshahi D, Rodriquez-Luna D, et al. Prediction of haematoma growth and outcome in patients with intracerebral haemorrhage using the CT-angiography spot sign (PREDICT): A prospective observational study. *Lancet Neurol.* 2012;11:307–314.

39. Gladstone DJ, Aviv RI, Demchuk AM, et al. Effect of recombinant activated coagulation factor VII on hemorrhage expansion among patients with spot sign-positive acute intracerebral hemorrhage: The SPOTLIGHT and STOP-IT randomized clinical trials. *JAMA Neurol.* 2019;76:1493–1501.

40. Sprigg N, Flaherty K, Appleton JP, et al. Tranexamic acid for hyperacute primary IntraCerebral Haemorrhage (TICH-2): An international randomized, placebo-controlled, phase 3 superiority trial. *Lancet* 2018;391:2107–2115.

41. Meretoja A, Yassi N, Wu TY, et al. Tranexamic acid in patients with intracerebral haemorrhage (STOP-AUST): A multicentre, randomised, placebo-controlled, phase 2 trial. *Lancet Neurol.* 2020;19:980–987.

42. Steiner T, Weitz JI, Veltkamp R. Anticoagulant-associated intracranial hemorrhage in the era of reversal agents. *Stroke* 2017;48:1432–1437.

43. Frumkin K. Rapid reversal of warfarin-associated hemorrhage in the emergency department by prothrombin complex concentrates. *Ann. Emerg. Med.* 2013;62:616–626.

44. Aiyagari V, Testai FD. Correction of coagulopathy in warfarin associated cerebral hemorrhage. *Curr. Opin. Crit. Care* 2009;15:87–92.

45. Ferreira J, DeLosSantos M. The clinical use of prothrombin complex concentrate. *J. Emerg. Med.* 2013;44:1201–1210.

46. Steiner T, Poli S, Griebe M, et al. Fresh frozen plasma versus prothrombin complex concentrate in patients with intracranial haemorrhage related to vitamin K antagonists (INCH): A randomised trial. *Lancet Neurol.* 2016;15:566–573.

47. Purrucker JC, Haas K, Rizos T, et al. Early clinical and radiological course, management, and outcome of intracerebral hemorrhage related to new oral anticoagulants.

JAMA Neurol. 2016;73:169–177. Gerner ST, Kuramatsu JB, Sembill JA, et al. Association of prothrombin complex concentrate administration and hematoma enlargement in non-vitamin K antagonist oral anticoagulant-related intracerebral hemorrhage. *Ann. Neurol.* 2018;83:186–196.

48. Baharoglu MI, Cordonnier C, Al-Shahi Salman R, et al. Platelet transfusion versus standard care after acute stroke due to spontaneous cerebral haemorrhage associated with antiplatelet therapy (PATCH): A randomised, open-label, phase 3 trial. *Lancet* 2016;387:2605–2613.

49. Marinkovic I, Strbian D, Pedrono E, et al. Decompressive craniectomy for intracerebral hemorrhage. *Neurosurgery* 2009;65:780–786.

50. Ferro JM, Crassard I, Coutinho JM, et al. Decompressive surgery in cerebrovenous thrombosis: A multicenter registry and a systematic review of individual patient data. *Stroke* 2011;42:2825–2831.

51. Yao Z, Ma L, You C, He M. Decompressive craniectomy for spontaneous intracerebral hemorrhage: A systematic review and meta-analysis. *World Neurosurg.* 2018:110:121–128.

CHAPTER FIFTY NINE

TREATMENT OF
VASCULAR MALFORMATIONS

ARTERIOVENOUS MALFORMATIONS: EARLY RECOGNITION
AND TREATMENT

Early descriptions of brain arteriovenous malformations (AVMs) were based on
their appearance uncovered during surgical exploration. The first report of a
spinal AVM was provided by Gaupp in 1888. He described the lesion as a
"hemorrhoid of the pia mater" [1]. That same year D'Arcy described an arterial
angioma of the angular gyrus at autopsy. The patient presented with right
hemiplegia and later died of intracranial hemorrhage [2].

During the first half of the twentieth century, as neurosurgical indications
increased and cerebral localization improved, cranial surgery became more
common. Surgeons identified vascular lesions and began to attempt their
removal. Fedor Krause, in 1908, and Sir Charles Balance, in 1921, independently identified an AVM while performing intracranial explorations for epilepsy [3]. They found large cortical veins and ligated them. In both cases,
blockage of venous drainage led to catastrophic bleeding. Hemorrhage was
controlled by packing the wound with gauze, which was left in place but later
removed during reexploration. Neurologic deficits improved over time.

Considering the available technology, resection was not a viable treatment
option at that time, so radiotherapy was attempted. American-born Vilhelm
Magnus (1871–1929), the preeminent neurosurgeon in Norway at the time,
reported the results of radiotherapy for an AVM diagnosed in 1913. The

patient had right-sided Jacksonian seizures. Exploratory craniotomy identified an arteriovenous "angioma" of the left central lobule. Instead of attempting resection, Magnus performed a decompressive craniectomy. The patient was then treated with radiotherapy. The bulging at the decompression site improved, and the seizures decreased in frequency and eventually stopped [4].

Harvey Cushing and Walter E. Dandy

Harvey Cushing described the first successful removal of a vascular malformation in 1927 [5]. This patient had first presented to Cushing in 1924 when he performed a craniotomy to remove a presumed meningioma [6]. Significant bleeding developed when the bone flap was elevated and was controlled by placing muscle fragments over bleeding points. The bleeding was so significant that Cushing attributed the patient's survival to the large amount of muscle available from a nearby case of a leg amputation, and the ability to perform blood transfusion, which at that time was obtained from a donor during surgery. After obtaining better visualization of the lesion, Cushing deemed removal to be too risky, so instead performed a subtemporal decompression. The patient awoke hemiplegic and aphasic but improved before discharge. He was treated with X-rays. Three years later he returned to Cushing with recurring symptoms. At this surgery, Cushing noted that the lesion had "degenerated." Using clips and electrocautery he performed the first successful resection of an AVM. He noted that the five-centimeter lesion, which consisted of a tangle of pulsating arterioles at the first operation, had become "largely thrombosed and transformed into a multitude of small bloodless shreds. It was found that the central lesion could be easily separated from the adjacent normal-looking cortex." The patient awoke hemiplegic and aphasic and improved but without the full recovery that followed his first surgery. While Cushing was encouraged that surgical resection might be possible following radiotherapy, he did not advocate removal of these lesions in their "active state." Rather, decompressive surgery followed by radiation therapy with the treatment effect monitored by serially assessing the cranial bruit was his favored treatment plan [6].

Walter E. Dandy, a former resident of Cushing, gained experience with vascular malformations during the 1920s at John Hopkins Hospital in Baltimore, Maryland [7]. Many terms were used to describe AVMs, depending on whether they were thought to contain arterial or venous predominance. Dandy noted that these terms described the superficial appearance of the lesions but that a common pathologic process led to different appearances. He referred to these lesions as "arteriovenous aneurysms" and published criteria for their recognition: "first and foremost, marked fulness and enlargement of the veins of exit; second, an increased size and tortuosity of the artery entering the snarled mass of vessels" [8].

In 1922, Dandy, attempted surgery for a right-sided arteriovenous aneurysm with drainage through Sylvian and Rolandic veins in a young man with epilepsy [8]. Initially, the sylvian vein was ligated and divided. He then attempted to undermine the vascular malformation, but this was impossible from that angle, so he shifted his dissection more medially, beginning with ligating and dividing the main draining Rolandic vein. He had difficulty ligating this engorged vessel: "in this instance the knot could be slipped down only step by step because of the pressure within the vein." A few minutes after ligation and division, the Rolandic vein burst, which Dandy attributed to increasing arterial pressure with the outflow occluded. Tamponade was attempted without success, until the carotid artery was ligated in the neck. The patient survived only a few hours after surgery [8].

Proximal ligation of arterial feeders was used in subsequent surgeries. Dandy ligated the left vertebral artery to treat a bilateral cerebellar arteriovenous aneurysm following a suboccipital decompression. After ligation, bulging of the decompression site improved as did cerebellar signs. The bruit heard previously over both temples also lessened. Craniotomy in another epilepsy patient showed a large AVM. Dandy performed a decompression and then ligated the ipsilateral carotid artery with an elastic to cause gradual occlusion. The patient had no seizures for one year after treatment, but seizures recurred, increased in frequency, and returned to preoperative frequency [8].

In 1928, Dandy resected an AVM without intraoperative complications. A 51-year-old man initially presented in coma attributable to a right parieto-occipital cerebral hemorrhage. Ventriculography showed a defect in the right post-rolandic cortex, likely from a prior hemorrhage. A craniotomy was performed and the AVM was identified anterior to a cystic cavity left by the prior hemorrhage. The lesion was removed after ligating the superficial vessels including three "fair-sized" feeders. Although this was an early surgical success, the patient died six days postoperatively from a slowly progressive intraventricular hemorrhage [8].

Cushing and Dandy published their respective series of patients. They each reported data on the etiology, presentation, natural history, pathology, and their preferred treatment options. Cushing was uncertain as to whether AVMs were developmental but had the potential to progress over time or were neoplasms. He favored the hypothesis that they were developmental [6]. Dandy concluded that these lesions were most likely congenital [8].

During the early days of AVM surgery, most patients presented with Jacksonian seizures involving the motor cortex. Without motor seizures, cerebral localization to guide a craniotomy would not have been possible. Seizures could begin at any age. Many patients did not develop symptoms until after age 30. Transient motor or sensory abnormalities often followed convulsions. For Dandy, a patient presenting with stereotypic seizures occurring over a prolonged period of time without any progression most likely had an AVM. The development of a sudden focal neurologic deficit with later improvement over time was suggestive of rupture and hemorrhage. Signs or symptoms of elevated intracranial pressure were uncommon in Dandy's series [8]. Cushing noted the importance of auscultation for a bruit as an important component of the physical examination. Additional physical exam findings that were utilized in diagnosis included increased vascularity of the scalp, carotid artery hypertrophy, and secondary cardiac hypertrophy. Ophthalmic findings such as papilledema and nonpulsating exophthalmos were occasionally noted.

The reports of Cushing and Dandy began to define the natural history of AVMs. Seizures and symptoms and signs often progressed over time. Approximately 40 percent of patients with AVMs presented with brain hemorrhage. Intracranial hemorrhage was the most common cause of death. Dandy noted that these lesions often extended and ruptured into a ventricle. Dandy and Cushing also each described the histopathology of these lesions. Dandy described vessels of varying diameters with varying degrees of irregular intimal thickening leading to weakness in the vessel walls. He found thrombi throughout multiple vessels in a given sample. He hypothesized that as veins thrombose, the decreased outflow strained the abnormal vessels causing increased risk of rupture and intracranial hemorrhage [8].

Dandy understood that the only way to cure AVMs was to ligate the feeding artery(s) or extirpate the vascular mass. He acknowledged the high risk of attempting these treatments, depending on the lesion location. An alternative strategy was proximal ligation of the major feeding artery – carotid or vertebral – to improve the signs and symptoms. Proximal ligation was less likely to cause permanent neurologic sequelae but also unlikely to cure. Dandy recognized that successfully treating these vascular lesions would not necessarily stop seizures, but might be associated with fewer convulsions that were more easily controlled [8].

Cushing favored craniectomy followed by radiotherapy. Decompressive treatments were followed by improvement in preoperative symptoms in some patients. Removal of the bone overlying the lesion was thought to allow better penetration of radiation. The treating clinician could follow the bruit to assess treatment response. Cushing wrote: "The surgical history of most of the reported cases shows not only the futility of an operative attack upon one of these angiomas but the extreme risk of serious cortical damage which it entails" [6].

Herbert Olivecrona

Herbert Olivecrona (1891–1980) singlehandedly founded Swedish neurosurgery [9]. He was born in July 1891 in Visby, Sweden, the son of a district court judge and a countess. His brother was a noted Swedish legal scholar. He began studying medicine at the University of Uppsala in 1909. He then transferred to the Karolinska Institute as an assistant in pathology, graduating in 1918. Olivecrona received a fellowship from the American-Scandinavian Foundation in 1919. This allowed him to perform experimental work at Johns Hopkins in Baltimore where he worked with Harvey Cushing. Olivecrona was offered a residency and to be Cushing's foreign assistant on the condition that he work for a year at Pierre Marie's clinic in Paris. Due to financial reasons, Olivecrona declined and returned to Sweden, where he established the first neurosurgery program at Serafimer Hospital in the 1920s. After further consultation with Cushing, Olivecrona improved his skills, and in 1930 was promoted to assistant surgeon in chief, allowing him to establish a 50-bed neurosurgery department. Olivecrona's clinic became a mecca where many came for training. In 1935, he became the first professor of neurosurgery at the Karolinska Institute, the first chair of neurosurgery in Europe. Olivecrona was a pioneer in the creation of surgical techniques for AVMs and aneurysms. In 1955, Olivecrona was elected a member of the Royal Swedish Academy of Sciences. He retired from the Karolinska in 1960 [9].

Olivecrona and Johannes Riives reported a series of AVMs in 1948 [10]. They found that they were not rare. The increased frequency of vascular malformations in this series was attributed to the use of arteriography beginning in 1932. Using arteriography, they were able to describe the patterns of feeding vessels from both the intracranial and extracranial circulation. Olivecrona described the characteristic wedge shape of these lesions with deep feeders at the apex along with the presence of aneurysms within the lesions. Few vascular malformations underwent serial arteriography, but in a case with interval imaging over 10 years, growth of the lesion was shown along with increased caliber of the feeding and draining vessels. This series included the first description of successful resection of an AVM in its active stage. This posterior fossa lesion was removed in 1932, and the patient was able to return to work after surgery [10]. In 1934, they treated a man with a large right posterior frontal AVM. At surgery the lesion was considered inoperable. Roentgen therapy was given without improvements. In the intervening 10 years, the patient's condition worsened and the lesion increased in size. In 1944, a second surgery was performed after ligation of the right internal carotid artery. After ligating the superficial feeding vessels, Olivecrona circumferentially deepened the dissection until only the veins held it attached and the lesion could be tilted out of the cavity. Only at this point was the draining vein ligated and divided. The patient woke up hemiplegic with some postoperative recovery [10].

With increased use of arteriography, Olivecrona was able to follow AVMs over time. Based on serial imaging, he concluded that Roentgen therapy was unlikely to be effective. He described the dangers of carotid ligation. Two patients developed hemiplegia following ligation that became permanent when the ligature was not removed in time. In those patients who tolerated ligation, he stated that "in none of the cases ... could it be said with any certainty that the spontaneous course of the illness was changed." Based on this experience, Olivecrona concluded that the choice was to remove the lesion or leave it alone. Among the 29 patients in whom removal was attempted, three died, a mortality rate of 10.7 percent. One died of uncontrolled hemorrhage, one of postoperative bleeding, and one of meningitis from opening the frontal sinus. Postoperative improvement in seizures was more common in patients with a shorter preoperative duration of symptoms [10].

MIDDLE AND SECOND HALF OF THE TWENTIETH CENTURY

Interest increased in the hemodynamic effects of AVMs. More resections were performed. In 1949, Gösta Norlén, a Swedish neurosurgeon who worked with Olivecrona, published a series of patients who had AVM resections [11]. He routinely performed angiography following these resections. He noted that feeding arteries that had been dilated and tortuous prior to resection regained their normal size and configuration within two to three weeks following resection. Peripheral vessels that had limited filling in the presence of the AVM often showed improved filling with contrast postoperatively [11].

High flow in AVMs was posited to "steal blood" away from other vascular territories [12]. As diagnostic imaging improved, a better understanding of the natural history was reached. A report from the the Cooperative Study of Intracranial Aneurysms and Subarachnoid Hemorrhage analyzed results from 549 AVMs [13]. Sixty-eight percent of the AVMs had bled. The peak age of hemorrhage was 15–20 years; more than half of the ruptured AVMs bled by age 30. Hemorrhage was fatal in 10 percent of patients [13].

Other studies concluded that the risk of hemorrhage from AVMs was 2–4 percent per year [14]. Although the risk of hemorrhage was increased after AVM rupture, by six months post-bleed, that risk had decreased and was similar to the risk of bleeding from non-ruptured AVMs [15]. The high morbidity and mortality associated with AVM rupture was confirmed by Duke Samson and Hunt Batjer [16]. In their series, each hemorrhage was associated with a 10–15 percent risk of mortality and 20–30 percent additional risk of serious morbidity. These natural history studies confirmed that AVMs were dangerous lesions with significant potential for rupture with substantial risk of morbidity after rupture [16].

Technologic advancements in anesthesia, diathermy, vessel clips, and blood transfusions contributed to better surgical outcomes. One of the most import-ant advances was the introduction of the binocular operating microscope into neurosurgery. Theodore Kurze was the first to use the operating microscope in a cranial procedure. He used the device to remove a vestibular schwannoma in a five-year-old boy in Los Angeles in 1957 [17]. One of the earliest and most successful devotees of the microscope was Gazi Yasargil, a Swiss neurosurgeon who used the microscope for anastomoses and surgery on aneurysms and AVMs [18].

He improved the operating microscope to increase efficiency and visualization and developed micro-instruments. Yasargil was able to perform microsurgical resection of 14 AVMs in 1969 with excellent results [19]. Most early case reports and series of AVM resections were on superficial lesions; deeper lesions were often considered inoperable. In 1976, Yasargil successfully resected AVMs of the corpus callosum (18 of the anterior and middle and 10 of the splenium), using microsurgical techniques with no reported operative mortality and minimal morbidity [20]. Yasargil published his series of 414 AVM patients [21]. He detailed the pre- and postoperative neurologic status, operative techniques, and anesthetic management. The use of the sitting position for infratentorial AVMs was discussed, and, reassuringly in his series, no instances of air embolism occurred [21].

One of the most skilled and prolific neurosurgeons who operated on many brain and spinal AVMs and fistulas was Roberto Heros of the University of Miami. Roberto C. Heros was born in 1942 in Havana, Cuba [22]. After Communist takeover in 1960, he left Cuba for exile. He was a paratrooper platoon commander during the Bay of Pigs invasion and was captured. After serving two years in prison, Heros was released as a result of an exchange with the US government. He attended medical school at the University of Tennessee where he graduated in 1968. Heros had his internship and his first-year general surgery residency at the Massachusetts General Hospital (MGH) in Boston and then served in the US Air Force as a major for two years. He completed his neurosurgery residency at MGH, Harvard Medical School, and then moved to the University of Pittsburgh. He moved back to MGH in 1980 to become director of cerebrovascular surgery. Heros moved through the academic ranks at Harvard to reach full professorship. In 1989 he moved to the University of Minnesota as the Lyle A. French Professor and Chairman of the department of neurosurgery. Heros moved to the University of Miami in 1995 as professor, co-chairman, and program director of the department of neurosurgery and the founding director of the University of Miami International Health Center [22]. He attracted many AVM and aneurysm patients from Central and South America to Miami for surgery. In 1982, Heros described angiographic criteria to determine if mesial temporal lesions were operable and described transcortical approaches to these difficult AVMs [23].

The advent of functional MRI in the early 1990s allowed neurologists and neurosurgeons to localize gray and white matter connections in relation to

AVMs. Based on information obtained from this new technology, the authors chose the appropriate treatment modality to protect eloquent brain function [24]. Flow-directed embolization with silicone particles was performed in 1960 with decreased flow through the AVM and a good clinical outcome [25]. Conventional radiotherapy and later stereotactic radiosurgery were used to treat some AVMs. Continued evaluation of radiosurgery showed that while it could obliterate AVMs, this was a progressive process that occurred over two to three years after treatment.

With the advent of these new nonsurgical treatment options and improvements in surgical techniques, it became increasingly important to evaluate and predict surgical outcomes. One such early schema, devised by Alfred Lussenhop and Thomas Gennarelli in 1977, graded AVMs from I to IV based on the number of named arterial feeders but did not consider the location of the lesion with regard to function of the surrounding tissue [26]. A more robust grading scheme was described in 1986 by Robert Spetzler and Neil Martin [27]. This classification, used to predict surgical morbidity and mortality, was based on lesion size, whether the lesion was in eloquent brain, and the presence or absence of deep venous drainage as a marker of deep location or extension. Robert Spetzler was one of the most skilled and prolific neurosurgeons who operated on aneurysms and AVMs during the later years of the twentieth century [28]. Spetzler was born in Stierhöfstetten, near Würzburg in Germany where his parents had been evacuated due to World War II. He moved with his parents at age 11 to the United States. He received his bachelor of science degree in 1967 from Knox College after attending a year of community college in Illinois. He spent a year at the Free University of Berlin and then matriculated at Northwestern Medical School, graduating in 1971. His neurosurgical residency was at University of California at San Francisco where he was mentored by Charles Wilson. In 1983, Spetzler was named chair of the division of neurological surgery at the Barrow Neurological Institute in Phoenix, Arizona, where he spent the remainder of his surgical career. The Spetzler Collection of operative videos is a historical archive that documents his approach to difficult AVMs and aneurysms [29].

Reviews of the natural history of AVMs showed that once a malformation bled there was a high risk of rebleeding and poor outcome. A general consensus developed that AVMs that had bled should be treated aggressively when feasible. Many AVMs presented because of headache or seizures (they ache, shake, or break). The malformations that were diagnosed by neuroimaging but had not bled had a much lower risk of bleeding and had a substantial risk of treatment complications [30]. Controversy surrounded whether these lesions should be treated with embolization, surgery, or radiotherapy or left alone until they showed signs of bleeding. To assess whether aggressive treatment (surgical resection, embolization, or radiotherapy) was indicated to treat AVMs that had not bled, the Randomized Trial of Unruptured Brain Arteriovenous Malformations (ARUBA) compared the risks of stroke or death in patients who were managed medically with those who had these interventions. The study was stopped early after interim analysis showed a superiority of medical treatment [31]. In individual AVM patients, many features, including location, size, and vascular features; the patient's age, clinical findings, comorbidities, and wishes; and the experience and capabilities of the treating physicians and treatment center, are weighed in deciding on treatment.

CAVERNOMAS

Cavernous angiomas and their surgical removal were described by Dandy in 1928 [32]. He characterized these as slow-growing lesions that carried risk of intermittent hemorrhage. Clinical symptoms varied with location and he favored surgical resection. Descriptions of cavernous angiomas (also called cavernomas and cavernous malformations) and their surgical removal began to appear in the mid-twentieth century. Cavernomas contained large sinusoidal vascular spaces without significant intervening brain parenchyma and were often surrounded by a capsule.

In 1948, Wilder Penfield and Arthur Ward described the calcified nature of some cavernomas and their association with seizures [33]. Heavily calcified cavernomas, while showing hemosiderin staining, were less likely to be associated with clinically significant hemorrhage. In one report, a 33-year-old woman was evaluated for headaches and papilledema. Electroencephalography was used to localize this lesion along with angiography and ventriculography. The mass excised was described as well encapsulated, noninvasive, and with very few blood vessels entering the capsule [34]. Multiple cavernomas were more common in those with a family history. An increased frequency of multiple cavernomas was found within Mexican-American families. Daniele Rigamonti, who was working in the US Southwest at the time, played an important role in elucidating family histories and genetic studies. Rigamonti obtained his medical degree from the Catholic University in Rome and completed his neurosurgery internship and residency at Mt. Sinai Hospital in New York [35]. He received his neurovascular fellowship training at the Barrow Neurological Institute in Phoenix, Arizona. He then moved to Johns Hopkins where he became the inaugural Salisbury Family Professor in Neurosurgery. Rigamonti first recognized the importance of genetic factors in the development of cerebral vascular malformations. He contributed to codifications of their imaging characteristics, and his research provided information on the natural history of developmental venous anomalies, cavernous malformations, and capillary telangiectasias. Genetic analysis implicated the CCM family of genes in multiple cavernomas

[36]. Surgery was performed mostly in cavernomas that had bled and were well circumscribed and close to the pial surface. Brainstem lesions, especially pontine lesions, were often quite disabling after bleeds. They could be removed if they abutted on the pial or fourth ventricular surface. Treatment for hemorrhagic lesions in inaccessible brain areas was attempted with radiosurgery, but this treatment was controversial and often limited to inoperable lesions with a history of multiple hemorrhages [37].

DEVELOPMENTAL VENOUS ANOMALIES

Lesions consisting only of venous structures were occasionally identified as a cause of brain bleeding and local edema [38]. These lesions were called "venous hamartomas" and "venous angiomas." When it was recognized that these lesions represented a congenital abnormality of venous drainage, the preferred designation was developmental venous anomalies (DVAs). Because some veins were absent or underdeveloped, accessory and anomalous venous structures developed to aid drainage of blood from areas within the brain. The anomaly consisted of a collection of dilated medullary veins that converged and drained into an enlarged transcortical or subependymal collector vein. One or more large central draining veins was usually conspicuous. The vein walls could become thick and hyalinized. When MRI became widely available, DVAs were the commonest vascular malformation found. DVAs were often associated with cavernous angiomas. By further compromising venous drainage, neurosurgical removal often caused important complications and was found to be nontherapeutic. Experience showed that these lesions should not be treated surgically or by radiosurgery.

CAROTID CAVERNOUS FISTULAS

In 1809, Benjamin Travers described the first case of pulsating exophthalmos [39]. He treated a pregnant 34-year-old woman who, after several days of headache, developed the sudden onset of left eye pain. She had proptosis, ophthalmoplegia, venous congestion around the orbit, and an audible bruit. Compression of the temporal, maxillary, and angular arteries had no effect on the symptoms, but compression of the ipsilateral common carotid artery led to near resolution of the bruit. He ligated the left carotid artery. While still in the operating theater she noted a decrease in pain and the bruit was no longer audible. By the fifth post-operative day, her proptosis decreased [39].

By the middle 1930s, the anatomical basis of the pulsating exophthalmos was attributed to development of a fistula between the internal carotid artery (ICA) and the cavernous sinus. Compression or ligation of the nuchal carotid artery was explored but often led to adverse neurological signs. Wallace Hamby and

W. James Gardner showed that intracranial ligation of the ICA was a potential treatment of pulsating exophthalmos [40]. Dandy analyzed the results of 800 traumatic and spontaneous carotid cavernous fistula (CCF) cases reported in the literature. He concluded that partial or complete ligations of the cervical CCA or ICA led to "capricious" results. In cases of cure of the CCF, Dandy posited that resolution was due to the formation of thrombi in the fistula and not due to isolation of the CCF from the circulation [41]. He reported the first two cases of intracranial ICA clip ligation as treatment following unsuccessful cervical carotid ligation [41].

In 1965, Parkinson described the direct surgical approach to the cavernous sinus to treat CCFs. Dwight Parkinson was born in Boise, Idaho; his early schooling was in Utah [42]. He matriculated at Dartmouth College and then McGill Medical School where he had contact with neurosurgeons Wilder Penfield and William Cone. Parkinson then served as a battalion surgeon in World War II. After the war he had a general surgery residency at Dartmouth and a neurosurgery residency at the Mayo Clinic in Rochester, Minnesota, where he was closely mentored by Grafton Love. He was offered a post in Canada, and, in 1950, Dwight Parkinson was the first qualified neurosurgeon to arrive in Winnipeg, Manitoba. He collaborated with Arthur Child, an experienced neuroradiologist, to create a neurosurgery and neuroscience program. He played a leading role in developing one of the earliest neurosurgical training programs in Western Canada. Parkinson became the first president of the Canadian Neurosurgical Society in 1965 [42].

Parkinson's first patient was a 29-year-old man who developed a right CCF after head trauma [43]. The right common carotid artery (CCA) was ligated. After worsening symptoms, ligations of the right ICA and external carotid artery (ECA) were performed nine years later. The left ECA and branches were then ligated, as were any bleeding points exposed via a right orbital incision. Symptoms persisted. In 1956, a right transfrontal craniotomy was performed and an ICA of normal size was visualized and clipped [43]. Parkinson later introduced a lateral transdural approach to the cavernous sinus; surgery was performed with the heart exposed and the great vessels of the aortic arch occluded. "Hemorrhagic flooding" with arterial blood developed after incising the cavernous sinus. Cardiac arrest was induced with clearing of the field. The cavernous ICA then became clearly visible and was ligated, packed with muscle, and divided. The heart was restarted and the patient awoke at his neurologic baseline. He had respiratory difficulties postoperatively and then died of a cardiopulmonary complication three days later [43].

Because carotid ligation and open surgical measures had shown limited success, alternative methods were explored. Muscle emboli were used. Fedor Andreevitch Serbinenko and his Russian colleagues reported using plastic tubes and string attached to the muscle embolus to guide the muscle to the fistulous site and allow adjustments [44]. Sean Mullan at the University of Chicago induced thrombosis using both open wire and copper electric stimulation [45]. He placed the wire during open craniotomy into the intracavernous ICA, thrombosing the fistula with preservation of the artery. A stereotaxic thrombosis was also successful in cases where direct surgery was not an option [45]. Serbinenko continued to devise endovascular treatments. He developed catheter-mounted balloons and later detachable balloons that were used to occlude intracranial vessels at the point of the fistula [44]. Gerard Debrun, a French neuroradiologist who later worked in London and Chicago, modified these techniques and devised detachable balloons filled with silicon [46]. By gradually inflating these balloons and monitoring ICA blood flow, he could occlude the fistula and optimize blood flow. He reported 17 cases of post-traumatic CCF treated with this technique. Among these, 12 patients had preservation of carotid blood flow [46]. Coils and liquid embolic materials began to be used to close the fistulas by both transarterial and transvenous routes with success [47]. In some instances, transfemoral transvenous routes to the cavernous sinus were not feasible and transvenous access was gained through the orbit using fluoroscopic guidance.

NOTES AND REFERENCES

1. Gaupp J. Casuistische Beitrage zur pathologischen anatomie des ruckenmarks und seiner haute. II. Hemorrhoiden der pia-mater spinalis in gebiete des lendenmarks. *Beitrage zur pathologishen Anatomie und zur allgemeinen Pathologie* 1888;2:510–524.

2. Worster-Drought C, Carnegie Dickson WE. Venous angioma of the cerebrum: Report of a case with necropsy. *J. Neurol. Psychopathol.* 1927;8(29):19–22.

3. Campbell H, Ballance C. A case of venous angioma of the cerebral cortex. *Lancet* 1922;199(5132):10–11.

4. Fodstad H, Ljunggren B, Kristiansen K. Vilhelm Magnus: Pioneer neurosurgeon. *J. Neurosurg.* 1990;73(3):317–330.

5. Harvey Cushing's initial experience with brain aneurysms is described in Chapter 18. Two detailed biographies describe the main life events and accomplishments of Harvey Cushing: Fulton J. *Harvey Cushing: A Biography – The Story of a Great Medical Pioneer.* Springfield, IL: Charles C. Thomas, 1946; and Bliss M. *Harvey Cushing: A Life in Surgery.* New York: Oxford University Press, 2007.

6. Cushing H, Bailey P. *Tumors Arising from the Blood-Vessels of the Brain: Angiomatous Malformations and Hemangioblastomas.* Springfield, IL: Charles C. Thomas, 1928.

7. The career and accomplishments of Walter Dandy are discussed in Chapter 56 and in Fox WL. *Dandy of Johns Hopkins.* Baltimore, MD: Williams and Wilkins, 1984.

8. Dandy WE. Arteriovenous aneurysm of the brain. *Arch. Surg.* 1928;117(2):190–243.

9. Ljunggren B. Herbert Olivecrona: Founder of Swedish neurosurgery. *J. Neurosurg.* 1993;78(1):142–149.

10. Olivecrona H, Riives J. Arteriovenous aneurysms of the brain, their diagnosis and treatment. *Arch. Neurol. Psychiatry* 1948;59(5):567–602.

11. Norle G. Arteriovenous aneurysms of the brain; report of ten cases of total removal of the lesion. *J. Neurosurg.* 1949;6(6):475–494.

12. Murphy JP. *Cerebrovascular Disease.* Chicago: Year Book Medical Publishers, 1954, pp. 73–105.

13. Perret G, Nishioka H. Report on the cooperative study of intracranial aneurysms and subarachnoid hemorrhage. Section VI. Arteriovenous malformations. An analysis of 545 cases of cranio-cerebral arteriovenous malformations and fistulae reported to the cooperative study. *J. Neurosurg.* 1966;25(4):467–490.

14. Fults D, Kelly DL Jr. Natural history of arteriovenous malformations of the brain: A clinical study. *Neurosurgery* 1984;15(5):658–662. Graf CJ, Perret GE, Torner JC. Bleeding from cerebral arteriovenous malformations as part of their natural history. *J. Neurosurg.* 1983;58(3):331–337. Ondra SL, Troupp H, George ED, Schwab K. The natural history of symptomatic arteriovenous malformations of the brain: A 24-year follow-up assessment. *J. Neurosurg.* 1990;73(3):387–391.

15. Crawford PM, West CR, Chadwick DW, Shaw MD. Arteriovenous malformations of the brain: Natural history in unoperated patients. *J. Neurol. Neurosurg. Psychiatry* 1986;49(1):1–10.

16. Samson D, Batjer HH. Preoperative evaluation of the risk/benefit ratio for arteriovenous malformations of the brain. In Wilkins RH, Rengachart SS (eds.), *Neurosurgery Update II.* New York: McGraw-Hill, 1991, pp. 121–133.

17. Theodore Kurze, MD, interviewed by Peter J. Jannetta, MD. YouTube. Available at www.youtube.com/watch?v=AOUZG3VajBk.

18. The career of Gazi Yasargil is discussed in Chapter 56 on aneurysms. Stienen MN, Serra, C, Stieglitz LH, Krayenbühl N, Bozinov O, Regli L. UniversitätsSpital Zürich: 80 years of neurosurgical care in Switzerland. *Acta Neurochir. (Wien)* 2018;160(1):3–22. Tew JM. M. Gazi Yaşargil: Neurosurgery's man of the century. *Neurosurgery* 1999;45 (5):1010–1014. Yasargil MG, Vise WM, Bader DC. Technical adjuncts in neurosurgery. *Surg. Neurol.* 1977;8:331–336.

19. Yasargil MG. *Microsurgery Applied to Neurosurgery.* Stuttgart: Georg Thieme, 1969, pp. 105–119.

20. Yasargil MG, Jain KK, Antic J, Laciga R. Arteriovenous malformations of the splenium of the corpus callosum: Microsurgical treatment. *Surg. Neurol.* 1976;5(1):5–14. Yasargil MG, Jain KK, Antic J, Laciga R, Kletter G. Arteriovenous malformations of the anterior and the middle portions of the corpus callosum: Microsurgical treatment. *Surg. Neurol.* 1976;5(2):67–80.

21. Yasargil MG. *Microneurosurgery, vol. III B: AVM of the Brain, Clinical Consideration, General and Special Operative Techniques, Surgical Results, Nonoperated Cases, Cavernous and Venous Angiomas, Neuroanesthesia.* New York: Georg Thieme Verlag Stuttgart, 1988.

22. Past honored guests: Robert C. Heros. 2005. Congress of Neurological Surgeons. Available at www.cns.org/meetings/past-honored-guests-detail/roberto-c-heros.

23. Heros RC. Arteriovenous malformations of the medial temporal lobe. Surgical approach and neuroradiological characterization. *J. Neurosurg.* 1982;56(1):44–52.

24. Latchaw RE, Hu X, Ugurbil K, Hall WA, Madison MT, Heros RC. Functional magnetic resonance imaging as a management tool for cerebral arteriovenous malformations. *Neurosurgery* 1995;37(4):619–625; discussion 625–626.

25. Luessenhop AJ, Spence WT. Artificial embolization of cerebral arteries. Report of use in a case of arteriovenous malformation. *JAMA* 1960;172:1153–1155. The use of

embolic particles to treat intracranial vascular lesions is discussed in detail in Chapter 56 on treatment of aneurysms.

26. Luessenhop AJ, Gennarelli TA. Anatomical grading of supratentorial arteriovenous malformations for determining operability. *Neurosurg.* 1977;1(1):30–35.

27. Spetzler RF, Martin NA. A proposed grading system for arteriovenous malformations. *J. Neurosurg.* 1986;65(4):476–483.

28. Robert F. Spetzler. Wikipedia. Available at https://en.wikipedia.org/wiki/Robert_F ._Spetzler. Past honored guests: Robert F. Spetzler. 1994. Congress of Neurological Surgeons. Available at www.cns.org/meetings/past-honored-guests-detail/robert-f-spetzler.

29. Spetzler collection. *Operative Neurosurgery* 2019 Oct;17(4):339.

30. van Beijnum J, van der Worp HB, Buis DR, et al. Treatment of brain arteriovenous malformations: A systematic review and meta-analysis. *JAMA* 2011;306:2011–2019. Wedderburn CJ, van Beijnum J, Bhattacharya JJ, et al. on behalf of the SIVMS Collaborators. Outcome after interventional or conservative management of unruptured brain arteriovenous malformations: A prospective, population-based cohort study. *Lancet Neurol.* 2008;7:223–230.

31. Mohr JP, Parides MK, Stapf C, Moquete E, et al. Medical management with or without interventional therapy for unruptured brain arteriovenous malformations (ARUBA): A multicentre, non-blinded, randomised trial. *Lancet* 2014;383 (9917):614–621.

32. Dandy WE. Venous abnormalities and angiomas of the brain. *Arch. Surg.* 1928;17:715–793.

33. Penfield W, Ward A. Calcifying epileptogenic lesions; hemangioma calcificans; report of a case. *Arch. Neurol. Psychiatry* 1948;60(1):20–36.

34. Schneider RC, Liss L. Cavernous hemangiomas of the cerebral hemispheres. *J. Neurosurg.* 1958;15(4):392–399.

35. Professorships: Daniele Rigamonti. Johns Hopkins University. Available at https:// professorships.jhu.edu/chair/daniele-rigamonti-md-facs/.

36. Rigamonti D, Hadley MN, Drayer BP, Johnson PC, et al. Cerebral cavernous malformations: Incidence and familial occurrence. *N. Engl. J. Med.* 1988;319 (6):343–347. Batra S, Lin D, Recinos PF, Rigamonti D. Cavernous malformations: Natural history, diagnosis, and treatment. *Nat. Rev. Neurol.* 2009;5(12):659–670.

37. Steiner L, Karlsson B, Yen CP, Torner JC, et al. Radiosurgery in cavernous malformations: Anatomy of a controversy. *J. Neurosurg.* 2010;113(1):16–21; discussion 21–22.

38. Truwit C. Venous angiomas of the brain: History, significance, and imaging findings. *Am. J. Radiol.* 1992;159:1299–1307. Crawford JV, Russell DS. Cryptic arteriovenous and venous hamartomas of the brain. *J. Neurol. Neurosurg. Psychiatry* 1956:19(1):1–11.

39. Travers, B. A case of aneurism by anastomosis in the orbit, cured by the ligature of the common carotid artery. *Med. Chir. Trans.* 1811;2(1):420–421.

40. Hamby WB, Gardner WJ. Treatment of pulsating exophthalmos with report of two cases. *JAMA Surgery* 1933;27(4):676–685.

41. Dandy WE. The treatment of carotid cavernous arteriovenous aneurysms. *Ann. Surg.* 1935;102(5):916–926.

42. Dwight Parkinson, MD, interviewed by Jock McBeath, MD. YouTube. Available at www.youtube.com/watch?v=VpzIIbeHRmU.

43. Parkinson, D. A surgical approach to the cavernous portion of the carotid artery. Anatomical studies and case report. *J. Neurosurg.* 1965;23(5):474–483.

44. The career and contributions of Fiódor Andreevitch Serbinenko is discussed in Chapter 56 on aneurysms. Arutiunov AI, Serbinenko FA, Shlykov AA. Surgical treatment of carotid-cavernous fistulas. *Prog. Brain Res.* 1968;30:441–444.

45. Mullan S. Treatment of carotid-cavernous fistulas by cavernous sinus occlusion. *J. Neurosurg.* 1979;50(2):131–144.

46. Debrun G, Lacour P, Caron JP, Hurth M, et al. Detachable balloon and calibrated-leak balloon techniques in the treatment of cerebral vascular lesions. *J. Neurosurg.* 1978;49(5):635–649.

47. Halbach VV, Higashida RT, Hieshima GB, Hardin CW, et al. Transvenous embolization of dural fistulas involving the cavernous sinus. *AJNR Am. J. Neuroradiol.* 1989;10 (2):377–383.

PART IV

STROKE LITERATURE, ORGANIZATIONS, AND PATIENTS

CHAPTER SIXTY

STROKE ORGANIZATIONS, JOURNALS, AND BOOKS

At the midpoint of the twentieth century there were no organizations devoted solely to stroke, and no stroke-oriented journals. In 1954, the American Heart Association (AHA) sponsored a cerebrovascular disease meeting held in Princeton, New Jersey. The attendees at this first conference were mostly internists and cardiologists. A second conference was held in January 1957. The preface to the Second Conference on Cerebrovascular Diseases noted that "because of the massive size of the subject, certain facets were not fully covered in the first meeting. For this reason and, as research activity in cerebral vascular disease has intensified, it was deemed wise to make plans for a second conference" [1].

The National Institutes of Health (NIH), a major focal point of medical research in the United States, also acknowledged the paucity of research and knowledge about stroke and its treatment. Two component organizations of the NIH – the National Institute of Neurological Diseases and Blindness and the National Heart Institute – appointed an ad hoc committee entitled the Joint Council Subcommittee on Cerebrovascular Diseases. This committee functioned from 1961 to 1972 as the NIH focal point for planning and funding subsequent Princeton conferences on cerebrovascular diseases and for initiating cerebrovascular disease survey reports that were published at five-year intervals [2].

Responding to an increased interest in stroke, the AHA appointed an ad hoc committee called the Coordinating Committee for a Nationwide Stroke Program. This group first met in March 1964 under the chairmanship of Irving Wright, a cardiologist and a professor of medicine at Cornell University in New York City. This committee was formed to identify interest and expertise in the field of stroke and to sponsor this activity securely within the bosom of the American Heart Association. In January 1967 the committee became the Stroke Council of the American Heart Association. The Stroke Council succeeded in convincing the AHA to sponsor publication of a journal dedicated to stroke and to sponsor meetings dedicated to the topic of cerebrovascular disease. The first edition of *Stroke* was published in 1970 under the editorship of Clark Millikan of the Mayo Clinic. *Stroke* was published every other month until 1988 when editions appeared monthly [3].

The Stroke Council of the AHA partnered with the Canadian Heart Foundation and Stroke Society, the section on cerebrovascular diseases of the American Association of Neurological Surgeons, and the American Neurological Association to plan and sponsor international meetings dedicated to stroke and cerebrovascular diseases. The first such international meeting took place in February 1976 in Dallas, Texas, the then new home of the AHA. About 350 attendees crowded the small meeting rooms and halls. These international stroke meetings were held each winter since then, usually in southern cities in the United States.

During the mid-1980s, members of the AHA Stroke Council and other physicians who had a major clinical and/or research interest in cerebrovascular disease debated whether to form a new stroke organization that could support and fund meetings and a journal. They ultimately decided to remain under the auspices of the AHA but urged the AHA to devote more resources and autonomy to *Stroke*. In 1998, the American Stroke Association became an independent component of the AHA.

In the United States, the National Stroke Association (NSA) was founded in 1984 in Colorado as a nonprofit organization that focused all of its efforts and resources on stroke. The NSA sponsored stroke clubs throughout the United States. These clubs were attended by former stroke patients and their families and had educational and service functions. In 2019, the National Stroke Association announced that it would be dissolved and its activities folded into the American Stroke Association.

NATIONAL AND INTERNATIONAL ORGANIZATIONS AND PUBLICATIONS

During the last decades of the twentieth century, many international stroke organizations were formed and became active. In Canada, the Heart and

Stroke Foundation became Heart and Stroke. In Europe, the European Stroke Council was formed and published the first edition of *Cerebrovascular Diseases* in 1990. The first European Stroke Conference (ESC) met in May 1990 in Dusseldorf; there were about 800 attendees. ESC meetings occurred annually in different European countries. The largest attendance was in London in 2013: 4,600 attendees. A second organization, the European Stroke Initiative, was composed of representatives of the different European countries. In 2007, the European Stroke Organization (ESO) was formed. The ESO began to publish the *European Stroke Journal*. The ESO holds summer school sessions each year to help educate and train European neurologists and other physicians about stroke.

The World Stroke Organization (WSO) was established in 2006 through the merger of two other organizations: the International Stroke Society and the World Stroke Federation. The WSO is composed of more than 60 societies representing 85 different countries. The WSO began publishing the *International Journal of Stroke* in 2006. The first conference jointly sponsored by the ESO and WSO met in the Philippines in 2019. The first World Stroke Conference was in Kyoto, Japan, in 1989. The 11th World Conference was held in Montreal in 2018. World stroke conferences are also now sponsored by the WSO.

Stroke organizations have been formed in many countries and regions throughout the world: The Japanese Stroke society was formed in 1975; the Chinese Stroke Association was established in 2014; the Indian Stroke Association met first in 2002; the Korean Stroke Society was formed in 1995 and began publishing the *Journal of Stroke* in 1995; and the Stroke Society of Australasia was formed in 1989. Stroke-related organizations and meetings were eventually organized in almost every country in the world. These societies sponsor education, meetings, and often publications in their respective countries. There are now 51 stroke-related journals, and this does not include primarily neurological journals, which also publish reports and reviews about cerebrovascular disease topics [4].

NOTES AND REFERENCES

1. Millikan C. Preface. In Wright IS, Millikan C (eds.), *Cerebral Vascular Diseases. Transactions of the Second Conference Held under the Auspices of the American Heart Association, Princeton NJ January 16–18, 1957*. New York: Grune & Stratton, 1958.
2. A review of the formation of the American Heart Association Stroke Council and the NIH stroke committees is contained in Caplan LR. The Stroke Council and the Young Investigator award. *Mayo Clinic Proceedings* 1989;64:125–128.
3. Caplan LR. Journal *Stroke*: Origin and evolution. *Stroke* 2020;51:1025–1026.
4. OMICS International (www.omicsonline.org) is an Open Access publisher and international conference organizer.

CHAPTER SIXTY ONE

PROMINENT STROKE PATIENTS

The history of the world has undoubtedly been altered by stroke. Many important leaders in science, medicine, and politics have had their productivity cut prematurely short by stroke. Some of the world-renowned artists, musicians, authors, actors, and sportsmen also suffered severely debilitating or fatal strokes.

Political Figures

The notion that an exceptional man had a legendary death is often questioned, since common health conditions like stroke are widely shared. The health status of political leaders is concealed, especially when the illness is perceived as stigmatizing. No doubt people would be indignant at the thought of having brought and left in power a mentally disabled leader.

Two important political leaders during the early twentieth century, Vladimir Lenin and Woodrow Wilson, had intellectual impairment owing to strokes while they were at the helms of their countries at critical times in history. Lenin, at age 52 years, had sudden onset of dysarthria and right hemiparesis. An observer noted that "often as he spoke, the worlds were slurred and he paused several times like a man who had lost the thread of his argument." Wilson, the architect of the League of Nations, had a series of small strokes that left him pseudobulbar and with left hemiparesis at a time when he was ardently working for world peace and cooperation [1].

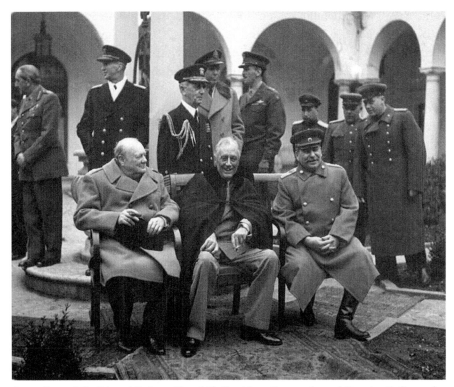

61.1. From left, Prime Minister Churchill, President Roosevelt, and Premier Stalin at the 1945 Yalta conference to discuss plans for a post–World War II planet. Source: https://en .wikipedia.org/wiki/File:Yalta_Conference_(Churchill,_Roosevelt,_Stalin)_(B%26W).jpg. Public domain.

At the Yalta conference, February 4–11, 1945, President Franklin D. Roosevelt of the United States, Soviet Union Premier Joseph Stalin, and British Prime Minister Winston Churchill met to discuss how post–World War II Europe should be organized (Figure 61.1). All three men died within the next two decades. President Roosevelt died two months after the Yalta conference due to a hemorrhagic stroke. Premier Stalin died eight years later, also due to a hemorrhagic stroke. Finally, Prime Minister Churchill died 20 years after the conference because of complications of stroke. The subsequent deterioration of these three leaders of the most powerful countries of the world had varying degrees of historical significance. Churchill's resignation following his illness led to Britain's mismanagement of the Egyptian Suez crisis and a period of mistrust with the United States. Roosevelt was still president and Stalin still premier at their times of passing, so their deaths carried huge political ramifications. The early death of Roosevelt may have exacerbated post–World War II miscommunication between America and the Soviet Union, which may have precipitated the Cold War [2].

In a study entitled "Stroke and the American Presidency," the authors listed eight American presidents who had strokes since 1846: John Quincy Adams,

John Tyler, Millard Fillmore, Andrew Johnson, Chester Arthur, Woodrow Wilson, Franklin D. Roosevelt, and Richard M. Nixon. Survival time from the last stroke was greater than one month in only president, John Tyler. Some of the presidents who developed strokes had unhealthy lifestyles. Chester Arthur was obese and got little exercise. Roosevelt was a heavy smoker and had severe uncontrolled hypertension. Andrew Johnson may have abused alcohol. Nixon represents the first president to be on scientifically validated prophylaxis, that is, warfarin. He was also the first president to be considered for a controlled therapeutic trial in acute stroke and the first to have had an advanced directive regarding terminal care [3]. President Dwight D. Eisenhower had nonfatal strokes while in office. He made arrangements with Vice President Nixon on what would happen if he couldn't do his duties as president. This idea became the basis of the Twenty-fifth Amendment: "If a president dies or resigns, the vice president takes over and then he appoints a new vice president" [4]. Finally, in 2000, former President Gerald Ford began slurring his words during a TV interview [5].

Some other world leaders who had strokes follow [6].

Margaret Thatcher, the first female British prime minister, also known as "The Iron Lady," died of a stroke on April 8, 2013 [7]. Yasser Arafat was the leader of the Palestine Liberation Organization. He received the 1994 Nobel Peace Prize for working for peace with Israeli leaders. He died of a massive brain hemorrhage on November 11, 2004 [8]. John A. Macdonald, the first prime minister of Canada, died of a stroke on June 6, 1891 [9]. The second prime minister of Canada, Alexander Mackenzie, also died of a stroke on April 17, 1892 [10]. Catherine the Great, the most renowned and the longest-ruling female leader of Russia, reigned from 1762 until 1796. Her reign is known as Russia's golden age. She died of a stroke on November 6, 1796 [11]. Isambard Kingdom Brunel, one of the most famous figures of the Industrial Revolution in Britain, died of a stroke on September 15, 1859 [12]. Samuel de Champlain, French explorer and the founder of New France and Quebec City, died of a stroke on December 25, 1635 [13]. Shirley Chisholm, the first Black American congresswoman, died of stroke on January 1, 2005 [14]. Arial Sharon, the prime minister of Israel, was left unconscious after a series of cerebrovascular events [15]. Indian prime minister Atal Bihari Vajpayee had a stroke in 2009 that impaired his speech [16].

Medical Pioneers

William Harvey, the anatomist and physiologist who discovered blood circulation, died of a cerebral hemorrhage at Roehampton in the house of his brother Eliab on June 3, 1657, aged 79 years [17]. Marcello Malpighi, discoverer of capillaries and the microscopic anatomy of the lungs, kidneys, and spleen, died of an apoplectic right hemiplegia [18]. Edward Jenner, "the father of immunology" and the inventor of the smallpox vaccine by using cowpox pus, died of a stroke on January 26, 1823. His work is said to have "saved more lives than the work of any other human" [19]. Louis Pasteur, known for his discoveries of the principles of vaccination, microbial fermentation, and pasteurization, had a stroke at the age of 46 years, leading to left hemiparesis. He rehabilitated himself and many of his greatest scientific achievements came after his stroke. He later had multiple debilitating strokes and died on September 28, 1895, at the age of 72 years [20]. Elizabeth Blackwell was the first woman to receive a medical degree in the United States as well as the first woman on the UK Medical Register. She died of a stroke on May 31, 1910 [21]. Daniel Williams was an American heart surgeon who performed one of the first successful open-heart surgeries in the United States and also founded the Provident Hospital in Chicago, the first African American–owned and operated hospital in America. He died of a stroke on August 4, 1931 [22].

Three important figures in twentieth-century neurology – Russell DeJong, the first editor of the journal *Neurology*; Raymond Escourolle, the French neuropathologist; and Houston Merritt, longtime Columbia professor, writer of *Merritt's Neurology*, and codeveloper of the antiepileptic drug phenytoin – were severely disabled by multiple strokes in their later years [23–25].

Jill Bolte Taylor is an American neuroanatomist, author, and an inspirational public speaker. She had a large cerebral hemorrhage following rupture of an arteriovenous malformation in 1996, at the age of 37, and underwent major brain surgery. Her subsequent eight-year recovery influenced her work as a scientist and a speaker and was the subject of her 2006 book *My Stroke of Insight: A Brain Scientist's Personal Journey*. She gave the first TED talk that ever went viral on the internet, after which her book became a *New York Times* bestseller and was published in 30 languages [26].

Scientists and Inventors

Alexander von Humboldt, a naturalist and explorer whose quantitative work on botanical geography laid the foundation for the field of biogeography, died of a stroke on May 6, 1859 [27]. John Logie Baird, the Scottish inventor of television, died of a stroke on June 14, 1946 [28]. Dorothy Hodgkin is best known for developing crystallography of biochemical compounds. Her work in the determination of the molecular structure of penicillin and vitamin B_{12} brought her the 1964 Nobel Prize for Chemistry. She died of a stroke on July 29, 1994 [29]. Henry Ford, the American industrialist and business magnate, founder of the Ford Motor Company, and chief developer of the assembly line technique of mass production, died of a cerebral hemorrhage on April 7, 1947 [30].

Authors

Charles Dickens, the greatest novelist of the Victorian period, died of a stroke. He had a slight stroke in 1869. His family doctor, Frank Beard, sent him to a consultant who advised him to reduce his workload. On June 8, 1870, at dinner, Dickens stood up and collapsed, was diagnosed with apoplexy, and died on the next day. The stroke was attributed by some to his opium use as a painkiller [31]. Anne Morrow Lindbergh was an acclaimed author whose books and articles spanned the genres of poetry and nonfiction. She was also the first licensed female glider pilot in the United States. She died of a stroke at age 94 on February 7, 2001 [32]. Bram Stoker, the Irish author of the 1897 Gothic novel *Dracula*, died of a stroke on April 20, 1912 [33]. Louisa May Alcott, the author of the popular novels *Little Women*, *Little Men*, and *Jo's Boys*, died after a stroke at the age of 55 on March 6, 1888 [34]. The Pulitzer prize–winning author Edith Wharton also died of a stroke [35].

Actors and Directors

Charlie Chaplin was a British comedian, actor, and filmmaker. He moved to America and became a famous actor known worldwide for his tramp character in silent films. He died of a stroke on December 25, 1977, aged 88 [36]. Grace Kelly, a Golden Globe and Oscar-winning actress, died in a crash resulting from a stroke [37]. Luke Perry, an American actor famous for his role in the teenage drama *Beverly Hills, 90210*, died of a stroke on March 4, 2019 [38]. Gene Kelly was an actor and dancer who transformed the Hollywood musical in 1950s with his dancing style and modern choreography. The 1952 musical *Singin' in the Rain* with his famous dance partnering an umbrella around a lamp post is often considered the "greatest musical ever made." He died of a stroke on February 2, 1996 [39]. Claudette Colbert, Broderick Crawford, Edwin Booth, and Ralph Richardson are some of the other famous actors who died following a stroke [6]. *Game of Thrones* star Emilia Clarke suffered complications of her brain aneurysms in 2011 and then in 2013 (see below).

Akira Kurosawa was a Japanese film director and screenwriter. He is widely regarded as one of the most important and influential filmmakers in the history of cinema. His films have influenced many Hollywood filmmakers, including Steven Spielberg and Martin Scorsese. He died of a stroke on September 6, 1998 [40]. George Cukor, a famous American director, died of stroke on January 24, 1983 [41]. Federico Fellini, a famous Italian filmmaker, also had multiple strokes leading to his death (see below).

MUSICIANS

Johann Sebastian Bach was one of the most prolific composers of the Baroque period. His 20 children featured many musicians and composers. He is known for instrumental compositions such as the *Brandenburg Concertos* and the *Goldberg Variations* and for vocal music such as the *St. Matthew Passion* and the *Mass in B minor*. He died of a stroke after having several prodromal episodes of near blindness on July 28, 1750 [42]. Felix Mendelssohn, German composer and pianist, is among the most popular composers of the Romantic era. Some of his best-known works include his Overture and incidental music for *A Midsummer Night's Dream*, the Italian Symphony, and the Scottish Symphony. He died of a stroke on November 4, 1847 [43]. Giuseppe Verdi was the dominant Italian composer of the nineteenth century. Born the same year as Richard Wagner, both composers created unique styles of opera that are still central to the opera repertory today. Verdi's works remain renowned for their melodies and theatrical style. He died of a stroke on January 27, 1901 [44]. Sergei Prokofiev was a Russian Soviet composer, pianist, and conductor. As the creator of acknowledged masterpieces across numerous music genres, he is regarded as one of the major composers of the twentieth century. His works include the March from *The Love of Three Oranges*, the suite *Lieutenant Kije*, the ballet *Romeo and Juliet*, and *Peter and the Wolf*. Prokofiev died of a brain hemorrhage at the age of 61 on March 5, 1953, the same day as Joseph Stalin. He had lived near Red Square, and for three days the throngs gathered to mourn Stalin, making it impossible to hold Prokofiev's funeral at the headquarters of the Soviet Composer's Union. His coffin had to be moved by hand through back streets in the opposite direction of the masses of people going to visit Stalin's body [45]. Thelonious Monk, one of the greatest jazz musicians of all time and one of the first creators of modern jazz and bebop, was born in 1917 in Rocky Mount, North Carolina. When he was four, his parents moved to New York City, where he spent the next five decades of his life. Monk began studying classical piano when he was eleven. Alongside Charlie Parker and Dizzy Gillespie he explored the fast, jarring, and often improvised styles that later become synonymous with modern jazz. In 1957, the Thelonious Monk Quartet, which included John Coltrane, began performing regularly in New York. They enjoying huge success and went on to tour the United States and made appearances in Europe. In 1964, Monk became one of four jazz musicians ever to grace the cover of *Time* magazine. On February 5, 1982, he had a major brain hemorrhage, slipped into a coma, and died two weeks later at age 64 [46].

SPORTS FIGURES

Ben Hogan, considered one of the greatest golfers in history, died of a stroke on July 25, 1997 [47]. Kirby Puckett, a famous Major League baseball center fielder, died of a stroke on March 6, 2006 [48]. Sam Snead, one of the top golfers in the world for almost four decades, died of a stroke on May 23, 2002 [49]. Bill Sharman, National Basketball Association guard best known for his time with the Boston Celtics in the 1950s, partnered with Bob Cousy in what some consider the greatest backcourt duo of all time. He is credited with introducing the morning shootaround, and was a 10-time NBA champion. He died of a stroke on October 25, 2013 [50]. Raymond van Schoor was a Namibian cricketer. He collapsed while batting at Wanderers Cricket Ground on November 15, 2015, and was admitted to a hospital after a stroke. He died five days later at the age of 25 [51].

In the following, the stroke histories of some of these individuals are examined in detail. Some strokes had devastating consequences for not only the individuals themselves but the nations that they led and the world. Treatment options were very limited in the past. We also share the journey of recovery following stroke of a young and popular actor, Emilia Clarke.

Lenin's Stroke

In Figure 61.2, the man who set fire to St. Petersburg in October 1917 and plunged Russia into chaos wears his cap as a great proletarian leader, sadly struck by stroke. In his wheelchair, he seems stiffened, thus betraying his hemiplegia. It is the summer of 1923, and Lenin is just a shadow of his former self. Historians believe that Lenin's serious health problems dated back to 1921, when the Russian civil war ended and the country was gripped by famine and devastation. Lenin began to have chronic headaches, insomnia, and fainting spells. He was then 51 years old and had difficulty maintaining his usual pace of work. He wrote to Alexei Maximovich Gorky, "I am so tired, I do not want to do anything at all" [51].

On April 23, 1922, on the advice of one of the German doctors called to his bedside, he had surgery to remove a bullet lodged near his neck since the 1918 attack. The operation went well, but on May 22 Lenin had a stroke. The relationship with neck surgery is relevant in the context of stroke. Stricken with hemiplegia on his right side, he also had difficulty speaking. He was examined again and a test of syphilis returned negative. He gradually recovered at Gorky Manor and continued to be informed of the work of the Politburo and Sovnarkom through Stalin, who regularly visited him [52].

Propaganda showed him still active, reading the newspaper (Figure 61.3). In December, he had a second stroke that marked the end of his political career and paralyzed his right side. In March 1923, a third stroke left him speechless. Lenin died on January 21, 1924, at the age of 53. Although then the doctors suggested that the origin of his health problems was linked to the two bullets left in his body after the 1918 conspiracy, the direct cause of death is hardly in

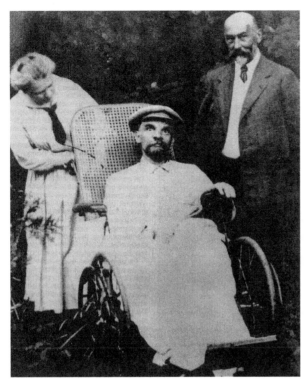

61.2. Vladimir Ilyich Ulyanov (Lenin)'s last photo. He had had three strokes at this point and was completely mute. https://rarehistoricalphotos.com/vladimir-lenin-last-photo-1923/.

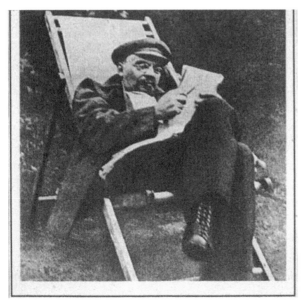

61.3. Lenin at his home in Gorki in August 1922. From *Moscow News*, April 22, 1990.

doubt today. Autopsy showed that Lenin's repeated strokes were due to severe atherosclerosis of his carotid and cerebral arteries, which were found to be almost blocked. During the autopsy, a doctor found that when he struck one of those arteries with a surgical forceps, it made a mineral sound, as if calcification had fossilized it. The large blood vessels supplying Lenin's brain were stiffened by atheroma plaques, and were in a way petrifying [53].

But what could have caused such damage to a man in his early fifties, with a healthy lifestyle? Lenin did not smoke and forbade people to light a cigarette in his presence; he drank moderately and was not obese. Furthermore, an article published by the journal *Human Pathology* concluded that the large size of Lenin's brain lesions and their location hardly corresponded to what is normally caused by neurosyphilis [54].

Lenin's father, Ilya Ulyanov, died of a stroke at the age of 54 – almost the same age as his illustrious son. Three of Lenin's siblings also died of cardiovascular disease, indicating a genetic predisposition to atherosclerosis. A genetic mutation causing arterial calcifications could also be a possible cause [55]. An inherited lipid disorder could also be a possibility [55]. Mystery still surrounds the death of the Bolshevik leader and organizer of the 1917 Soviet revolution, Vladimir Lenin. Many of the documents regarding his death remain classified.

WOODROW WILSON'S STROKE

This is a war to end all wars.
—Woodrow Wilson

Let us return, however to the League of Nations. To create an organization which is in a position to protect peace in this world of conflicting interests and egoistic wills is a frighteningly difficult task.
—Hjalmar Branting

Woodrow Wilson's idea of peace was the League of Nations, an international organization to maintain world peace by settling disputes without bloodshed. In January 1919, at the Paris Peace Conference that ended World War I, the US president, Wilson, persuaded the leaders from France, Great Britain, and Italy to come together with the leaders of other nations to draft a Covenant of League of Nations. While his idea got international support, it was vehemently opposed in his own country by the US Congress [1,56,57].

Wilson then embarked on a very strenuous national tour of the country to sell the idea directly to the general public on August 22, 1919, against the strong advice of his doctor. Wilson was to cover 8,000 miles in 22 days and would give two or three speeches every day. The tour took serious toll on his health [1,56,57]. Previously, in 1906, at the age of 50, Wilson woke up one morning blind in his left eye, which was attributed to a left ophthalmic artery occlusion, possibly from left carotid artery disease. The attack was transient and his vision gradually improved [1,58].

As the tour began in 1919, the president began to have severe headaches that increased in both duration and intensity. On the return leg of this tour, his headaches became even more debilitating and he grew unusually restless. Suddenly, he developed a weakness on the left side of his face. The tour was cut short and he began his journey back to Washington. He developed a stroke that had more severe clinical signs a week later. As described by his second wife, Edith Bolling Galt Wilson [1],

> At 11, on Sunday morning, September 28, 1919, the train pulled its heavy way into Washington ... all the rest of the day my husband wandered like a ghost between the study at one end of the hall and my room at the other. The awful pain in his head that drove him relentlessly back and forth was too acute to permit work or even reading ... the next day, the third since our return, the President seemed a little better. I had been sleeping fitfully, getting up every hour or so to see how my husband was.... At 5 or 6 in the morning I found him sleeping normally, as it appeared. Relieved, I dozed off again until after 8. This time I found him sitting on the side of the bed trying to reach a water bottle. As I handed it to him, I noticed that his left hand hung loosely. "I have no feeling in that hand. Will you rub it? But first help me to the bathroom," he said. He moved with great difficulty, and every move brought spasms of pain; with my help he gained the bathroom. It was so alarming that I asked if I could leave him long enough to telephone the doctor. He said yes, and hurrying into my room, I reached Dr. Grayson at his house. While on the phone, I heard a slight noise and rushing into my husband's apartment I found him on the bathroom floor unconscious.

The only treatment available at that time was rest. The president was to be released from all disturbing problems during the days of nature's efforts to repair the damage done [1]. His illness was concealed by his wife. She acted as a barrier between Wilson and the outside world. Every document had to go through her. She decided what was important for the president. She was a secret president running a bedside government that excluded even Wilson's staff, the Cabinet, and the Congress. Wilson, on the other hand, became very rigid and would not acquiesce or compromise to any changes in the treaty concerning the League of Nations proposed by the Senate. The treaty was ultimately rejected [1,59].

Wilson's personality changes could have been a result of his cerebrovascular disease. The League was initially his idea and during the period of his illness, he himself led to its downfall. The League of Nations was eventually formed without the United States as a member. While it met with success in certain areas, it could not prevent World War II [1].

WINSTON CHURCHILL'S STROKES

During his nation's "darkest hours" in World War II, Prime Minister Winston Churchill inspired the United Kingdom. Recall his famous statement that called for worldwide resistance against Axis forces and the National Socialist regime: "We shall defend our island whatever the cost may be; we shall fight on the beaches, landing grounds, in fields, in streets and on the hills. We shall never surrender."

But the strains of war showed even on the man called Britain's Bulldog. He had a slight heart attack in December 1941 while at the White House with his most important ally, Franklin D. Roosevelt. After the war, during the summer of 1949, Churchill visited the South of France to rest and enjoy painting in the French Riviera. While there, he suddenly lost sensation in his right arm and right leg. This incident was handled with a reassuring commentary: "He contracted a chill while bathing." He rapidly recovered and returned to England [60].

In June 1953, at a dinner, Churchill gave a speech, but then couldn't continue discussion and slumped back in his chair; he appeared weak on his left side. The next day, after conducting a Cabinet meeting, he was driven to Chartwell, his country home in Kent. This stroke was consistent with small vessel pathology. This was his second hypertension-related lacunar stroke; the first was in 1949. He did not stay down for long, and in December 1953, he went to Bermuda to meet with President Dwight Eisenhower, who was not aware of Churchill's strokes [61–64].

The news blackout during these tense, Cold War times was maintained. The nation's press barons agreed to keep the secret. Churchill's physician, Lord Moran, his staff, and family also kept hidden other events, including "mini-strokes" he had had in 1950 and 1951. In 1952 a fleeting speech disturbance suggested a spasm or partial occlusion of the artery supplying the speech center of the brain. By then, both the right and left sides of Churchill's brain were affected by atherosclerosis and hypertension [61–64].

Recognizing that he was slowing down both physically and mentally, Churchill retired as prime minister in 1955, but remained in parliament until 1964. After multiple attacks effected certainly by alcohol, cigars, depression (the "black dog"), and the stress of war, on January 15, 1965, at the age of 90 years, the Lion was struck by his last stroke. He died nine days later, and was mourned by millions at a massive state funeral, televised worldwide, to say farewell to the man who may have done more than any other to stop the Nazis [61–64].

CHARLES DICKENS'S STROKE

In 1868, the novelist Charles Dickens, while walking to the house of his friend John Forster, noticed that "he could read only the halves of the letters of the shop doors that were on his right as he looked" [65,66]. He had the same problem again on March 21, 1870, as described by Forster: "He told us that as he came along, walking up the length of Oxford-street, the same incident had recurred as on the day of a former dinner with us, and he had not been able to read, all the way, more than the right-hand halves of the names over the shops." Dickens's friends were amazed at the peculiarity of the symptoms and by Dickens's explanations. These quotes seem to describe a hemianopia or a form of spatial neglect [67].

On April 18, 1869, in the middle of a grueling, albeit lucrative tour of public readings, Dickens fell ill and wrote to his doctor, Frank Beard, who rushed to Dickens, canceled the tour, and brought him back to London, to be seen the next day by Sir Thomas Watson. Watson wrote, "After unusual irritability, [Dickens] found himself, last Saturday or Sunday, giddy, with a tendency to go backwards and to turn round.... He had some odd feeling of insecurity about his leg and did not drag his leg. Also, he spoke of some strangeness of his left hand and arm; missed the spot on which he wished to lay that hand." Watson concluded that Dickens "had been on the brink of an attack of paralysis of his left side, and possibly of apoplexy." These fears were confirmed the next year when, at dinner, Dickens stood and collapsed to his left. Apoplexy was diagnosed and Dickens died the next evening without having regained consciousness. No necropsy took place. Dickens had had signs of heart disease, perhaps precipitated by renal disease, for several years, and in 1866 he was prescribed iron, quinine, and digitalis. Watson also noted signs of cardiac enlargement [68].

Dickens was apparently a regular reader of *The Lancet*, and his novels often described medical conditions. Despite repeated, unpleasant indications of serious disease, Dickens denied his symptoms (anosognosia is a common occurrence after right hemispheric strokes) [69].

FEDERICO FELLINI'S STROKE

Federico Fellini was born on January 20, 1920, in Rimini, in the region of Emilia- Romagna, in Italy. Fellini's output as a filmmaker was vast, having directed a total of 22 films. Notable among these are *La Strada* (1954), *La Dolce Vita* (1960), *8½* (1963), and *Amarcord* (1973). He received countless awards, including four Academy awards for *La Strada* (1956) (including best foreign film) [70].

In Chandler's biography, Fellini is quoted as saying, "Heart trouble and strokes run in my family." These conditions suggest a possible familial dyslipidemia or even hereditary prothrombotic state. In 1993, he went to Switzerland to undergo myocardial revascularization [70].

After the coronary bypass, Fellini went to Rimini to recover in a resort hotel, where he had his first stroke in August 1993 [71,72]. He was 73 years old. He had a sudden-onset neurological deficit with severe left sensory-motor hemiplegia, left inferior quadranopsia, and left spatial neglect. A CT scan performed at Rimini Hospital one week after the stroke showed an extensive area of infarction in the posterior temporoparietal regions of the right cerebral hemisphere. In the follow-up he was confused at night, suggesting a form of spatial delirium. Fellini was then transferred to the San Giorgio Hospital in Ferrara. In an interview with the journalist Charlotte Chandler, he said, "It's terrible when the mind is going as fast as ever, faster, and the body will no longer take orders from it. It's like being trapped in someone else's body. Now I understand I am a missing person. I've lost myself." During the follow-up after his first stroke, Fellini had complete neuropsychological testing by Cantagallo and Della Sala [73]. This evaluation, which was published in 1984, concluded that he had left visuomotor neglect, which persisted for two months, neglect dyslexia, and extrapersonal neglect but preserved insight [74]. During this period, his wife, Giulietta Masina, was diagnosed with metastatic brain tumors due to lung cancer, for which there was no surgical treatment. Fellini's clinical condition worsened rapidly, with swallowing problems and depression. While being prepared for discharge from hospital in October 1993, he had a second major stroke and died on October 31, one day after he and his wife, Giulietta Masina, celebrated their fiftieth wedding anniversary.

EMILIA CLARKE'S STROKE

Game of Thrones star Emilia Clarke had to deal with complications of her brain aneurysms in 2011 and then 2013 [75]. On the morning of February 11, 2011, Clarke was about to work out with her trainer when she "started to feel a bad headache coming on. ... Meanwhile, the pain – shooting, stabbing, constricting pain – was getting worse. At some level, I knew what was happening: my brain was damaged." She was eventually helped to Whittington Hospital in the United Kingdom, where an MRI of her head revealed that she had a subarachnoid hemorrhage. Clarke had emergency surgery to repair the artery [75].

Clarke wrote,

> I remember being told that I should sign a release form for surgery. Brain surgery? I was in the middle of my very busy life – I had no *time* for brain surgery. But, finally, I settled down and signed. And then I was unconscious. For the next three hours, surgeons went about repairing my brain. This would not be my last surgery, and it would not be the worst. I was twenty-four years old. [75]

This first surgery was "minimally invasive," lasting about three hours. Clarke wrote how she managed to get through these two weeks, making good progress. Shortly thereafter, another issue emerged. When she was asked to say her name, she couldn't remember it. Granted her full name is Emilia Isobel Euphemia Rose Clarke, she was aphasic. The aphasia disappeared after about a week. As she described, one month after the surgery, she was able to leave the hospital and soon resume her acting career [75].

One caveat was that the doctors had discovered a smaller aneurysm on the other side of her brain, and it could "pop" at any time. The doctors said that it could remain dormant and harmless indefinitely [75]. Fast forward to 2013, when she had a brain scan in New York City to do a routine check on her other aneurysm, and the doctors, found that the growth on the other side of her brain had doubled in size and that they should "take care of it" [75].

The doctors first tried another minimally invasive procedure to fix the aneurysm to prevent it from bursting. However, when things went awry and she began bleeding inside her head, an emergent open surgery was necessary. The recovery from this was much more intense [75].

She explained that she eventually fully recovered, except possibly that "what it robbed me of is good taste in men." Her experience has inspired her to develop with others a charity called SameYou that provides treatment for people recovering from brain injuries and stroke [75].

NOTES AND REFERENCES

1. Friedlander WJ. About three old men: An inquiry into how cerebral arteriosclerosis has altered world politics. *Stroke* 1972;3:467–473. Available at www.ahajournals.org/doi/abs/10.1161/01.str.3.4.467.

2. Ali R, Connolly ID, Li A, Choudhri OA, Pendharkar AV, Steinberg GK. The strokes that killed Churchill, Roosevelt, and Stalin. *Neurosurg. Focus* 2016 Jul 1;41(1):E7.

3. Meschia J, Safirstein BE, Biller J. Stroke and the American presidency. *J. Stroke Cerebrovasc. Dis.* 1997;6(3):141–143.

4. Profiles of Aphasia: Dwight D. Eisenhower. National Aphasia Association. 2017. Available at www.aphasia.org/stories/aphasia-eisenhower/.

5. Loyola Medicine. Ten U.S. presidents have suffered strokes. Newswise. February 15, 2013. Available at www.newswise.com/coronavirus/ten-u-s-presidents-have-suffered-strokes.

6. Famous people who died of a stroke. On This Day. Available at www.onthisday.com/people/cause-of-death/stroke#google_vignette.

7. Margaret Thatcher (British prime minister). On This Day. Available at www.onthisday.com/people/margaret-thatcher.

8. Yasser Arafat (Palestinian leader). On This Day. Available at www.onthisday.com/people/yasser-arafat.

9. John A. Macdonald (prime minister of Canada). On This Day. Available at www.onthisday.com/people/john-a-macdonald.

10. Alexander Mackenzie (2nd prime minister of Canada). On This Day. Available at www.onthisday.com/people/alexander-mackenzie.

11. Catherine the Great (Empress of Russia). On This Day. Available at www.onthisday.com/people/catherine-the-great.

12. Isambard Kingdom Brunel (engineer). On This Day. Available at www.onthisday .com/people/isambard-kingdom-brunel.

13. Samuel de Champlain (French explorer). On This Day. Available at www.onthisday .com/people/samuel-de-champlain.

14. Shirley Chisholm (1st Black congresswoman). On This Day.com. Available at www .onthisday.com/people/shirley-chisholm.

15. Ariel Sharon. Wikipedia. Available at https://en.wikipedia.org/w/index.php?title= Ariel_Sharon&oldid=995418061.

16. Atal Bihari Vajpayee. Wikipedia. Available at https://en.wikipedia.org/w/index.php? title=Atal_Bihari_Vajpayee&oldid=996555661.

17. Gregory A. William Harvey, English physician. In: *Encyclopædia Britannica*. Available at www.britannica.com/biography/William-Harvey.

18. Marcello Malpighi. Wikipedia. Available at https://en.wikipedia.org/w/index.php? title=Marcello_Malpighi&oldid=996719034.

19. Edward Jenner (physician and scientist). On This Day. Available at www.onthisday .com/people/edward-jenner.

20. Louis Pasteur (bacteriologist). On This Day. Available at www.onthisday.com/people/ louis-pasteur.

21. Elizabeth Blackwell (physician). On This Day. Available at www.onthisday.com/ people/elizabeth-blackwell.

22. Daniel Williams (heart surgeon). On This Day. Available at www.onthisday.com/ people/daniel-williams.

23. Gilman S. Russell N. De Jong, 1907–1990. *Ann. Neurol.* 1991;29(1):108–109.

24. Hauw J-J. In memoriam Dr. Raymond Escourolle (1924–1984). *Acta Neuropathol.* 1984 Jun 1;65(2):89.

25. Neurologist H. Houston Merritt is dead. *JAMA* 1979 Feb 23;241(8):784.

26. Jill Bolte Taylor. Wikipedia. Available at https://en.wikipedia.org/w/index.php? title=Jill_Bolte_Taylor&oldid=998568807.

27. Alexander von Humboldt (naturalist and explorer). On This Day. Available at www .onthisday.com/people/alexander-von-humboldt.

28. John Logie Baird (inventor of television). On This Day. Available at www.onthisday .com/people/john-logie-baird.

29. Dorothy Hodgkin (chemist). On This Day. Available at www.onthisday.com/people/ dorothy-hodgkin.

30. Watts S. *The People's Tycoon: Henry Ford and the American Century.* Random House, 2006.

31. Charles Dickens (novelist). On This Day. Available at www.onthisday.com/people/ charles-dickens. and https://hekint.org/2017/03/04/the-medical-journey-of-charles-dickens/.

32. Anne Morrow Lindbergh (aviator and author). On This Day. Available at www .onthisday.com/people/anne-morrow-lindbergh.

33. Bram Stoker (novelist). On This Day. Available at www.onthisday.com/people/bram-stoker.

34. Louisa May Alcott (author). On This Day. Available at www.onthisday.com/people/ louisa-may-alcott.

35. Edith Wharton (Pulitzer prize–winning novelist). On This Day. Available at www .onthisday.com/people/edith-wharton.

36. Charlie Chaplin (comedian, actor and filmmaker). On This Day. Available at www .onthisday.com/people/charlie-chaplin.

37. Grace Kelly (actress). On This Day. Available at www.onthisday.com/people/grace-kelly.

38. Luke Perry (actor). On This Day. Available at www.onthisday.com/people/luke-perry.

39. Gene Kelly (actor and dancer). On This Day. Available at www.onthisday.com/people/gene-kelly.

40. Akira Kurosawa (film director and screenwriter). On This Day. Available at www.onthisday.com/people/akira-kurosawa.

41. George Cukor (director). On This Day. Available at www.onthisday.com/people/george-cukor.

42. Johann Sebastian Bach. Wikipedia. Available at https://en.wikipedia.org/w/index.php?title=Johann_Sebastian_Bach&oldid=998372010.

43. Felix Mendelssohn (composer and pianist). On This Day. Available at www.onthisday.com/people/felix-mendelssohn.

44. Giuseppe Verdi (composer). On This Day. Available at www.onthisday.com/people/giuseppe-verdi.

45. Sergei Prokofiev. Wikipedia. Available at https://en.wikipedia.org/w/index.php?title=Sergei_Prokofiev&oldid=999020472.

46. Thelonius Monk. Biography.com. Available at www.biography.com/musician/thelonious-monk.

46. Ben Hogan (golfer). On This Day. Available at www.onthisday.com/people/ben-hogan.

47. Kirby Puckett (MLB center fielder). On This Day. Available at www.onthisday.com/people/kirby-puckett.

48. Sam Snead (golfer). On This Day. Available at www.onthisday.com/people/sam-snead.

49. Bill Sharman (NBA guard). On This Day. Available at www.onthisday.com/people/bill-sharman.

50. Raymond van Schoor. Wikipedia. Available at https://en.wikipedia.org/w/index.php?title=Raymond_van_Schoor&oldid=984934224.

51. Lerner V, Finkelstein Y, Witztum E. The enigma of Lenin's (1870–1924) malady. *Eur. J. Neurol.* 2004;6:371–376.

52. Kaplan G P, Petrikovsky B M. Advanced cerebrovascular disease and the death of Vladimir Ilyich Lenin. *Neurology* 1992;1:241–245.

53. Vinters H, Lurie L, Mackowiak PA. Vessels of stone: Lenin's "circulatory disturbance of the brain." *Hum Pathol.* 2013;10:1967–1972.

54. St Hilaire C, Ziegler SG, Markello TC, Brusco A, Groden C, et al. NT5E mutations and arterial calcifications. *N. Engl. J. Med.* 2011;364:432–442.

55. Kaplan GP, Petrikovsky BM. Advanced cerebrovascular disease and the death of Vladimir Ilyich Lenin. *Neurology* 1992;42(1):241–245.

56. Wilson embarks on tour to promote League of Nations. History.com. Available at www.history.com/this-day-in-history/wilson-embarks-on-tour-to-promote-league-of-nations.

57. American Presidents: Woodrow Wilson 28th US President. YouTube. Available at www.youtube.com/watch?v=2wsrF6SsIoU.

58. Striner R. The surprising evidence that Woodrow Wilson was suffering from a brain malfunction before the stroke that crippled him. History News Network. Available at http://historynewsnetwork.org/article/155787.

59. Markel H. When a secret president ran the country. PBS NewsHour. 2015. Available at www.pbs.org/newshour/health/woodrow-wilson-stroke.

60. Scadding JW, Vale JA. Winston Churchill's acute stroke in June 1953. *J. R. Soc. Med.* 2018;10:347–358.

61. Scadding JW, Vale JA. Winston Churchill: His first stroke in 1949. *R. Soc Med.* 2018;9:316–323.

62. Werring DJ. Winston Churchill's cerebrovascular disease: Small vessels with big implications. *J. R. Soc. Med.* 2018;9:314–315.

63. Scadding JW, Vale JA. Winston Churchill: Acute ataxic stroke in June 1955 with excellent recovery. *J. R. Soc. Med.* 2019;6:226–235.

64. Scadding JW, Vale JA. Winston Churchill: Two mild left hemisphere strokes, finger gangrene and syncope in 1959. *R. Soc. Med.* 2019;7:278–291.

65. McManus IC. Charles Dickens: A neglected diagnosis. *Lancet* 2001 Dec 22–29;358 (9299):2158–2161.

66. Forster J. *The Life of Charles Dickens*, edited by JWT Ley. London: Cecil Palmer, 1928.

67. Ellis AW, Young AW, Flude BM. Neglect and visual language. In Robertson IH, Marshall JC (eds.), *Unilateral Neglect: Clinical and Experimental Studies*. Hove: Lawrence Erlbaum Associates, 1993, pp. 233–255.

68. Bowen WH. *Charles Dickens and His Family*. Cambridge: W. Heffer and Sons, 1956.

69. Parkin AJ. *Explorations in Cognitive Neuropsychology*. Hove: Psychology Press, 1996.

70. Chandler C. *I Fellini*. New York: Cooper Square Press, 1995.

71. Dike CC, Baranoski M, Griffith EEH. Pathological lying revisited. *J. Am. Acad. Psychiatry Law* 2005;33:342–349.

72. Chiu HC. Neurology of the arts. *Acta Neurol. Taiwan* 2009;18:132–136.

73. Cantagallo A, Della Sala S. Preserved insight in an artist with extrapersonal spatial neglect. *Cortex* 1998;34:163–189.

74. Dieguez S, Assal G, Bogousslavsky J. Visconti and Fellini: From left social neorealism to right-hemisphere stroke. In Bogousslavsky J, Hennerici MG (eds.), *Neurological Disorders in Famous Artists – Part 2*. Front. Neurol. Neurosci. Basel: Karger 2007, 22:44–74.

75. Clarke E. A battle for my life. *The New Yorker*. March 21, 2019.

INDEX

Aaslid, Rune, 330–332
ABCD2 score, 359–361
Abciximab in Emergent Stroke Treatment Trial II
    (AbESTT-II), 461–462
Abercrombie, John, 48–49, 52, 142–144, 175
Abernathy, John, 529–530
Abu Ali Al-Hossein Ibn Sina (Avicenna), 10–11
    on stroke, 14–16
Abu Bakr Muhammed Ibn Zakria AlRazi (Rhazes),
    11–12, 14–15
Ackerman, Robert Harold, 347, 479–481
actors and directors, stroke in, 614
acute chest syndrome, 220–221
acute neonatal stroke, 383
acute stroke-ready hospitals, 393–394
Adamkiewicz, Albert Wojciech, 85–86, 240
Adams, Francis, 8
Adams, John Quincy, 611–612
Adams, Raymond
    on basilar artery occlusion, 129–130
    Caplan and, 283–285
    Princeton Conferences and, 413–414
    on stroke and coma, 269–270, 399
    on transient ischemic attacks, 131–132
Adams, Robert J., 332–333
Addison, Thomas, 58
Aesculapius, 3–4
agraphia, early research on, 76–78
Aicardi, Jean François Marie, 380–381, 383
Akbar Mahomed, Frederick, 465–467
Alajouanine, T., 241–242
à la poupée technique, 56
Alauddin Abu al Hassan Ali ibn Hazmi (Ibn
    AlNafis), 12–13
Albers, Greg, 554–555
Alberta Stroke Program Early CT Score
    (ASPECTS), 309–311
Albucasis. See AlZahrawi, AlQasim Khalaf Ibn
    AlAbbas (Albucasis)
Alcott, Louisa May, 614
alexia, early research on, 76–78
alirocumab, 475
alkaptonuria, 212
Allyn, William, 226
alteplase, 496–497

AlZahrawi, AlQasim Khalaf Ibn AlAbbas
    (Albucasis), 12–13, 15–16
Alzheimer, Alois, 122–124
Amarenco, Pierre, 356, 359–361, 475
American Society of Neuroimaging, 333–334
Aminoff, Michael, 244
AMPA antagonists, excitotoxicity and channel
    blockers, 483
Anatomical Plates of the Bones and Muscles Reduced from
    Albinus, for the Use of Students in Anatomy, and
    Artists (Hooper), 56–57
anatomical research
    by Bright, 58–59
    by Carswell, 57–61
    by Cruveilhier, 45, 59
    early history of, 22–24
    Foix's contributions to, 251–258
    history of, 55–57
    by Hooper, 56–57
    print technology and, 56
Anatomie des centres nerveux (Dejerine-Klumpke), 73
Anatomie pathologique du corps humain (Cruveilhier),
    376–381
Ancient Greece
    medical culture in, 3–4
    particulate theory in, 211
Anderson, Carl, 340–341
Anderson, Craig, 582
Anderson, William, 221–222
Andrew, Maureen, 384–385
aneurysms. See intracerebral aneurysm (ICA);
    subarachnoid hemorrhage (SAH)
angioplasty
    carotid artery, 537–538, 541–546
    intracranial arteries, 546–549
Angrist, A., 134–135
animal rights movement, neurorehabilitation and,
    519–522
anterior cerebral artery (ACA)
    Foix's research on, 254–255
    Moyamoya syndrome and disease, 193–196
anterior choroidal artery (AChA)
    anatomy, 84–90
    Foix's research on, 255–257
anti-apoptotic agents, 481–482

anticoagulants. *See also specific drugs, e.g.*, heparin
    clinical trials involving, 415, 421–422
    direct oral anticoagulants, 442–446
    intracerebral hemorrhage and reversal of,
        583–584
    transient ischemic attacks and, 131–132
Antiphospholipid Antibodies and Stroke Study
        (APASS), 207
antiphospholipid antibodies and syndrome,
        206–207
antiplatelet therapy
    glycoprotein IIb/IIIa antagonists, 461–462
    intracerebral hemorrhage and reversal of,
        583–584
    overview of, 455–462
    phosphodiesterase inhibitors, 456–458
    thienopyridines, 458–461
Antiplatelet Trialist's Collaborative, 418–419
antithrombotics
    clinical trials of, 413
    heparin and, 431–432
aorta
    border zones, spinal cord ischemia and, 242–243
    spinal cord ischemia and, 240–242
The Aphorisms of Hippocrates, 3–4
apixaban, 444–445
apoplexy
    Areteus of Cappadocia on, 7–8
    in children, 374–375
    defined, 358
    early writings about, 14, 157–158
    Hippocrates's description of, 4–5
    history of research on, 42–53
    Morgagni's description of, 38–40
    Paul of Aegenia on, 8
Arafat, Yasser, 612
*Archiv für pathologische Anatomie und Physiologie und
        für klinische Medizin* (*Archives of Pathological
        Anatomy and Physiology and of Clinical Medicine*),
        95
ARCOS (Auckland Regional Community Stroke
        Study), 366
Areteus of Cappadocia, 7–8
Aring, Charles D., 261, 263–264
Aristotle, 211
    on stroke, 14
ARISTOTLE trial, 444–445
Arneson, Barry, 287
arterial dissection, 188–192
arterial systems and arteries. *See also specific arteries*
    anatomy, 84–87
    artery of Adamkiewicz, 85–86
    artery of Bernasconi and Cassinari, 87
    artery of Percheron, 86–87
arterial tortuosity syndrome, 222–223
arteriosclerosis
    Osler's work on, 100–101
    Virchow's research on, 96–97

arteriovenous malformations, 167–169. *See also*
        cavernous malformations (cavernomas)
    carotid cavernous fistulas, 599–601
    Cushing on, 591–593
    Dandy on, 591–593
    developmental venous anomalies, 599
    early recognition and treatment, 590–591
    Olivecrona's work in, 593–595
    spinal cord infarction and arteriovenous fistulas,
        243–244
    surgical management of, 591–593, 597
    twentieth-century research on, 595–598
arteritis, early research on, 84–85
Arthur, Chester, 611–612
artificial radioactivity, positron emission
        tomography (PET) and, 340–341
aspirin
    anticoagulants vs., 439–440
    Antiplatelet Trialist's Collaborative, 418–419
    cilostazole and, 457–458
    clinical trials and controversy over, 415–418
    clopidogrel (Plavix) vs., 459–460
    clotting prevention by, 449
    dipyridamole and, 455–457
    hemostasis and, 202–203
    and myocardial infarction, 449
    as preventive for thrombosis, heart attack, and
        stroke, 447–453
    production of, 449–450
    stroke prevention and, 452–453
    TIAs and, 131–132
Asplund, Kjell, 365–366
Asymptomatic Carotid Atherosclerosis (ACAS) trial,
        332–333, 536–537
Asymptomatic Carotid Surgery Trial (ACST), 537
ATACH (Antihypertensive Treatment of Acute
        Cerebral Hemorrhage) trial, 582
atherosclerosis, blood lipids and, 471–475
Atherosclerosis Risk in Communities (ARIC)
        study, 365–369
atrial fibrillation
    anticoagulants and, 421–422, 437–438, 444–445
    brain embolism and, 274
    electrocardiography and, 354
Auer, Ludwig, 404
authors, stroke in, 614
Averroes. *See* Ibn Ahmad Ibn Rushd, Mohammed
        (Averroes)
Avery, Oswald Theodore, 213
Avicenna. *See* Abu Ali Al-Hossein Ibn Sina
        (Avicenna)

Babinski, Joseph Jules Francois Félix, 67–68, 75, 299
Babinski-Nageott syndrome, 67–68, 75, 127–128
Bach, Johann Sebastian, 615
Bacon, Francis, 26, 38
Bailey, Percival, 167–169
Baird, John Logie, 613

Baker, A. B., 397
Baker, Donald, 328–329
Balance, Charles, 590–591
Banker, Betty, 376–380
Banks, Gordon, 287
Banting, Fredrick G., 318, 469–470
Barber, Philip, 309
Barinagarrementeria, Fernando, 180–181, 183–185
Barnard, Robin, 244
Barnett, Henry Joseph Macaulay, 416–417,
    422–423, 533–534
Baron, Jean-Claude, 347–348, 479–481
Barritt, D. W., 437–438
Barrows, Lawrence, 438
Barsan, Bill, 496–497
Basch, Samuel Siegfried Karl Ritter, 465–467
basilar artery occlusion, 129–132
    fibrinolytic infusion, 551–552
    warfarin and, 439
Bastian, Henry Charlton, 239
Bateson, William, 212
Batjer, H. H., 595
Bayer company, 449–450
Bayle, Francois, 44, 109
Beach, Kirk, 331
Beatles, computed tomography and, 305 308
Beck, Claude, 398
Becker, D. P., 400–401
Beecher, Henry, 397, 399
Beevor, Charles Edward, 82–83
Beevor's sign, 83
Benedikt, Moritz, 69–70
Benedikt syndrome, 127–128
Berg, Paul, 213–214
Bernasconi, Vittorio Luigi, 87
Bertina, Roger, 203–204
Bertrand, Ivan, 252
Best, Charles H., 318, 429–430, 469–470
beta-blockers, 467
Bierman, William, 516
Bigelow, W. G., 485–487
Billau, Alfons, 494–495
Binswanger, Otto, 122–124
Binswanger disease, 122–124, 216–218
Biumi, Francesco, 144, 562–563
Bizzozero, Giulio, 202
Black, James, 467
Blackwell, Elizabeth, 612–613
Blane, Gilbert, 144
Bleich, Howard, 285
Bloch, Felix, 313
Bloch, Konrad, 471–472
blood disorders
    antiphospholipid antibodies and syndrome,
        206–207
    brain hemorrhage with, 208
    clinical research on, 201–203
    early studies, 200–201

factor V Leiden, 203–204
    hyperhomocysteinemia, 205–206
    inherited thrombophilias, 203
    prothrombin gene mutation, 204
blood-letting, practice of, 25–26
blood lipids, 471–472
blood pressure
    intracerebral hemorrhage and control of, 582
    stroke and, 465–467
Boehinger-Ingelheim Pharmaceuticals, 456–457
Bond, J. P., 355–356
Bonetus, Theophilus, 38
Bonita, Ruth, 366
Booth, Edwin, 614
border-zone ischemia, 112–113
Borel, Cecil, 402–404
Born, Gustav Victor Rudolf, 455–457
Botticelli, Sandro, 22
Bottomley, Paul, 319–320
Bouchard, Charles, 158–159
Bousser, Marie-Germaine, 179, 183–185, 216–218,
    508–509
Boyle, Robert, 32–33
Boyle's law, 32–33
brachial plexus palsy, 73–74
brain, anatomy and vasculature of, 31 36
Brain, Russel (Lord), 102
Brain Attack Coalition (BAC), 393–394
brain function, PET imaging studies, 347–348
brain injury, diagnosis and management,
        neurocritical care and, 399–405
brainstem. See also specific conditions, e.g., lateral
        medullary infarction
    early research on, 45–46, 75–79
    Foix's research on, 253–254
    posterior circulation research, 127–128
    vasculature, 87
brain-time continuum, 479–481
brain tumors, early research on, 60–61
Bramwell, Byrom, 240–242
BRAVO trial, glycoprotein IIb/IIIa antagonists, 462
Bright, Richard, 58–59, 99–101, 142–144, 465–467
Bright, William, 144
Bright's disease, 58
Brink, R. A., 435–436
Brissaud, Édouard, 251
British Doctors Study, 366
Broderick, Joe, 163, 372, 422, 496–497
Brooks, Barney, 570
Brott, Tom, 163, 372, 422–423, 496–497, 545–546
Brown, Michael S., 472–475
Brownell, Gordon, 344–345
Brozovic, Milica, 430–431
Bruce, A. N., 101–103
Bruckmann, Helmet, 495–496
Brunel, Isambard Kingdom, 612
Buchan, Alastair, 309, 479–481
Buchner, Johann Andreas, 448

Budd-Chiari syndrome, 110
Bumke, O., 103
Burrows, Gregory, 49–50

Cairns, Hugh, 534
calcium channel blockers
    excitotoxicity and, 482–483
    subarachnoid hemorrhage, 148–149
Call, Greg, 196–197
Call-Fleming syndrome, 196–197
Canadian Cooperative Study Group trial, 416
Canadian Pediatric Ischemic Stroke Registry,
    182–183, 384–385
Candelise, Livia, 420–421
candidate gene studies, stroke genetics and, 214–215
The Canon of Medicine (al-Qanun fi'l tibb) (Avicenna),
    10–11, 15–16
Cantu, Carlos., 180–181
Caplan, Louis R.
    carotid artery disease research and, 115–116
    Harvard Cooperative Stroke Registry and, 371
    lacunar infarct research and, 121–124, 271–272
    life and work of, 280–290
    thrombolytic therapy research and, 495–496
    vascular imaging and, 497–500
cardiac computed tomography, 356
cardiac magnetic resonance imaging, 356
cardiopulmonary disease
    subarachnoid hemorrhage and, 149–150
    thrombolytic therapy and, 492–493
cardiopulmonary resuscitation, neurocritical care
    and, 398
cardiovascular disease
    anticoagulant therapy and, 437–438
    blood liipids and, 471–475
    hypertension and, 466–467
    imaging and function, 352–356
    intensive care units and mortality reduction in,
        398–399
CARESS trial, 332–333
"carotico-vertebral" stenosis, 129–130
carotid angiography, 570–571
carotid artery disease
    acute carotid stroke mechanisms, 114–115
    arterial dissection, 189–190
    chronic eye ischemia, 232–233
    diagnosis of, 530
    Fisher's research on, 269, 273
    hemodynamic vs. embolic mechanisms, 113–114
    historical research on, 109–113
    mid-twentieth-century research on, 111–113
    pulse palpation and auscultation, 115–116
    stenosing and nonstenosing lesions,
        116–117
    surgical management of, 529–538
    Wepfer's research on, 43
carotid artery surgery
    asymptomatic patients, 536–537

early history of, 529–533
    endarterectomy vs. stenting, 537–538
    intracranial aneurysms, 564
    ligature and clamping, 564–565
    recent developments in, 533–534
    severity of stenosis and, 534–536
carotid bruit, early descriptions of, 65
carotid cavernous fistula, 530, 599–601
Carotid Revascularization Endarterectomy versus
    Stenting Trial (CREST), 537–538, 545–546
Carrea, Raul, 531
Carswell, Robert, 56–61
Case Histories (Rufus of Ephesus), 7
Cas9 (CRISPR-associated protein 9), 214
Casserio, 34
Cassinari, Valentino, 87
catastrophic antiphospholipid syndrome (CAPS),
    207
Catherine the Great, 612
CAVATAS stent trial, 545
cavernous malformations (cavernomas), 169–170
    carotid cavernous fistula, 530
    research on, 598–599
    spinal cord infarction and, 245–246
cellular intervention, neuroprotection and, 484–485
cellular targets, neuroprotective interventions,
    481–482
Celsus, Aurelius Cornelius, 6
cerebellar hemorrhage, 134–135
cerebral amyloid angiopathy (CAA), 151–152,
    163–164
    genetics, 223
cerebral anemia, 102–103
cerebral angiography (CA)
    arterial dissection, 190
    carotid artery imaging, 530
    cerebral vein and dural sinus thrombosis,
        177–179
    early developments in, 110–111
    fibromuscular dysplasia, 192–193
    pediatric stroke and, 380–385
    subarachnoid hemorrhage, 144–145
cerebral autosomal dominant arteriopathy with
    subcortical infarct and leukoencephalopathy
    (CADASIL), 124, 216–218, 508–509
cerebral autosomal recessive arteriopathy with
    subcortical infarct and leukoencephalopathy
    (CARASIL), 124, 218–219
cerebral blood flow (CBF)
    energy metabolism and, 342–344
    Harvey's discovery of, 25–29
    imaging studies, 338–349
    neuroprotection and improvement of, 484–485
    physiology of, 338–340
    posterior circulation research, 127–128
    spinal cord infarction and, 240
cerebral embolism, Virchow's research on, 96–97
cerebral glucose utilization, PET research and, 344

cerebral hemorrhage
    Aring and Merritt's research on, 263
    Fisher's research on, 272–273
cerebral hyperemia, 102–103
cerebral leukodystrophy, 219–220
cerebral vein and dural sinus thrombosis (CVDST),
        174–185
    cerebral angiography, 177–179
    computed tomography, 179
    diagnosis, 176–177
    early research on, 175–176
    imaging studies, 181–182
    ISCVT study on, 183–185
    recent research on, 182–183
Cerebral Venous Sinus Thrombosis Study Group,
        182–183
cerebral venous thrombosis
    anticoagulant therapy for, 437–438
    blood disorders and, 200–201
    in children, 378–385
    decompressive hemicraniectomy, 511
    direct oral anticoagulant therapy, 511–512
    factor V Leiden, 203–204
    heparin in management of, 429–430, 506–509
    low-molecular-weight vs. unfractionated
        heparin, 510
    prothrombin gene mutation, 204
    thrombolytic and endovascular treatment,
        510–511
    treatment of, 505–512
Cerebri anatome cui accessit nervorum descriptio et usus
    (The Anatomy of the Brain and Nerves), 34
cerebrovascular accident (CVA), defined, 359
cerebrovascular disease
    cardiac imaging and function and, 352–356
    in children, 380–385
    eye involvement in, 234–235
    PET imaging studies, 347–348
    Princeton Conferences and classification of, 414
    spinal cord infarction and, 238–246
    thrombolytic therapy in, 495–496
    visual loss and, 226–235, 268–269
cervical artery dissection, 273–275
CGS19755 NMDA antagonist, 482–483
Chabriat, Hugues, 218
Champlain, Samuel de, 612
CHANCE trial (clopidogrel and aspirin), 459–460
channel targets, neuroprotection and, 482–483
Chao, W. H., 530
Chaplin, Charlie, 614
Charcot, Jean-Martin, 74–75, 81–82, 119
    on intracerebral hemorrhage, 158–159
    textbooks by, 103
Chargaff, Erwin, 213, 430
Charles, Arthur F., 429
Charpentier, Emmanuelle, 214
Cheyne, John, 46–47, 133, 142–144, 158–159
Chiari, Hans, 110, 530

Chiari malformations, 110
childhood hemiplegia, 380–385. See also pediatric
    stroke
Childs, T., 134–135
Chimowitz, Mark, 421–424, 547–549
Chinese Acute Stroke Trial (CAST), 419
Chisholm, Shirley, 612
cholesterol
    atherosclerosis and, 471–472
    lipoprotein metabollism and, 472
    statins and reduction of, 475
chronic adhesive arachnoiditis, spinal cord infarction
        and, 245–246
chronic eye ischemia, 232–233
Chung, C.-S., 135–136
Chung, M.-F., 239–240
Churchill, Winston, 611–623
cilostazole, 457–458
Circle of Willis, 34
circulation of blood
    cerebral blood flow imaging, 338–349
    Harvey's discovery of, 25–29
    posterior circulation research, 127–128
    spinal cord infarction and, 240
Clarke, Emilia, 622–623
Claude syndrome, 127–128
clinical trials in stroke research. See also specific trials
    anticoagulant trials, 415, 421–422
    antiplatelet collaborative trials, 418–419
    aspirin trials, 415–418, 452–453
    evidence-based medicine and, 420–421
    heparin trials, 415, 429–430
    intracranial intervention procedures, 423–424
    neuroprotection trial protocols, 484–485
    overview of, 413–424
    Princeton conferences, 413–414
    surgical trials, 422–423
    thrombolytic trials, 422
    warfarin trials, 438–440
clopidogrel (Plavix), 459–460
Clopidogrel and Aspirin versus Aspirin Alone for
        the Prevention of Atherothrombotic Events
        (CHARISMA) trial, 459–460
Clopidogrel versus Aspirin in Patients at Risk of
        Ischemic Events (CAPRIE) trial, 459–460
Clot Lysis Evaluation of Accelerated Resolution of
        Intraventricular Hemorrhage (CLEAR-III)
        trial, 403
CLOTBUST trial, 332–333
clotting. See also blood disorders
    animal studies of, 435–436
    antiplatelet therapy, 455–462
    aspirin's inhibition of, 449
    clinical research on, 201–203
    early research on, 45, 95–96, 200–201
coagulation
    animal studies of, 435–436
    clinical research on, 201–203

coarctation of aorta, spinal cord lesions, 241–242
Cochrane, Archie, 420–421
Cochrane Stroke Group, 420–421
Coga, Arthur, 33
Cogswell, Mason, 563
Cohn, Alfred, 353
Colbert, Claudette, 614
Cole, F., 162
Cole, William, 44–45, 358–359
collagen 4A1 (COL4A1) syndrome, 220
collateral circulation
    carotid artery disease, 111–115
    early research on, 34
Collen, Désiré, 493–495
Coller, Barry Spencer, 461–462
Collins, Francis S., 214
Collip, James B., 318, 469–470
coma, stroke and, 271
    diagnosis and management, neurocritical care
        and, 399–405
comprehensive stroke center (CSC), 393–394
Compston, Alistaire, 83
computed tomography (CT)
    brain injury assessment and, 399–401
    cardiac CT, 356
    cerebral vein and dural sinus thrombosis,
        177–179, 181–182
    EMI Mark I development, 307–308
    evolution of, 308–309
    history of, 304–311
    intracerebral hemorrhage, 163
    subarachnoid hemorrhage, 144–145
computed tomography angiography (CTA),
        132–137, 302–303
    arterial dissection, 190
    development of, 309–311
Conley, John, 530
connective tissue, inherited disorders of, 222–223
Connors, Buddy 547
constraint-induced movement therapy (CIMT),
        519–522
Cooke, John, 47–48
COOLAID trial, 485–487
Cooley, Denton, 532–533
Cooper, Astley, 58, 238–239, 529–530, 563
Cooperative Clinical Study of Anticoagulant
        Therapy in Cerebral Thromboses and
        Transient Ischemic Attacks, 415
Cooperative Study of Intracranial Aneurysms and
        Subarachnoid Hemorrhage, 168–169, 595
Cope, Freeman Winder, 313–316
Cormack, Allan M., 305–308
corticosteroid therapy, intracerebral hemorrhage,
        577–578
Coulter, John S., 516
coumadin, synthesis of, 437–438, 442–446
coumarin, isolation and synthesis, 436–437
Courville, Cyril, 379–380

Crafoord, Clarence, 429–430
craniotomy
    arteriorvenous malformations, 590–591
    intracerebral hemorrhage, 579–580
Craven, Lawrence L., 449
Crawford, Broderick, 614
Crick, Francis, 213
CRISPER (clustered regularly interspaced short
        palindromic repeats), 214
Crompton, M. R., 147–149
Crowell, Robert, 348
Cruveilhier, Jean, 45, 56, 59, 94–96, 120, 176–177,
        376–381
Cukor, George, 614
cupping, practice of, 26
Curie, Marie, 340–341, 355–356
Curie, Pierre, 340–341, 355–356
Cushing, Harvey, 60–61, 138–142, 167–169, 564,
        566, 591–593
Cushing-McKenzie clip, 566–569
cyclic guanosine monophosphates (cGMP), vascular
        pathology and, 456–457

dabigatran etexilate, 443–445
Dahlbäck, B., 203–204
Dalsgaard-Nielsen, T., 370
Dalziel, John, 397
Damadian, Raymond, 313–318
Dana, Charles Loomis, 103, 133, 159
Dandy, Walter, 167–169, 298–299, 304–305, 397,
        566–568, 591–593, 595–599
Darwin, Charles, 212
data banks and registries of stroke research, 370–372
Davalos, A., 497
Davis, Steve, 422, 493, 497
Dawber, Thomas, 364–365
Deaver, George, 518
DeBakey, Michael, 532–533
Debrun, Gerard, 600–601
Dechambre, Amedée, 120
decompressive hemicraniectomy, 400–401
    arteriovenous malformations, 590–591
    cerebral venous thrombosis, 511
    intracerebral hemorrhage, 584–585
    for malignant hemispheric stroke, 404
deferoxamine, intracerebral hemorrhage
        management, 578
defibrillation, neurocritical care and, 398
A Definition of Irreversible Coma (Adams, Schwab,
        Denny-Brown, and Beecher), 399
De humani corporis fabrica (Vesalius), 22–24
Dejerine, Jules Joseph, 72–79, 239–240
Dejerine-Klumpke's paralysis, 73–74
Dejerine-Roussy syndrome, 74–76
Dejerine-Sottas disease, 74–75
Dejerine-Thomas olivopontocerebellar atrophy,
        74–75
Dejong, Russell, 612–613

delayed cerebral infarction (DCI), 147–149

Del Zoppo, Greg, 401–402, 495–496

Demchuk, Andrew, 309

De medicina (Celsus), 6

Denier, André, 355–356

Dennis, Martin, 420–421

Denny-Brown, Derek, 132, 283–285, 399

2-deoxyglucose (DG), PET research and, 344

Derdeyn, Colin, 423–424, 547–549

Derouesné, Christian, 120–121

De sedibus et causis morborum per anatomen indagatis (Morgagni), 38–40, 55

DESTINY trial, 404

DeVeber, Gabrielle, 182–183, 383–384

developmental venous anomalies (DVAs), 170–171, 599

De Vries, Linda, 384

DeWitt, Dana, 288

DeWood, Marcus, 493

diabetes
    Areteus of Cappadocia on, 7–8
    early research, 467–469
    insulin and, 469–470
    Osler's work on, 100
    stroke and, 467–471

Diagnosis of Stupor and Coma (Plum and Posner), 399

diaschisis theory, 347–348

Di Chiro, Giovanni, 243–244

Dickens, Charles, 614, 620–621

Die Infantile Cerebrallähmung (Infantile Cerebral Paralysis) (Freud), 378

Diemer, N. H., 479–481

diffusion-weighted imaging (DWI), 320–322

Diggs, Lemuel, 220–221

digital subtraction angiography (DSA), 145, 302–303

dipyridamole, 456–457

direct oral anticoagulants (DOACs), 442–446, 511–512
    intracerebral hemorrhage and reversal of hematoma expansion, 583–584

disconnection syndrome, early research on, 76–78

Diseases of the Brain and Nervous System Together with a Concise Statement of the Diseased Appearance of the Brain and Its Membranes (Bright), 58

Diseases of the Spinal Cord (Bramwell), 240–242

diving medicine, ultrasound research and, 327

DNA, genetics research and, 213

"doctrine of signatures," 447–449

Doidge, Norman, 520–521

Doll, Richard, 534

Donaghy, Raymond M. P., 569–570

Donnan, Geoffrey, 422, 493, 497

dopaminergic agents, stroke rehabilitation, 525

Doppler, Christian Andreas, 325–326

Doppler effect, 325–326
    echocardiography and, 355–356

Doppman, J. L., 243–244

Dos Santos, Cid, 531

Dott, Norman, 565–566

Doudna, Jennifer, 214

Douglas, Stuard, 420–421

Drake, George Charles, 416–417, 534, 568–569

Dreser, Heinrich, 449–450

Drinker, Philip, 397

Dupuytren, Guillaume, 59

dural arteriovenous fistulas (DAVFs), 151–152, 171

dural venus sinus thrombosis, warfarin and, 440

Durand-Fardel, Maxime, 120

Duret, Henri, 65, 81–82, 129

Duret hemorrhages, 81–82, 133–134

Dussik, Friedrich, 326

Dussik, Karl Theodore, 326

Dutrochet, René, 211

Duvernoy, Henry M., 87

Duvernoy, Maurice, 87

DWI or CTP Assessment with Clinical Mismatch in the Triage of Wake-Up and Late Presenting Strokes Undergoing Neurointervention with Trevo (DAWN) trial, 557–558

Eastcott, H., 531

Easton, J. Donald, 421–422

Ebers Papyrus, 447, 562–563

echocardiography, 355–356

edaravone, 483–484

Edelman, Robert, 321

Edinburgh stroke group, 420–421

Edison, Thomas, 304

Edler, Inge, 355–356

edoxaban, 444–445

Ehlers, Hertha, 379–380

Eichengrün, Arthur, 449–450

Einhäupl, Karl Max, 179, 183–185, 507, 509

Einthoven, Willem, 353

Eisenhower, Dwight D., 437–438, 612

electrocardiography, development of, 353–354

electroencephalography, 598–599
    early research in, 327

electrolyte abnormalities, subarachnoid hemorrhage, 149–150

electrothrombosis, 573–574

Eloy, Fernand, 458–459

embolism
    anticoagulant therapy for, 437–438
    atrial fibrillation and, 274
    blood disorders and, 200–201
    carotid artery disease and, 111–114
    early research on, 50–51, 65–66
    embolic device filters, 544
    heparin efficacy in, 431–432
    Osler's work on, 100–101
    placental, 380–385
    strokes and, 114–115
    ultrasound detection of, 327
    Virchow's research on, 96–97

emergency medicine, stroke management and, 497–500
EMI Mark I CT, 307–308
encephalitis subcorticalis chronica progressive (ESCP), 122–124
Endo, Akira, 472–475
endocrine abnormalities, subarachnoid hemorrhage, 149–150
endovascular therapy (EVT)
    cerebral venous thrombosis and, 510–511
    early history, 551–552
    evolution of, 553–554
    intracerebral aneurysm, 570–574
    ischemic stroke, 551–558
    mechanical thrombectomy, 555–558
    randomized controlled trials involving, 552–553
    stent retrieval, 554–555
    treatment time window expansion, 557–558
Endovascular Treatment for Small Core and Anterior Circulation Proximal Occlusion with Emphasis on Minimizing CT to Recanalization Times (ESCAPE) trial, 556–557
energy metabolism, cerebral blood flow and, 342–344
ENGAGE trial, 444–445
Ensor, Frederick, 449
epidemiology of stroke, 364–367
    early research on, 51–53
epidural hemorrhage, early research on, 49
EQUATOR website, 420–421
Erichsen, John E., 240
Escourolle, Raymond, 612–613
ESCPE NA-1 trial, 484–485
European Carotid Surgery Trial (ECST), 535
European Cooperative Acute Stroke (ECASS) trials, 308–309, 422
    thrombolytic therapies, 497
European Society of Neurosonology and Cerebral Hemodynamics (ESNCH), 333–334
European Stroke Prevention Studies (ESPS-1 and ESPS-2), 418, 457
Evelyn, Kenneth, 266
evidence-based medicine, 420–421
evolocumab, 475
evolution, genetics and, 212
excitotoxicity, neuroprotection and, 482–483
Experiments in Plant Hybridization (Mendel), 212
"Experiments upon the Blood and Lymph of the Terrapin, and the Origin of the Fibrin Formed in the Coagulation of the Blood" (Howell), 427–429
Extending the Time for Thrombolysis in Emergency Neurological Deficits with Intra-Arterial Therapy (EXTEND-IA) trial, 556–557
extracranial cervical vertebral arteries (ECVAs), 190
extracranial to intracranial artery bypass (EC-IC bypass), 569–570

eye, cerebrovascular disease and. *See also* visual loss, vascular disease and
    chronic eye ischemia, 232–233
    early research, 226
    Fisher and Hollenhorst's research on, 228–230, 268–269, 275–276
    giant cell arteritis, 234–235
    Gowers's research on, 226–229
    ischemic optic neuropathy, 234–235
    retinal vascular spasm, 233–234
    Russell's research on, 230–232

Fabricius, Johannes, 38, 42
Fabry, Johannes, 221–222
Fabry's disease, 221–222
factor VIII, 202–203
factor V Leiden disease, 203–204
factor Xa, new oral anticoagulants (NOACs) and, 443–445
Fallopius, Gabriel, 34, 38
familial hypercholesterolemia, 473–474
family history, genetics, 150–151
Fang, Henry, 414, 438
al-Farabi, 10–11
Fay, Temple, 401
Feigin, Valery, 367
Feldman, R. L., 547
Fellini, Federico, 614, 621–622
Ferbert, Andreas, 495–496
Ferguson, Robert, 541–542
Ferrand, J., 119–120
Ferriero, Donna, 384
Ferro, José, 182–185, 509
fetal circulation, pediatric stroke and, 376–380
fibrin, 201–203, 491
fibrinogen, 200–201, 491
fibrinolytic infusion, 551–552
fibromuscular dysplasia (FMD), 192–193
Fields, William Straus, 266, 272–275, 416–417, 532–533
Fieschi, Cesare, 422, 497
Fillmore, Millard, 611–612
Fisher, C. Miller
    anticoagulant trials and, 415
    on arterial dissection, 189–190
    on basilar artery occlusion, 129–130
    Caplan and, 283–285, 288
    carotid artery disease research, 109, 111–113, 115–117, 530
    on cerebellar hemorrhage, 134–135
    on coma, 399
    on delayed cerebral infarction and vasoconstriction, 147–149
    early research by, 36
    Foix compared with, 258
    on hypertension and intracerebral hemorrhage, 160–162
    lacunar infarct research by, 120–121

life and career of, 265–276
Princeton Conferences and, 413–414
on reversible cerebral vasoconstriction syndrome,
196–197
on thalamic hemorrhages, 135–136
on transient ischemic attacks, 359–361
on visual loss in vascular disease, 228–230
warfarin research and, 438
Fitch, T. S., 551–552
Fizeau, Armand Hippolyte Louis, 325–326
Flaenius, Rufus, 562–563
Fleming, David, 529–530
Fleming, Marie, 196–197
Flemming, K. D., 169–170
flow-directed embolization, arteriovenous
malformations, 596–597
fluid abnormalities, subarachnoid hemorrhage,
149–150
fluid-attenuated inversion recovery (FLAIR)
imaging, 320–322
2-[F[18]] fluoro-2-deoxy-D-glucose (FDG) PET,
344, 349
focal ischemic stroke models, 479–481
cellular targets, 481–482
Foerster, O., 103
Foix, Charles, 83–84, 101, 129, 251–258
Foix-Alajuanine syndrome, 258
Foix, Chavany, Marie syndrome, 258
Ford, Frank, 378–379
Ford, Gerald, 611–612
Ford, Henry, 613
For One without a Doctor (Man la Yahduruhu al-Tabib)
(Rhazes), 11–12
4VO stroke model, 479–481
Foville, Achille Louis, 68–69
Foville syndrome, 127–128
Fowler, Joanna, 344
Framingham Study, 364–365, 471–475
Frankel, Mike, 496–497
Franklin, D. L., 326
Franklin, Rosalind Elsie, 213
Fraser, J. S., 175–176
free radical hypothesis, neuroprotection and,
483–484
Frei, E. H., 570–571
fresh frozen plasma (FFP), intracerebral hemorrhage
and reversal of hematoma expansion, 583–584
Freud, Sigmund, 378
Froin, George, 141
frontal artery sign, 115–116
Froriep, Robert, 95–96
Fukutake, Toshio, 218–219
Fulton, John, 339–340
Furlan, Anthony, 232–233, 422, 495–496
Fuster, Valentin, 116–117

gadolinium compounds (Gd-DPTA), MRA and,
321–322

Gaines, Ken, 496–497
Galen, 562–563
Circle of Willis and, 34
on circulation, 29
Greco-Roman medical tradition and, 7
humoral theory of, 25, 37
on stroke, 14
Galvani, Luigi, 353
Garcin, Marie Mathieu Jean Raymond, 174,
176–177, 241–242, 380–381
Garland, Hugh, 241–242
Garrod, Archibald E., 212
Gaupp, J., 590–591
Gautier, Jean-Claude, 230–232
Geiger-Muller tube, 341–342
Genentech, 495
general paralysis of the insane (GPI), 122–124
gene therapy, 213–214
genetics. See also specific genetic disorders
early research on, 211–214
intracerebral aneurysm and, 150–151
key developments in stroke genetics, 214–215
stroke and, 211–223
Gennarelli, Thomas. A., 597
genome-wide association studies (GWAS), stroke
genetics and, 214–215
genomics, 214
The Genuine Works of Hippocrates, 3–4
Germany, ischemic stroke management in, 401–402
Geschwind, Norman, 76–78, 283
giant-cell arteritis, 234–235
Gillilan, Lois Adele, 86
Ginsberg, Myron, 481, 484–485
Glasgow Coma Scale, 401–402
glimepride, 470
glitazones, 470
global ischemic stroke models, 479–481
cellular targets, 481–482
excitotoxicity and channel targets, 482–483
glycoprotein IIb/IIIa antagonists, 461–462
Golden, Gerry, 381
Goldstein, Joseph, 472–475
Gortner, Ross A., 435–436
Gould, D. B., 220
Gowers, William, 101–102, 109–110, 159, 226–229,
239–240
Goyal, Mayank, 554–555
Grades of Recommendation Assessment,
Development, and Evaluation (GRADE)
System, 420–421
gradient echo (GRE) sequencing, 320–322
granulocyte-colony stimulating factor (G-CSF),
525–526
gray-scale imaging, development of, 328
great spinal artery, 85–86
Greco-Roman medical tradition, 6–8
Greenberg, Steve, 163–164
Griffith, Frederick, 213

Grotta, Jim, 422, 496–497
growth factors, stroke rehabilitation, 525
Gruentzig, Andreas, 541
Gruner, J., 241–242
Gubler, Adolphe, 68–69
Guglielmi, Guido, 573–574
Guillain, Georges., 241–242
Guillain-Barré syndrome, 399–400
Gull, Withey, 144
Guyatt, Gordon, 420–421
"Guy's Triumvirate," 58
Guyton, Arthur, 466–467

Hackam, D. G., 116–117
Hacke, Werner, 396–405, 422, 495–497, 500–501
Hakim, Antoine, 479–481
Haley, Clark, 422, 496–497
Halliday, Allison, 422–423, 537
Haly, Abbas, 14–15
Hammond, William A., 103
Handbook on Diseases of the Nervous System (Beevor), 82–83
Handbuch der Physiologie (*Handbook of Physiology*) (Muller), 94–95
Hankey, Greame, 420–421
Hanley, Daniel F., 396, 402–405, 580–581
Hardy, Godfrey Harold, 212
Hardy-Weinberg equilibrium, 212
Harrison, Tinsley R., 101
Hart, Robert, 421–422
Harvard Cooperative Stroke Registry, 371
Harvey, William, 24, 612–613
    circulation research of, 25–29
    early life and training, 26–27
Hayreh, Sohan S. S., 234–235
HeADDFIRST trial, 404
Hedges, Thomas Reed, Jr., 232–233
Heiss, Wolf-Dieter, 348, 479–481
hematology, pediatric stroke and, 384–385
hematoma expansion, 163
    intracerebral hemorrhage and control of, 581–585
hematoma resolution, intracerebral hemorrhage, 579–581
hemicraniectomy. *See* decompressive
    hemicraniectomy
hemorrhagic stroke
    early descriptions, 14–15, 57–62
    early research on, 60–61
hemostatic agents, intracerebral hemorrhage, 582–583
Hennerici, Michael., 130–131, 497
heparin
    antidote development, 430
    clinical trials involving, 415, 429–430
    discovery and production of, 427–429
    efficacy of, 431–432
    history of research on, 427–433
    isolation and synthesis of, 436–437

low-molecular-weight variant, 430–432, 510
    venous thrombosis and, 429–430, 506–509
"Heparin and Thrombosis of Veins Following
    Injury" (Murray and Best), 429–430
hepatotoxicity, direct oral anticoagulants and, 443–444
Hereditary Cerebral Haemorrhage with
    Amyloidosis (HCHWA), 223
Hereditary Endotheliopathy with Retinopathy,
    Nephropathy and Stroke (HERNS), 219–220
hereditary vascular retinopathy (HRV), 219–220
heredity, early research on, 211–214
heroin, production of, 449–450
Heros, Roberto C., 244, 596
Herrick, James, 220–221
Hertz, Hellmuth, 355–356
Hess, Robert M., 145–147
Heubner, C. F., 436–437
Heubner, Johann Otto, 84–85, 376–377
Heubner's arteritis, 245
Heyman, Albert, 414, 438
Heynecker, Herb, 495
Hier, Dan, 287
Highly Effective Reperfusion Evaluated in Multiple
    Endovascular Stroke Trials (HERMES)
    collaboration, 556–557
Hill, Leonard, 339–340
Hill, Michael, 309, 484–485
Hillemand, P., 253–255
Hiller, Friedrich, 103
Hippocrates, 6–8, 142–144, 157–158, 358, 478–479
Historia anatomica de puella sine cerebro nata (Wepfer), 43
Hobbes, Thomas, 26
Hobson, Robert, 422–423, 545–546
Hodgkin, Dorothy, 613
Hodgkin, Thomas, 57–62
Hodgkin's disease, 57–62
Hoff, Julian T., 577–578
Hoffman, E. J., 345–347
Hoffmann, Felix, 449–450
Hogan, Ben, 615–616
Hollenhorst, Robert, 112, 230, 232–233
Holt, Luther Emmett, 378
Holt, T. Emmett, 429
Holter, Norman Jeff, 354
Homer, 3–4, 157–158
homocysteine, atherothrombosis and, 205–206
homocystinuria, 222–223
Hooke, Robert, 33, 211
Hooper, Robert, 56–57
Hope, James, 56
Horner's syndrome, 232–233
Horsley, Victor, 563–564
Horton, Bayard Taylor, 235
Hounsfield, Godfrey N., 305–308
Hounsfield scale, 307–308

Howell, William Henry, 427–429, 434–435
HTRA1 gene, CARASIL and, 218–219
Hultquist, G. T., 111
human extrinsic plasminogen activator, 494–495
Human Genome Project, 214
humoral theory, 25–26
Hunt, James Ramsay, 110
Hunt, William, 145–147
Hunt and Hess SAH classification, 145–147
Hunter, John, 45, 93–94, 144, 563
Hunter, William, 93–94, 167–169
Hutchinson, E. C., 129–130
Hutchinson, Jonathan, 234–235
Hutinel, V. H., 175–176
hydrocephalus, 33
    subarachnoid hemorrhage and, 149–150
3-hydroxy-3-methylglutaryl-coenzyme A (HMG-
    CoA) reductase inhibitor, hyperlipidemia and,
    472–475
hypercoagulation, blood disorders and, 200–201
hyperhomocysteinemia, 205–206
hyperlipidemia
    stroke risk and, 471–475
    treatment of, 472–475
hypertension
    early research on, 99–101
    fibromuscular dysplasia, 192–193
    intracerebral hemorrhage and, 163–165
    stroke and, 465–467
    treatment of, 466–467
hypertensive encephalopathy, early research on,
    38–40
hypotension, spinal cord ischemia and, 242–243
hypothermia
    history of, 478–479
    neuroprotection and, 485–487
    stroke management and, 401
Hypothermia after Cardiac Arrest trial, 401

Iadecola, Constantino, 479–481
Ibn Ahmad Ibn Rushd, Mohammed (Averroes),
    12–13, 15–16
Ibn AlNafis. See Alauddin Abu al Hassan Ali ibn
    Hazmi (Ibn AlNafis)
Ibn Qayyam Al-Juzziya, 10
Ibsen, Bjørn, 397
Ichord, Rebecca, 384
ICTuS 2 trial, 485–487
idarucizumab, 445
Iles, Thomas, 31
image-based stroke therapy, 499
Imhotep, 562–563
inborn errors of metabolism, 212
induced hypothermia, traumatic brain injury and,
    401
infection, childhood hemiplegia and, 378–380
inflammation, early research on, 94–96
Ingram, Vernon, 220–221

Ingvar, David H., 343, 479–481
Ingvar, Martin, 479–481
inherited thrombophilias, 203
Institute of Applied Physiology and Medicine
    (IAPM), 327, 329
insulin
    discovery of, 318, 469–470
    resistance, 470–471
intensive care units (ICUs), neurocritical care and,
    391–392, 396–399
    ischemic stroke in, 401–402
INTERACT (Intensive Blood Pressure Reduction
    in Acute Cerebral Hemorrhage) trial, 582
intermittent cerebral claudications, 110
internal medicine
    early textbooks on, 99–101
    textbooks on, 101
international normalized ratio (INR), anticoagulants
    and, 442–446
International Pediatric Stroke Study (IPSS), 383–385
International Stroke Genetics Consortium (ISGC),
    215–216
international stroke organizations and publications,
    608–609
International Stroke Trial (IST), 419
International Study on Cerebral Vein and Dural
    Sinus Thrombosis (ISCVT), 183–185, 509
interventional radiology, heparin use in, 432–433
intervertebral disk material, spinal cord infarction
    and, 245
intraarterial thrombolysis, 500–501
intracerebral aneurysm (ICA)
    demography, epidemiology, family, and genetic
        information with, 150–151
    early research on, 144
    early treatment of, 563–568
    electrothrombosis, 573–574
    endovascular treatment, 570–574
    microneurosurgery, 569–570
    recognition of, 562–563
    surgery and clipping, 567–569
    twentieth-century research on, 138–142
intracerebral hemorrhage (ICH)
    anticoagulant/antiplatelet reversal, 583–584
    blood pressure control, 582
    critical care of, 402–404
    decompressive hemicraniectomy, 584–585
    early research on, 38–40, 46–47, 157–158
    hematoma expansion control, 581–585
    hematoma resolution, 579–581
    hemostatic agents, 582–583
    hypertension and, 163–165, 466–467
    imaging studies, 163
    nineteenth- and early twentieth-century research
        on, 158–159
    Osler's work on, 100–101, 159
    parenchymal effects, 577–578
    treatment overview, 577–585

intracerebral hemorrhage (ICH) (cont.)
   Wepfer's research on, 43–44, 158–159
intracranial arteries
   angioplasty and stenting, 546–549
   Bayle's research on, 44
   dissections, 191–192
   early research on, 65–66
   Moyamoya syndrome and disease, 193–196
   surgery on, 529–538
   thrombolytic therapy for occlusion in, 495–496
   transcranial ultrasound of, 330–332
   Wepfer's research on, 43
intracranial hemorrhage
   arteriovenous malformations and, 595–598
   bleeding disorders and, 208
   early research on, 49–50
   endovascular therapy, 552–553
intracranial intervention procedures, clinical trials
   of, 423–424
intracranial pressure (ICP) monitoring, 400–401
   intracerebral hemorrhage, 577–578
intracranial venous occlusion, 151–152
Intraoperative Computed Tomography–Guided
   Endoscopic Surgery for Brain Hemorrhage
   trial, 404
intravenous thrombolysis, 308–309
"The Invisible College," 32
Irons, Ernest, 220–221
ischemic optic neuropathy, 234–235
ischemic stroke
   cellular targets, 481–482
   early research on, 51–53
   endovascular treatment for, 551–558
   global vs. focal models, 479–481
   hypothermia and, 478–479, 485–487
   noncardioembolic ischemic stroke, 415
   pediatric stroke and, 382–383
   penumbra imaging of, 321–322, 348, 479–481
   transcranial Doppler ultrasound imaging of, 332
   treatment of, 401–402
ISIS-2 clinical trial, 419
Islam, medical contributions from, 10–14
Isler, Werner, 381–382
Itano, Harvey, 220–221
Ito, U., 479–481
Iyer, Sriram, 541–542

Jackson, David, 398–399, 404–405
Jeffray, James, 62
Jellinger, Kurt, 163–164
Jenner, Edward, 612–613
Jennett, Bryan, 400–401, 579–580
Johnson, Andrew, 611–612
Johnson, Edward, 430–431
Joint Study of Extracranial Arterial Occlusion, 533
Joliot, Jean Frédéric, 340–341
Joliot-Curie, Iréne, 340–341
Jones, Ronald, 505–506

Jones, Terry, 347
Jonson, Ben, 32
Jordan, M. B., 437–438
Jorpes, Erik, 429
Joslin, Elliott Proctor, 467–469
Joutel, Anne, 218
Jovin, Tudor, 554–555
Joyner, Claude, 329
Joyner, C. R., Jr., 355–356

Kadyi, Henryk, 85–86, 240
Kalbag, R. M., 176–177
Kallman, Heinz, 341–342
Kang, S. S., 205–206
Karp, Herb, 438
Kase, Carlos, 365
Kaste, Markku, 422, 497
Kearns, Thomas, 232–233
Kearns-Sayre syndrome, 222
Kees, G., 568–569
Kelly, Gene, 614
Kelly, Grace, 614
Kenealy, Lori, 521–522
Kennedy, Sean, 399–400, 404–405
Kerber, C. W., 171
Kety, Seymour S., 342–344
King, Edmund, 33
Kirino, T., 479–481
Kirkham, Fenella, 382–384
Kirkland, Thomas, 45–46
Kistler, Phillip, 147–149, 288, 497–500
Kjellberg, Raymond. 400–401, 404
Klumpke, Augusta Marie, 73–79
Kolbe, Hermann, 448
Kolisko, Alexander, 84–90
Kornberg, Roger D., 214
Kornyey, S., 134, 160
Koroshetz, Walter, 497–500
Korotkov, Nikolai, 100
Krahn, A. D., 354
Kraig, Richard, 479–481
Kraus, Walter, 101
Krause, Fedor, 590–591
Krayenbühl, Hugo, 111, 177–179
Krev interaction trapped 1 (KRIT1) gene, 169–170
Krusen, Frank Hammond, 515–516
Kubik, C., 129–132
Kuhl, David, 344–345
Kurland, Leonard, 370
Kurosawa, Akira, 614
Kurze, Theodore, 595–596
Kussmaul, A., 109
Kwiatkowski, Tom, 496–497

lacunar infarcts (lacunes)
   early research on, 119–124
   Fisher's work on, 271–272
   neuroimaging of, 122

pathology, 120–121
  white matter pathology, 122–124
Laennec, René, 352–356
L'Anatomie pathologique du corps humain
  (Cruveilhier), 59–60
Lancet (journal), 26
Landouzy, Louis Théophile Joseph, 74–75
Landouzy-Dejerine syndrome, 74–75
Landry, Jean Baptiste-Octave, 69
Lane, Steven, 316–317
Langhorne, Peter, 420–421
Lapresle, Jean, 241–242
Lassen, Niels A., 343, 347–348
lateral medullary infarction, early research on, 64–68
lateral tegmental hematomas, 134
Lauterbur, Paul, 315–318
Lawrence, Ernest, 341
laws of heredity, 212
lazaroids, 483–484
learned paralysis, stroke rehabilitation and, 523–524
Le Blon, Jacob Christoph, 56
leech therapy, 26
Lenin, Vladimir, 610, 616–618
Leonardo da Vinci, 22
Lev, Michael, 310
Levine, Steve, 496–497
Levy, David, 496–497
Lewandowsky, M., 103
Lewis, Thomas, 354
Liber almansoris (Rhazes), 11–12
Lidell, John A., 50–52, 158–159
Lima, Almeida, 299–300
Lindbergh, Anne Morrow, 614
Lindbergh, John, 327
Lindley, Rickard, 420–421
Link, Karl Paul Gerhard, 435–437
lipohyalinosis, 120–121, 271–272
lipoprotein metabolism, 472
lithography, anatomical atlases and, 56
Locke, John, 32, 44–45, 358–359
Loeb, C., 359–361
Logue, Valentine, 244, 567–569
Lombroso, Cesare, 380–381
Long, Don, 402–404
Louis, Pierre C. A., 57–61
Lower, Richard, 32–34
low-molecular-weight heparin, 510
  development of, 430–432
Luessenhop, Alfred J., 570–571, 597
Lundberg, Nils, 400–401
lupus anticoagulant (LA), 206–207
lupus erythematosus, 206–207
Lyden, Pat, 422, 485–487, 496–497
Lyme borreliosis, spinal cord infarction and, 245

Macdonald, John A., 612
Macewen, William, 579
Mackenzie, Alexander, 612

Maclagan, Thomas John, 448–449
Macleod, Colin Munro, 213
Macleod, J. J. R., 318, 469–470
Maffrand, Jean-Pierre, 458–459
magnetic resonance angiography (MRA), 132–137
  arterial dissection, 190
  discovery of, 321
magnetic resonance imaging (MRI)
  arteriovenous malformations, 596–597
  cardiac, 356
  cerebral vein and dural sinus thrombosis, 181–182
  clinical applications, 319–320
  early research, 313–316
  evolution of, 309, 313–322
  first human scans, 316–317
  intracerebral hemorrhage, 163
  perfusion imaging and, 309–311, 321–322
  posterior circulation and, 132–137
  stroke and cerebrovascular disease and, 320–322
Magnus, Vilhelm, 590–591
Maimonides (Moses ben Maimon), 12–14
Mallord, John, 319–320
Malpighi, Marcello, 37–38, 200–201, 612–613
man-in-the-barrel syndrome, 112–113
Mansfield, Peter, 316–318
Manual of Diseases of the Nervous System (Gowers),
  226–229
Marcet, A., 66–67
Marfan syndrome, 222–223
Marie, Pierre, 119–120, 251–253
Markus, Hugh, 332–333
Marlowe, Christopher, 32
Marriott, Henry, 354
Masur, Henry, 402–404
MATCH trial, clopidogrel vs. asprin in, 459–460
Matteucci, Carlo, 353
Mayfield, Frank. H., 568–569
Mayfield-Kees clip, 568–569
Mayo Clinic
  stroke data bank and registry at, 370
  stroke epidemiology research at, 367
McCarty, Maclyn, 213
McClintock, Barbara, 212–213
McCormack, L. J., 192–193
McCormick, William F., 169–171
McCully, Kilmer, 205–206
McDevitt, Ellen, 414
McDonald, R. Loch, 147–149
McKinney, William Markley, 327
McKissock, Wylie, 134–135, 579
McLean, Jay, 427–429
McNealy, D. E., 399–400
McNutt, Sarah J., 376–377
mechanical thrombectomy, 432–433, 555–558
Medical Compendium in Seven Books (Paul of
  Aegenia), 8
medical textbooks, early editions of, 103
medulla, arterial supply, 85

melodic intonation therapy (MIT), 524–525
"Memoir on the Curability of Cerebral Softening"
    (Dechambre), 120
Mendel, Gregor, 212
Mendelow, Alexander David, 579–580
Mendelssohn, Felix, 615
meninges, spinal cord infarction and, 245
MERCI (Mechanical Embolus Removal in
    Cerebral Ischemia) trial,
    553–554
Merritt, H. Houston, 263, 370, 413–414, 612–613
metabolic syndrome
    insulin resistance and, 470–471
    stroke risk and, 467–471
Metaphysics (Aristotle), 10–11
metformin, 470
methylenetetrahydrofolate reductase (MTHFR),
    homocysteine metabolism, 205–206
Meyer, John Sterling, 493
Michelangelo, 22
microneurosurgery, intracerebral aneurysm,
    569–570
microsurgical neuroanatomy, 88–89
midbrain lesions, early research on, 69–70
middle cerebral artery (MCA)
    dissection, 190–191
    Foix's research on, 253–254
    Moyamoya syndrome and disease, 193–196
    occlusion, endovascular therapy for, 551–553
    pediatric occlusion, 380–385
Middle Cerebral Artery Embolism Local
    Fibrinolytic Intervention Trial (MELT),
    552–553
Middle East, medical contributions from, 10–14
Middlemore, R., 226
migraine, brain ischemia and, 274–275
Millard, August, 68–69
Millard Gubler syndrome, 68–69, 127–128
Miller, J. D., 400–401
Miller Fisher variant (Guillain-Barré syndrome), 258
Millikan, Clark, 131–132, 413–415, 438
Mills, Charles A., 103
Mills, Edward, 269–270
Milton, John, 26
Minimally Invasive Surgery Plus rt-PA for ICH
    Evacuation (MISTIE) trials,
    403–404, 579–581
Minkoff, Larry, 316–317
Minot, George Richards, 467–469
mirror neurons and mirror box therapy,
    523–524
Mistichell, Domenico, 45–46
Mitchell, N., 134–135
mitochondrial myopathy, encephalopathy, lactic
    acidosis and stroke-like episodes (MELAS), 222
mitochondrial pore inhibitors, 481–482
MK-801 NMDA antagonist, 482–483
mobile stroke unit (MSU), 394

Moehring, Mark, 331
Moersch, F. P., 188–189
Mohr, Jay P., 112–115, 286, 288, 371, 421–424,
    497–500
Molins, Mahels, 531
MONICA (Monitoring of Trends and
    Determinants in Cardiovascular Disease) study
    (WHO), 365–366
Moniz, Egas, 318
    aneurysm and hemorrhage research, 168–169,
        567–569
    cerebral angiography development and, 110–111,
        144–145, 305, 530
    thrombosis research, 177–179
Monk, Thelonius, 615
monogenic stroke conditions, 216
Monro-Kellie doctrine, 49–50
Morawitz, Paul Oskar, 202
Morbid Anatomy of the Human Brain (Hooper),
    56–57
*Morbid Anatomy of the Human Uterus and Its
    Appendages* (Hooper), 56–57
Morgagni, Giovanni Battista
    on anatomy, 55
    on aneurysm, 562–563
    on arterial dissection, 188–189
    on intracerebral aneurysm, 144
    on pathology, 37–41, 93
    on subarachnoid hemorrhage, 142–144
Morgan, Thomas Hunt, 212–213
Mori, Etsuo, 495–496, 551–552
Mosso, Angelo, 339
Motulsky, Arno G., 473
Moyamoya syndrome and disease, 193–196
Muhammad (prophet), 10–14
Mullan, Sean, 600–601
Mullani, N. A., 345–347
Müller, Johannes Peter, 94–95, 200–201
Müller, Paul Herman, 318
Multicenter Randomized Clinical Trial of
    Endovascular Treatment for Acute Ischemic
    Stroke in the Netherlands (MR CLEAN),
    556–557
multimodal computed tomography (MCT),
    309–311
multiorgan system failure, critical care units and,
    398–399
multiple sclerosis, early research on, 62
Murphy, William, 468
Murray, D. W. Gordon, 429–430
muscle emboli, carotid cavernous fistula closure,
    600–601
Museum anatomicum (Sandifort), 55
musicians, stroke in, 615
myocardial infarction, aspirin and, 449
myoclonus epilepsy ragged red fibre syndrome, 222
*My Stroke of Insight: A Brain Scientist's Personal
    Journey* (Taylor), 612–613

Nageott, Jean, 67–68, 75
National Health and Nutrition Examination Survey
    (NHANES), 366
National Institute of Neurological Diseases
    (NINDS)
    CT development and, 308–309
    Stroke Data Bank, 287–288, 371
    stroke scale, 497
    thrombolytic therapy trials, 496–497
Nelson, Thomas, 101
nephrology, early research on, 58
nerinetide, neuroprotection trials with, 484–485
neurocritical care. See also stroke centers
    birth of, 404–405
    brain injury diagnosis and management and,
        399–405
    comatose patient, 399
    decompressive craniectomy for malignant
        hemispheric stroke, 404
    defibrillation and cardiopulmonary resuscitation,
        398
    induced hypothermia, 401
    intracerebral hemorrhage, 402–404
    ischemic stroke treatment, 401–402
    overview, 396–405
    positive pressure mechanical ventilation, 397
    post-operative and respiratory units, 397
NeuroCritical Care (Hacke), 404–405
NeuroFlo devis, 484–485
The Neurological Examination of the Comatose Patient
    (Fisher), 399
neurology
    Dejerine's contributions to, 74–75
    early textbooks on, 101–103
neuroplasticity, stroke rehabilitation and, 518–525
neuroprotection
    cellular and vascular intervention, 484–485
    cellular targets, 481–482
    excitotoxicity and channel targets, 482–483
    free radicals and, 483–484
    global vs. focal ischemic stroke models, 479–481
    history of, 478–479
    hypothermia and, 485–487
    overview of, 478–484
neurorehabilitation, 518–525
neurosonology societies, 333–334
Newell, David, 331–332
Newkirk, Ingrid, 520–521
new oral anticoagulants (NOACs), 443
Newton, Isaac, 56
Newton, T. H., 171
Nexletol, cholesterol reduction and, 475
Nicolesco, J., 253
NINDS-SiGN GWASD study, 215–216
NINDS stroke scale (NIHSS), 497
Nishioka, H., 168–169
Nissl, F., 122–124
Nixon, Richard M., 612

NMDA antagonists, excitotoxicity and channel
    targets, 482–483
NMR Specialties company, 315–316
Nobel Prize, controversies over, 318
Nogueira, Raul, 554–555
nonaneurysmal subarachnoid hemorrhage, 151–152
noninvasive brain stimulation (NIBS), 522–523
noradrenergic agents, stroke rehabilitation, 525
Nordisk Insulin Laboratory, 470
Norlén, Gösta, 595
North American Consortium of Acute Brain Injury
    (NACABI), 403
North American Symptomatic Carotid Surgery
    (NASCET) trial, 332–333, 422–423, 534–536
NOTCH3 gene, CADASIL and, 218
nuclear magnetic resonance (NMR),
    313–316
Nurses Study, 366
Nymman, Gregor, 44

Observationes anatomicae ex cadaveribus eorum, quos
    sustulit apoplexia, cum exercitatione de eius loco
    affecto (Wepfer), 43
Observations on the Structure of the Intestinal Worms of
    the Human Body (Hooper), 56–57
Occlusion of the Internal Carotid Artery (Fisher), 112
Of the Causes and Signs of Acute and Chronic Disease
    (Areteus of Cappadocia), 7–8
Ojemann, Robert, 116–117, 147–149, 189–190,
    273–275
Okazaki, H., 223
Oldendorf, William, 306–307
Olivecrona, Hebert, 568–569, 579, 593–595
Olszewski, J., 122–124
Ommaya, A. K., 243–244
On Apoplexy (Cooke), 47–48
On the Cerebral Circulation (Burrows), 49–50
one-and-a-half syndrome, 275–276
On the Names of the Parts of the Human Body (Rufus
    of Ephesus), 7
On the Origin of Species by Means of Natural Selection
    (Darwin), 212
ophthalmic artery, vascular disease and, 112
ophthalmoscopy, development of, 226
Oporinus, Johannes, 22–24
Oppenheim, Gustav, 163–164, 223, 239–240
Oppenheim, Herman, 103
oral antihyperglycemics, 470
Osler, William, 99–101, 159, 268, 377, 456
Otis, Shirley, 495–496
otitic hydrocephalus, 175–176
Otsuka Pharmaceutical Company, 457–458

Pacheco, Alex, 520–521
Paracelsus, 447
paralysis
    Areteus of Cappadocia on, 7–8
    Hippocrates's description of, 4–5

paramedian pontine reticular formation (PPRF), 69
Para-Operational Device (POD), 570–571
Paraphrase of Rhazes, 21–22
paraplegia, Areteus of Cappadocia on, 7–8
Paré, Ambroise, 529–530
Parillo, Joseph, 402–404
Parkinson, Dwight, 600
particulate theory, in ancient Greece, 211
Paslubinskas, A., 192–193
Pasteur, Louis, 612–613
*Pathological Anatomy: Illustrations of the Elementary
    Forms of Disease* (Carswell), 57–61
"Pathological Observations in Hypertensive
    Cerebral Hemorrhage" (Fisher), 160–162
pathology
    atlases of, 55–56
    early research on, 37–41
Patrono, Carl, 417–418
Pauling, Linus Carl, 220–221
Paul of Aegenia, 8
Pavalakis, S. G., 222
pediatric stroke, 374–385
Penfield, Wilder, 266–267, 598–599
Pennica, Diane, 495
penumbra imaging, in ischemic stroke, 321–322,
    348, 479–481
Penumbra Pivotal Stroke Trial, 553–554
Penumbra reperfusion catheter and separator,
    553–554
People for Ethical Treatment of Animals (PETA),
    520
Percheron, Gerard, 86–87
perfusion imaging, 309–311, 321–322, 347–348
    thrombolytic therapy and, 499
peri-hematoma edema, intracerebral hemorrhage,
    577–578
perimesencephalic hemorrhages, 151–152
Perret, G., 168–169
Perry, Luke, 614
Pessin, Michael, 114–115, 288, 495–496
Pestel, Maurice, 174, 176–177
Peterson, Frederick, 377–378
Petit, Jean Louis, 563
Petito, Carol, 479–481
Peto, Richard, 418–421
Petty, William (Sir), 32
Phelps, Michael, 345–347
N-tert-butyl-α-phenylnitrone (PBN), 483–484
phlebitis
    Cruveilhier's theory concerning, 59–60
    early research on, 94
phosphodiesterase (PDE) inhibitors, 456–458
physical medicine, and stroke rehabilitation
    evolution and expansion of, 518
    history of, 515–518
    melodic intonation therapy, 524–525
    mirror neurons and mirror box therapy, 523–524
    noninvasive brain stimulation (NIBS), 522–523

pharmacological agents, 525
    polio epidemic and, 516–517
    robotics, 525
    stem cell therapy, 525–526
    whole -person approach to, 517–518
*Physical Medicine: The Employment of Physical Agents
    for Diagnosis and Therapy* (Krusen), 516
physicians, stroke in, 612–613
*The Physiology and Pathology of Cerebral Circulation:
    An Experimental Research* (Hill), 339
The Physiology and Pathology of Circulation (Basch),
    465–467
Pickering, George, 230–232, 531
Piepgras, David, 244
pioglitazone, 470
Piria, Raffaele, 448
plaque formation, carotid artery disease, 116–117
plasma exchange therapy, 399–400
plasmin, 491
platelet aggregation
    antiplatelet therapy, 455–462
    aspirin and, 415–418, 449
Plum, Fred, 399–400, 479–481, 533–534
pneumoencehpalography, 298–299, 304–305,
    566–568
Poeck, Klaus, 495–496
Poirier, Jacques, 120–121
poliomyelitis epidemic, rehabilitation medicine and,
    516–517
political figures, stroke in, 610–612
polymerase chain reaction (PCR), 213–214
pons, arterial supply, 85
pontine hematoma, 133–136
pontine lesions, early research on, 68–69
Poppin-Blalock clamp, 564–565
positive pressure mechanical ventilation, 397
positron emission tomography (PET)
    basic principles of, 341–342
    cerebral blood flow imaging, 338–349
    and cerebral glucose utilization, 344
    cerebrovascular disease and brain function
        imaging, 347–348
    early research on, 340–341
    evolution of scanners, 344–347
    2-[F[18]] fluoro-2-deoxy-D-glucose (FDG), 344,
        349
    global and focal stroke models and, 479–481
    limitations of, 349
    and radioactive isotopes, 343
"Positron Imaging in Ischemic Stroke Disease Using
    Compounds Labelled with Oxygen 15: Initial
    Results of Clinicophysiologic Correlations"
    (Ackerman), 347
Posner, Jerry , 399
posterior cerebral artery (PCA), Foix's research on,
    253–254
posterior circulation
    basilar artery occlusion, 129–130

pathologic and imaging studies, late 20th century, 132–137
transient ischemic attacks and, 131–132
vascular lesions, 128–132
vertebrobasilar disease, 127–128, 133–136
posterior inferior cerebellar artery (PICA) syndrome, early research on, 65–66
postoperative and respiratory critical care units, 397
Poungvarin, N., 577–578
power motion Doppler (PMD), 331
Practice of Physic (Willis), 34
Pragmatic Ischemic Thrombectomy Evaluation (PISTE) trial, 556–557
prasugrel (Efient), 460–461
PRECISE stent, 544
pregnancy
cerebal vein and dural sinus thrombosis and, 174–185
spinal cord infarction and, 245
venous thrombosis in, 505–506
"Preliminary Report on Postoperative Treatment with Heparin as a Preventive of Thrombosis" (Crafoord), 429–430
presidents, stroke in, 611–612
PREVAIL clinical trial, heparin efficacy in, 432
Prieto, A., 400–401, 404
primary stroke centers (PSCs), 393–394
Princeton Conferences on Cerebrovascular Diseases, 413–414
print technology, anatomic atlases and, 56
PROACT trial, endovascular therapy, 552–553
The Prognostics (Hippocrates), 3–4
Prokofiev, Sergei, 615
Prolyse in Acute Cerebral Thromboembolism trials (PROACT I and II), 501
pronethalol, 467
prophetic traditions (sunnah), 10–14
propranolol, 467
proprotein convertase subtilisin/kexin type 9 (PCSK9), cholesterol reduction and, 475
prostacyclin, aspirin and, 415–418
prothrombin complex concentrates (PCCs), intracerebral hemorrhage and reversal of hematoma expansion, 583–584
prothrombin gene mutation, 204
prothrombin time test, 202–203
pro-urokinase therapy, 501
pseudotumour cerebri, cerebal vein and dural sinus thrombosis and, 180–181
pseudoxanthoma elasticum, 222–223
Puckett, Kirby, 615–616
pulmonary embolism
anticoagulant therapy for, 437–438
urokinase and streptokinase therapy, 493
pulmonary thrombosis
heparin in management of, 429–430
Virchow's research on, 96–97

pulse palpation and auscultation, carotid artery disease, 115–116
Pulsinelli, Bill, 479–481
Purcell, Edward, 313
Purdon, Martin, J., 175–176

Quain, Richard, 376–381
Quick, Armand James, 202–203
Quinke, Heinrich Irenaeus, 141
Quran, 10–14
Qureshi, Adnan, 582

Rabi, Isidor, 313
radioactive isotopes, PET research and, 343
radionuclides, cerebral blood flow imaging, 338–349
Radner, Stig, 300–301
Raichle, Marcus, 345–347
Ramachandran, V. S., 523–524
ramollissements (softenings)
brainstem circulation and, 129
in early research, 48–53, 56–57
hemorrhage and, 57–62
lacunar infarcts and, 120
Randomization of Endovascular Treatment with Stent-Retriever and/or Thromboaspiration versus Best Medical Therapy in Acute Ischemic Stroke Due to Large Vessel Occlusion Trial (RESILIENT), 556–557
Randomized Trial of Unruptured Brain Arteriovenous Malformations (ARUBA), 597–598
Raybaud, Charles, 383
Raymond's syndrome, 69
Reaven, Gerald, 470–471
rebleeding
arteriovenous malformations, 597–598
subarachnoid hemorrhage, 145–147
ReCCLAIM Trials, 485–487
recombinant DNA, 213–214
recombinant pro-urokinase (rpro-UK), endovascular therapy with, 552–553
recombinant tissue plasminogen activator (rt-PA), 401–404, 483–484, 493–500
recurrent artery of Heubner, 84–85
regional cerebral blood volume/regional cerebral blood flow (rCVB/rCBF), 321–322
rehabilitation. *See* physical medicine, and stroke rehabilitation
Reid, John, 328–329, 355–356
Reinhardt, Benno Ernst Heinrich, 95
Reivich, M., 130–131
RE-LY trial, 444–445
renal artery, fibromuscular dysplasia, 192–193
Reports of Medical Cases, Selected with a View to Illustrate the Symptoms and Cure of Diseases by a Reference to Morbid Anatomy (Bright), 58
respiratory critical care units, 397
retinal vascular spasm, 233–234

retinal vasculopathy, 219–220
retinal vasculopathy and cerebral leukodystrophy
    (RVCL), 219–220
Revascularization with Solitaire FR Device vs. Best
    Medical Therapy in the Treatment of Acute
    Stroke Due to Anterior Circulation Large
    Vessel Occlusion Presenting within Eight
    Hours of Symptom Onset (REVASCAT) trial,
    556–557
reversible cerebral vasoconstriction syndrome
    (RCVS), 196–197
Revive stent retriever, 554–555
rFVIIa, intracerebral hemorrhage, 582–583
Rhazes. *See* Abu Bakr Muhammed Ibn Zakria
    AlRazi (Rhazes)
rheumatic fever, 448–449
Rhoton, Albert Loren, Jr., 88–89
Rich, Charles, 189–190
Richardson, E. P., 283–285
Richardson, Ralph, 614
Riella, Anthony, 383
Rifkin, Daniel, 494
Rigamonti, Danielle, 598–599
Riives, J., 594
Rijken, Dingeman, 494
Ringelstein, Berndt, 495–496
RING finger 213 (*RNF213*) gene, Moyamoya
    syndrome and disease, 195–196
Rinkle, Gabriel, 150–151
Ripley, H. R., 192–193
RISC trial, 417–418
risk factors for stroke, 364–367
    diabetes and metabolic syndrome, 467–471
    hyperlipidemia, 471–475
    hypertension, 465–467
Riva-Rocci, Scipione, 100
rivaroxaban, 444–445
Rizzolatti, G., 523–524
Roach, Steven, 383
Rob, Charles., 531
Roberson, Glenn, 147–149
robotics, stroke rehabilitation and, 525
ROCKET-AF trial, 444–445
Roderick, L. M., 434–435
Röentgen, Wilhelm Conrad, 304
Rokitansky, Carl von, 110
Roosevelt, Franklin D., 466–467, 516–517, 611–623
Ropper, Allan, 396, 399–400, 404–405
Rosenblum, W. I., 162
rosiglitazone, 470
Ross Russell, Ralph, 179, 230–232
Rostan, Léon, 48, 60–61
Rothberger, Carl, 354
Rothenberg, Steven, 570–571
Rothwell, Peter, 420–421
Roubin, Gary, 542–545
Roussy, Gustave, 74–75, 252–253, 299
Roy, Charles, 339

Royal Society of London, 32
Rufus of Ephesus, 7
Rusk, Howard, 517–518
Russel, David, 333–334
Russell, W. Ritchie, 397
Rutherford, Ernest, 341–342

Sachs, A. L., 414
Sachs, Bernard, 377–378
Sackett, David, 420–421
Safar, Peter, 398, 401
Sahs, Adolph, 438
SAINT trials 1 and 2, 483–484
salicyclic acid, 448
Samson, Duke., 595
Sandercock, Peter, 420–421
Sandifort, Eduard, 55
Sandok, Burton, 192–193
Sanofi company, 458–459
SAPPHIRE trial, carotid stenting, 544
Sapporo criteria, antiphospholipid syndrome,
    206–207
Saryan, Leon, 315–316
Satran, Richard, 244–246
Saver, Jeff, 554–555
Sayre, G., 188–189
Schafer, Edward, 353
Schaffer, A. J., 378–379
Schalit, I., 254–255
Scheel, L. D., 436–437
Scheinberg, Peritz, 113–114, 414, 438
schistomiasis, spinal cord infarction and, 245
Schmidt, Alexander, 200–201
Schmidt, Carl, 342–343
Schoeffel, Eugen Wilhem, 436
Schoene, W. C., 122–124
Schofield, Frank, 434
Scholz, W., 223
Schroeder, Collin, 437–438
Schwab, Robert, 399
scientific method, evolution of, 26
scientists and inventors, stroke in, 613
Scott, David A., 429
Seelig, R., 400–401
Seldinger, Sven-Ivar, 112–113, 145, 301–302, 530
selective serotonin reuptake inhibitors (SSRI),
    stroke rehabilitation, 525
Selhorst, John, 233–234
Selim, Magdy, 578
Sémiologie des affections du système nerveux (Dejerine-
    Klumpke), 73
Senator, H., 67
Senefelder, Alois, 56
Sepetka, Ivan, 573–574
*Sepulchretum sive anatomia practica ex cadaveribus morbo
    denatis* (Bonetus), 38
Serbinenko, Fiódor Andreevitch, 570–571, 600–601
Serres, Antoine Étienne Augustin, 48

Servetus, Michael, 29
Seshadri, Sudha, 365
Shakespeare, William, 26, 32
Sharman, Bill, 615–616
Sharon, Ariel, 612
Shaw, Louis, 397
Sheehan, H. L., 175–176
Shennan, T., 188–189
Sherman, David, 421–422
Sherrington, Charles, 339, 343
Sherry, Sol, 492–493
Shick, R., 131–132
Sicard, Jean Athanase, 251, 253, 297–298
sickle cell disease, stroke and,
        220–221, 332–333
    pediatric stroke, 380–385
Siekert, Robert, 131–132
Siesjö, Bo K., 343, 479–481
Silver Spring monkeys, 519–522
Simpson, Roy, 379
Singer, S. J., 220–221
Singhal, Aneesh, 196–197
single photon emission computed tomography
        (SPECT), 344–345
SITS-MOST Registry, 498
Skinhøj, Erik, 343
Slack, Warner, 285
Smith, W. K., 435–436
Snead, Sam, 615–616
softening of brain, early research on,
        46–49
Sokoloff, Louis, 344
Solitaire stent, 554–555
Solitaire with the Intention for Thrombectomy as
        Primary Endovascular Treatment for Acute
        Ischemic Stroke (SWIFT PRIME) trial,
        556–557
Sottas, Jules, 74–75
Spence, D. J., 116–117
Spence, William T., 570–571
Spencer, Merrill P., 327, 329
Spencer's curve, 329
Spenser, Edward, 26, 32
Spetzler, Robert, 597
sphygmomanometer, 100, 465–467
Spielmeyer, W., 479–481
Spiller, William Gibson, 239–240
spinal cord, vasculature of, 85–86
    aorta and ischemia of, 240–242
    arteriovenous fistulas and malformations,
        243–244
    causes, 244–246
    hypotension and aortic border zones,
        242–243
    lesions, 60
    vascular disease and, 238–246
Spinoza, Baruch, 26
sports figures, stroke in, 615–616

SPOTLIGHT ("Spot Sign" Selection of
        Intracerebral Hemorrhage to Guide
        Hemostatic Therapy) trial, 582–583
Srinavasan, K., 180–181
STAIR clinical trial guidelines, 484–485
Stalin, Joseph, 611–623
Stam, Jan, 507–509
Stansfield, Fredrick Ross, 175–176, 505–506
statins
    cholesterol reduction with, 475
    early research on, 472–475
Steinheil, S. O., 167–169
stem cell therapy, stroke rehabilitation and,
        525–526
stenting
    carotid artery, 537–538, 541–546
    intracerebral aneurysms, 573–574
    intracranial arteries, 546–549
    stent retrieval, 554–555
    Wallstent development, 543
Stenting versus Aggressive Medical Therapy for
        Intracranial Arterial Stenosis (SAMMPRIS),
        423–424, 547–549
STICH (Surgical Trial in Intracerebral
        Haemorrhage), 579–580
Stoker, Bram, 614
Stone, Edward, 447–448
Stopford, John Sebastian Bach, 85, 129
STOP-IT (The Spot Sign for Predicting and
        Treating ICH Growth) trial, 582–583
Strandness, Eugene, 328–329
streptokinase thrombolytic therapy, 492–493
stroke. *See also* pediatric stroke; surgical
        management, of stroke; *specific conditions, e.g.,*
        subarachnoid hemorrhage
    aspirin and prevention of, 452–453
    clinical features of, 14
    data banks and registries, 370–372
    defined, 358–359
    epidemiology and risk factors, 364–367
    etiology and localization, 14–15
    Hippocrates's description of, 4–5
    neuroprotection against, 478–484
    prominent patients, 610–623
    risk factors, 364–367, 465–471
    severity and prognosis, 16
    terminology, 358–361
    writings about, 14
stroke centers, 393–394, 497–500. *See also*
        neurocritical care
Stroke Data Bank, 287–288, 371
stroke nurses, 393
stroke organizations, journals, and books
    national and international organizations and
        publications, 608–609
    United States, 607–608
Stroke Prevention by Aggressive Reduction in
        Cholesterol Levels (SPARCL) trial, 475

Stroke Prevention in Sickle Cell (STOP) program, 332–333

stroke units, establishment of, 391–392

Strully, K. J., 531–532

subarachnoid hemorrhage (SAH)
 cellular and vascular intervention in, 484–485
 delayed cerebral infarction and vasoconstriction, 147–149
 early research on, 46–47, 142–144
 Fisher's work on, 272–273
 Hippocrates's description of, 4–5
 imaging studies of, 144–145
 intracranial artery dissection, 191–192
 natural history and rebleeding, 145–147
 nonaneurysmal, 151–152
 Osler's work on, 100–101
 sequelae and complications, 149–150
 twentieth-century research on, 138–142
 Wepfer's research on, 43–44

subclavian artery disease, 273

subclavian steal syndrome, 130–131

subcortical arteriosclerotic encephalopathy, 122–124

Sudlow, Cathie, 420–421

sulfonylureas, 470

surfer's myelopathy, spinal cord infarction and, 245–246

surgical management, of stroke, 422–423, 529–538
 intracerebral aneurysm, 567–569
 microneurosurgery, 569–570

susceptibility weighted imaging (SWI), 320–322

Sussman, B. J., 551–552

Suzuki, Jiro, 193–196

Swank, Roy, 266–267

Swedish Aspirin Low-Dose Trial (SALT), 417–418

Sweet, William, 344–345

sweet clover disease, 435–436

Sydenham, Thomas, 32, 44–45, 358–359

Sydney criteria, antiphospholipid syndrome, 206–207

Symon, Lindsay, 347–348, 479–481

Symonds, Charles, 138–142, 175–176, 534

systematic review, clinical stroke trials and, 418–419

Tabulae anatomica sex (Vesalius), 22–24

Takemi, Taro, 354

target windows
 endovascular therapy, 557–558
 ischemic stroke models and, 479–481

Taub, Edward, 519–522

Taveras, Juan Manuel, 301–302

Taylor, Jill Bolte, 612–613

Teasdale, Graham, 579–580

tenecteplase (TNKase), 500

Ter-Pogossian, M. M., 345–347

Tesla, Nicola, 319–320

A Text-book of Physiology for Medical Students and Physicians (Howell), 427–429

Textbook of Medicine (Osler), 99–101

thalamus
 hemorrhage, 135–136
 vasculature of, 86–87

Thatcher, Margaret, 612

therapeutic hypothermia (TH). *See* hypothermia

thiazide compounds, hypertension management and, 466–467

Thieffry, Stéphane, 380–381

thienopyridines, 458–461

Thomas, André, 74–75

Thomson, John, 57–61

thorotrast, research using, 111

THRACE (Thrombectomie des artères cerebrales) trial, 556–557

thrombectomy, 432–433, 555–558

thrombi and thrombosis. *See also* cerebral vein and dural sinus thrombosis
 antiphospholipid antibodies and syndrome, 206–207
 antiplatelet therapy and, 455–462
 Aring and Merritt's research on, 263
 in children, 378–385
 Cole's early research on, 44–45
 factor V Leiden, 203–204
 heparin efficacy in, 431–432
 hyperhomocysteinemia, 205–206
 inherited thrombophilias, 203
 ischemic stroke management and, 401–402
 Virchow's research on, 96–97

thrombin, 491
 coagulation and, 201–203
 new oral anticoagulants (NOACs) and, 443

thrombo-endarterectomy, 531

thrombolytic therapy (thrombolysis), 401–402, 491–501
 cerebral venous thrombosis and, 510–511
 clinical trials involving, 422
 emergency medicine and, 497–500
 endovascular devices and, 553–554
 image-based therapy, 499
 intraarterial thrombolysis, 500–501
 streptokinase, 492–493
 tenecteplase (TNKase), 500
 tissue plasminogen activator (tPA), 493–500
 vascular imaging and, 497–500

'The Thromboplastic Action of Cephalin' (McLean), 427–429

thrombosis, carotid cavernous fistula closure, 600–601

thromboxane A2, 417–418

Tibbul-Nabbi (the Medicine of the Prophet), 10–14

ticagrelor (Brilinta), 460–461

ticlopidine (Ticlid), 458–459

Tillett, William Smith, 492–493

time-averaged maximum mean flow velocities (TAMM), 332–333

time is brain algorithms, 497

tissue factor research, 201–203

tissue plasminogen activator (tPA)
    clinical trials of, 422
    endovascular therapy with, 552–553
    as thrombolytic therapy, 491, 493–500
tissue window theory, neuroprotection and, 482
Titian, 22
TO-ACT, cerebral venous thrombosis therapy,
    510–511
Toni, D., 497
Tonnellé, M. L., 176–177
Toole, James F., 327, 332–333, 422–423, 438,
    536–537
Tournier-Lasserve, Élisabeth, 217
Traité du ramollissement du cerveau (Durand-Fardel),
    120
tranexamic acid, intracerebral hemorrhage and, 583
Tranexamic Acid for Hyperacute Primary
    Intracerebral Hemorrhage (TICH-2) trial, 583
transcranial direct current stimulation (tDCS),
    522–523
transcranial Doppler ultrasound (TCD)
    arterial stenting and, 544
    development of, 330–332
    pediatric stroke and, 382–383
    subarachnoid hemorrhage and, 149
transcranial magnetic stimulation (TMS), stroke
    rehabilitation and, 522–523
transesophageal echocardiography (TEE), 355–356
transient ischemic attacks (TIAs)
    arterial dissection, 190–191
    carotid artery disease and, 113–114
    clinical trials involving, 415
    posterior circulation and, 131–132
    terminology of, 359–361
    warfarin for management of, 438–440
    Willis's description of, 35–36
transient monocular blindness, carotid artery disease
    and, 113–114
"Transient Monocular Blindness Associated with
    Hemiplegia" (Fisher), 112
transtentorial herniation, 511
transthoracic echocardiography (TTE), 355–356
trauma
    arterial dissection, 190
    subarachnoid hemorrhage, 151–152
traumatic brain injury (TBI)
    induced hypothermia, 401
    management of, 400–401
Travers, Benjamin, 530, 599
"Treatise on Diseases II and III" (Hippocrates),
    157–158
Trevo stent retriever, 554–555
TREX1 gene, retinal vasculopathy and cerebral
    leukodystrophy, 219–220
triphasic perfusion computed tomography, 310–311
Troubles de la motilité (Dejerine-Klumpke), 75–79
"Tumour Detection by Nuclear Magnetic
    Resonance" (Damadian), 314–315

Turan, Tanya, 423–424
2VO stroke models, 479–481
Tyler, John, 611–612

Über das farbige Licht der Doppelsterne und einiger
    anderer Gestirne des Himmels (On the Coloured
    Light of the Binary Stars and Some Other Stars of
    the Heavens) (Doppler), 325–326
ultrasound
    cerebrovascular imaging with, 325–334
    clinical trial diagnoses, 332–333
    duplex system, 328–329
    early principles and research, 325–326
    echocardiography and, 355–356
    neck vessel imaging using, 327–329
    training and standardization, 333–334
    transcranial ultrasound of intracranial arteries and
    brain, 330–332
United States, stroke organizations, journals and
    books in, 607–608
urokinase
    endovascular therapy with, 552–553
    intracerebral hemorrhage and, 403

Vajpayee, Atal Bihari, 612
Valsalva, Antonio, 37–38, 55
Van Calcar, Jan Stephan, 21–22, 151–152
Van Crevel, Hans, 507–508
Vane, John, 416, 451–452
van Gijn, Jan, 150–151, 420–421
van Schoor, Raymond, 615–616
varicella-zoster virus infection, spinal cord infarction
    and, 245–246
Varolio, Costanzo, 44
vascular anatomy. See also arterial systems and
    arteries
    arterial systems and single arteries, 84–87
    Beevor's work on, 83
    Duret's work in, 81–82
    Foix's work on, 83–84
    microsurgical neuroanatomy, 88–89
    posterior circulation and vascular lesions, 128–132
    twentieth-century research on, 81–89
vascular Ehlers-Danlos syndrome, 222–223
vascular intervention
    neuroprotection and, 484–485
    stroke management and, 497–500
vasculitis, spinal cord infarction and, 245–246
vasoconstriction
    pediatric stroke and, 380–385
    retinal vascular spasm, 233–234
    reversible cerebral vasoconstriction syndrome,
    196–197
    subarachnoid hemorrhage, 147–149
vasospasm, delayed cerebral infarction and, 147–149
Velaquez, A. C., 570–571
Velpeau, Alfred, 570
venography, development of, 309–311

venous lesions, 170–171
venous thromboembolism (VTE)
    anticoagulant therapy for, 437–438
    blood disorders and, 200–201
    in children, 378–385
    decompressive hemicraniectomy, 511
    direct oral anticoagulant therapy, 511–512
    factor V Leiden, 203–204
    heparin in management of, 429–430, 506–509
    low-molecular-weight vs. unfractionated
        heparin, 510
    prothrombin gene mutation, 204
    thrombolytic and endovascular treatment,
        510–511
    treatment of, 505–512
ventriculography, 298–299, 304–305
Verdi, Giuseppi, 615
vertebral artery dissection, 191
vertebrobasilar disease
    early studies, 127–128
    hemorrhages, 133–136
    vascular lesions within posterior circulation,
        128–132
    warfarin and, 439
vertical shift theory, 399–400
Vesalius, Andreas
    anatomical research by, 21–24, 26–27, 55,
        127–128
    circulation research and work of, 37, 38
Vesling, 34
Vieusseux, Gaspard, 66–67
Viñuela, Fernando, 573–574
Virchow, Rudolph Ludwig Karl
    anatomical atlases, 45
    on arteriovenous malformations, 167–169
    on cerebral embolism, 96–97
    experimental pathology and, 94–97
    on phlebitis, 59–60
    on thrombosis and embolism,
        200–201, 491
Virchow's triad, 200–201
visual loss, vascular disease and, 226–235, 268–269.
    See also eye, cerebrovascular disease and
vitamin K antagonists. See anticoagulants
Vitek, Jiri, 541–542
Vitesse Intracranial Stent Study for Ischemic Stroke
    Therapy (VISSIT) trial, 549
vivisection, Harvey's experiments in, 25–29
Vollständiges Lehrbuch der Steindruckerey (A Complete
    Course of Lithography) (Senefelder), 56
Volpe, Joseph, 384
Von Basch, Samuel, 100
Von Dusch, T., 176–177
Von Helmholtz, Hermann, 226
Von Hösslin, R., 175–176
von Humboldt, Alexander, 613
Von Kummer, R., 497
Vulpian, Edmé Félix Alfred, 72, 81–82

Wallace, Alfred Russel, 212
Wallenberg, Adolph, 64–68, 128–132, 465–467
Wallenberg syndrome, 64–68, 127–128
Waller, Augustus, 353
Wallis, John, 32
Wallstent, 545
    arterial stenting and, 543
Walton, John, 479–481, 533–534
Warach, Steven, 321
Ward, A., 598–599
Wardlaw, Joanna, 122, 420–421
warfarin
    clinical trials of, 421–422
    dipyridamole and, 457
    early human trials of, 437–438
    intracerebral hemorrhage and reversal of,
        583–584
    research and development of, 434–440
    stroke management and, 438–440
    transient ischemic attacks and, 131–132
Warfarin-Aspirin Recurrent Stroke Study
    (WARSS), 439
Warfarin-Aspirin for Symptomatic Intracranial
    Disease (WASID) trial, 132, 439–440
Warlow, Charles Picton, 420–421, 535
Washington, George, 26
Watson, James D., 213
Waugh, John, 316–317
WEAVE registry trial, 549
Weber, G., 111
Weber, Hermann David, 69–70
Wechsler, Israel S., 103
Weimar, Willem, 494–495
Weinberg, Wilhelm, 212
Weissmann, August, 212
Welch, Francis, 226
Wells, Ibert, 220–221
Wepfer, Johann Jakob
    on anatomy, 34, 44–45
    on intracerebral hemorrhage, 43–44
    on posterior circulation, 127–128
    on ramollissements (softening), 52
    on subarachnoid hemorrhage, 142–144
Wharton, Edith, 614
Whipple, George, 468
Whisnant, Jack, 131–132, 367, 370, 439
Wieloch, Tadeus, 479–481
Wiggers, Carl, 398
Wilkins, Maurice, 213
Williams, Daniel, 612–613
Willis, Thomas, 24–29, 31–36, 37, 44–45, 376,
    478–479
willow leaves, aspirin and, 447–449
Wilmut, Ian, 213–214
Wilson, S. A. Kinnier, 101–103, 162–163
Wilson, Woodrow, 610–612, 618–619
Wingspan stent system, 547–548
Winstein, Carolee, 520

Winterberg, Heinrich, 354
Winterkorn, Jacqueline Marjorie Schuker, 233–234
Wintermark, Max, 309–311
Wojak, J. C., 547
Wolf, Alfred, 344
Wolf, Philip, 365
Wolf, Steve, 520
Wolff, Harold, 413–414
Wong, Lawrence, 331
Wood, Ernest, 301–302
Woolf, A. L., 176–177
World Health Organization (WHO)
    aspirin controversy and, 416
    MONICA study by, 365–366
    stroke definition, 358–359
Wray, Shirley, 230–232
Wren, Christopher, 32–34

Wright, C. R., 449–450
Wright, Irving, 413–414

Ximelagatran, 443–444
X-ray imaging, of brain, early research
    using, 304

Yadav, Jay, 541–542, 544
Yaşargil, Mahmut Gazi, 569–570, 595–596
Yates, P. O., 129–130, 162
Yodh, S. B., 570–571

Zervas, Nicholas, 147–149, 399–400, 404–405
Zeumer, Herman, 495–496, 500–501, 551–552
Zimmerman, Harry, 241–242
Zoll, Paul, 398
Zülch, Klaus Joachim, 242–243